*F*or me, the process of dealing with having cancer, facing major surgery, and undergoing chemotherapy and radiation was much easier knowing that I could come out of it perhaps cured and with pretty much the same body. You go into it very frightened. Part of the terror is not knowing exactly what you are going to look like. It was comforting to know that I had options.

*A lot of positive things have come out of this year, particularly how I view life and treat other people. I am more sensitive, but I live with much less illusion that I have control over my life. Loss of control was very difficult for me. I always thought I could manage everything. Breast cancer has a way of bringing you up short and making you face reality. You never really have control. I was the epitome of the self-contained woman who didn't really need anybody or anything. I could do everything for myself. I didn't need support. I found out through this that I do need support and I tell people that I need it now. It has become a very freeing experience.*

*Once cancer is brought into the equation, it makes life more real. I have no idea what percentage of the remainder of my life is left. I have learned to treasure the experiences that I have, good or bad, because I learn and grow from them. I have learned to treasure the people who are in my life and to tell them today.*

**—Debbie,**
who had a lumpectomy and
partial breast reconstruction, is one of the
fourteen women who tell their stories in
A WOMAN'S DECISION

# A WOMAN'S DECISION

## Breast Care, Treatment & Reconstruction

*3rd edition*

Karen Berger and
John Bostwick III, M.D.

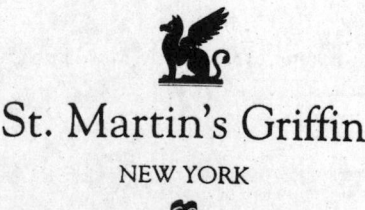

St. Martin's Griffin

NEW YORK

This book presents current scientific information and opinion. It does not provide advice concerning specific diagnosis and treatment of individual cases. The authors and publisher will not be responsible or liable for actions taken as a result of the opinions expressed in this book.

ISBN 0-312-18229-5

First published in the United States by Quality Medical Publishing.

10 9 8 7 6 5 4 3

To our mothers

**Bobbie Friedman** and **Dorothy Bostwick**

who have been an unwavering source
of support and inspiration

# FOREWORD

This remarkable and informative book blends the perspectives of patients with breast cancer and the physicians who treat them. In contrast to many other diseases affecting women, breast cancer requires treatment decisions that involve not only the physical malady but the quality of life as well. These quality-of-life issues are influenced by familial, social, cultural, emotional, and spiritual variables that are very personal and unique to each woman. In view of this, medical and surgical decisions must integrate the perspectives of both the patient and her physicians. Thus listening skills, empathy, sensitivity, and a willingness to accept the patient as a partner in treatment planning are a must for physicians. The patient, in turn, needs to be familiar with medical terminology and be well informed about treatment options and their potential impact on her life, both physically and emotionally. The bottom line in the decision-making process is this: do the benefits outweigh the risks for a given combination and sequence of treatments after taking into account all the available options?

This invaluable book should be read by every physician who sees women with breast diseases. It provides unique and valuable insights into women's perspectives about breast cancer, including their fears, emotional needs, and desire for the information that is critical to assuming a responsible decision-making role in their own treatment and rehabilitation. Every woman who has breast disease or who is at risk for developing breast cancer will benefit greatly by reading this informative and well-illustrated book. The voices of women and their loved ones that permeate these pages will help others face the trauma associated with this disease and cope with the decisions that must be made knowing that they do not face this crisis alone. These pages offer a woman a better understanding of the complex choices she faces and thus reduce her anxieties. She can also learn about the option of breast reconstruction, the different operations available for breast restoration, and the associated risks and benefits. Such a factual, realistic, and no-nonsense information base is the best way to deal with these issues, for it allows a woman to act knowledgeably in selecting her physicians and in making the treatment decisions that are right for her.

I want to compliment Karen Berger and John Bostwick on their significant and unique contribution to the literature. Karen Berger is a leading medical publisher and writer who has devoted years to working with women with breast cancer. This book reflects her desire "to educate women about the treatment alternatives available to them so that they can more effectively influence their own destinies and play an active role in their own health care." Dr. John Bostwick is one of the foremost breast reconstructive surgeons whose extensive experience working with breast cancer patients is well known. His care and compassion for patients are evident throughout this book. These authors have written a meaningful and easily understood text to help women deal with the fear and reality of breast cancer by enabling them to become informed participants in the treatment-planning process. They have succeeded admirably. This book will enhance the understanding and trust between those who are afflicted with breast diseases and those who care for them.

**Charles M. Balch, M.D., F.A.C.S.**
*President and Chief Executive Officer,*
*City of Hope National Medical Center;*
*Clinical Professor of Surgery, University of*
*Southern California, Los Angeles, California;*
*Former Professor and Head, Division of Surgery*
*and Anesthesiology, The University of Texas*
*M.D. Anderson Cancer Center, Houston, Texas*

# ACKNOWLEDGMENTS

A book progresses through many stages and numerous revisions during its evolution. Initially the authors struggle in isolation while committing their thoughts to paper. Transforming their rough manuscript into a published book, however, requires the assistance of others. Our book was no exception. Although this is a third edition, the writing process was as intense as if it were a new creation. All aspects of the book were carefully reexamined, and most chapters were rewritten to incorporate the latest information in a field that has become increasingly complex and dynamic.

Enormous progress has been made in breast cancer diagnosis and therapy, and we wanted this new edition to reflect these major advances. For a time, our book seemed to be a moving target that shifted its direction at every turn. Each day brought news of dramatic new developments and promising new genetic therapies to shrink tumors, disrupt cell growth, and interfere with cell signals. These amazing discoveries led to chronic last-minute changes with no end in sight. Ultimately, as all authors must, we relinquished the manuscript, ever hopeful that it was as current as the publishing process allows. Most likely we would still be revising the manuscript had it not been for the assistance of numerous experts who contributed their time and knowledge to help finalize this writing project. We were fortunate to have the advice of medical experts, skilled editors, and sensitive friends and associates. With their guidance and encouragement, we brought the book to a conclusion. We have many people to acknowledge and to thank for their contributions.

A debt of gratitude is due to Michelle Leaman, who helped distribute our latest survey to 900 breast cancer survivors throughout the United States. The results of this survey form the basis for much of the material presented. She also was instrumental in contacting different agencies and support organizations for resources and information. Thanks to Michelle we have a book that reflects the needs, hopes, and desires of a broad spectrum of women throughout the United States.

Special thanks are also due to the following individuals and organizations for soliciting breast cancer patients throughout the country to participate in this survey and/or provide us with valuable resources and suggestions that would be of interest to our readers. We would like to note their contributions here:

**Alex E. Denes, M.D.**
St. John's Mercy Medical Center
St. Louis, Missouri

**Lois Howland, R.N., B.S.N.**
Cancer Information Center, Barnes-Jewish Hospital
St. Louis, Missouri

**Amy Langer**
Executive Director, National Alliance of Breast Cancer Organizations
    (NABCO)
New York, New York

**Michele Nobs, R.N., B.S.N, O.C.N.**
St. John's Mercy Medical Center Breast Cancer Support Group
St. Louis, Missouri

**Judy Perotti**
Director of Patient Services, Y-ME National Breast Cancer Organization
Chicago, Illinois

**Lynn P. Stadnyk, R.N., M.A., L.P.C.**
Oncology Counselor, Department of Surgery
St. Luke's Hospital
St. Louis, Missouri

We would especially like to thank the many women who responded to our surveys. They took time to answer our questions because they desired to help other women and because they had a statement to make about their experiences. We received hundreds of letters and phone calls from them. Their response was both gratifying and helpful in formulating our ideas. Their words not only inspired us but taught us how to improve this edition to better meet the needs of breast cancer patients.

Lois Howland also played an important role in helping us formulate a complete guide to the breast cancer support and information resources available throughout the country. She checked and rechecked telephone numbers, addresses, and facts and helped rewrite descriptions of the various agencies offering assistance. Her input has been enormously helpful in making our book responsive to our readers' needs. We would also like to express our appreciation to Norbert Krämer, a dear publishing colleague, who encouraged us and who helped gather information on the network of international breast cancer support groups.

Much of the tone and focus of this book was derived from the emotion-packed interviews we had with the women and men who allowed us to record their feelings about and experiences with breast cancer and reconstruction. Particular thanks are reserved for the women and men whose stories are recorded here. They allow us to relive their experiences with them and in so doing to learn from them. Even though the names and personal details of these individuals have been changed to protect their privacy, their feelings and experiences reflect their real-life encounter with breast cancer and breast reconstruction.

We would like to pay special tribute to Arvella Carter, whose legacy of courage and spirituality stands as a lasting tribute to her memory.

Several chapters include major contributions from others, and we wish to acknowledge these experts here. Among the contributors are:

**Kenneth J. Arnold, M.D.**
Assistant Professor of Clinical Surgery
Washington University School of Medicine
St. Louis, Missouri

**John M. Bedwinek, M.D.**
Medical Director, Department of Radiation Oncology
St. Joseph Health Center
St. Charles, Missouri

**Benjamin A. Borowsky, M.D.**
Associate Professor of Internal Medicine
Washington University School of Medicine
St. Louis, Missouri

**Roger S. Foster, Jr., M.D.**
Chief of Surgical Services, Crawford Long Hospital and
Wadley Glenn Professor of Surgery, Emory University School of Medicine
Atlanta, Georgia

**Mary Ellen Hawf,** R.N., O.C.N.
Head Nurse/Case Manager, Inpatient Oncology Unit
Missouri Baptist Medical Center/BJC System
St. Louis, Missouri

**Jacob Klein,** M.D.
Assistant Professor of Clinical Obstetrics and Gynecology
Washington University School of Medicine
St. Louis, Missouri

**Lynne A. McCain,** B.S.N., R.N.
Patient Educator/Patient Counselor
Section of Plastic and Reconstructive Surgery, The Emory Clinic
Atlanta, Georgia

**John S. Meyer,** M.D.
Chief Pathologist Emeritus and Director of Laboratories
St. Luke's Hospital and
Visiting Professor of Pathology
Washington University School of Medicine
St. Louis, Missouri

**Barbara S. Monsees,** M.D.
Professor of Radiology and Chief of Breast Imaging Section
Mallinckrodt Institute of Radiology
Washington University School of Medicine
St. Louis, Missouri

**Gary A. Ratkin,** M.D.
Clinical Associate Professor of Medicine
Washington University School of Medicine and
Missouri Baptist Cancer Center
St. Louis, Missouri

**William C. Wood,** M.D.
Joseph Brown Whitehead Professor and Chairman
Department of Surgery, Emory University School of Medicine
Atlanta, Georgia

These experts wrote the sections detailing their respective roles as internist, gynecologist, radiologist, general surgeon, radiation oncologist, medical oncologist, oncology nurse, and plastic surgery nurse and also reviewed, revised, and even rewrote the information presented on these topics in Chapter 5, "Breast Lumps and Other Breast Conditions," and Chapter 6, "Breast Cancer Facts and Treatment Options." Recognition is also due to Mimi Greenberg, who allowed us to reprint excerpts on the patient's responsibilities from her book entitled *Invisible Scars*. The contributions from these experts have resulted in a comprehensive update on current breast cancer therapy and breast reconstruction technique that is unavailable elsewhere in a single book for the general public.

Some of our contributors merit special recognition for their assistance in critiquing the entire manuscript, writing or revising sections as requested, and obtaining much-needed resource material. Drs. Gary A. Ratkin, John M. Bedwinek, Roger S. Foster, Jr., William C. Wood, John S. Meyer, and Barbara S. Monsees always took time out of their busy schedules and overwhelming patient loads to help. No request was too great, although we asked them to write and rewrite many times. Dr. Ratkin was one of those individuals. He critiqued the previous edition carefully and provided us with valuable suggestions that have shaped our writing. He alerted us to many of the exciting developments going on in breast cancer research and therapy and to the promising work on monoclonal antibodies and angiogenesis that were incorporated with his guidance. He also wrote sections on new chemotherapy and hormonal therapy drugs and expected side effects, bone marrow transplantation and cell seeding techniques, among others. Drs. Bedwinek, Foster, and Wood carefully read and critiqued the previous edition and our current revision, making valuable recommendations and supplying answers to significant questions. Whenever we realized that some topic had not been covered or that a new therapy was being touted, we called on them to supply missing data and write the necessary explanatory material. They helped us to refocus the discussion on local therapy for breast cancer to present a more balanced view of options now available to women that emphasizes breast conservation and preservation techniques as well as the new "designer" estrogens, the role of monoclonal antibodies, and the new drugs and genetic therapies that are revolutionizing breast cancer treatment today. They also wrote definitive sections on current treatment approaches, axillary node and sentinel node biopsy, conservative surgery and irradiation, breast cancer trials with tamoxifen, and skin-sparing mastectomy. Dr. Meyer was enormously helpful in explaining the latest breast cancer research and the role of the pathologist in diagnosing breast cancer. The female author's frequent calls to him requesting information on oncogenes, *HER-2/neu*, *BRCA1*, and *BRCA2*, among other topics, were always met with a patient explanation in understandable terms. His translation of a complex topic gives our readers the benefit of this highly scientific knowledge that is so crucial to their lives. Although she was overwhelmed in planning a major breast imaging center, Dr. Monsees still took the time to totally rewrite her chapter on mammography and provided new information on the latest imaging methods, image-guided biopsy techniques, and sentinel node biopsy. Her contribution helps highlight the valuable role that breast imaging plays in early detection and diagnosis of breast cancer.

We also want to thank Mary Ellen Hawf, R.N., O.C.N., who described the role of the oncology nurse and how she helps the patient, and Lynne A. McCain, B.S.N., R.N., who described how the plastic surgery nurse ministers to the breast reconstruction patient's physical and emotional needs. These nursing professionals provided a major service for breast cancer patients and their families by informing them of the excellent nursing resources that are available to support them through this trying experience.

In addition to the experts who contributed to our book, a number of professionals in this field have reviewed the manuscript, provided input, and assisted us in gathering resource materials. In particular, they reviewed the new information on breast cancer research, breast cancer diagnosis and treatment, breast implants, and breast reconstruction. We would like to acknowledge the encouragement and assistance of Rosemary Locke, Dr. Charles Balch, Dr. Gerald Pitman, Dr. Bahman Teimourian, Dr. Ian T. Jackson, Fay Schenkman, Linda Saslow, and Joan Swirsky, R.N., M.S. Joan, who was involved in revising her excellent book on breast cancer and a new exciting book on lymphedema, as well as other writing projects, still found the time to share her considerable expertise with the female author, particularly in the area of nutrition.

Drs. William C. Wood and the surgical oncology group at Emory, including Drs. Toncred Styblo, Douglas Murray, Grant Carlson, George Daneker, and Charles Staley set a standard for us; they represent the type of quality care that this book is all about. Drs. Jack Culbertson, Grant Carlson, Glyn Jones, and Robert Wood also made major contributions. Thanks are also due to the plastic surgery residents, physician assistants, and dedicated nursing staff of the Emory University–Affiliated Hospitals and the Plastic Surgery Section of the Emory Clinic.

The editing skills of Carolita Deter were an invaluable asset. She polished our prose and offered critical suggestions for shaping and reworking the manuscript. Despite her protestations that the book really didn't need her help, Carolita accepted this assignment because the female author prevailed on her friendship. She read our chapters, making valuable editorial and stylistic suggestions and bringing her incredible skill to bear on our writing. We are both grateful for the care she lavished on our book. Her efforts on our behalf have greatly enhanced this writing effort.

This manuscript would never have been completed had it not been for the efforts of the outstanding team at Quality Medical Publishing. Nancy Ladousier, Suzanne Murat, and Karen Kierath tirelessly transcribed tapes from the interviews and typed and retyped the manuscript because they cared about the project. Esha Gupta, Leslie Wagner, and Barbara Lopez-Lucio searched the literature and the Internet to provide us with the latest information on new developments and to ensure that all references were current. Additional assistance came from Beth Campbell-Blethroad, who read and critiqued chapters, and Kathy Jenkins, who proofread the manuscript. Katherine Spakowski deftly managed and coordinated the publishing project, checking and reviewing the pages and helping to ensure a quality publication. Judy Bamert helped to organize the book's illustrations, Susan Trail produced the artistic layout, and Billie Forshee arranged for the book's scheduling, production, and manufacture. Doug Wilmsmeyer, Cindy Meilink, Tom Mastroianni, and Retta Petzel provided the marketing support so necessary for any publishing project. David Berger used his considerable computer skills to fine-tune our cover design and help us determine the ideal color scheme and look for our book. Other staff members of Quality Medical Publishing also provided support and expertise throughout this endeavor. Their assistance and encouragement were deeply appreciated, as was the cooperation and assistance of Cathy McCrary, who effectively coordinated the Atlanta half of this endeavor.

William Winn created the new drawings for this book. Diane Beasley's cover design has given this third edition a new face. As always her design manages to capture the essence of a book.

Our friends, relatives, and associates shared our concerns and were an ongoing source of support. Vicki Sharp, a prolific writer and breast cancer survivor, encouraged us throughout the process. Anitra Sheen and Dr. Jack Sheen were always positive and encouraging. Anitra, a talented writer, took time from her novel to offer insightful comments and to help the frustrated female half of the writing team refocus the first chapter and craft a new first paragraph that reflects the book's expanded coverage. Jeff Friedman, a poet and skilled editor, reviewed the manuscript and wrote the back cover copy. Harriet Kopolow is a true friend who the female half of our writing team has always valued; her support was pervasive, as was that of Ann Smith Carr, Pat Simons, Marilyn Ratkin, Colleen Randall, Vicki Friedman Diane Feldman, Dr. Joel Feldman, Joan Foster, Joanna Hart Matthews, Audrey Lenharth, and Marjorie Jackson. Dr. Jessica Lewis was one of the reasons the book was written; it meant a great deal to know that she believed in the project and in the authors.

Our final appreciation belongs to our spouses, Phil and Jane, and our children, David and Andrew, and Mary and John, who understood our feelings about this subject, allowed us the freedom to explore them, and encouraged us in the process.

**Karen Berger**
**John Bostwick III**

# CONTENTS

Appendices

## NOTE:
## THE GENDER PROBLEM

In writing this book, we were confronted with the
dilemma of which gender pronouns to use to refer to the
surgeons and plastic surgeons we discussed. Because all of the
patients in this book are female and are referred to as she,
we decided to avoid confusion and use the male
pronoun for all the doctors in this book.

# Our Purpose in Writing

Today, women diagnosed with breast cancer have more and better options for treatment, preservation, and reconstruction of the breast. No longer is the choice reduced to saving a life or saving a breast. Now the choices are more promising, but they are also more complex. Current diagnostic methods and medical and surgical therapies allow women to make their own decisions based on available information about the effectiveness of treatment, risk factors, and possibilities for breast restoration. In this context, access to reliable, balanced information becomes increasingly important. This new edition is written to fill that need. Our purpose is to provide our readers with the latest information and to assist them in understanding and evaluating the many factors that will influence a decision that will profoundly affect their lives.

Options now available to women include local therapy that focuses on optimal cancer removal with simultaneous breast preservation or reconstruction and systemic therapy using new chemotherapy and hormonal therapy regimens. Breast-conserving surgery with irradiation has become a widely accepted and increasingly appealing option for most women with early breast cancer. It offers excellent cancer treatment with survival rates equivalent to those for mastectomy. Mastectomy operations have also been modified and improved. Many women who require or choose mastectomy can now have skin-sparing procedures for breast removal followed by immediate breast reconstruction.

Women and their families are far better educated about their health than they were a mere 15 years ago. Vast resources are readily available to them. Logging onto the Internet can yield a wealth of information on a wide variety of topics. Breast cancer is covered in abundant detail. In fact, the array of available materials can be overwhelming. The challenge lies in sorting through this data to glean the information that is pertinent, meaningful, and appropriate for you. Our goal is to give women and their loved ones an overview of current health issues, new developments, and approaches to breast cancer diagnosis, treatment, and rehabilitation. Armed with this information they can take control of their health, their lives, and their destinies.

This third edition reflects the transformation in breast cancer therapy. When we wrote the first edition 15 years ago, our primary emphasis was on mastectomy and breast reconstruction. At that time total breast removal was the most effective therapy for local treatment of breast cancer, and we wanted to let women know that breast restoration was available to them. The second edition was written as breast-conserving surgery was gaining more advocates. The current revision represents the changing face of breast cancer diagnosis and treatment and the exciting new developments on the horizon.

This book describes the diversity of choices increasingly available to women. It includes routine self-inspection tips, guidelines for mammography, descriptions of commonly occurring breast problems, breast cancer risk factors, as well as updates on hormone replacement therapy and the so-called designer estrogens. Recent research developments and therapeutic approaches to breast cancer are fully explored. Image-guided biopsy techniques, sentinel node biopsy, breast-conserving surgery and irradiation, skin-sparing mastectomy, and promising drug therapies for breast cancer prevention are among the many topics that now share the spotlight with breast reconstruction.

Even so, breast reconstruction remains a major focus, and this edition continues to offer a comprehensive, yet understandable account of this topic for women who wish to explore this option. All aspects of breast reconstruction are covered. Why do women seek breast restoration? Who is a candidate? What is the correct timing for this surgery? What is the best method for breast reconstruction? What are the risks and benefits? What are the facts about breast implants? Answers to these frequently asked questions and many others are combined with personal accounts of women who have had their breasts restored. Pain, recuperation, and expense are issues of primary concern to any woman contemplating elective surgery, and these have been dealt with in detail. We itemize the costs, risks, and benefits and describe and illustrate the different reconstructive techniques available. We try to present all sides of this topic from an unbiased perspective. Clearly, breast reconstruction is not for every woman. Many will not wish to undergo further surgery, pain, or expense. But for those who are interested, we provide a source of current, reliable information to enable them to make an educated decision.

This is not intended to be a medical text. We are speaking as professionals, but the scope of our book extends far beyond statistical analysis or scientific explanations of tumor behavior. Rather, we address the concerns of women confronting their fears of breast malignancy and monitoring their breasts. We believe that women with breast problems need to take a commonsense approach in dealing with physicians and the treatments they prescribe. We try to provide a personal, yet medically accurate account.

Readers will find these pages liberally sprinkled with medical terms. Care has been taken to define these words, not to eliminate them. We are not proponents of medical jargon, just realists who respect the intelligence of our readers. Despite doctors' best efforts to give their patients understandable explanations, it is only natural for them to rely heavily on the communication tools they routinely use. For a woman to feel fully in control, she must familiarize herself with this terminology if she is not to be frustrated in her efforts to learn more about her condition and to communicate more fully with her physicians. We strongly believe that it is important for women to understand the language they will encounter during the treatment process.

Because breast cancer touches so many people's lives, the audience for this book is a broad one. Since the first edition was published in 1984, over 1 million women have developed breast cancer. Now the alarming news is that it will strike one out of eight women during her lifetime. For the female half of our writing team, these statistics have come home. She notes with each passing year that breast cancer is an intimate reality for more and more relatives and friends. She feels that she is writing this book for herself, to answer all of those questions that have always worried and haunted her. The physician half of our writing team sees the need for such a book to help answer patient questions. Over the years he has seen significantly greater numbers of women in search of breast reconstruction; alarmingly, many of these women are in their thirties and forties, far younger than the patient population he was treating a mere 15 years ago. Both of us wish to reach the more than 2 million women in the United States today who have had mastectomies or lumpectomies and the more than 180,000 women each year who develop breast cancer in this country. We want these women to know about the options for breast cancer treatment and breast reconstruction and to understand that a diagnosis of breast cancer does not necessarily equate with permanent breast loss or disfigurement.

This book is also directed at women who are disease free. If they know that lumpectomy and irradiation and breast reconstruction are available, they might be less prone to procrastinate seeking medical attention for suspected breast problems. Early detection remains the key to survival. Women need to understand the critical importance of mammography, breast self-examination, and physician examination.

We are also writing for men, not because they will suffer from breast cancer (the incidence of breast cancer among men is 1% that of women), but because they will know, love, work with, and live among women who have had this experience. Perhaps this knowledge will sensitize them to the psychological and physical concerns that this disease generates.

Much of the information in this book is drawn from 15 years of research, over 2000 questionnaires, hundreds of letters and comments received from our readers, and numerous interviews with men and women. We principally surveyed women who had lumpectomies and mastectomies for breast cancer and asked them to relate their feelings about and experiences with this disease, their methods for coping, as well as their subsequent therapy and rehabilitation. We asked women to supply us with questions that they wanted answered and issues that they would like to see addressed.

It was apparent that the women who responded to our surveys had invested considerable time pondering our questions and had answered thoughtfully. They painstakingly recorded their thoughts on the backs of pages, typed extra sheets, wrote letters, and attached articles and reading lists that they thought would assist us. They even e-mailed their responses and articles to us. Especially gratifying for us were communications received from women who had read the first two editions of this book; they graciously described the book's impact on their lives and provided suggestions for revision.

These women's responses prompted us to make critical changes in the tone and direction of the book. Because of them, we have carefully reexamined all of the information in existing chapters, adding, rewriting, and amplifying as we went along and significantly updating this material. We have also updated the Appendix to include current information on support services, patient education resources, and informed consent.

Since our last literary excursion, many new developments have occurred in breast cancer research and therapy. Despite the numerous books and articles on the general health issues related to breast disease, our surveys indicate that many women remain woefully ignorant of them. Therefore we have interwoven basic information on these subjects throughout. Of particular interest are expanded sections on new tests and therapies for diagnosing and treating breast cancer, sentinel node biopsy, methods for breast cancer staging, criteria for choosing lumpectomy with irradiation, the latest chemotherapy and hormonal therapy regimens, and updates on ongoing clinical trials to investigate promising new treatments for breast cancer prevention. In addition, we have greatly expanded the discussion of breast cancer genetics and the breast cancer genes (*BRCA1* and *BRCA2*), adding new information on the ethical dilemmas associated with genetic testing. We have also placed greater emphasis on the social, psychological, and wellness issues confronting the breast cancer patient. Consequently, the chapter on breast cancer and its effect on relationships has been expanded to include more input from men and single women and greater attention to the practical realities of daily life. In our surveys and interviews we probe the strategies others have used to help them cope with dating, sex, communication, making new acquaintances, and building lasting relationships. Their solutions are surprising, creative, and always inspiring.

Finally, we have totally updated the chapters on breast reconstruction to incorporate the numerous advances that have taken place in the past 15 years and to respond to women's questions about breast restoration. All of the currently available reconstructive techniques, from the simplest to the most complex, are described in detail and accompanied by numerous photographs and drawings of the procedures and the anticipated results, as our readers proposed. In view of the mounting demand for immediate breast reconstruction, this topic has been explored in depth. We have added information on endoscopic techniques, filler reconstruction after lumpectomy and partial mastectomy, and new free flap procedures. We have also completely rewritten the chapter on breast implants to provide the scientific documentation to put this topic into perspective.

The concluding chapter of the book has always been cited by our readers as being particularly helpful to them in understanding the possibilities and limitations of breast reconstruction. It captures conversations with breast reconstruction patients throughout the country. In this edition six new interviews have been added to reflect the latest reconstructive techniques. These women poignantly explain their motivations for seeking breast reconstruction. They candidly discuss such diverse issues as dating and sex after breast cancer, postsurgical depression, and the doctor/patient relationship. All of these women freely share the details of their surgery as well as their intense feelings about it and about the breast cancer experience.

Breast cancer is a complex and terrifying disease. It attacks a woman's self-confidence, her physical being, and her very life. It affects friends, family, and acquaintances alike. It does not discriminate. Wealth, power, and privilege offer no protection against its assault. Knowledge, however, is the common defense that unites all women. It is the secret to overcoming fear and regaining control. Early detection is still the key to long-term survival.

It is our hope that this book will educate women about the full spectrum of options available for dealing with breast cancer, thereby empowering them with the strength and understanding required to confront this life-threatening disease. Many exciting developments are taking place in breast cancer research and therapy that offer new hope for improved quality of life and for a potential cure. Equipped with this knowledge, women will be able to more effectively influence their own destinies and play an active role in their own health care.

# BREAST ANATOMY AND PHYSIOLOGY

How much do most women really know about their breasts? Most likely very little. Unless they develop breast problems, they usually are not motivated to learn about the inner structure of this intimate female body part. Yet women need to be more familiar with the normal anatomy and physiology (function) of their breasts if they are going to be able to recognize the earliest and most treatable signs of breast cancer. With this knowledge, they will not be so frightened every time they notice a breast change. This chapter provides that information in a simple and straightforward manner. It offers women a baseline for evaluating their own health care requirements. Additionally, it provides assistance for women interested in performing breast self-examination, a crucial routine for proper breast surveillance.

The breast is a mound of glandular, fatty, and fibrous tissue located over the pectoralis muscles of the chest wall and attached to these muscles by fibrous strands (Cooper's ligaments). The breast itself has no muscle tissue, which is why exercises (often vigorously engaged in by teenagers intent on enlarging their breasts) will not build up the breasts. A layer of fat surrounds the breast glands and extends throughout the breast. This fatty tissue gives the breast a soft consistency and gentle, flowing contour. The actual breast is composed of fat, glands (with the capacity for milk production when stimulated by special hormones), blood vessels, milk ducts to transfer the milk from the glands to the nipples, and sensory nerves that give feeling to the breast. These nerves extend upward from the muscle layer through the breast and are highly sensitive, especially in the regions of the nipple and areola, which accounts for the sexual responsiveness of some women's breasts. Because the breast is made up of tissues with differ-

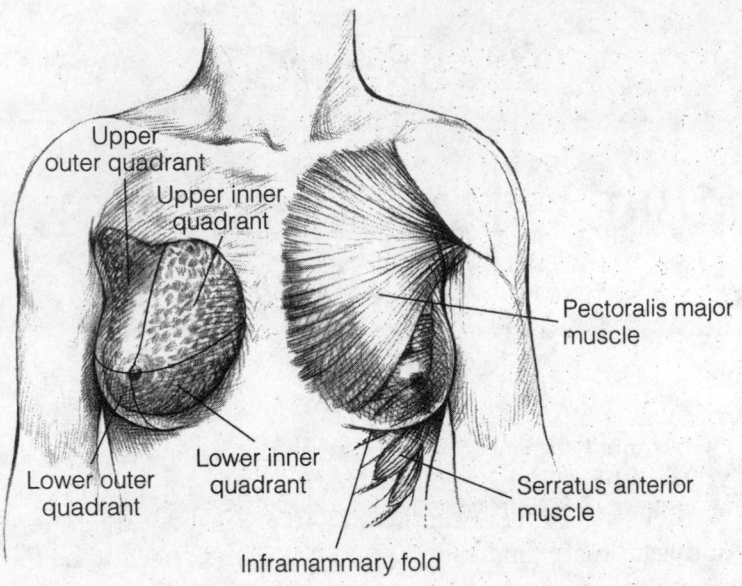

ent textures, it may not have a smooth surface and often feels lumpy. This irregularity is especially noticeable when a woman is thin and has little breast fat to soften the contours; it becomes less obvious after menopause, when the cyclic changes and endocrine stimulation of the breast cease and the glandular tissue softens. Estrogen supplements after menopause can cause continued lumpiness. The breast glands drain into a collecting system of ducts that go to the base of the nipple. The ducts then extend through the nipple and open on its outer surface. In addition to serving as a channel for milk, these ducts are often the source of breast problems. Experts now believe that most breast cancer begins in the lining of the ducts and sometimes the milk glands. Benign fibrocystic changes also originate in these ducts.

The ducts end in the nipple, which projects from the surface of the breast, and are a conduit for the milk secreted by the glands and suckled by a baby during breast-feeding. There is considerable variation in women's nipples. In some the nipple is constantly erect; in others it only becomes erect when stimulated by cold, physical contact, or sexual activity. Still other women have inverted nipples. Surrounding the nipple is a slightly raised circle of pigmented skin called the areola. The nipple and areola contain specialized muscle fibers that make the nipple erect and give the areola its firm texture. The areola

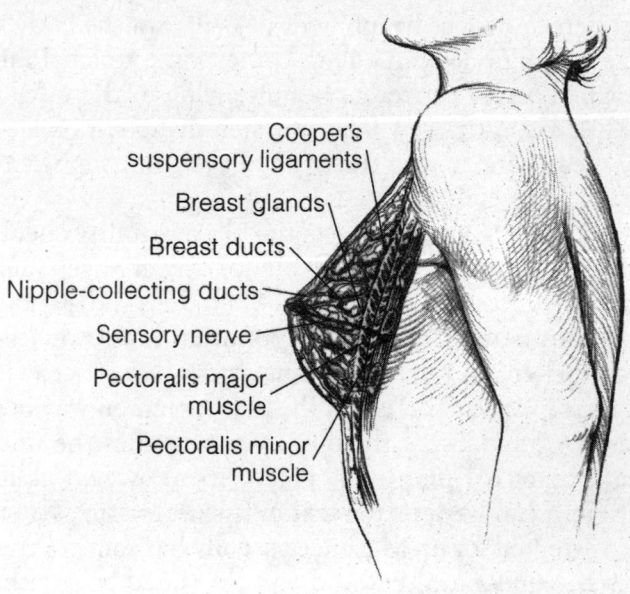

Cooper's
suspensory ligaments
Breast glands
Breast ducts
Nipple-collecting ducts
Sensory nerve
Pectoralis major
muscle
Pectoralis minor
muscle

also contains Montgomery's glands, which may appear as small, raised lumps on the surface of the areola. These glands lubricate the areola and are not symptoms of an abnormal condition.

Beneath the breast is a large muscle, the pectoralis major, which assists in arm movement; the breast rests on this muscle. (Portions of three other muscles are also found under the lower and outer portions of the breast.) Originating on the chest wall, the pectoralis major extends from deep under the breast to attach on the upper arm. It also helps form the axillary fold, created where the arm and chest wall meet. The axilla (armpit) is the depression behind this fold. Removal of the pectoralis major muscle, as was formerly done during a radical mastectomy (an operation rarely performed anymore), left a considerable deformity: the chest had a hollowed-out appearance under the collarbone, the skin was tight and drawn over the rib cage, and the axillary fold and axilla were missing.

A rich system of blood vessels supplies nutrients and hormones to the breast. Because blood flow is increased during the menstrual cycle, pregnancy, and sexual stimulation, the breasts become engorged.

Fluid exits the breast through the venous network of the bloodstream and the lymphatic channels. The lymphatics are small vessels that carry tissue fluid away from the breast, where it passes through a system of filters known as lymph nodes. As part of the body's immune system, the lymph nodes can enlarge in response to local infection or tumor. Trapped breast cancer cells multiplying in these lymph nodes also can cause them to swell. The two main lymph drainage areas are under the breastbone and in the axilla. Enlarged lymph nodes in the axilla usually can be felt.

In examining a woman's breasts the physician first checks the appearance of the skin and nipple-areola for any changes such as dimpling, nipple inversion, or crusting. He then feels the glandular tissue of the breast to detect suspicious or unusual lumps or thickenings. (Despite the beneficial value of mammograms [breast x-ray films], the physical breast examination is still the most common way of detecting breast masses.) In addition, the physician examines the underarm to determine if there is lymph node enlargement. When breast cancer spreads, it often can be detected first in the underarm. Thus a patient who is being treated for breast cancer usually has some of these lymph nodes from the underarm removed and examined by a pathologist to see if the cancer has spread to them and if so to what extent. Removal of the lymph nodes can accentuate the depth or hollow appearance of the armpit.

Each woman's breasts are shaped differently. Individual breast appearance is influenced by the volume of a woman's breast tissue and fat, her age, a history of previous pregnancies and lactation, her heredity, the quality and elasticity of her breast skin, and the influence of breast hormones.

The breast is responsive to a complex interplay of hormones that causes the breast tissue to develop, enlarge, and produce milk. The three major hormones affecting the breast are estrogen, progesterone, and prolactin, which cause glandular tissue in both the breast and uterus to change during a woman's menstrual cycle. Because of reduced hormonal levels the breasts are less full for 1 to 2 weeks after menstrual flow; therefore it may be easier to detect breast lumps during this time. Reduction of hormonal levels is also responsible for the breast's return to its prepregnant state after breast-feeding is concluded.

The cells lining the small lobular ducts of the breast change with each menstrual cycle. They grow under the influence of estrogen early in the cycle, and in the latter part of the cycle they replicate their DNA and divide under the influence of progesterone and estrogen. This process continues through the onset of menstruation until, with declining levels of estrogen and progesterone, a number of cells equal to those that have been divided is destroyed. By this process the cells of the terminal lobular ducts are essentially replaced with each menstrual cycle in young women. This process of cell loss and renewal slows as a woman approaches menopause. After menopause, the terminal lobular ducts atrophy, cell renewal all but ceases, and the lobules atrophy unless supplemental hormones are given. The process of cell renewal in the breast lobules during the reproductive years is reminiscent of a similar process in the endometrium (lining of the uterus). It provides a continually fresh cell population ready to undergo growth and development in preparation for lactation during pregnancy. Proliferation and turnover of cells in the lobular breast ducts are particularly rapid in women below age 35, especially in the teens and twenties. Radiation exposure should be minimized during these younger years because the risk of inducing cancer is high when cells are proliferating.

Some women have a large amount of breast tissue and/or breast fat and thus have large breasts. Others have a small, but normal amount of breast tissue with little breast fat and thus have small breasts. After weight loss, pregnancy, or menopause, many women experience a decrease in breast size and volume. If the skin does not have sufficient elasticity, the breasts also can appear to droop or sag. The size of a woman's breasts often influences whether they will sag. The larger the breasts, the more likely they are to succumb to the constant force of gravity. This sagging appearance (ptosis) often accompanies the aging process, particularly if the breast size decreases.

Few women have completely balanced breasts; one side is often larger or smaller, higher or lower, or shaped differently than the other side. The underlying chest wall may also be asymmetric. Breast asymmetry is normal, even though some women are not aware of it unless it is pointed out to them.

Breast shape and appearance change as a woman ages. In the young woman the breast skin is stretched and expanded by the developing breasts. The breast in the adolescent is usually hemispherical, rounded, and equally full in all areas. As a woman gets older, the top side of the breast tissue settles to a lower position, the skin stretches, and the shape of the breast changes. After menopause, with the decrease of hormonal activity, the composition of the breast changes: the amount of glandular tissue decreases and fat and ductal tissues become the predominant components of the breast. Reduction in glandular volume can result in further looseness of the breast skin.

Skin quality influences breast shape. Even though breast skin contains special elastic fibers, there is much natural and hereditary variation in the amount of elasticity and thickness of each individual's breast skin. Some women have thicker skin with considerable elasticity or stretch. They tend to have tighter and firmer breasts longer than women who have thinner skin with less elasticity. Women with very thin skin may even develop stretch marks, or striae. These marks are actual tears of the deeper layers of the thin skin and usually indicate a lack of elasticity.

Few women realize the large area of their chest that is actually covered by breast tissue; it may extend from just below the collarbone to the level of the sixth rib and from the edge of the breastbone to the underarm area. A portion of the breast even reaches into the armpit region. The breast also has mobility on the chest wall because of loose fibrous (fascial) attachments to the underlying muscles. This breast motion is limited and the breasts are given support by special ligaments known as Cooper's ligaments. When a breast is removed, these ligaments, their fascial attachments, some lymph nodes from the armpit area, and sometimes even the underlying muscles are removed. Thus the deformity created encompasses much more than a missing breast, and for breast reconstruction to be successful, it must fill in or restore all of these areas.

# 3

# BREAST SELF-EXAMINATION

Breast self-examination (BSE) can save a woman's life. Many women are so fearful of finding a breast lump they avoid checking their breasts; this neglect can prove to be foolishly dangerous. It may even allow cancer to go undetected and spread outside the local breast tissue, thus decreasing the chance for cure and long-term survival. Periodic breast examinations are important for early detection of breast cancer, which ranks second to lung cancer as the most frequent cause of cancer death in women. Statistics reveal that most breast cancers are first discovered by women themselves. If more women practiced routine BSE and became familiar with the normal feel of their breasts, the incidence of death from breast cancer could possibly be reduced by as much as 18% because BSE-detected tumors usually are discovered when the tumor is in its early, more curable stages. In addition to checking her own breasts, a woman should have her gynecologist, internist, or family physician examine them at least once a year.

BSE is clearly an essential part of a woman's health care. It is easy to learn and perform, does not require a special setting, and can be incorporated into any woman's normal routine. BSE is basically a "familiarity exercise" that helps acquaint a woman with the look and feel of her breasts and their normal cyclic changes, making it easier for her to detect breast changes early, when treatment is most likely to be effective. As a result of early detection of breast cancer, a less extensive operation may be needed.

Many women are puzzled by their breasts' natural lumpy texture and question their ability to find a small lump within this irregular breast tissue. Initially it may be difficult to differentiate between normal and abnormal breast tissue. A woman may even want to ask her doctor to go through the procedure with her the first time. He can examine her breasts, tell her what he feels and why, and help her to understand what she is looking for. Eventually, with monthly inspection, she will feel more comfortable and knowledgeable about this process.

Some women have fibrocystic changes that give their breasts a lumpy texture and confound their attempts at BSE. These lumps frequently shrink and swell with the menstrual cycle. Women with fibrocystic breasts should identify the ordinary bumpy areas of their breasts so that they can monitor cyclic changes and thus discover any new, distinct lumps.

Ideally, BSE should be conducted once a month. If a woman is still menstruating, she should inspect her breasts approximately 7 to 10 days after the beginning of menstruation, when they are not swollen and tender. If she is no longer menstruating, she should still perform regular monthly examinations; the first day of each month is often an easy-to-remember schedule. Monthly BSE should also remain a part of a woman's routine after she has had a mastectomy or lumpectomy or after breast reconstruction.

## HOW TO DO BSE

BSE consists of visual inspection and palpation (feeling).

### Visual Inspection

To examine your breasts visually, stand in front of a mirror in a well-lighted room and carefully observe all sides of your breasts for unusual characteristics. Any differences in the size or shape of your breasts should be noted. You are looking for discharge from your nipples, sudden nipple inversion (if your nipples were previously erect), a skin rash, scaling, redness, puckering, or dimpling. Some women may notice that they have prominent veins in their breasts. This condition, in itself, is not cause for alarm if it is the normal state of a woman's breasts. Changes in the appearance of these veins are important. If you notice any of these variations in your breast appearance, you should immediately report them to your doctor.

To identify any changes in the shape of your breasts, observe yourself in three positions: (1) straightforward with your hands at your sides, (2) hands raised and clasped behind your head with hands pressed forward, and (3) hands pressed firmly on your hips with shoulders and elbows pulled forward. As you assume the last two positions, you should be able to feel your chest muscles tense. The outline of your breasts should have a smooth curve in all positions.

## Visual Inspection

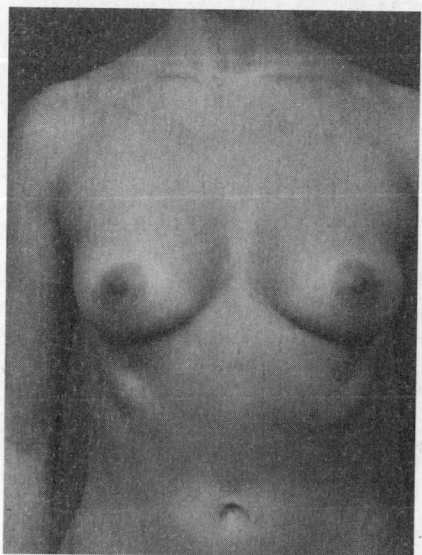

Stand straightforward with your hands at your sides.

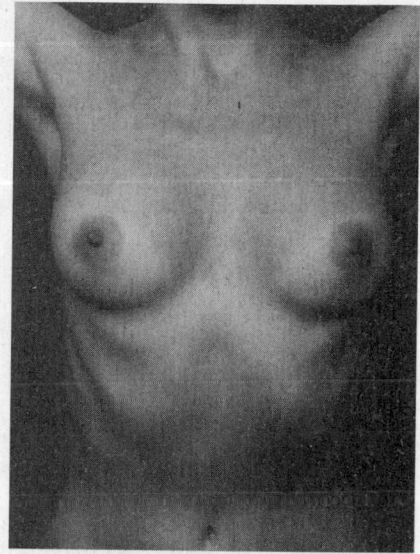

Raise your hands and clasp them behind your head with your hands pressed forward.

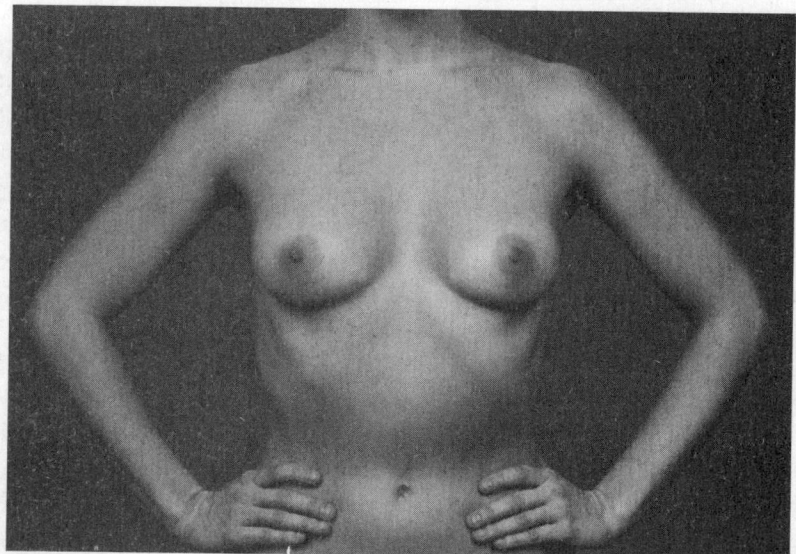

Press your hands firmly on your hips with your shoulders and elbows pulled forward.

If you have had a mastectomy or lumpectomy or breast reconstruction, you must also observe the breast scar for any sign of new swelling, lumps, redness, or color change. Although redness may be caused by chafing from your undergarments or your prosthesis, it should be reported to your doctor.

## Palpation (Feeling)

The most important part of the examination, feeling your breasts, can be done while you are standing or lying down. There is no need to be embarrassed about feeling your breasts; this is a normal part of a woman's health care.

Many women prefer the privacy of the shower for this inspection. The soap and water make their skin feel slippery, and their fingers can glide smoothly over their breasts, making it easier for them to detect any textural changes underneath.

If palpation is performed while standing, begin the inspection by raising your left arm and using the flat, cushioned part of your fingers of your right hand (not the fingertips) to feel your left breast. Place your fingers at the outer edge of your breast and slowly press or compress the breast tissue gently down to the chest wall beneath.

Several patterns can be used for examining your breasts. With one, the strip pattern, you start at the top of your chest and palpate your breasts in a vertical pattern, carefully compressing the breast tissue, strip by strip, until all breast tissue has been inspected. With another pattern, you examine your breasts by moving your fingers in small circles around your breast, gradually working toward the nipple. Still another pattern approaches the breast as if it were a circle divided into wedges (sometimes referred to as the "wedge" pattern). Then you examine your breast wedge by wedge, working from the outer portion of your breast toward the nipple until the whole breast is examined. Which pattern you choose is not important. What is important is selecting one, using it consistently, and allowing yourself enough time for a thorough and deliberate examination. With all of these patterns, be sure to palpate the entire breast region and the areas above the breast and under the collarbone and the underarm, including the armpit itself. Sometimes lumps are discovered in this area. You are looking for any thickening, masses, swollen lymph nodes, or unusual lumps under the skin and especially a change from previous examinations. They might feel like firm, distinct bumps. Repeat this examination on your right side.

## Palpation

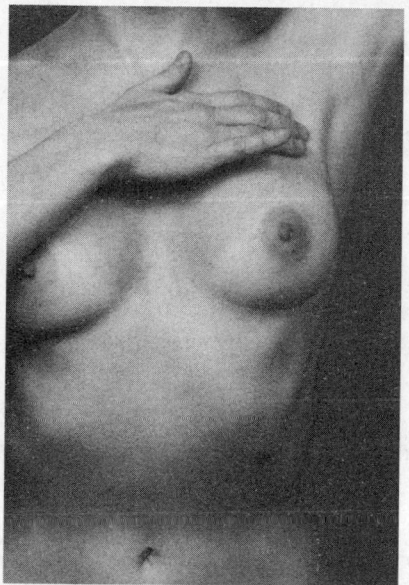

Place your fingers at the outer edge of your breast and slowly compress the breast tissue.

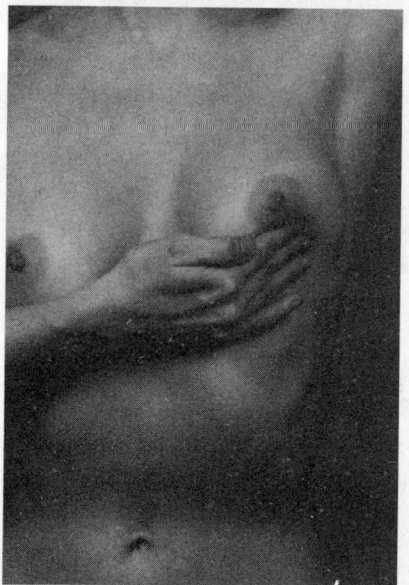

Move your fingers in small circles, working toward the nipple.

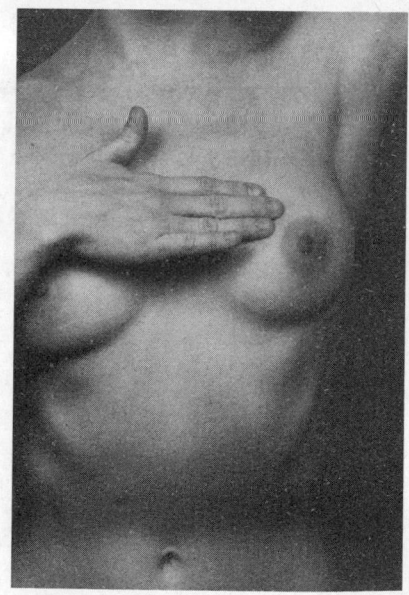

Check the entire breast and underarm, including the armpit.

## Palpation Patterns

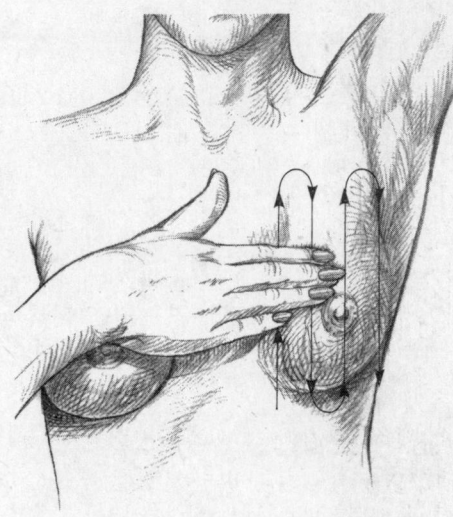

Vertical pattern

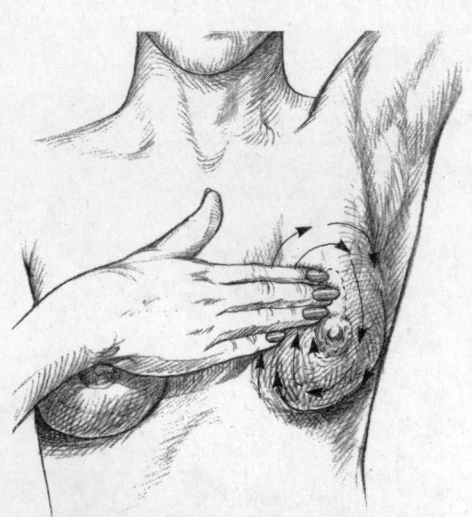

Circular pattern

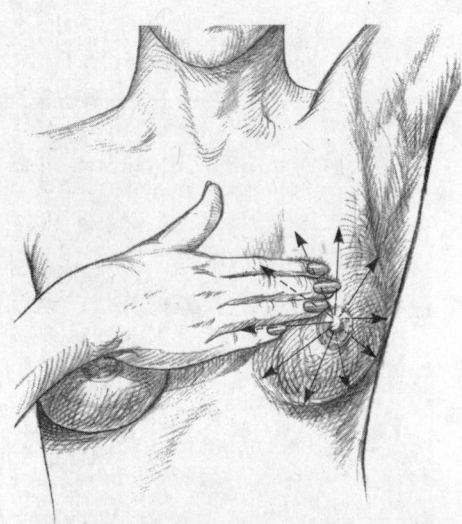

Wedge pattern

If you have had a mastectomy, a lumpectomy, or breast reconstruction, you should feel your chest area, paying close attention to the scar and tissue surrounding it. Raise your arm on the unoperated side (or opposite side if you have had bilateral surgery) and using your opposite hand place three or four fingers at the top of the scar. Press gently using the circular motion described previously. Inspect the entire length of the scar. You are looking for lumps, bumps, hard spots, or thickenings. As with your breasts, familiarity with your scar will make it easier for you to recognize any changes and report them to your physician.

If you perform the inspection while lying down, lie flat on your back with your left arm over your head and a pillow or rolled towel under

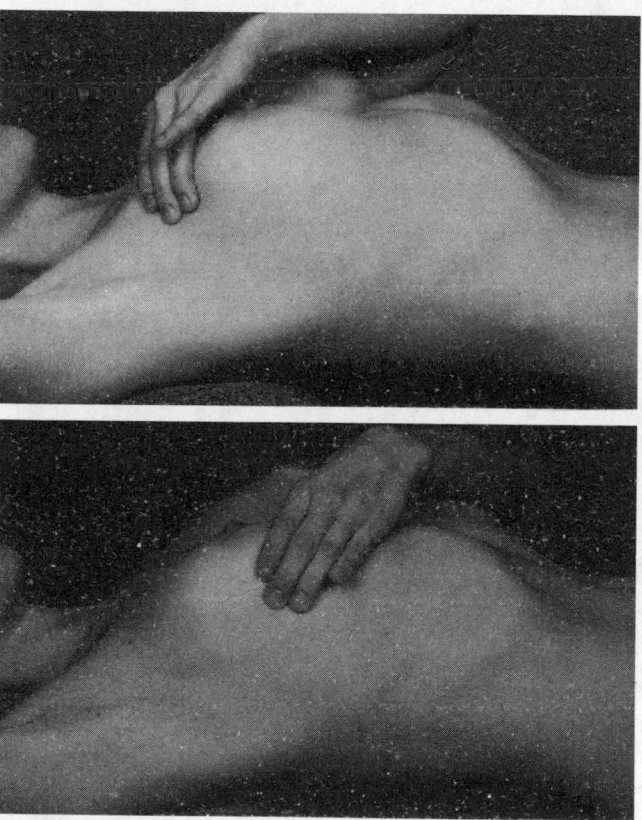

Breast self-examination while lying down

your left shoulder. This position flattens your breasts and makes it easier for you to examine them. Use the same strip, circular, or wedge pattern described previously and repeat the procedure on your right breast.

Remember, most women's breasts have a bumpy texture and the upper, outer portion is usually the lumpiest. The best way to discover abnormal breast lumps is to know what is normal for your breasts; then if a problem develops, you can spot it immediately. Essentially what you are looking for are persistent lumps that do not disappear or change size after menstrual cycles. These are dominant lumps, appearing suddenly and persisting. Abnormal breast lumps will vary in size, firmness, and sensitivity. They may be hard or irregular with sharp edges. Still others appear as thickened areas with no distinct outlines. Some lumps are painful and tender. Pain and/or tenderness is not ordinarily a sign of breast cancer, however, and may simply indicate the development of a breast cyst. Sometimes natural underlying anatomic structures such as breast glands, breastbone, or ribs can be mistaken for lumps. A firm ridge in the lower curve of each breast is normal. Don't worry about making a mistake. *Suspected lumps should always be reported to your doctor. It never hurts to be wrong, but it can be fatal to ignore a cancer.*

Whether you perform BSE while standing or lying down, the important point is to make the decision to do a self-inspection each month. Any breast changes, unusual pain or tenderness, or lumps you discover should be investigated further by your doctor. Along with your monthly BSE, you should have regular checkups by your family physician, internist, or gynecologist. A breast examination should be a routine part of your yearly office visit. The American Cancer Society recommends the following guidelines for the detection of breast cancer in asymptomatic women:

- Women 20 years of age and older should perform monthly BSE.
- Women 20 to 39 should have a physical examination every 3 years by a health care professional (such as a physician, physician assistant, nurse, or nurse practitioner).
- Women 40 and older should have a physical examination of the breast every year by a health care professional.
- Women 40 years of age and older should have a yearly mammogram.

Most breast lumps are benign, but for those that are malignant, mammography, BSE, and physician surveillance will ensure early detection and a significantly higher cure rate.

# MAMMOGRAPHY AND OTHER BREAST IMAGING METHODS FOR EARLY DETECTION AND DIAGNOSIS

BARBARA S. MONSEES, M.D.

Mammography (x-ray examination of the breast) is the single most sensitive method for early detection of breast cancer. Yet, surprisingly, despite extensive media coverage about the value of screening mammography, many women still fail to take advantage of this lifesaving diagnostic tool. It is estimated that 40% of women between ages 40 and 49, 35% of women between ages 50 and 64, and 46% of women older than 65 have not had a mammogram in the past 2 years. Fear of finding that their worst suspicion is confirmed, apprehension that radiation exposure from mammography may cause the very breast cancer it seeks to detect, fear of possible breast loss from mastectomy, concerns about the costs of this test, and lack of support by their physician often deter women from having mammograms taken. These fears may prove to be a woman's worst enemy.

Many well-documented studies have demonstrated that women who have routine mammography have a lower death rate from breast cancer than those who do not. When properly performed and interpreted, mammography has the potential to detect approximately 85% to 90% of breast cancers. Cost deterrents have also been addressed through mandated insurance coverage in most states, Medicare coverage, and the availability of low-cost screening mammography. *Most masses detected on mammograms are benign.* Of the cancerous tumors detected by mammograms before they are large enough to be felt, many can be cured, most by a lumpectomy with irradiation without a mastectomy. Furthermore, the radiation delivered during mammography is so small that the benefits of detecting a possible tumor far outweigh the theoretical risk of developing breast cancer.

Basically there are two types of mammograms: screening mammograms and diagnostic mammograms.

## SCREENING MAMMOGRAMS

Screening is the process of evaluating healthy people with no symptoms to detect early signs of disease. A baseline screening mammogram provides a record of normal breast tissue appearance against which later changes can be compared. Once a baseline has been established, routine screening mammograms are used to find possible abnormalities. Further workups may then be necessary to determine the significance of the findings. Although mammograms are extremely effective in finding most breast cancers, they cannot provide a definitive diagnosis; that can only be done by a biopsy (see Chapter 5).

Mammography is a highly sensitive method for detecting breast cancer, but it is not perfect. For this reason, a woman should not request a screening examination if she suspects that she has a breast lump or other signs or symptoms suggestive of breast cancer. A mammogram interpreted as normal in that circumstance may offer false assurance that breast cancer is not present. Therefore, if a lump or area of breast thickening is present, a woman should seek the advice of her personal physician and possibly a breast surgeon. When there is a suspected sign or symptom of breast cancer, a diagnostic mammogram is warranted for full evaluation.

## DIAGNOSTIC MAMMOGRAMS

A diagnostic mammogram is used to evaluate a woman in any of the following situations: when a lump or thickening has been felt, when a screening mammogram reveals a potential problem (such as a shadow) that requires further investigation, when she has breast implants, or when she has a personal history of breast cancer. Physical examination of the breasts performed as part of a diagnostic evaluation can be correlated with the mammographic findings. Specially tailored views may be ordered to better assess an area of abnormality found on either mammography or physical examination. Preferably, the diagnostic examination should be monitored by a radiologist, which adds to the cost. If the radiologist feels it is appropriate, an ultrasound evaluation may be used as an adjunct to the diagnostic mammogram.

The diagnostic mammogram may demonstrate that a palpable abnormality (one that can be felt) is a characteristically benign or malignant lesion and therefore determine whether a biopsy is warranted. It may also confirm a lesion that is considered indeterminate, meaning that only biopsy can determine whether it is benign or malignant. The mammogram may also detect another abnormality at a different location in the same breast or in the opposite one. Therefore women over the age of 30 scheduled to have a biopsy should first have a mammogram to determine if another suspicious area requires attention. Women over 30 who are having breast surgery should also have a mammogram before the operation.

The location, character, and extent of disease seen on a mammogram can often be helpful in determining if a woman is a good candidate for lumpectomy or breast-conserving surgery. If a biopsy is positive, a postoperative mammogram may be ordered to see if other tumors are present in the breast that would dictate mastectomy rather than breast-conserving therapy.

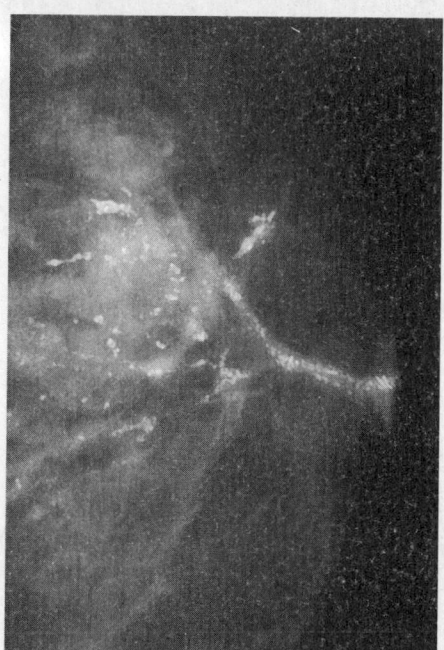

Screening mammogram showing microcalcifications with malignant appearance. (These appear as small white dots in a branching pattern.)

## SCREENING RECOMMENDATIONS

When should a woman have her first mammogram and how often should she have follow-up mammograms? Much media attention and public confusion has been generated over conflicting reports about the value of screening mammography for women in their forties. Fortunately, this controversy has now been resolved. The American Cancer Society has revised its guidelines to recommend annual screening for women beginning at age forty. This decision is based on the following evidence:

- "One in 66 women in their forties will develop breast cancer.
- About 18% of all breast cancers occur in women in their forties
- 13% of the 44,000 women expected to die of breast cancer during 1998 will be in their forties.
- Results from the most recent meta-analysis (a compilation of many studies) of all eight randomized clinical trials found 18% fewer deaths from breast cancer among women in their forties who had mammography.
- Results from two individual randomized clinical trials in Sweden found fewer deaths from breast cancer in women in their forties undergoing screening mammography. In one study, breast cancer deaths in this age group were reduced by 44%; in the other study they were reduced by 36%.
- Breast cancers found by mammographic screening of women in their forties were smaller and at an earlier stage (with less spread to lymph nodes or other organs) than cancers found in women not having mammography."

"The American Cancer Society believes that the benefits of yearly mammography for women in their forties and older outweigh the impact of occasional false positive results leading to biopsy of noncancerous abnormalities and the economic cost of these examinations."

For women over age 50, there is no debate about the benefit of yearly mammograms, which are recommended by both the National Cancer Institute and the American Cancer Society. Mammograms are most effective for women in this age group since their breasts are not as dense and abnormalities can be more readily identified. A woman's gynecologist or family physician usually arranges for this test to help monitor her health care. The incidence of breast cancer rises between the ages of 50 and 74, and screening mammograms become especially important.

Like any test, however, mammography should be used appropriately, and regular mammograms are not routinely advised for young women under the age of 30 who are not at high risk. Young girls and teenagers have the highest theoretical risk of developing a radiation-induced breast tumor and also have an extremely low risk of having breast cancer. Also, younger women's breasts are denser, making it more difficult to distinguish a mass or dense spot or early breast cancer on a mammogram. Therefore the benefit of routine screening mammography in younger women is low.

Women with a close family member who has had premenopausal breast cancer may be advised to begin earlier screening, perhaps as early as age 25 to 30. The recent discovery of specific genes that carry a very high risk of breast cancer for affected women is hopeful as well as frightening. If a woman has a family history suggestive of familial breast cancer, she should consider genetic counseling. Such a family history may be suspected if a close relative such as a mother or a sister has breast cancer. Multiple affected family members, particularly with bilateral breast cancer (both breasts) or diagnosis at an early age, and/or a family history of ovarian cancer may also indicate such a predisposition. A genetic tendency for breast cancer can also be inherited through the father's side of the family. Since men rarely have breast cancer, relatives that might point to a significant family history include the paternal grandmother or paternal aunts.

## THE EXAM

Mammogram units have compression plates to thin and flatten the breast to a uniform thickness. Adequate compression not only improves the quality of the breast images, but also lowers the x-ray dose to the breast. During a typical examination two or three views are taken of each breast, one with the breast squeezed between two angled plates and one more with the breast squeezed between two horizontal plates. More than one view of each breast is necessary to unfold the overlapping breast densities seen on the film.

Some women complain of discomfort from the squeezing necessary to pull the breast tissue away from the chest wall and compress it between the plates for the x-ray films. However, this process takes only a few seconds for each exposure. The entire examination usually takes less than 5 minutes. Many women have no problem at all.

Women who complain of breast tenderness should consider delaying the test until after their period or early in the monthly cycle (if they are still menstruating) or a time when their breasts are less tender. Mammograms may also be delayed for a few weeks after a breast operation because the breast compression may prove uncomfortable. As with any test or procedure, the ability to tolerate pain and discomfort varies among individuals. Most admit, however, that any pain associated with mammography is short lived and the benefits far outweigh the momentary discomfort.

## WHERE TO GET YOUR MAMMOGRAM

Many women wonder where to go to ensure they get a high-quality mammogram. Screening mammography may be performed in a breast diagnostic center, at a radiology office, at a physician's office, or on a mobile mammography unit. Federal law dictates that any mammography facility has to meet certain minimum standards delineated in the Mammography Quality Standards Act. All facilities should be certified by the Food and Drug Administration. Before making a decision about where to go, you should consult with your personal physician.

Asking the following questions may help you determine the quality of a facility:

*How many mammograms are taken each day?*

If 20 or more mammograms are performed per day, there is a higher likelihood that the technologist and radiologist will be experienced.

*Does the facility have a film processor expressly devoted to developing mammograms or does it develop other x-ray films in the same processor?*

Film processors used for chest or bone x-ray films are not likely to result in top-quality mammograms.

*Is the person who takes the mammograms a dedicated registered mammography technologist or does he or she take other types of x-ray films as well?*

The more experienced the technologist, the greater the likelihood that this professional will do a better job of breast positioning and thus obtain better quality images.

### *Is the radiologist who reads the mammograms specially trained to do so?*

The radiologist should be board certified and should have taken specific training courses in mammography. A radiologist who specializes in breast imaging is likely to be more experienced in interpreting the findings.

If you have found a good facility, try to return there year after year; that strategy will make it easier to compare current with older films. If you switch facilities, try to bring your old films for comparison.

## WHAT ARE THE COSTS?

Because of widespread recognition of the importance of breast x-ray films, many hospitals, clinics, and medical centers are offering low-cost screening mammograms ranging from $50 to $150, and many states require insurance carriers to cover the expenses of this test. Additionally, Medicare now pays for annual mammograms. Insurance carriers and Medicare should reimburse for both screening and diagnostic mammography when indicated. To find the least expensive source for mammograms, a woman can compare prices by calling the American Cancer Society's national toll-free number, 800/ACS-2345, to request a list of low-cost, quality mammography facilities in her local area.

## MAMMOGRAPHY IN SPECIAL CIRCUMSTANCES
### Augmentation Mammaplasty

Breast implants can affect the quality of the mammogram and the radiologist's ability to detect breast cancer. Because the implant is opaque to x-rays, any breast tissue underlying the implant cannot be seen on the films. If a woman is at higher risk for developing breast cancer because of her family history, she should discuss this matter with her plastic surgeon prior to undergoing augmentation.

Extra views can be obtained to compensate for the inability to "see through" the implant. Most helpful are the so-called implant displacement views that allow visualization of the breast after the breast tissue has been gently pulled in front of the implant. Implant displacement views provide better visualization if the implant has been placed under rather than over the chest wall muscle (submuscular position),

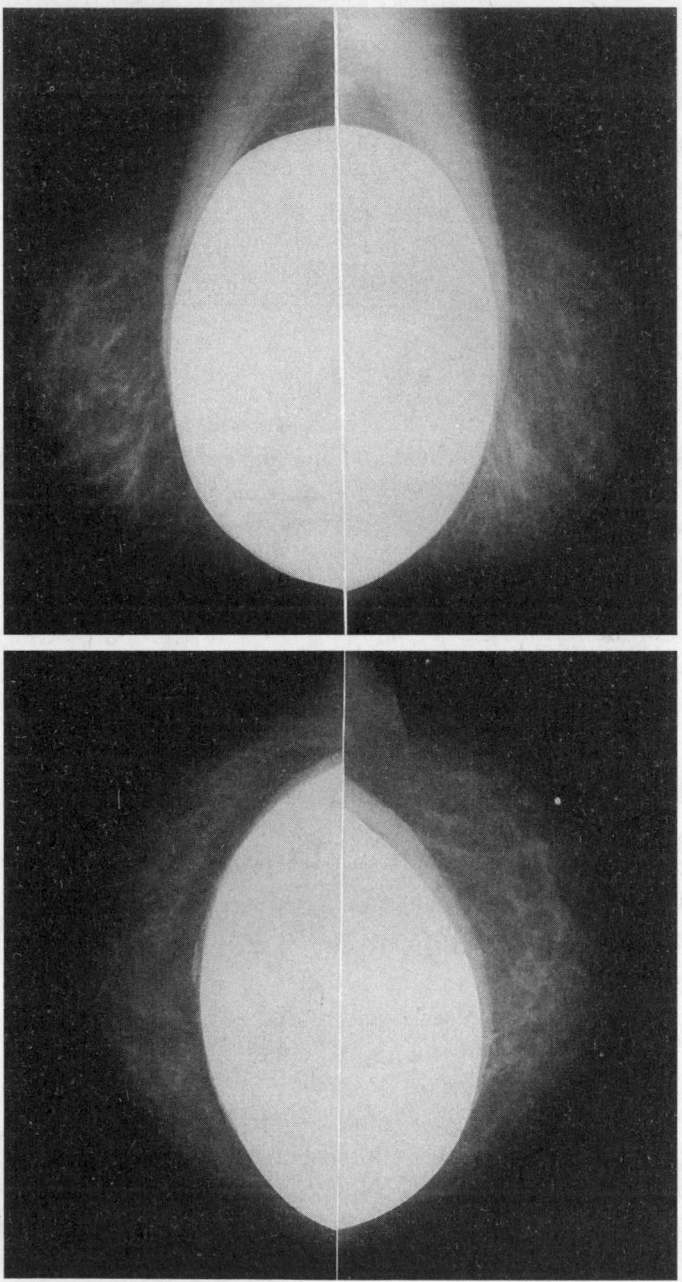

Full mammographic views of both breasts in two routine projections
of a patient with subpectoral breast implants

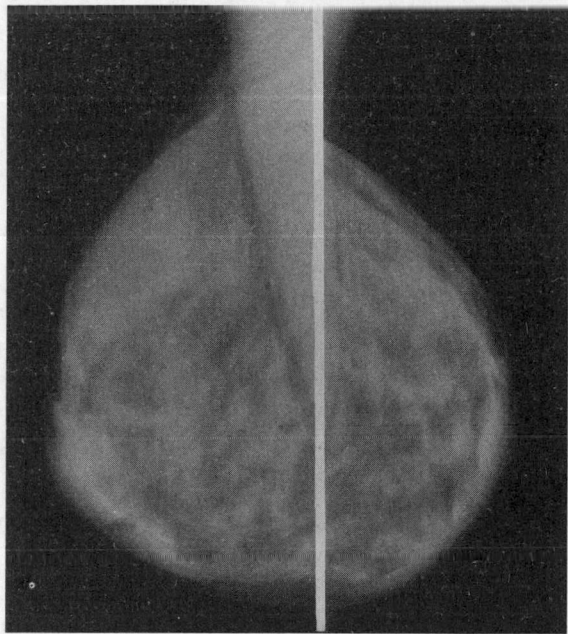

Special implant displacement view of breast with implant

if a smaller implant has been used, and if the breast has remained soft. Women should notify the technologist if they have breast implants before having a mammogram taken. The pressure on the breast during mammography will not break or rupture a breast implant. If the facility does not routinely obtain displacement views in all women with implants, the woman should go elsewhere for her mammogram.

## Reduction Mammaplasty

Women who have had breast reduction should also inform the radiologic technologist of this before a mammogram is taken. Although scarring from breast reduction is sometimes seen on the mammogram, it does not usually present a problem for radiographic interpretation. Unless an implant has been placed in the breast at the time of reduction, no special views are necessary. Routine screening mammography as suggested by the American Cancer Society is recommended. If an implant has been placed at the time of reduction, then the woman should have implant displacement views appropriate for mammography in women with breast implants.

If a woman is contemplating having reduction or augmentation mammaplasty, a preoperative mammogram should be obtained to screen for breast cancer if the woman is over the age of 30 to avoid missing a nonpalpable breast problem. This should be discussed with the plastic surgeon prior to the surgery.

## After Mastectomy

A woman who has had a mastectomy for breast cancer needs routine surveillance of the opposite breast to screen for breast cancer. Mammography should be performed every year following the initial diagnosis, regardless of the patient's age. Women often ask if they need mammograms taken on the mastectomy side. Some facilities obtain special chest wall views to examine for recurrence in the skin or muscle of the chest wall. There is no evidence that such views can change the outcome by earlier detection of recurrences on the chest wall. However, if a woman or her physician can feel a nodule on the chest wall, views of that area can be helpful in evaluation and may determine the need for a biopsy. If a woman has had a mastectomy and subsequent reconstruction, yearly mammography of the opposite breast is warranted to screen for breast cancer. However, as in the case of a woman who has had a mastectomy with reconstruction, mammography of the reconstructed breast is not necessary because no breast tissue remains on the mastectomy side. If a problem develops in the reconstructed breast, special views of the region can be obtained and are often useful in evaluation. Ultrasonography may also be used under these circumstances.

## After Breast-Conserving Surgery and Irradiation

A woman who has undergone lumpectomy and radiation therapy must have meticulous follow-up mammograms of the treated breast. Yearly screening of the opposite breast is adequate, but mammographic follow-up of the treated breast may be done at more frequent intervals. If a new abnormality (such as a mass or area of microcalcifications) is found on the mammogram or felt to be present on physical examination, then biopsy may be necessary to determine if there is a recurrence in the treated breast.

# OTHER IMAGING MODALITIES
## Ultrasonography

Ultrasonography is an extremely useful adjunct to mammography, but it is not a substitute or match for mammography in detecting small cancers and therefore should not be used for routine screening. Its ability to differentiate a breast mass containing fluid (a cyst) from a solid mass (a benign or malignant tumor or other finding) offers distinct benefits. If a mammogram discloses the presence of a rounded mass in the breast that cannot be felt, an ultrasound scan is often obtained. If the mass is a simple cyst containing fluid, then biopsy is not necessary. With the use of ultrasound guidance, the fluid can be drained from a breast cyst if desired. In most instances, however, unless the cyst is painful or large (greater than 2 cm or approximately 1 inch), aspiration is usually not warranted. However, if the cyst is not a simple cyst but exhibits irregularities, then biopsy may be recommended.

Ultrasonography has undergone many advances in recent years and may be useful in a variety of other circumstances. The ultrasound characteristics of a palpable abnormality can often indicate whether a

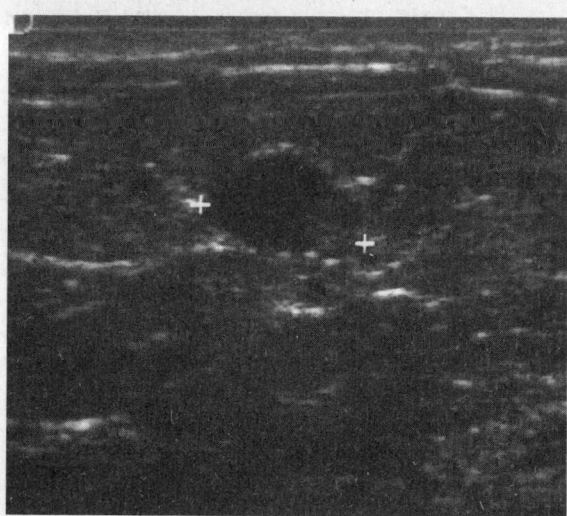

Ultrasound scan of small breast mass shows a tiny solid mass attached to the wall of a breast cyst. This patient will require a breast biopsy.

lesion is more likely to be benign or malignant. It can also be used to assess a patient with the signs or symptoms of infection or a patient with breast implants to evaluate a lump or the integrity of the implants. However, as is true of mammography, this test is not tissue specific and biopsy is often warranted for a definite diagnosis. Ultrasonography, however, can be effectively used to guide special procedures in the breast (image-guided biopsy), such as fine-needle aspiration or core biopsy.

## Techniques With Occasional Application

Computed tomography (CT) is rarely useful in breast imaging. Magnetic resonance imaging (MRI) is under investigation for its value in evaluating breast tissue and in detecting breast cancer in patients with extremely dense breasts on mammograms or in very high-risk patients such as women known to carry a breast cancer gene. It may also have a role in assessing the extent of disease within the breast in patients with a diagnosis of breast cancer. MRI is extremely useful in evaluating the integrity of breast implants. Special breast coils are needed to adapt the equipment for breast evaluation and can detect over 90% of breast implant ruptures. Positron emission tomography (PET) is still considered experimental and is being assessed in some centers for its usefulness in evaluating the axillary lymph nodes and the extent of metastatic disease. It may also prove useful in the search

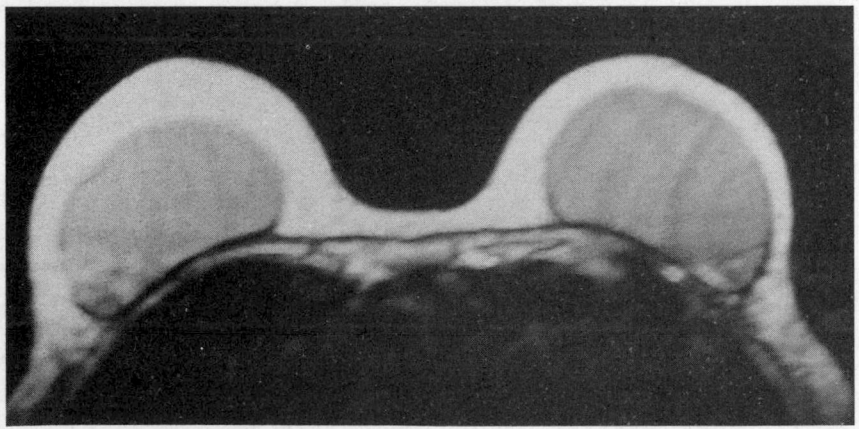

MRI scan of the chest of a woman with bilateral breast implants

for a primary breast cancer and in estimating the response to systemic therapy such as chemotherapy or hormone therapy.

Scintimammography, a nuclear medicine technique, has received FDA approval and is being used clinically in practices across the United States. Unfortunately, although "safe," its effectiveness in detection and diagnosis has not been well studied and its clinical role is questionable. It is much less reliable when used to evaluate smaller breast lesions, those most likely to result in early detection "cures," and therefore its efficacy is doubtful.

## IMAGE-GUIDED BIOPSY

Image-guided biopsy represents one of the most exciting developments in breast biopsy and reflects the increasing use of minimally invasive surgery in different areas of the body. The imaging methods used are ultrasound guidance (mentioned above) and stereotactic guidance. (The stereotactic unit is a variation of a mammogram unit in which two images are obtained at different angles.) Identifying an imaged abnormality on both views allows a computer to calculate and indicate the accurate placement of a needle into the lesion. For small breast lesions that cannot be felt, image-guided biopsy enables cells or small pieces of tissue to be removed from the area of abnormality with a high degree of accuracy. If the biopsy yields a definitive benign diagnosis, then open surgical biopsy may be avoided. If a definitive malignant diagnosis is made, then the woman can begin discussion regarding her treatment options before she has surgery. These image-guided biopsy techniques are no longer considered experimental and are used routinely in practice.

### Sentinel Node Biopsy

Sentinel node biopsy, which is currently under investigation, is a new and very promising technique for lymph node evaluation. The sentinel lymph node (the first draining node or nodes) is biopsied to determine whether or not the tumor has spread. Two different methods are used for localizing the sentinel node. One approach involves injecting blue dye in the region of the breast cancer and following the dye to the sentinel node. Alternatively, a radioisotope can be injected near a tumor to localize the lymph nodes using nuclear medicine cameras and hand-held probes. Once identified, the sentinel node is removed and sent to the pathologist for evaluation. If it is negative for tumor, then other nodes do not need to be evaluated because the sentinel node status is a good indicator of whether the tumor has spread. This new biopsy technique may replace standard axillary lymph node dissection in women with newly diagnosed breast cancer, thereby virtually eliminating some of the associated problems and complications (such as lymphedema) that have sometimes been associated with axillary lymph node dissection (see Chapter 5).

The growing incidence of breast cancer demands women's attention. Breast cancer currently accounts for 32% of new cancers and 19% of cancer deaths among women in the United States. Any test that can facilitate early detection and improve the chance of surviving this disease merits consideration. Mammography is such a test; in most cases it is capable of detecting breast cancer as long as 1 to 4 years before it can be felt on physical examination. However, as with most tests, mammography is not infallible and may fail to find 15% of breast cancers, particularly in younger women, underscoring the complementary role of mammography and breast physical examination. Routine breast physical examination by a skilled examiner, breast self-examination, and routine screening mammography currently represent the most effective way to monitor women for breast cancer and to ensure detection in its earliest stages with the best chance for cure or long-term survival.

Adjunctive techniques such as ultrasonography and MRI are helpful in characterizing abnormalities detected on mammography or by clinical breast examination. Image-guided biopsy and sentinel node biopsy represent the latest advances in minimally invasive approaches to diagnosis. Image-guided biopsy is highly accurate, commonly used, and well tolerated. Sentinel node biopsy is still being evaluated but shows great promise for lymph node assessment.

# BREAST LUMPS AND OTHER BREAST CONDITIONS

When a woman discovers a breast lump, she naturally fears that she has breast cancer. Fortunately, most breast lumps are benign and are not related to breast cancer. Nevertheless, these conditions can cause a woman and her family considerable anxiety. Her breasts also may be painfully uncomfortable because of breast engorgement or inflammation. Although many women immediately equate breast pain with cancer, most tender lumps are not malignant. Lumpy breasts, however, can be a problem and may make it difficult for a woman or her doctor to detect possible breast tumors. Awareness of commonly occurring benign breast conditions is therefore extremely valuable information for alleviating unwarranted fears and assisting a woman in early detection of a cancer if it does occur.

Although breast cancer occurs in women of all ages and the incidence among younger women has risen, one of the important factors in predicting whether an isolated breast lump is a cancer is the person's age. Less than 3% of breast cancers occur in women under the age of 35. Most breast cancers develop after menopause. When a woman in her thirties or forties finds a lump, it is more likely to be a simple cyst filled with fluid than a cancer. Less than one third of breast cancers occur in women under the age of 50. After menopause, benign breast conditions occur less frequently and the incidence of breast cancer rises; thus any lump is viewed with more concern.

## BENIGN BREAST CONDITIONS
### Fibroadenomas

When lumps are found in the breasts of teenagers and women in their twenties, they are almost always benign. The most common benign breast lump found in this age group is a firm, rounded, rubbery tumor known as a fibroadenoma. Fibroadenomas are not related to and are not precursors of breast cancer. Surgical removal of these tumors is usually recommended.

### Fibrocystic Breasts

It is normal for many women in their childbearing years to notice that their breasts swell and become painfully tender before their menstrual periods. Along with this swelling the breasts often develop a lumpy texture that in some cases become a permanent breast characteristic. Although this lumpy condition reflects normal changes within the glandular tissue and milk ducts of the breast, it is commonly described as fibrocystic disease. Calling this condition a disease is inappropriate and unnecessarily frightening to women since these physiologic changes occur in at least half of all North American women and are particularly common in women from age 20 to menopause. Because they occur during a time when a woman has a high level of female hormones, they are related to the response of the breast to those hormones. After menopause, fibrocystic activity usually subsides as a result of a woman's reduced hormonal levels. Women taking hormones after menopause may note a persistence of fibrocystic activity and breast fullness.

The symptoms of fibrocystic change frequently vary with a woman's monthly cycle and are often associated with breast pain, which may be constant or may be accentuated when her breasts are swollen. Breast tenderness further increases a woman's anxiety that a tumor may be present even though diffuse pain and tenderness are rarely manifestations of breast cancer. The soreness also can prevent a careful breast examination by the woman herself or by her physician.

Fibrocystic breasts usually feel "bumpy" because of cysts, irregularities, or thickened areas; some of these lumps are indistinguishable from tumors. These fibrocystic changes are not believed to be precancerous, but they may produce noticeable breast lumps that can be confused with cancer or even obscure the diagnosis of a small cancer. The newer image-guided biopsy techniques have further reduced the need for operations for fibrocystic disease.

Fibrocystic change is usually managed without surgery if the doctor confirms that no other breast condition is present. Because it is a chronic condition, it may require surveillance over a long period by both the woman and her doctor, including regular breast self-examination, physician follow-up and examination, mammograms, ultra-

sound studies, aspiration of cysts, and biopsies of lumps that persist af
ter aspiration.

In addition, some experts believe that caffeine can accentuate the
symptoms of fibrocystic breasts and recommend that women with this
problem try to avoid caffeine-containing substances such as colas,
coffees, teas, and chocolates. Some women notice a significant improvement in breast tenderness after abstinence from these foods,
whereas others notice no change in their breasts. Vitamin E in a daily
dosage of 800 IU (international units) is believed by some to lessen
the symptoms of fibrocystic change in some women, although controlled studies have demonstrated no benefit from vitamin E. In ex-
ceptionally severe cases the doctor can prescribe danazol (Danocrine)
or tamoxifen (Nolvadex) to control the pain and swelling. These
drugs are rarely indicated, however, because of undesirable side effects, expense, and lack of efficacy.

### Nipple Drainage

Nipple discharge is usually not caused by cancer. The only nipple dis-
charges that are significant are those that are bloody and those that
occur spontaneously without manipulating or squeezing the nipple.
(It is normal to be able to express or squeeze a small amount of fluid
from the nipples.) A discharge of blood or serum, however, can indicate the presence of cancer and should never be ignored. The doctor
can take a sample of the nipple discharge by spreading a thin layer of
fluid on a glass slide and send it to the pathologist for examination under the microscope; definitive diagnosis, however, can only be made
by biopsying the involved duct.

Small benign tumors within the nipple ducts (ductal papillomas)
as well as fibrocystic changes or inflammation can be the source of
drainage. Sometimes a localized infection within a duct can cause
persistent drainage. Treatment occasionally involves removal of the
source of the drainage within the ductal system. The doctor also may
order some hormonal studies of the blood to identify other benign
causes of nipple discharge.

### Calcifications

Calcifications are calcium deposits in the breast that can only be detected by mammography. These deposits are common in the breasts of
women over the age of 50 and in a smaller percentage of younger
women. Calcifications are associated with benign or noncancerous

conditions and most likely represent degenerative changes in a woman's breasts subsequent to aging of the breast arteries, old injuries, inflammations, or common benign conditions such as fibrocystic changes. Calcifications may be large and coarse (macrocalcifications) or tiny (microcalcifications).

Sometimes minute particles of calcium are discovered on mammograms. Although these microcalcifications can be an indication of precancerous changes or of breast cancer itself, this is not usually the case and a woman should not panic if these are diagnosed. Microcalcifications are common in breast tissue and most (over 80%) are benign and are not markers of breast cancer.

A woman who has numerous scattered microcalcifications in both breasts is not likely to have cancer. Of more concern is a cluster of microcalcifications in one breast, especially if it is new; this may be the earliest finding indicating intraductal cancer. Grouped or clustered microcalcifications are perhaps the most significant secondary sign of malignancy, frequently suggesting the presence of a breast cancer. The probability of malignant disease increases with the degree of irregularity in the shapes of the microcalcifications as well as their size variations. Calcifications can also be noted after breast operations such as breast reduction and breast reconstruction. Most calcifications seen on mammography are benign.

Currently, mammography cannot accurately distinguish between some benign and malignant microcalcifications; therefore, in those cases, biopsy is needed for a definitive diagnosis and to rule out the possibility of breast cancer. A new density in the breast visible on two mammographic views should also be investigated. If a questionable abnormality is discovered on a woman's first mammogram, the doctor may sometimes delay biopsy for several months and then take another mammogram to see if the findings are stable or have changed. Usually, however, unless the findings indicate a very low level of suspicion about possible malignancy, this abnormality needs to be positively identified by the pathologist after a biopsy.

A woman who is concerned about a lump in her breast should insist on appropriate and prompt evaluation that leads to a definitive diagnosis. The process of evaluation ordinarily should last no more than a month or 6 weeks. Sometimes, however, particularly when the woman is young, this process may be complicated by several forces operating in divergent directions. Breast cancer is rare in women under age 35; nevertheless, it does occur, even in women in their early twenties. Cancers in young women are generally faster growing than those in older women and early diagnosis is critical. However, because a lump in a young woman's breast is usually not malignant, the physician may be less likely to suspect breast cancer. He may have referred other patients to surgeons with negative findings. Furthermore, some health maintenance plans penalize primary care physicians for excessive referrals to specialists. Mammography is less effective in detecting cancer in the breasts of young women than older women. *A negative mammogram in such a case does not rule out cancer; in fact, it may be worrisome unless it actually reveals a benign condition.* Reevaluation of the mass at a different stage of the menstrual cycle and needle aspiration for fluid (cyst) or to obtain cells for microscopic examination are appropriate measures. If a benign diagnosis is not established by these or other measures within 6 weeks, the patient should have a biopsy (minimally invasive if possible).

## DIAGNOSIS AND MANAGEMENT

Assuming that a breast problem is detected on a mammogram or that a woman finds a lump in her breast, what can she expect when she visits her doctor? The procedure varies, depending on her symptoms and her doctor's preferences. Some physicians will refer her to a surgeon immediately, whereas others might prefer to examine her first. A medical history is always taken.

It is important to understand that referral to a general surgeon or surgical oncologist does not necessarily mean that a biopsy will be done. Surgeons do not just operate; they are skilled in examining breast lumps, discussing and advising women about commonly occurring breast conditions and breast disease, and helping to detect and treat cancer at an early stage.

As a preliminary step, when a lump is first detected, the physician can use several noninvasive (nonsurgical) diagnostic tools. The doctor may suggest that the woman have diagnostic mammography or ultrasonography, in which sound waves are used to evaluate lumps. Ultrasonography is less specific and less dependable for detecting breast abnormalities than mammography and therefore is not as effective for screening. Unlike mammography, ultrasonography usually does not detect microcalcifications or identify very small cancers. However, it is particularly useful for distinguishing a simple cyst from a solid lump. It is also useful for examining younger women who have normally glandular breasts. The most frequently used and reliable nonoperative diagnostic test is mammography. Magnetic resonance imaging (MRI), a technique that does not use radiation, may be useful in some diagnostic situations. Its applications are evolving. (More detailed information on mammograms and other imaging modalities is provided in Chapter 4.)

Breast examination and mammography are complementary diagnostic tools. Mammography alone without breast examination is inadequate. Sometimes even obvious breast lumps will not show up on x-ray examination; this is more often the case when the woman is under 40 years old and her breasts are relatively dense. A mammogram is a very valuable diagnostic tool, however, because it can indicate a breast abnormality at a very early stage before it can be felt and while it is still small and curable. It cannot, however, positively identify a calcification or a mass as cancerous; this can only be done through a biopsy of the area for examination under a microscope. A biopsy is done after all appropriate imaging tests have been completed.

### Needle Aspiration

When there is a palpable lump in the breast that feels like a cyst, it is usually drained (aspirated) with a thin needle. Occasionally the doctor may tell the patient to return to his office after her next menstrual cycle so that he can reexamine her breast before doing needle aspiration. Tissue that shrinks and then swells again before her next cycle could indicate a cyst or an area of fibrocystic change (both are benign and not related to cancer).

Needle aspiration is a method for determining if a breast mass is cystic or solid. It is a simple and relatively painless procedure that can be done in the surgeon's office. A surgical biopsy may be avoided if the lump disappears after the fluid has been withdrawn from the suspected cyst. The doctor may want to send the fluid for analysis to a pathologist, especially if it is bloodstained. If no fluid is aspirated, the lump could be a fibroadenoma, a fibrocystic change, or a cancer. Most cysts are benign; breast cancer is usually a solid tumor.

If the fluid is bloody or if a mass cannot be aspirated, further investigation is warranted to rule out the possibility of breast cancer regardless of the findings on mammography. In these cases the surgeon removes the lump or samples a portion of the lump so that a specific diagnosis of the tissue can be made by a pathologist. This sampling is called a biopsy and can be performed by needle aspiration or surgery.

Stereotactic or ultrasound-guided needle biopsy may be done when an abnormality is seen on the mammogram but cannot be felt.

## Fine-Needle Aspiration Biopsy

JOHN S. MEYER, M.D.

Fine-needle aspiration biopsy (FNAB) is a method for making a definitive diagnosis of breast carcinoma without an incision or surgical procedure. This approach uses a narrow-gauge needle (similar to or smaller than the type employed to draw blood) that is attached to a syringe. The mass is localized (located) by touch, and the needle is introduced into it as the syringe plunger is drawn back to produce negative pressure, thereby drawing cells and fluid into the needle. Several repeat passes of the needle are necessary to obtain a satisfactory sample. A local anesthetic may be used during the procedure to prevent discomfort. From a few to over 100,000 cells may be obtained in a drop or two of fluid. The cells are deposited on glass slides, stained, and examined microscopically. Interpretation is similar to that for Papanicolaou (Pap) smears. Malignant cells are recognized by their large abnormal nuclei (centers) and disorderly relationships one to another.

Aspiration biopsy in lieu of formal surgical biopsy can be done in the doctor's office, often without the need for anesthesia, and the results can be available so that a decision on therapy can be reached prior to surgery. A number of studies have shown accuracy to be very high when cancer is diagnosed with FNAB; only about 1 in 1000 such diagnoses have been in error. Fibroadenoma (a benign tumor discussed earlier in this chapter) may rarely be indistinguishable from carcinoma in needle aspiration biopsies, and premalignant changes accompanying fibrocystic breasts can at times be confusing to the cytopathologist. For the most part, however, a positive aspiration cytologic diagnosis of cancer can be considered equivalent to a diagnosis by formal biopsy.

FNAB is not as accurate, however, when the results are negative, indicating that no cancer is present. There are several reasons for this diminished reliability. One is the possibility of missing the tumor with the needle. This risk increases as the tumor size becomes smaller. The other reason is that some breast carcinomas have small nuclei with minimal abnormalities, and these cells are difficult to distinguish from cells of fibroadenomas or other benign conditions. Therefore cytopathologists err on the side of caution in diagnosing carcinoma and in certain cases may withhold diagnosis, recommending surgical biopsy for further clarification. If a suspicious lump persists after a negative needle biopsy, a surgical biopsy is necessary for definitive diagnosis.

FNAB may also be indicated when the physician is uncertain about the existence of a breast mass or a mammogram shows a focus of uncertain significance. In this situation the suspicious area can be examined by FNAB to help exclude the possibility of carcinoma. If the FNAB is positive, a diagnosis may be made at an early stage in the evolution of the disease.

Although FNAB is often sufficient for diagnosis of cancer, it is not sufficient for complete classification of the cancer type. The structural pattern of the cancer cannot be ascertained and the cancer cannot be graded by standard pathologic criteria. Estrogen and progesterone receptor assays can be done if several slides are specially prepared for this procedure. FNAB is sufficient for diagnosis prior to lumpectomy or mastectomy. It is not recommended prior to neoadjuvant chemotherapy (chemotherapy prior to definitive surgical removal of the tumor). Neoadjuvant chemotherapy often produces significant tumor shrinkage that can prevent adequate grading and assessment of estrogen and progesterone receptor status when FNAB is used. These results can be obtained instead from a small open incisional or core-needle biopsy.

## Core-Needle Biopsy

Core-needle biopsy uses a cutting-type needle (somewhat larger than the needle used for FNAB) to remove a sample of the breast mass for microscopic examination. A core of tissue 1 mm in diameter ($\frac{1}{32}$ inch) and 1 to 2 cm ($\frac{3}{8}$ to $\frac{3}{4}$ inch) long is obtained with each pass of the needle. This quantity of tissue is sufficient for histologic grading, estrogen and progesterone receptor analysis, and assay for *HER-2/neu* and other molecular entities for genetic studies of the cancer cells. The role of this type of needle biopsy is to make a reasonably definitive diagnosis without a formal operation on a fairly large breast tumor.

## Stereotactic and Ultrasound-Guided (Minimally Invasive) Biopsy

One of the newer methods for biopsying suspicious areas that can be seen on mammograms but cannot be felt is called minimally invasive or closed-needle biopsy. This technique combines FNAB or core-needle biopsy with three-dimensional computer imaging (stereotactic guidance) or with ultrasonography. It allows a needle to be introduced into a lesion that is ultrasonically or mammographically visible. (See Chapter 4 for additional information on minimally invasive biopsy.) This nonoperative or minimally invasive technique requires only a small incision and is performed under local anesthesia with minimal recovery time. Although both biopsy methods are used in some centers, the core-needle biopsy method is becoming a more common approach because specific diagnoses can be made from exact tissue samples that can be evaluated by standard methods in most pathology departments.

Stereotactic-guided and ultrasound-guided core-needle biopsy techniques are sufficiently accurate for diagnosing small tumors less than ½ inch in diameter. These tumors need not be palapable. By this means, the great majority of breast lesions, both benign and malignant, can be identified. If the lesion is benign, excisional surgery is unnecessary. If malignant, the surgeon can plan the definitive operation with full knowledge of the nature of the cancer. Multiple samples (4 to 20 cores) may be used to maximize the accuracy of this procedure. Some techniques remove larger amounts of breast tissue and may require stitches to close the incision.

When stereotactic guidance is used, computer-assisted mammography equipment maps the precise location of the lesion or suspicious area. Then the needle can be inserted through the skin and into the lesion, which is accurately pinpointed on the three-dimensional x-ray image. Either cells or samples of tissue are removed and sent to the pathologist for evaluation. This technique, however, requires expensive specialized machinery and the skilled use of this equipment by a radiologist or surgeon to position the needle and collect the samples. Its advantages are a smaller incision with a shorter recovery period for the patient. New technology permits even smaller samples to be identified and removed with increasing accuracy.

As mentioned in the previous discussion on fine-needle and core-needle biopsy, false negative results may occur since the needle may miss the malignant lesion (that is why multiple samples are often suggested to improve accuracy) or may not yield sufficient tissue or cells for a diagnosis. This technique is becoming more widely used and is available in most major cities and large teaching hospitals.

## Surgical Biopsy

A more specific and definitive procedure is known as a surgical biopsy. This method requires a small incision in the skin; the surgeon then directly identifies the lump and either removes the entire lump (excisional biopsy) or a representative sample (incisional biopsy). This open biopsy is the most reliable method for obtaining a specific diagnosis of a breast lump or of a suspicious area that is discovered on mammography. It can be done under local anesthesia; however, some surgeons and patients prefer general anesthesia.

When calcifications or suspicious abnormalities are seen on a mammogram but are not palpable, an open biopsy can be performed after preoperative needle localization. Needle localization is usually done under local anesthesia. The clinician performing the needle localization may use a film image, stereotactic equipment, or ultrasound equipment to insert a small needle into the breast pointing toward the lesion. Then a wire with a hook on the end is passed through the needle and positioned so that it rests where the calcification, density, or suspicious area has been seen. The wire (and sometimes the needle) is left in the breast when the patient goes to the operating room to guide the general surgeon when he performs the open biopsy. Sometimes, after inserting a needle, some dye is placed on the suspicious area to help the surgeon localize the area. This is called *dye localization*. After the incision is made for the biopsy, the surgeon follows the wire or needle and removes the area of tissue surrounding the wire and/or the area containing the dye. The tissue is then sent to the radiology department where it is x-rayed to determine that the correct area has been removed. Once the accuracy is confirmed, the specimen is sent to pathology for evaluation. To be sure that all of the calcifications or suspicious areas have been removed, in some cases the patient may need a follow-up mammogram 3 to 6 months later.

When a surgical biopsy is recommended, the surgeon is concerned that the suspicious area or lump may be malignant. Plans must be made before the biopsy to consider the options for treatment if the lump proves cancerous. It is possible to diagnose the lump and do a lumpectomy or mastectomy in one operation (a one-step procedure) or remove the lump and delay treatment to allow the patient time to consider her options (a two-step procedure).

If her doctor recommends a surgical biopsy to clarify the diagnosis of her lump, a woman should ask questions about this procedure in advance so that she fully understands what is involved. She should also ask her doctor if he recommends a one-step or two-step procedure.

One-step procedures are requested by some women who have already decided that if they have breast cancer they prefer a mastectomy or lumpectomy and axillary dissection. These women, having already made a decision for therapy, may select a one-step procedure to avoid the anxiety-filled interval between the diagnosis of cancer and the surgery to treat that disease. They should also consider immediate breast reconstruction as part of this one-stage procedure. One-step procedures are usually done under general anesthesia after the biopsy. The woman remains on the operating table while the tissue specimen is sent to the pathologist for a frozen section analysis. The pathologist places the specimen on a chuck (holder) and secures it in a microtome (slicer); it is frozen and then cut into thin slices of tissue, which are placed on glass slides, stained, and examined under the microscrope. With this technique the pathologist is able to make an immediate determination as to whether the lump is benign or malignant. Although frozen section examination is more expensive than routine histologic examination, this expense is more than justified by the large savings realized by avoiding a second surgical procedure. Occasionally the pathologist cannot make a specific diagnosis based on these findings. If the report indicates that the lump is benign, the incision is closed and the woman is returned to the recovery room. If malignancy is diagnosed in the one-step approach, the doctor will proceed with the mastectomy or lumpectomy with lymph node removal during this one-step procedure.

The two-step procedure allows a woman with breast cancer time to investigate her options and make an informed decision. She may wish to obtain a second opinion and explore the different types of therapy available for treating her cancer and for possible breast reconstruction. In a two-step procedure the biopsy and treatment are done at separate times. The biopsy usually can be done on an outpatient basis under local anesthesia or even by fine-needle aspiration in the office. The pathologist then performs a "definitive histologic study," which takes longer but the results are easier to read than a frozen section. In addition to the standard staining techniques used for the definitive histologic study, other staining methods can be used to help make a correct diagnosis. Some of the methods employ immunohistochemistry, which enables the detection of specific molecular entities. These can include estrogen and progesterone receptors and "oncogene" products (*HER-2/neu* [see Chapter 6] and epidermal growth factor receptor) and proteins specific for proliferative cells (e.g., Ki-67). The latter studies are useful for determining hormonal responsiveness, growth rate, and prognosis of cancer. This definitive histologic study takes approximately 24 hours. At its completion the pathologist is able to make a final report.

A woman should also ask about the length and location of the biopsy scar. Many times these scars are short and can be hidden around the outer edge of the areola, placed in inconspicuous areas of the breast, or planned to facilitate a future incision for lumpectomy or mastectomy and reconstruction. Such scars often are practically invisible once they have faded, but the final appearance depends on how a person heals.

A woman who detects a breast lump either during self-inspection or after physician examination should constantly keep in mind the most significant fact that countless women overlook: not all lumps are cancerous. Eighty percent of all breast lumps are benign. If a calcification or suspicious area is detected on a mammogram, she should not panic. Again, most of these problems are not associated with cancer. She should not hesitate to have her doctor examine her and determine what needs to be done. Early detection and conclusive identification can ensure a better chance for cure if a cancer is present and can quickly alleviate a woman's needless fears if the breast condition is benign.

# BREAST CANCER FACTS AND TREATMENT OPTIONS

B reast cancer typically strikes healthy women in their prime years. Disbelief and shock are natural responses of women faced with this shattering experience. Frequently they are as worried about the loss of a breast as about the presence of cancer. To them "cancer" is a word, a general medical entity that strikes other people, whereas a breast is a personal and intimate body part and its loss directly threatens them in many ways.

Breast cancer is the most common cancer occurring in U.S. women today. (The incidence of breast cancer in men is only 0.5%.) The American Cancer Society reports that one out of every eight women in the United States will develop breast cancer in her lifetime, and it is the second most common cause of death from cancer for women in the United States between the ages of 15 and 75. (Because of smoking, lung cancer, a much less treatable form of cancer, has become the most common cause of cancer death in women.) Breast cancer treatment now costs an estimated $3.5 billion per year in the United States; that represents 1% of the total health care budget or 0.15% of the gross national product. This year alone over 180,000 U.S. women will develop breast cancer. For many of these women, attempts to treat their disease and save their lives will also result in partial or complete breast loss. Information about cancer, its prognosis, and the options for therapy is necessary before they can make informed and enlightened decisions about their future.

## NATURAL HISTORY OF BREAST CANCER

Breast cancer usually originates in the drainage ducts of the mammary glands and is called ductal carcinoma. This is the most common type of breast cancer and occurs in 70% to 80% of all cases. In most other instances it originates in the mammary or milk glands (called breast lobules) and is called lobular carcinoma.

A type of breast cancer previously considered uncommon, intraductal carcinoma or ductal carcinoma in situ, has been diagnosed with increasing frequency with more widespread use of mammography for screening. Recent reports indicate that 15% to 20% of all breast cancers being diagnosed currently are intraductal; these cancers are usually very small, often less than 1 cm (or less than ½ inch in diameter), and may be too soft and small to be felt. They usually are detected by mammography, thus underscoring the importance of this test for early detection. Intraductal cancers are not invasive but, if left untreated, may develop into invasive cancer. When intraductal cancers are found at this early stage, the prognosis for cure and long-term survival is excellent. A special type of intraductal cancer, known as Paget's disease of the nipple, is characterized by a rash on the nipple associated with underlying cancer; this may be only intraductal cancer or it may be intraductal and invasive ductal cancer.

Breast cancer does not appear overnight. It is not precipitated by injury or a bump to the breast. Instead, it is thought to be a gradual process in which certain cells lining the ducts (the epithelial cells) change from normal cells showing an abnormal amount of growth (hyperplasia) to cells that are noticeably different from normal breast cells (atypical) but are not cancerous by definition. These atypical cells may eventually undergo further change and begin to regenerate themselves (autonomous growth), an uncontrolled growth that can extend through the cells lining the breast ducts. Thus breast cancer begins when a change in a breast duct cell gives that cell a growth advantage over other breast duct cells. The advantage may be a faster rate of cell division or a lower probability of cell death or both.

These cancerous cells initially grow inside the breast ducts (intraductal cancer) before they spread. If the cancer is discovered in the intraductal phase (or in situ), it has not yet spread outside the duct lining and potentially gained access to the rest of the body. When the intraductal carcinoma cells break through the outer lining of the breast ducts, the cancer is described as *invasive*. Once the cells become invasive, they can be picked up by the small lymph vessels of the breast and transported to the lymph nodes surrounding the breast, especially those present in the armpit or beneath the breastbone. The invasive tumor cells can also be picked up by the bloodstream or lym-

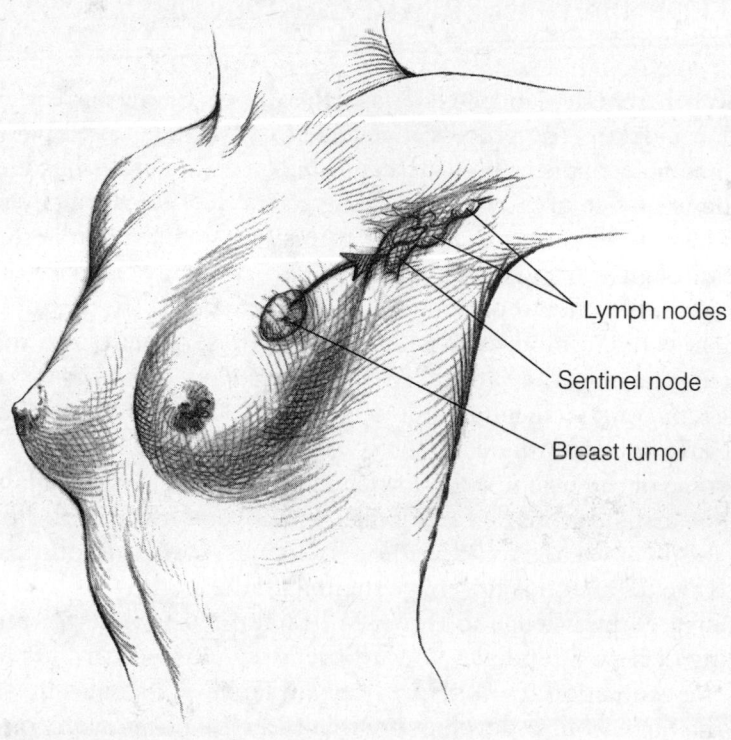

Lymph nodes

Sentinel node

Breast tumor

phatics and carried to other parts of the body. When tumor cells are carried or spread outside the breast to other parts of the body and continue to grow, the process is known as metastasis. New information indicates local growth factors that promote new blood vessel formation (angiogenesis) also lead to *metastasis*.

Since breast cancer develops from extremely small, microscopic cells, some experts believe that it often takes 4 to 10 years for the cancer to grow large enough to be felt as a mass or tumor. (Mammograms help identify breast cancers in their earliest stages before they can be felt.) These tiny cancer cells have the potential to become invasive and spread to other parts of the body before the tumor can be felt, accounting for the high mortality from breast cancer and the serious and sometimes unpredictable nature of this disease. This invasive potential is also the reason it is so important to identify the patient at high risk so that increased surveillance can allow breast cancer to be found in its earliest stages, before it has a chance to spread.

## DEVELOPMENTS IN BREAST CANCER GENETICS

JOHN S. MEYER, M.D.

Research in breast cancer genetics offers hope for new treatments aimed at blocking the process that makes cells cancerous. Investigation of the mechanisms by which cells become cancerous has identified the existence of growth-regulating genes that are normally present in all cells. These genes appear to play an important role during the years of growth and development but are normally dormant or relatively inactive once a person reaches adulthood. If these genes become activated, tumors can result. Because these genes play a role in producing cancers, they are called oncogenes ("onco" comes from the Greek root "onkos" meaning bump or tumor). Several of these oncogenes have been identified as factors causing breast cancer. The activity of some of these genes can now be measured in the clinical laboratory. For instance, breast carcinomas with overactivity of the *HER-2/neu* (also known as *erb B-2/neu*) or epidermal growth factor receptor (EGFR) genes are known to have rapid growth rates.

Increased knowledge in this area has also led to a better understanding of how a tendency toward breast carcinoma can be passed from one generation to another in certain families. Families in which more than one woman develops breast cancer are not uncommon, but in most instances probably do not represent inherited tendencies for breast cancer. The disease is sufficiently common to account for multiple instances in families by chance. For example, one would not assume that a family in which two or three members developed arthritis in later years necessarily had an inherited tendency toward that disease since arthritis is so common. If arthritis developed in childhood or the twenties or thirties in several members, a hereditary disease would more likely be suspected. The same applies to breast cancer. Whereas a mother and child or two sisters might develop breast cancer after age 50 by chance, if they developed the disease before age 50, a genetic breast cancer tendency would be more suspect. Recent studies of inherited breast cancer have begun to establish that the disease tends to occur at younger ages, even in the twenties, when breast cancer ordinarily is quite rare. Thus the probability of an inherited mutation becomes higher when affected women of a given family are relatively young.

The current challenge is to recognize women who carry a heritable breast cancer tendency. Two genes, *BRCA1* (breast cancer 1) and *BRCA2* (breast cancer 2), have been identified that, when changed or mutated, lead to an increased susceptibility to breast cancer. These two genes are thought to account for the majority of instances of breast cancer caused by inherited genetic errors. (Human cells have 46 distinct chromosomes.) *BRCA1* has been identified on the long arm of chromosome 17. Over 100 mutations have been identified. Some of these mutations change the protein product of this gene in such a way that it fails to perform its function of suppressing cell division. When both copies of this gene are mutated or lost, there is an increased risk of breast cancer, probably in the range of 50% to 75% over a lifetime. Some mutations appear more likely to allow the development of breast cancer than others. *BRCA1* is also associated with a 10% to 35% lifetime risk of ovarian cancer. The second breast cancer gene, *BRCA2*, is associated with a similar or slightly lower risk of breast cancer and an increased risk of ovarian cancer, but much less so than *BRCA1*. *BRCA2* is also associated with male breast cancer. *BRCA1* and *BRCA2* are both associated with prostate cancer.

Both of these genes are unusually large. Breast cancers have been associated with mutations at a number of sites in either gene without any strong predilection for the mutation to occur at a given site. Analysis of these large genes has to be very thorough to cover all the likely sites for mutation, and even then up to 33% of mutations may be missed on *BRCA1*. Spontaneous, noninherited defects in *BRCA1* have been identified in half of sporadic, noninherited breast cancers. The defect identified so far is the loss of a segment of chromosome 17 that contains the *BRCA1* gene. Since chromosomes are paired, if a normal *BRCA1* gene is missing from one chromosome 17 (loss of heterogeneity), production of a normal gene product is totally dependent on having a normal gene on the other chromosome 17. This implies that a mutation occurring in the remaining copy of the gene may lead to breast cancer.

The *BRCA1* and *BRCA2* genes are thought to belong to a class of cancer-related genes known as suppressor oncogenes. Rather than directly causing cancer, these genes produce substances that prevent cells from becoming cancerous. When both copies of a suppressor oncogene are missing or defective, cancer may occur. If a person has inherited only one rather than the normal two copies of a suppressor oncogene, damage to or loss of the remaining gene in a particular cell can cause cancer. A number of suppressor oncogenes have been identified, and many more will likely be discovered. Consequently, other genetic causes of a familial breast cancer tendency probably will be discovered in addition to the *BRCA1* and *BRCA2* genes. This knowledge can be valuable in targeting surveillance of women for detection of breast cancer to the groups with the highest risk.

More than 50 oncogenes have been identified, and at least several of them are implicated in breast carcinoma, indicating a breast duct cell can become cancerous by more than one pathway. Therefore it is not surprising that there are also different types of breast cancers and that these cancers vary in their growth rates and in their ability to invade and metastasize (grow in other parts of the body). Certain types have an excellent prognosis, even without chemotherapy or hormonal therapy, and others are more aggressive and have a poorer prognosis. Histologic assessment (microscopic analysis of cells and tissues) of breast cancer cell characteristics is helpful in determining whether the cancer might have spread. Growth rate measurements are also helpful in prognosis. Cancers with high rates of growth are more likely to produce recurrences within a few years of treatment than those with slow growth rates. (These new tests are discussed later in this chapter under prognostic factors and in Chapter 7.)

## Pros and Cons of Genetic Testing

For many woman, the identification of *BRCA1* and *BRCA2*, the so-called breast cancer genes, is welcome news. They are excited that this genetic breakthrough could pave the way for identifying the cause of breast cancer and ultimately the cure. Tests are now available to enable women to discover if they harbor these fateful genes. Women with breast cancer, women at high risk, and their families can potentially be tested to learn if they carry this indicator of heritable breast cancer. The problem is what to do with the information once they have it. Of even more concern is how their insurance companies, their managed care providers, their employers, their spouses and significant others, and they themselves will react to this information. Since there is no known method for preventing breast cancer, many women may see no clear benefit in knowing whether they are carriers of these genes. Prophylactic mastectomy, also called risk-reducing mastectomy, probably can reduce the risk somewhat. (In one Mayo Clinic study risk reduction was reported to be 90% effective.) If you test positive, it means you have a very high chance of getting breast cancer. Having that information in your medical record could have a detrimental effect on your insurance and employment. If you test negative, this may affect family dynamics with others who have tested positive for breast cancer. It isn't a simple issue. The experts offer no easy solutions. Consultation with a genetic counselor, however, may help clarify the issues and is recommended for women who are considering being tested.

In deciding whether to have *BRCA1* testing, women must weigh complex information about the potential benefits of testing against the limitations and possible risks of this new technology. Benefits of genetic testing include the potential for early detection and reduction of uncertainty. Limitations include uncertainties inherent in cancer risk figures, the absence of proven strategies for preventing cancer in carriers, and the fact that not all mutation carriers get cancer and noncarriers can still get cancer. Risks of genetic testing include the potential for discrimination in employment or in obtaining or retaining insurance, loss of insurance or employment, and adverse psychosocial consequences for oneself and one's family on learning one's genetic status.

Breast cancer survivors expressed the following views about the benefits, risks, and limitations of testing in responding to our surveys . Most important to all the women we surveyed was gaining genetic information as a means of learning about risks for their children and their relatives. The most important risks they identified were that the tests might not be accurate and that they might lose their health insurance as a result of a positive result indicating that they were carriers. As one woman related, "It's a terrible burden and dilemma. I know I should be tested. I owe it to my daughters and my nieces. But what happens if I test positive? I am terrified of the possible consequences. What assurances do I have that my test results will be kept confidential. I can't afford to lose my insurance or even my job. I just don't know what to do."

The potential for discrimination by health insurers on the basis of genetic status is perhaps one of the most serious risks of *BRCA1* and *BRCA2* testing. Recent studies also suggest that lack of health insurance may also be a significant barrier to participation in genetic testing programs. Moreover, the possibility of losing health insurance was cited by many of the women we interviewed as an important risk in being tested for the breast cancer genes. Concerns about insurance discrimination may also deter carriers of *BRCA1* and *BRCA2* mutations from sharing their mutation status with their providers and insurers and from undergoing potentially beneficial preventive interventions. Also, individuals who know their mutation status and deliberately withhold such information from insurance companies could risk the loss of their policy or coverage for an illness related to the mutation. Currently steps are under way in Congress to address the issue of discrimination in genetic testing; these may come to fruition in the near future. Individuals who lack health insurance also expressed concern about getting testing, fearful that they could not afford the cost of subsequent medical care that might be indicated if they tested positive. The results of genetic testing may also be useful to carriers in decision making about prophylactic mastectomy.

The cost of commercial genetic testing (estimated to range from $250 to $2500) was also deemed a deterrent for some individuals. Although some insurance companies may pay for testing and counseling services, patients are reluctant to request such payment because of concerns about future confidentiality and discrimination issues.

## GENETIC TESTING: INDICATIONS AND GUIDELINES
WILLIAM C. WOOD, M.D.

Testing for *BRCA1* and *BRCA2* genes can now be conducted using techniques that are sensitive for detecting mutation and for testing focal areas known to be at high risk for mutation. Such genetic testing should *only* be done after extended genetic counseling regarding the potential benefit of such genetic information or lack thereof. Established genetic screening services will include counseling as part of the package, and a patient will only be tested after extensive counseling with the patient and, if desired, family members. Because of polymorphisms (many different forms of the gene) and lack of sensitivity in detection of mutations, general screening of unselected populations for mutations in *BRCA1* and *BRCA2* is not appropriate. However, such screening may be worthwhile for certain high-risk groups such as Ashkenazi (Eastern European) Jewish women with any family history of breast cancer, in whom several specific mutations occur commonly. Those who have a sufficiently high risk of heritable breast cancer in whom such testing might be considered include those with multiple breast cancers in one family, some of which were diagnosed very early in life, and families in which both breast and ovarian carcinoma have occurred.

Women found to have a mutation of *BRCA1* or *BRCA2* can be monitored closely by mammography, clinical examination, and breast self-examination. Trials of medical prophylaxis (preventive therapy) are under way with agents such as tamoxifen to attempt to minimize the subsequent development of breast cancer. Prophylactic or preventive mastectomy with immediate reconstruction is also an option.

However, it is not recommended under ordinary circumstances, even for women who have mutations of these genes, because of concerns about removing two normal breasts that may never develop breast cancer when accepted breast cancer therapy today would usually recommend only removing the tumor if a breast cancer did develop. For women who are tested who do not have mutations identified, a high risk may still be present and even inherited. Although it is estimated that only about 5% of breast cancers arise from heritable causes and that BRCA1 and BRCA2 probably account for a majority of these, new breast cancer suppressor genes are expected to be identified in the future.

## RISK FACTORS

Some women are at higher risk of developing breast cancer than others. Age, family history, and previous breast cancer are three factors associated with high risk. (More information on risk factors is included in Chapter 15.)

### Age

A woman's age strongly influences her risk of developing cancer. Breast cancer is unusual before age 30. The largest number of breast cancers are detected in postmenopausal women between the ages of 50 and 70 years. A third of the cases occur in patients under the age of 50 and 25% in women over 65. As our population ages, however, a larger proportion of breast cancer cases will occur in women over 65. Any individual woman's risk is slightly higher with each year of age.

During the past 15 years, however, the breast cancer rate among women age 25 to 44 has increased, as it has in women of all ages. Our surveys and interviews confirm these findings. Many of the women we canvassed during the last 8 years were in their thirties and early forties with no previous family history of breast cancer. This increase in young women with breast cancer excludes the statistical increase resulting from better detection through mammography. Experts cite various reasons for the rise. Some point to late childbearing, fat in the diet, toxins in the environment, or some other unknown cause. Whatever the cause, it is crucially important that breast lumps in young women be thoroughly evaluated to rule out the possibility of cancer. This disease does occur in young women, and if a suspicious lump persists, it should be biopsied for definitive diagnosis.

### Family History

Having first-degree maternal relatives (mothers and sisters) who developed breast cancer increases a woman's risk by two or three times, with a lifetime risk of about 20%. If breast cancer developed before age 50, the risk is somewhat greater (30%). If the cancer was bilateral, the risk may approach 50%. Some women with these family histories have genetically identifiable heritable risk of breast cancer, such as women who have tested positive for BRCA1 or BRCA2 mutations. Other families simply have random occurrences of multiple sporadic cancers. Increasingly, laboratory testing can define which of these two situations accounts for a particular woman's family history.

### Previous Breast Cancer

When breast cancer occurs in one breast, the cumulative risk of a cancer in the other breast is about 14% for women younger than 50 years old with a first cancer. It is less, approximately 4%, for women older than 50. If the first was lobular carcinoma or if lobular carcinoma in situ was present, some experts once thought the risk of a second invasive breast cancer was somewhat greater. More recent studies, however, have not confirmed that there is a higher risk after lobular cancers than after ductal cancers. The risk of a second breast cancer is greater if the first cancer is diagnosed before age 50.

### Relative Risk Factors

Women in the following categories have a slightly increased risk of developing breast cancer:
- History of breast cancer in maternal or paternal grandmother, father's sister, or mother's sister.
- Excessive exposure to radiation, particularly before age 20. Currently used diagnostic x-ray examinations (even cumulatively) do not reach these levels. Women who underwent radiation therapy of the chest for previous malignancies such as Hodgkin's disease are included in this group.
- Early menarche (beginning of menstruation).
- Birth of first baby after age 30.
- Never having borne children (nulliparity).
- Late menopause.
- Obesity.
- Socioeconomic status. Women of higher socioeconomic status have a higher risk than poorer women.
- History of some types of fibrocystic change.

- Alcohol consumption. Studies suggest a possible link between alcoholic consumption even in moderate amounts and a woman's risk of breast cancer. Many experts recommend limited or no consumption.
- Race. Although the incidence of breast cancer is a little lower for black women than for white woman, once they get the disease, African-American women do not do nearly as well. In fact, their survival rate dropped by 14% in the 1980s, whereas the survival rate for white women actually increased during the same period. This may be attributed in part to socioeconomic status, education, and access to mammography and physician examination to ensure early detection, but there may also be other factors, perhaps dietary.
- Environmental factors. At this time no conclusive findings have linked environmental factors to an increased risk of breast cancer. However, there seem to be geographic "hot spots" for breast cancer or areas in the United States where there is a higher incidence of breast cancer than one would ordinarily suspect. For example, the high incidence of breast cancer on Long Island has been widely reported. Breast cancer rates are also lower in warmer climates, perhaps related to sun exposure.

## Diet and Nutrition

Although no connection has been found between a high fat diet and breast cancer, the National Academy of Sciences and many experts recommend reducing total fat intake from 40% of calories (average U.S. consumption) to 30% to try to reduce serious health problems. Generally, low fat diets are recommended to prevent excess fat, which is widely thought to be the primary culprit in heart disease. This applies particularly to saturated fats found in many cooking oils, butter, and animal fats and not to monounsaturated or polyunsaturated fats found in olive and canola oils. In the case of breast cancer a low fat diet is recommended because the female hormone estrogen accumulates in body fat. Conversion of steroid hormones to estrogen occurs in fat through action of the enzyme aromatase. Since estrogen has been found to be a "promoter" of breast cancer, it is believed that reducing body fat might prevent an overload of estrogen in the body and therefore a reduction of breast cancer risk.

A diet with less than 30% of calories from fat is usually recommended by nutritional experts. Some low fat foods include fruits, vegetables, whole grain products, beans, peas, and pasta. Look for the words, "fat free," not "low fat," on processed foods. Avoid oil, butter, and whole milk dairy products. Olive oil, canola, and peanut oil are healthy sources of fat in moderation. White chicken meat, white turkey meat, and veal are lowest in fat. When ground they can be substituted for meatballs or hamburger. For those who want to eat beef, top and eye round cuts are leanest; prime cuts have more fat than choice cuts of beef.

As far as a good diet is concerned, fruits and vegetables, if possible four or five times a day, are needed for vitamins and minerals. Protein helps healing. Carbohydrates are a good source of energy. Fats provide the body with fuel. To maintain a workable dietary regimen, a good rule of thumb is to eat three or four meals a day that contain a balance of protein, carbohydrates, and fat; drink six to eight glasses of water (unless you're on a fluid-restricted diet, in which case only two or three); and fill up on food with fiber (such as apples, bananas, berries, figs, dates, cherries, kiwi fruit, papaya, and pears) and vegetables (such as beans, chickpeas, cowpeas, parsnips, plantains, and potatoes). Other high fiber foods are bran, multigrain bread, brown rice, and millet. Barbecuing is to be avoided since it creates carcinogens.

## Estrogen Supplements and Estrogen Replacement Therapy

Because estrogen stimulates the growth of breast tumors, controversy exists over the advisability of taking estrogen in pill form, either as an oral contraceptive or for estrogen replacement therapy. Some studies suggest that women who started taking the pill in their teens may be at greater risk than women who started later or not at all. This may be because pills contained more estrogen when they were first marketed. Studies also indicate a slightly increased risk of breast cancer after 5 years of estrogen replacement therapy. This risk becomes even greater after 15 years. Because estrogen replacement therapy also reduces the risk of heart disease and osteoporosis, women who take estrogen live longer than those who don't. It is largely fear of breast cancer that fuels the debate about hormone replacement.

Most experts believe that estrogen replacement drugs should be avoided after breast cancer is detected and treated since they might accelerate cancer growth. This issue, however, is still under investigation and new estrogen drugs may significantly decrease these risks. Newer low-dose estrogen supplements and so-called designer estrogens are thought to have less risk. A new drug on the market that has generated much excitement among oncologists and other cancer experts is raloxifene (Evista). This estrogen is intended to counter the risk of osteoporosis without producing the detrimental effects of conjugated estrogens. Although experience with its use in humans is still limited, current studies would suggest that raloxifene has a low risk or even "no risk" of producing breast cancer and does not increase the risk of uterine cancer. Raloxifene may prove a viable alternative for woman who need hormone replacement therapy. Ongoing studies also suggest that raloxifene may have a possible benefit for breast cancer prevention, but additional long-term studies are needed to determine its potential role as a breast cancer combatant.

## BREAST CANCER STAGES

Once the diagnosis of breast cancer has been made, the stage of the breast cancer is determined to aid in making treatment decisions. Physicians classify the localization and spread of cancer in terms of stages. A basic element of staging is classifying the cancer as invasive, meaning it has the potential to metastasize (grow in other parts of the body), or noninvasive. Invasive breast cancer is graded from stage I to stage IV, and both treatment and prognosis are directly related to the stage of the cancer when detected. Unquestionably, it is best to discover the breast cancer before it becomes stage I (in its preinvasive form) and before it has spread beyond the breast ducts. Breast cancer in this preinvasive form is known as in situ cancer (in situ means in place), and if a woman's breast tissue is removed at this stage, invasive cancer can be prevented. If no treatment is undertaken, up to 40% of these women may develop a more serious invasive cancer.

Staging is determined by the size of the tumor, local extension to the chest wall or skin, the number and location of lymph nodes involved, and whether there are metastases in other areas of the body. To provide a more precise and standardized approach to staging, the TNM system has been developed: T stands for tumor size, N stands for nodal spread, and M stands for distant metastases. The TNM staging system ranks patients as having stage group TIS (tumor in situ, or noninvasive cancer) or stages 0 through IV, with stage IV indicating known distant metastases. Although there are various staging methods, the system devised by the American Joint Commission on Cancer Staging is now considered the standard method (see Appendix D for this classification system).

## Special Tests for Breast Cancer Staging

ROGER S. FOSTER, Jr., M.D.

Opinion differs as to what tests should be done before surgery to help stage breast cancer when the patient has no signs or symptoms that the cancer has spread beyond the breast and axilla. Experts agree that appropriate studies should be carried out for specific symptoms or any abnormal findings discovered on physical examination. There is also general agreement that patients with invasive cancer should have a chest x-ray film, a complete blood count, and a liver enzyme assay. Selected patients may need additional studies such as bone scans to rule out evidence of tumor spread to bone. At one time liver scans were commonly obtained, but experience has shown that they contribute very little to the care of most patients, and special scans of the liver usually are now done only if liver enzymes are abnormal, specific physical symptoms are present, or the patient has a more advanced stage of cancer.

## PROGNOSIS OF CANCER

The outcome, or prognosis, for a woman with breast cancer is related to the extent or spread of the disease at the time of diagnosis. Some experts believe that survival is directly related to the size of the tumor at the time of diagnosis. Those with small cancers (less than 1 cm, or less than ½ inch in diameter) have a 10-year survival rate of over 90%. Large tumors with direct extension to the chest wall or with skin involvement have a significantly worse prognosis.

The lymph nodes removed during axillary dissection are the best predictors of the course of the disease and outcome of the patient. The number of lymph nodes in each armpit (axillary) area varies. The nodes lying between the muscles and below the axillary vein are removed by the surgeon during axillary dissection and examined by the pathologist to determine if the breast cancer has spread to this area. The pathologist checks each of these lymph nodes carefully under the microscope. This process is time consuming; it may take several days before the final report is available. Patients with no involved or cancerous axillary lymph nodes (stage I) have a 65% to 75% likelihood of survival for 10 years. If one to three nodes are found to be cancer bearing (stage II), there is a 40% to 60% chance for 10-year survival. If more than four nodes are involved, there is less than a 25% possibility of survival for the next 10-year period. If any axillary nodes are involved, chemotherapy usually is recommended in an attempt to improve the chances of survival.

After pathologic identification of the tumor type, other microscopic studies of the cells can be conducted to determine whether they are likely to be aggressive. Additional information can be obtained by examining the tumor to determine histologic type. For instance, some cancers are of special histologic types, for example, tubular carcinomas and papillary carcinomas, and have a more favorable prognosis. Cell differentiation is also an indicator. Cancer cells that closely resemble normal mature breast cells are considered well differentiated and are associated with a better prognosis than poorly differentiated cancer cells that are less normal, or atypical, in appearance and have a less favorable prognosis because they are thought to be more aggressive. The prognosis is also less promising when tumor necrosis (areas of dead cells) is identified or when there is evidence of tumor invasion via the blood vessels or lymphatic vessels.

The microscopic appearance of the cancer is especially valuable in node-negative breast cancer. Measurement of how many cells are dividing or the degree of cell division ("nuclear grade") is a reliable indicator of risk of cancer recurrence in most pathology laboratories and is used as a standard measure of risk. The most aggressive cancers tend to have many cells dividing at the same time due to rapid growth. Less aggressive cancers tend to have very few cells dividing. Pathologists usually grade on a scale of 1 to 3 or 4, with the lower number being the best. Another microscopic feature being evaluated today and quantitated by new technology is the formation of new blood vessels or induction of new blood vessels by the tumor (angiogenesis). Angiogenesis is thought to facilitate metastasis to other parts of the body.

Measurement of the estrogen and progesterone hormone receptors on the tumor cells is also helpful in predicting prognosis and response to hormonal therapy. If laboratory evaluation shows the mass to be cancerous, hormone receptor tests will be run to determine if proteins that are called receptors are present. Estrogen and progesterone are female hormones that can affect breast cancer cell growth. When breast cancer cells have higher levels of receptors for these hormones (estrogen receptor positive, or ER+), that often indicates the tumor is slower growing and the prognosis is slightly better. It also suggests that this patient's tumor will probably respond favorably to hormonal manipulation. Hormone receptor tests help your doctors determine whether cancer cells might be destroyed or slowed by administering anti-estrogen or other anti-hormones or if chemotherapy will be more effective.

In addition to the microscopic description of the tumor and lymph nodes, a panel of tests may be used to better estimate a woman's risk of recurrent breast cancer. Despite the increasing ability to tailor risk estimates, most women with a breast cancer greater than 1 cm in diameter will benefit from treatment with chemotherapeutic or anti-estrogen drugs to lower the risk of local and distant tumor recurrence. The role of these and other new tests is not yet well established, but promising advances are being made in understanding the nature of changes in cells that make them cancerous.

A major thrust of breast cancer research seeks new markers that will improve the ability to predict a patient's prognosis and more important predict the outcome after specific therapy. A good deal of this research is focusing on growth rate measurements. Scientists have identified growth factors that are important in the transformation of hyperplastic (fast-growing) cells to those with atypical features to actual cancer cells. With such unlikely names as S-phase, ploidy, *HER-2/neu* oncogene, epidermal growth factor receptor, and cathepsin-D, these markers can tell physicians how the malignant cells are growing and how likely the cancer is to spread or recur. For example, measurement of the genetic material (DNA) in tumor cells enables the physician to determine the growth rate of cells (S-phase fraction) and whether or not the tumor cells contain normal or abnormal quantities of DNA (ploidy). Other potential markers are related to the genes in cells that influence cell behavior (the oncogenes mentioned earlier). In particular, scientists are studying the *HER-2/neu* oncogene and its protein products to see if they will aid in predicting response to chemotherapy. Current studies of families with multiple cases of bilateral breast cancer are focusing on analyzing their DNA for evidence of cancer-causing genes. Now women with a family history of breast cancer can be tested with success to identify the presence of these breast cancer genes.

Breast cancer remains a threat because of its unpredictable growth and potential to invade and spread to other parts of the body before the tumor can be detected. Death from breast cancer and virtually all symptoms are due to spread to other organs of the body such as the liver, lungs, bone, or brain. Research continues to seek the answer to why cancers invade and metastasize. Early detection is critical today, but an understanding of the basic nature of cancer will allow innovative treatments to prevent invasion or spread.

• • •

Even though cancer statistics can be quite frightening and information on oncogenes, DNA, and cell growth factors intimidating, it is important to remember that progress is being made. Recent American Cancer Society data suggest an improved 5-year survival rate for whites and blacks alike. This is exciting news and underscores the importance of early detection combined with the effectiveness of local and systemic therapy in influencing survival rates as well as improving the length and quality of life. The use of chemotherapy and/or hormonal therapy as part of the patient's initial treatment for breast cancer represents a significant advance in the care of cancer patients and is one method for improving the prospects of those women at high risk by preventing further spread or recurrence of their breast cancer. Tests are now available to allow the selection of patients who are at increased risk of recurrence and to use this information to help reduce that risk. Recent studies also indicate a possible survival advantage for adjunctive use of radiation to the chest wall for women with several positive nodes. There is much good news to report and recent genetic research suggests that the future holds promise for many new developments and advances in breast cancer treatment.

## LOCAL THERAPY: SURGERY AND RADIATION

Surgery with or without radiation therapy has always been considered the primary local treatment for breast cancer and the best means of eliminating cancer in the breast and in the adjacent lymph nodes. This is still the case, but the means for achieving this goal have changed dramatically over the years. Whereas cancer surgery once sought to remove as much tissue as possible to eradicate all local traces of malignancy and all possibilities for local recurrence, it now seeks to accomplish the same goal with less extensive surgery and without permanent breast loss. Although most women diagnosed with cancer were once treated with mastectomy, breast-conserving surgery with radiation therapy is now becoming the norm for many women whose cancers are detected early and are confined to a specific area of the breast. Large randomized studies and experience with outcomes have taught us that less radical surgery can provide equivalent survival for most women without the deformity previously associated with these operations. Mastectomies have also undergone transformation as new skin-sparing techniques have been introduced which, combined with immediate reconstruction, offer many women a viable and aesthetic alternative when a complete mastectomy is necessary. The good news is that women's breast cancer treatment options are expanding; now they can realistically expect less extensive surgery that does not compromise treatment or survival yet produces excellent cosmetic results. Women can now have the most appropriate treatment for their breast cancer and still have a breast either through lumpectomy and radiation therapy or skin-sparing mastectomy and immediate reconstruction.

Following is a discussion of local surgical therapies with and without radiation therapy that are used for breast cancer treatment. Although surgery of the breast and axillary lymph node dissection are commonly performed as a single procedure, in the interest of clarity, our discussion will treat these topics separately. We will start with an explanation of the regional lymph nodes, including axillary node dissection and sentinel node dissection. Then we will explore the range of surgical treatments from breast-conserving surgery and irradiation to the various mastectomies with and without immediate breast reconstruction. The role of adjunctive radiation therapy as a supplement to surgery will conclude our discussion of local therapy.

## Regional Lymph Nodes

JOHN M. BEDWINEK, M.D., and ROGER S. FOSTER, Jr., M.D.

When breast cancer becomes invasive, it can spread to the regional lymph nodes. The nodes most commonly involved with metastases are the axillary (armpit) lymph nodes. Less commonly, cancer may spread to the internal mammary lymph nodes just behind the ribs near the sternum (breast bone) or to the supraclavicular lymph nodes (above and below the collarbone).

Surgical removal of regional lymph nodes in breast cancer patients serves two purposes: diagnosis (or staging) and treatment by removing nodes containing cells that could proliferate. At the present time, for patients with an invasive breast cancer, the number of nodes containing cancer is the single most important prognostic indicator as to the probability of having microscopic cancers elsewhere in the body (micrometastases); these can then be treated to prevent a recurrence.

(See information on staging and prognostic factors earlier in this chapter.)

When the lymph nodes in the axilla are not involved by metastasis, the chance that the tumor will spread to other parts of the body in the future is decreased. When there are metastases to one or more lymph nodes, the risk for microscopic spread elsewhere in the body becomes higher. The greater the number of involved nodes, the greater the risk. The lymph nodes provide further information about the spread or extent of the cancer so that the course of the tumor can be predicted. This information on the involvement of the lymph nodes plus information on the size and character of the tumor are used in making therapeutic decisions. Knowing whether these nodes contain cancer helps the medical oncologist decide whether to recommend systemic therapy (chemotherapy and/or hormone therapy) and, if so, what kind of systemic therapy. Removal of level I and II lymph nodes also serves a therapeutic purpose. When these lymph nodes are excised, it is rare for cancer to recur in the axillary area.

Radiation therapy can also be used to treat the regional nodes if they are not enlarged. The effectiveness of radiation therapy is roughly equivalent to surgical removal of the nodes. Radiation therapy of the axillary nodes may be indicated when it is judged that no useful additional information will be gained by pathologic examination of the lymph nodes. Radiation therapy is also used when it is felt that there is high risk for spread to the lymph nodes over the collarbone (supraclavicular nodes) or behind the breastbone (internal mammary lymph nodes). There are fewer side effects when lymph nodes in these areas are treated by radiation rather than surgery. Radiation to the axilla combined with complete surgical axillary node removal should be avoided if possible because of the increased possibility of swelling (lymphedema) of the area. (The arm lymphatics also drain through the axilla.)

## Axillary Node Dissection

The most common drainage pathway for lymphatics in all portions of the breast is the axillary lymph nodes. Therefore the standard surgical procedure for evaluating these nodes, called an axillary node dissection, has been to remove the lymph nodes lying below the axillary vein and those between the major back muscle that attaches to the arm (latissimus dorsi) and the major chest wall muscles beneath the breast (pectoralis major and minor muscles). Axillary dissection to remove these lymph nodes can be performed in conjunction with standard modified radical mastectomy, with skin-sparing mastectomy and breast reconstruction, or with breast-conserving surgery when a partial mastectomy or lumpectomy is performed. Surgeons may refer to these axillary dissections as removal of level I and level II axillary lymph nodes. Ten or more lymph nodes are usually found by the pathologist in the excised tissue after this type of surgery.

### When Axillary Node Dissection May Not Be Necessary

Although the axillary node dissection has been a standard component of mastectomy and breast-conserving surgery and irradiation for years, there is a growing consensus among breast cancer specialists that a node dissection may not be necessary for many women. New data indicate that some women will benefit from chemotherapy whether their nodes are negative or positive. If knowing whether or not the nodes contain cancer will not change a woman's treatment, then there is no compelling reason for removing the nodes. Other women for whom a node dissection may not be necessary are those with nonpalpable, slow-growing tumors that are less than 1 cm in diameter. The likelihood of nodes being positive in these women is so low (less than 3% for tumors 0.5 cm or less) that a node dissection is probably not worthwhile.

### Sentinel Node Biopsy

For those women in whom a node dissection is required, there is a promising, but as yet unproved new procedure called a *sentinel node biopsy* in which only the first draining node or nodes are removed through a small incision instead of an entire node dissection. (See Chapter 4 for additional information on sentinel node biopsy.) When no tumor is found in the sentinel node or nodes, it is unlikely that other axillary nodes will contain breast cancer cells. Thus, in the future, we may be able to eliminate the axillary node dissection for those women who do not really need it and substitute sentinel node biopsy for those who do. This represents progress since a node dissection is a major surgical procedure that can cause discomfort, requires significant healing time, and can occasionally contribute to edema of the skin of the breast. *At this time, however, the axillary node dissection is still a standard component for mastectomy and breast-conserving surgery and irradiation for most women.*

## Breast-Conserving Surgery and Irradiation

JOHN M. BEDWINEK, M.D.

### *Lumpectomy*

Breast-conserving surgery and irradiation is an option for primary treatment of breast cancer that has become widely accepted and is used with increasing frequency. As its name implies, the chief advantage of this treatment approach in comparison with mastectomy is that a woman's natural breast is preserved. The surgeon removes only the cancerous lump along with a small margin of normal breast tissue. This procedure is referred to as a lumpectomy; it is also called tumorectomy or tylectomy. Sometimes the surgeon will remove the entire breast quadrant containing the tumor in an effort to reduce the possibility of local recurrence. This procedure is called a *quadrantectomy* and is cosmetically inferior to a lumpectomy since it can leave a significant deformity in the breast that may dictate a partial breast reconstruction during the same procedure or later. Fortunately, lumpectomy is just as safe as quadrantectomy provided that the surgical margins are "negative." (A pathologist examines the removed breast tissue under the microscope to judge whether or not the cancer cells come up to the edges of removed tissue. Painting the removed breast

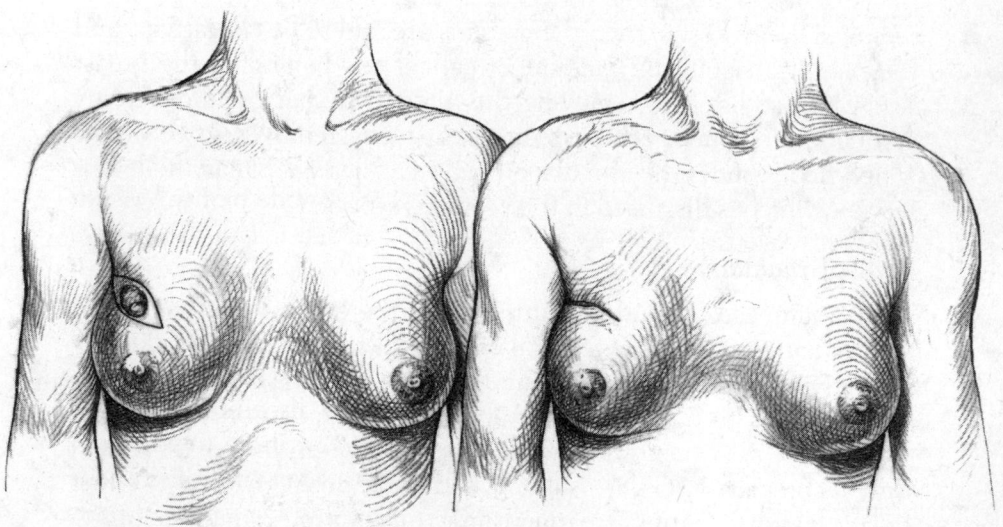

Lumpectomy

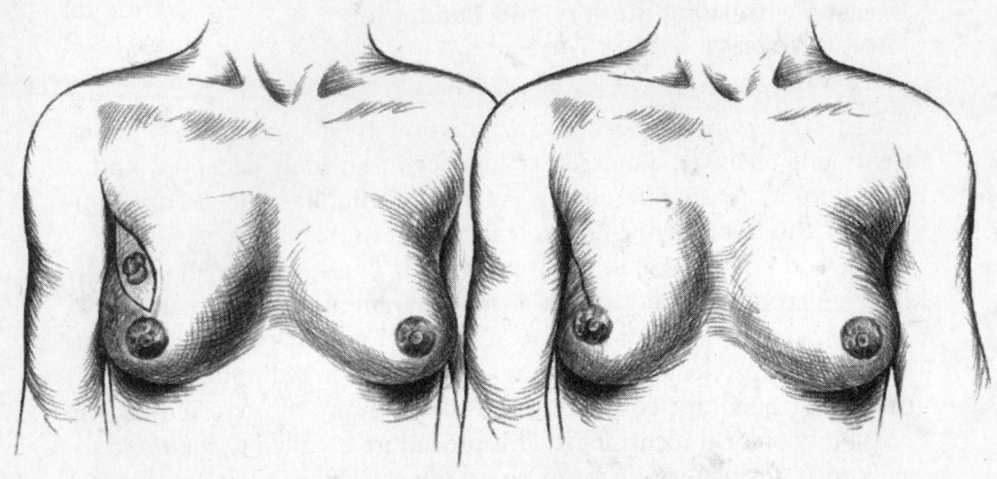

Quadrantectomy

tissue with India ink before the microscopic examination enables him to make this judgment accurately. If the cancer cells border the edge of the removed tissue, then the margins are said to be "positive," and there is a high risk that a significant amount of cancer is left behind in the patient's breast. If the cancer cells do not border the edge of the removed breast tissue, then the margins are said to be "negative," and the risk of a significant amount of cancer left behind in the breast is low.) In addition to removing the lump (whether by lumpectomy or quadrantectomy), the surgeon also usually removes some of the lymph nodes under the arm in a procedure called an axillary node dissection, which is discussed in the previous section.

### Breast Irradiation

After a lumpectomy and node dissection, the entire breast is treated with radiation to kill any residual cancer cells. The radiation therapy consists of a single daily treatment 5 days a week for a total of 25 to 28 treatments (5 to 6 weeks of therapy). A total radiation dose of approximately 5000 centiGray is delivered to the entire breast (centiGray, abbreviated cGy, is a unit of radiation dose). During the first 1 to 2 days of radiation, treatment may take 45 to 60 minutes to ensure accurate planning; however, subsequent radiation treatments should last only 10 to 15 minutes. Most women continue to work and lead normal lives during their radiation therapy.

After irradiation of the entire breast is completed, an additional radiation dose of approximately 1000 to 2000 cGy is usually applied only to the site from which the tumor was removed. This additional dose to the tumor site is referred to as the "boost" and is given to ensure that all residual cancer in that area is eradicated. The boost can be administered with a special type of external irradiation called an electron beam.

The radiation used in breast-conserving treatment does not cause hair loss, nausea, or any significant loss of energy. It does, however, cause a temporary reddening of the breast skin similar to a mild sunburn. This reddening usually occurs 3 to 4 weeks after radiation therapy is started and usually disappears by 2 weeks after its completion. In about 25% of the cases slight thickening of the skin and the breast occurs because of increased fluid in the skin (edema). This skin edema, if it occurs, results from the axillary node dissection, which severs the small lymph vessels through which breast fluid normally escapes. In 18 to 24 months these vessels regenerate, and the edema usually disappears. If node dissection can be avoided, as mentioned above, skin edema does not occur.

As beneficial as eliminating axillary node dissection would be, it would be even more ideal to be able to avoid breast irradiation. Investigators at Harvard University Medical School have tried to determine if there are certain women for whom irradiation after lumpectomy might not be necessary. They selected women with small tumors that were less than 1 cm in size and very slow growing for lumpectomy without irradiation. Unfortunately, many of them developed a recurrence in the breast, and the investigators concluded that even women with small slow-growing tumors need breast irradiation after lumpectomy. There is, however, another group of women who may not need irradiation. These are women with noninvasive cancers. If a cancer is detected before it penetrates the wall of the duct, it is said to be non-invasive. These noninvasive cancers, or intraductal cancers as they are sometimes called, rarely spread to lymph nodes or to other parts of the body; therefore axillary node dissection is definitely not indicated. The cure rate with simple mastectomy (mastectomy without node dissection) or with breast-conserving surgery and irradiation is greater than 95%. Although some of these intraductal cancers can be extensive (see below), many are limited to a small area in the breast. In some centers these limited intraductal cancers are being treated with lumpectomy only (no irradiation), and thus far the results seem to be equivalent to those for lumpectomy and irradiation. Whether or not patients with limited intraductal cancers need irradiation is still controversial, but at this time it would appear that some of these patients may be safely treated with lumpectomy only.

### Who Is a Candidate for Breast-Conserving Therapy?

In 1983, when the first edition of this book was being prepared, breast conserving surgery followed by irradiation was controversial, and many surgeons questioned whether it was as safe as mastectomy. By 1992, during the preparation of the second edition of this book, breast conserving surgery was no longer controversial and had become widely used as an acceptable alternative to mastectomy. Its safety had been proved beyond a doubt by the results of seven large randomized studies involving thousands of women. Nonetheless, most surgeons and radiation oncologists still thought that only certain women should be treated by breast-conserving surgery and irradiation. They used specific selection criteria such as tumor size, tumor location, and breast size to determine who was a candidate. Now, at the writing of the third edition of this book, many of these selection criteria are no longer important since breast-conserving surgery has become the standard of treatment for just about all women with stage I and II breast cancer. The long-term results of the randomized trials mentioned above continue to show that it is just as effective as mastectomy. For example, results of the recent NSABP (National Surgical Adjuvant Breast Project) Trial of Induction Therapy indicate that tumor size is no longer a limiting factor. If a tumor is of sufficient size that its removal by complete excision will leave a surgical defect that will mar the aesthetic result, *induction chemotherapy* (preoperative chemotherapy) may first be used to shrink the tumor to a size that can be well treated by breast-conserving therapy. This trial indicates that survival at 5 years is identical; even earlier data suggest that eventual survival may be even better with such therapy. Reports on local recurrence indicate an average recurrence of approximately 10% at 10 years. Thus there are very few medical reasons for not doing breast-conserving surgery and irradiation and these are listed below.

### Medical Reasons for Not Doing Breast-Conserving Surgery and Irradiation

**Pregnancy.** Radiation should not be delivered to the breast during pregnancy because of the potential for radiation exposure to the fetus. Even though the scattered radiation to the fetus is extremely low, fetal tissues are many times more susceptible to radiation than adult tissues. Small amounts of radiation to the developing embryo can cause congenital malformations, and small amounts to the fetus can increase the risk of cancer or leukemia. If a pregnant woman desires to save her breast, she can have lumpectomy and node dissection during the pregnancy and then have breast irradiation immediately after delivery of her child provided that her oncologist does not feel that the delay will compromise her treatment.

**Prior radiation therapy to the involved breast.** Women who have had radiation treatment of all or part of a breast for a prior malignancy (such as Hodgkin's disease) should not have breast conserving-surgery and irradiation for a cancer of that breast. The radiation that a given volume of tissue receives is additive, and the amount of radiation used for breast-conserving surgery and irradiation, when added to the previous radiation, may exceed the radiation tolerance of the breast tissue and thereby cause damage such as severe scarring or ulceration.

**Preexisting rheumatologic disorders.** The three main rheumatologic disorders are rheumatoid arthritis, lupus, and scleroderma. Women with scleroderma or lupus that involves the skin should have mastectomy since radiation in the setting of these disorders can increase the risk of severe scarring of the breast. Women with rheumatoid arthritis and most other forms of lupus, however, can be safely treated with breast-conserving surgery and radiation.

**Extensive intraductal component in which excision with negative margins would create a significant surgical deformity.** Occasionally an invasive breast cancer will be accompanied by a large amount of intraductual cancer. This intraductal portion, if it comprises more than 25% of the entire cancer and if it extends beyond the main cancer, is said to be extensive. The name applied to this situation is extensive intraductual component (EIC). Investigators at Harvard have shown that invasive cancer with EIC has a very high rate of recurrence if the margins are positive. For this reason, if the pathologist notes that EIC is present and the margins are positive, the surgeon must excise more breast tissue to achieve negative margins. If excising more breast tissue will create a significant surgical defect, the patient should strongly consider mastectomy and subsequent reconstruction instead of breast-conserving surgery and irradiation.

**Two cancers in the same breast.** Although this is a rare occurrence, occasionally a woman will have two separate cancers in one breast. If all of the following conditions are met, then the women can safely have breast-conserving therapy: (1) both of the cancers are within the same quadrant and can be removed through a single incision, (2) there is not an extensive intraductal component (see above), and (3) the excision margins are negative. If one or more of these conditions cannot be met, then the patient is better treated with mastectomy since the risk of recurrence in the breast after tumor excision and irradiation in this setting can be as high as 40%.

**Diffuse malignant microcalcifications seen on mammogram.** One of the ways a mammogram can detect a very early cancer is by showing tiny flecks of calcium. These tiny flecks of calcium are referred to as microcalcifications. If there are microcalcifications that have been proven by biopsy to be malignant and if these microcalcifications extend throughout a large area of the breast, this means that there are small amounts of cancer (usually intraductal cancer) extending widely throughout the breast. Under these circumstances the risk of recurrence following lumpectomy and irradiation is extremely high even if all the microcalcifications can be removed. It is recommended that these women have mastectomy.

**Rare patients with large locally advanced tumors or those with clinically apparent inflammatory breast cancer.** Many oncologists believe that patients with these more agressive or advanced cancers are not good candidates for breast conservation.

### Nonmedical Reasons for Not Doing Breast-Conserving Surgery and Irradiation

In addition to the medical reasons for not performing breast conservation and irradiation, there may be nonmedical reasons for choosing mastectomy instead of breast conservation.

**Lack of a strong desire for breast preservation.** Some women will say, "You're telling me that all I have to do to save my breast is to come in for a 15-minute radiation treatment once a day for 33 treatments. I'd come in for a 100 treatments to save my breast!" Other women, however, might say, "You mean I have to come in there every day, 5 days a week, for 6 weeks. I don't have time for that kind of foolishness. I'd rather have my breast off and get it over and done with!" Every woman is different and the above two comments probably reflect opposite ends of the spectrum. It is clear, however, that not every woman has a strong desire for breast preservation. There are some women who don't mind having one breast and don't mind wearing a prosthesis every day. For these women, mastectomy is the better option since it is quicker and easier, minimizes the local recurrence incidence and usually eliminates the need to have radiation treatments.

**Inability to get to and from a radiation center on a daily basis.** For some women, daily radiation treatments can be a real hardship because of logistical problems or a physical disability. A logistical problem might be lack of transportation or living a long distance from the radiation oncology center. An example of physical disability would be severe arthritis making it difficult, and even painful, to travel on a daily basis. Some patients with kyphoscoliosis (the humpback that is caused by osteoporosis) find it very painful to lie on a hard table (which is what patients have to do to get radiation treatments). For all of the above reasons, mastectomy may be a kinder and easier option than breast-conserving surgery and irradiation.

**Fear of radiation.** Some women have heard horror stories about radiation or remember a relative "who got burnt up by that cobalt." These fears, while they may not be based in reality, are very real and difficult to dispel. Such women may be psychologically better off to be treated by mastectomy.

**Fear of the cancer-producing breast.** Some women will view the affected breast as a cancer-forming organ and will experience continued anxiety unless rid of it. Obviously, for these women, mastectomy is the treatment of choice.

• • •

There are few medical reasons today for not doing breast-conserving surgery and irradiation, but physicians (surgeons and radiation oncologists) should be able to recognize these reasons when they exist. They should also realize that nonmedical reasons may be just as important, if not more important, than medical reasons. The future holds promise for eliminating lymph node dissection for many women. We may also be able to identify a subgroup of women for whom irradiation will not be needed.

## Mastectomy

The most dramatic change in breast cancer treatment in the past 10 years is that mastectomy (removal of the entire breast and often part of the underlying chest muscle) is no longer considered the only safe course. Large randomized studies have determined that the chances of survival are no better after a mastectomy than after a lumpectomy (see previous discussion).

There are, however, good reasons for choosing mastectomy, and for about 30% of women, mastectomy is the only sensible choice. A mastectomy is indicated for women with diffuse ductal carcinoma in situ (DCIS) or diffuse microcalcifications that are suspicious and prevent the detection of recurrent disease. It is also appropriate for women whose tumors have disseminated throughout the breast, whose tumors are large while their breasts are very small, or who have two or more separate tumors. Concerns about which procedure to choose often have as much to do with lifestyle and attitudes as they do with the therapy itself. A lumpectomy with radiation therapy requires a commitment of time to undergo the daily radiation treatments following surgery. A family history, genetic and ethnic status, personal preference, and fear of the cancerous breast or of the radiation itself are all factors that enter into the decision-making process. Even occupation plays a role, as in the case of the breast imager who chose mastectomy and reconstruction over lumpectomy because she didn't want to have to worry about her breasts in light of the breast disease she was seeing on a daily basis.

The goal of mastectomy is to surgically remove a woman's breast while the tumor is still confined to the breast area to minimize the possibility of local recurrence and before it has spread to other parts of the body. Several different types of surgical treatment are used for removing a woman's breast: radical mastectomy (a rarity today), modified radical mastectomy, and total or simple mastectomy.

### Radical Mastectomy

Radical mastectomy was introduced over a hundred years ago and was the first effective operation for local control of breast cancer at a time when breast tumors were usually discovered when they were large. Although this procedure effectively removed the breast cancer, it also left the woman with a large deformity after her breast, underlying chest wall muscles (pectoralis major and minor muscles), and axillary lymph nodes were all removed. The mutilating aspects of radical mastectomy and the early diagnosis of smaller breast cancers led to the development of the modified radical mastectomy, which preserves the pectoralis major muscle.

### Modified Radical Mastectomy

Today, radical mastectomy is rarely performed; the modified radical mastectomy with axillary dissection is the method *for total breast removal* chosen by most surgeons for operable breast cancer. It has been

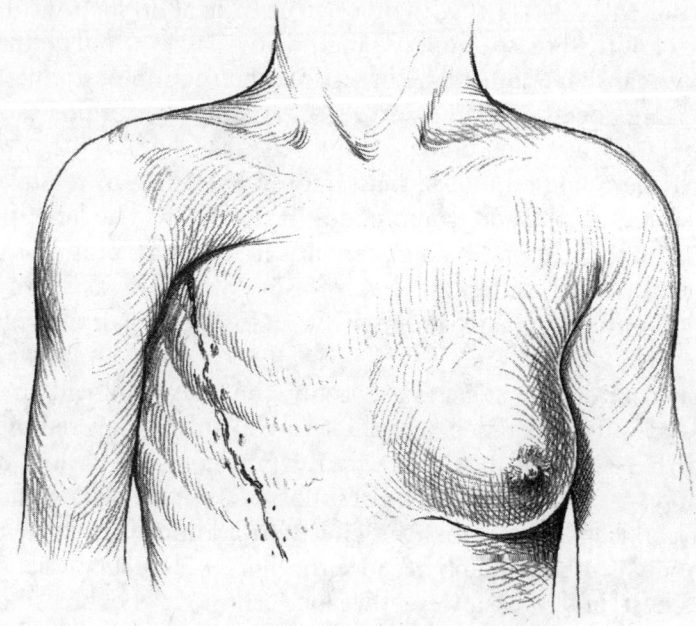

Radical mastectomy

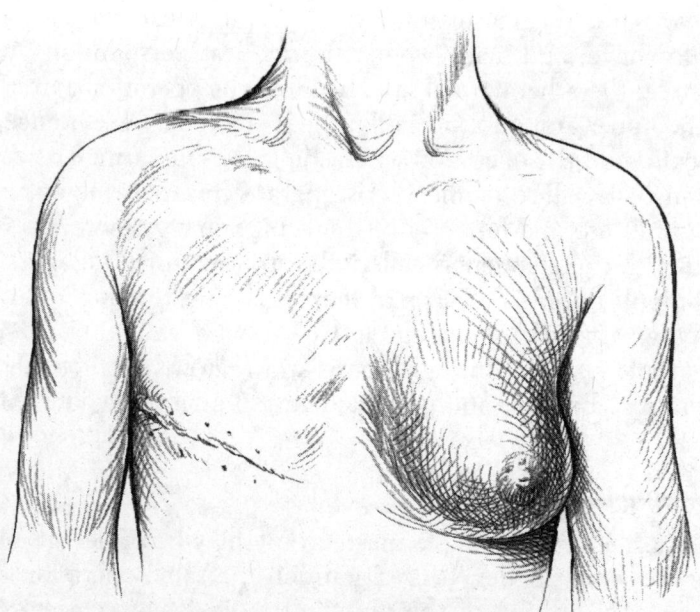

Modified radical mastectomy

shown that this operation is as effective as radical mastectomy for local control of the breast tumor. Women who want to avoid permanent breast loss can have immediate breast reconstruction performed during the same operation or delayed reconstruction performed as a separate operation at a later date.

With the modified radical mastectomy, the surgeon removes the breast, nipple-areola, and lymph nodes in the axilla. The largest chest wall muscle, the pectoralis major, remains intact. This muscle is located in the front of the chest and helps to support the breasts; preservation of this muscle greatly reduces the deformity resulting from the mastectomy.

After a modified radical mastectomy, the chest wall will not have a hollowed-out appearance, and the ribs will still be covered by muscle and therefore will not seem overly prominent. The loss of the breast and nipple will result in a chest flatness. A scar will extend horizontally or diagonally across the chest. In addition, the area of the mastectomy is usually numb because the nerves that supply sensation to the chest and breast were threaded through the breast tissue, which is now gone. The inside of the upper arm can also be numb because the nerves to this area that go through the axillary region may have to be removed with the axillary dissection. Many surgeons can now spare these nerves and reduce the numbness of the inner upper arm area. After the mastectomy, the armpit is usually deeper and harder to shave, and many women notice less perspiration on that side than on the other normal side. Because the operation extends beneath the upper arm into the axilla, the woman may experience temporary pain after the operation when she moves her arm. The general surgeon usually will recommend postoperative exercises to ensure the return of full use and function of the arm. Some women also report experiencing a phenomenon called phantom pain in the area of the missing nipple or breast. They may feel throbbing, tingling, numbness, or stabbing pains. These sensations are probably caused by the nerve endings that were cut during surgery and regrow incompletely after the operation. Exercise and pain medication might alleviate this discomfort.

### Total or Simple Mastectomy

A total mastectomy or simple mastectomy may be done without removing the lymph nodes. It is very much the same operation as the breast removal portion of the modified radical mastectomy. All or nearly all of the breast tissue is removed. Depending on the extent of the tumor in the breast, and also depending on whether or not the patient is to have immediate breast reconstruction, variable amounts of skin are removed. When no reconstruction is planned, the surgeon usually removes a relatively large amount of skin.

### Skin-Sparing Mastectomy
WILLIAM C. WOOD, M.D.

For patients who are to have mastectomy with immediate reconstruction, a skin-sparing mastectomy may be considered. This approach is only appropriate for those individuals who have *no tumor involvement of the skin area to be saved*. For women requiring mastectomy who are appropriate candidates for this skin-sparing approach, this operation provides the best cosmetic result. With this procedure, only the nipple and areola are excised as well as the overlying skin in those areas. If necessary, the incision extends to the side of the nipple and areola in a horizontal or vertical line approximately ½ to 1 inch to allow all of the breast and the lower axillary nodes to be removed. During the immediate breast reconstruction the skin envelope is then refilled to

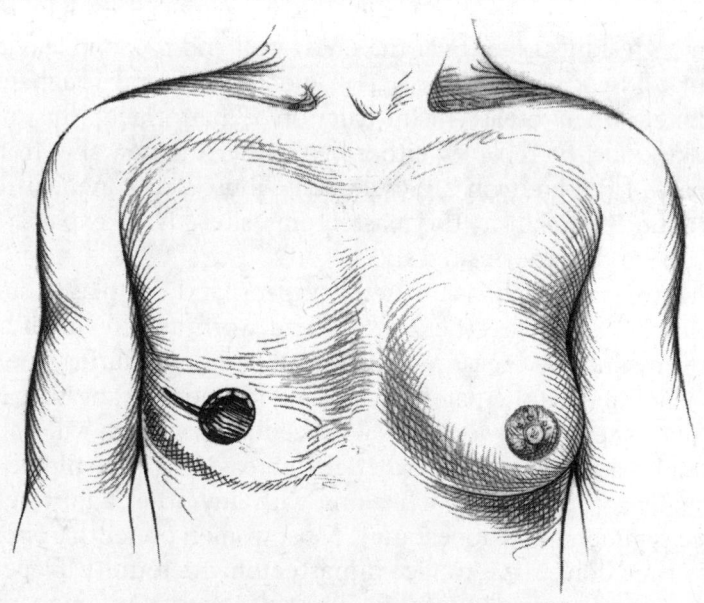

Skin-sparing mastectomy

provide a symmetric breast appearance that is very similar to the pre-mastectomy appearance. The appearance and symmetry are enhanced by preservation or recreation of the anatomic landmarks of the breast, such as the inframammary fold, the lateral breast line, and the cleavage line.

## Immediate Breast Reconstruction
WILLIAM C. WOOD, M.D.

Many surgeons who recommend a mastectomy for women with breast cancer also inform them of the option of breast reconstruction to rebuild their breasts and fill in the defects left from their cancer surgery. Immediate breast reconstruction has become an appealing option for women undergoing mastectomy, and they are choosing it with increasing frequency because it combines a safe and effective treatment for breast cancer with immediate breast restoration. Immediate breast reconstruction often permits a skin-sparing mastectomy to be performed (provided there is no tumor involvement in the skin), which requires less skin removal and sensory nerve division and produces shorter scars. By removing the breast and replacing the volume immediately, the skin that is not excised as a part of the cancer operation can then be used for the reconstruction. If the mastectomy is performed separately, more breast skin must be removed initially to create a smooth skin surface over the chest wall and to avoid leaving redundant folds of breast skin that would thicken and toughen over time. Later, when breast reconstruction is performed, the missing breast skin must be replaced either by transferring new skin from another part of the body on a muscle-skin (musculocutaneous) flap or by stretching the skin at the mastectomy site (tissue expansion) to make it expand to the desired size.

With this approach, the general surgeon and the plastic surgeon must closely coordinate their efforts and work as a team since the mastectomy and the breast reconstruction are done during one operation, which means the patient will have to undergo anesthesia only once. Since there is only one initial procedure, a woman will not have to wear a breast prosthesis or experience breast loss. The nipple-areola is usually reconstructed later along with any other adjustments to enhance symmetry and appearance. Most women prefer this approach because they don't have to face a mastectomy deformity. Depending on the reconstructive procedure chosen, the patient may need a blood transfusion. Therefore, as a precaution, most surgeons recommend that patients undergoing immediate breast reconstruction donate their own blood in advance (autologous donation) to avoid the need of receiving another's blood and the accompanying risks and concerns.

In the past some have expressed concern that breast reconstruction, particularly when done immediately, would make it difficult to examine the chest wall for recurrent disease. This has not proved to be the case. In most instances there is no contraindication to immediate reconstruction for patients with stage I or II breast cancer. However, women with stage III breast cancer (locally advanced) must have a combination of surgery, chemotherapy, and chest wall radiation therapy. Therefore, for these patients, it may be prudent to complete all therapy before pursuing breast reconstruction. Although patients with stage III breast cancer can safely have reconstructive surgery, some oncologists suggest that these very high-risk patients wait 1 to 2 years before proceeding with further surgery. An alternate approach is initial chemotherapy (neoadjuvant or induction) to shrink the tumor, followed by a mastectomy, immediate breast reconstruction, and follow-up radiation therapy. Cancer treatment should be the first priority, and any complication of reconstruction that would delay therapy should be avoided. For the majority of women facing mastectomy, however, immediate reconstruction is a welcome option that permits them to receive optimal treatment of their breast cancer without suffering the trauma of breast loss.

## Postoperative Irradiation

JOHN M. BEDWINEK, M.D., and WILLIAM C. WOOD, M.D.

In the past women who had mastectomies and were found to have positive axillary lymph nodes were given radiation therapy after surgery. The radiation was directed to the chest wall and to the lymph nodes above the collarbone and beneath the breastbone. It was thought that this postoperative radiation therapy would improve survival by killing any cancer cells not removed by the mastectomy. Radiation does, indeed, drastically reduce the likelihood of a local recurrence, that is, the reappearance of cancer on the chest wall or in the nearby lymph nodes. This prevention of a local recurrence does not necessarily improve the chances of cure, however, since most patients who have a local recurrence of cancer after a mastectomy also will develop distant metastases that radiation therapy does not prevent. Many studies have been conducted to test whether postoperative radiation will improve survival, and the results have been inconsistent. Some recent studies have shown that in combination with chemotherapy, radiation therapy for women with smaller tumors and fewer positive nodes produces improved survival. Many other studies, however, have shown a decrease in local recurrence but without the survival benefit.

Since there is no conclusive evidence today that for most breast cancer patients combining radiation therapy with mastectomy will improve the chances of cure, it is given only to women whose risk of having a recurrence is very high. These women have large breast tumors (5 cm, or 2 inches, or more), enlarged lymph nodes under the arm, many lymph nodes with cancer metastases, or tumors that extend outside the breast at the margin of the removed tissue and have invaded into the skin of the breast or into the pectoralis muscle underlying the breast. Postoperative radiation therapy is also recommended if extensive lymph node involvement is anticipated. For example, patients with the inflammatory variant of breast cancer are very commonly treated with radiation therapy. If there is a recurrent tumor on the chest wall after a mastectomy and radiation therapy has not previously been given, radiation therapy might commonly be used at that time after surgical removal of the recurrent cancer. For these women, keeping the risk of local recurrence minimal by adding radiation therapy is of definite benefit because a local recurrence is difficult to treat successfully and can cause unpleasant symptoms such as pain or bleeding. Postoperative radiation therapy for women with a high risk of recurrence continues to be the standard of care. Fortunately, the majority of patients who have a mastectomy today do not have a high risk of local recurrence, and postoperative radiation therapy is not usually needed.

## SYSTEMIC THERAPY: CHEMOTHERAPY, HORMONAL THERAPY, AND GENETIC THERAPY

Whereas surgery and radiation therapy seek local cancer removal in the breast and axilla, chemotherapy, hormonal therapy, and genetic therapy seek to interfere with the growth and spread of cancer to other parts of the body. As such, these therapies are often referred to as adjunctive because they supplement the effectiveness of surgery.

When a woman learns that she requires additional therapy after her surgery and/or possible radiation, this is often devastating news. The last thing she wants to deal with is another assault on her body with potentially toxic drugs. Most women have heard horror stories about the side effects associated with these therapies and dread the possibility of hair loss, nausea, and hot flashes, among others. As one woman we interviewed explained, "It is bad enough to have to face a cancer diagnosis, but the thought of losing my hair and throwing up was more than I could take. I actually screamed at my doctor and told him 'no way was I going to subject myself to that kind of torture.' I had had enough."

Chemotherapy and hormonal therapy, however, are essential life-saving treatments and integral to current breast cancer treatment regimens. Their long-term benefits should not be overlooked because of side effects that will pass relatively quickly, are often not as debilitating as feared, and are not permanent. A woman owes it to herself to seriously weigh the life-sustaining value of these therapies. Even though surgery will greatly reduce the risk of cancer spread, particularly if the cancer is detected in its earliest stages (in situ cancer), some risk still remains. Despite the increasing ability to tailor risk estimates, any woman with a breast cancer over 1 cm in diameter will probably benefit from treatment with chemotherapeutic or anti-estrogen (hormonal) drugs to lower her risk of recurrent tumor. If microscopic cancer cells are found in the lymph nodes or if the tumor has other bad prognostic signs, we know that cancer has a higher chance of being in other parts of the body. That is where systemic therapy takes over. Chemotherapy and hormonal therapy drugs travel through the bloodstream to attack cancer in distant sites, thereby significantly reducing the risk of recurrence by as much as one half and profoundly affecting the life span of women with breast cancer. Chemotherapy can also play a role preoperatively (neoadjuvant or induction chemotherapy) when used to shrink the tumor before surgery, often permitting a less extensive surgical procedure to be performed. (See Chemotherapy Induction Trials later in this chapter for more information on this topic.)

Monoclonal antibodies and anti-angiogenesis drugs that seek to shrink tumors and prevent growth of tumors that have spread also hold promise although they are investigational.

## Chemotherapy
GARY A. RATKIN, M.D.

Chemotherapy is the use of drugs to kill or damage cancer cells. Healthy tissue can be temporarily affected, thereby causing side effects, but usually recovers with the return of normal function. Although chemotherapy was first employed in patients with widespread metastatic cancer, a major advance in breast cancer management has been the use of chemotherapy to prevent the recurrence or spread of breast cancer. Adjuvant chemotherapy uses drugs to destroy cancer cells when they are present in a microscopic form.

Physicians now can conduct tests on breast masses to find those patients who are at high risk for spread or recurrence of breast cancer after surgery. An advanced stage (II or above) or microscopic features of the cancer cells in the biopsy may indicate a greater chance of cancer recurrence or spread in the future. Specialized tests to measure the cancer growth rate or test for genetic changes in the cancer cells can also assist in detecting those with an increased chance of recurrence. Chemotherapy or hormonal therapy is indicated for patients who are found to have this higher risk of metastasis.

Chemotherapy can also be effectively used in many woman whose breast cancer has recurred locally or spread widely throughout her body. It is frequently used when there is lung, liver, or bone marrow involvement. These drugs may be used when there is a low chance of response to hormonal therapy or when a patient is so ill that hormonal therapy will not work fast enough or be potent enough to deal with the illness. Combinations of chemotherapy with hormonal therapy or radiation are often used.

### Administration of Chemotherapy Drugs

Most chemotherapy is administered by intravenous injection. Few agents are available in pill form. Combinations of chemotherapeutic drugs have become standard for adjuvant therapy and for treatment of metastatic disease. In modern chemotherapy programs these drugs are administered in brief courses (8 months or less is typical) every 3 to 4 weeks, depending on the specific program. By giving the medications intermittently, the normal bone marrow and other areas of the body have a chance to recover.

It is important to start adjunctive chemotherapy as soon as possible after the patient has healed from surgery (usually within 4 to 6 weeks). More intensive treatment programs and other drug combinations for shorter periods of time (4 months is becoming more common in standard clinical practice) are under study. As a general rule, oncologists try to administer as much chemotherapy as safely as possible to get the best results with adjunctive regimens.

Some of the most frequently used medications for adjuvant chemotherapy include methotrexate, 5-fluorouracil (5-FU), cyclophosphamide, vincristine, doxorubicin, and prednisone. Three or more of these medications may be used in combination and are referred to by acronyms such as CAF or FAC (cyclophosphamide, Adriamycin, 5-FU); or CMF (cyclophosphamide, methotrexate, 5-FU).

**Chemotherapy Drugs Commonly Used for Adjuvant Therapy**

Cyclophosphamide (Cytoxan)
Methotrexate (often with calcium leucovorin)
5-Fluorouracil (5-FU)
Vincristine (Oncovin)
Prednisone
Doxorubicin (Adriamycin)

### Side Effects of Chemotherapy

Although chemotherapy is used to try to improve a woman's prognosis, normal tissues may be temporarily affected by these powerful drugs, which produce side effects. Four of the most common are nausea, vomiting, hair loss, and low blood counts. Other symptoms caused by chemotherapy might include interruption of the menstrual cycle, fatigue, mouth sores, tingling in the fingers and toes, and rarely diarrhea.

Much progress has been made in controlling the more serious or bothersome of these side effects. It is common to administer anti-nausea medications immediately prior to chemotherapy to prevent this side effect. Even hair loss, which is a widely publicized side effect of chemotherapy, does not occur with every drug. Patients are examined regularly to be certain that uncommon side effects such as bladder irritation or heart scarring (seen with cyclophosphamide) are not occurring. Doxorubicin can cause heart scarring, but it almost always occurs if a lifetime dose is given that goes beyond a "safe" limit.

Suppression of the bone marrow by chemotherapy is the most serious side effect experienced. Chemotherapy can temporarily lower the white blood count (neutropenia or leukopenia), placing the patient at increased risk of bacterial or fungous infection. Today, a growth factor (G-CSF-filgrastim [Neupogen] or GM-CSF-sargramostim [Leukine]) is often given with adjunctive chemotherapy to maintain an adequate white count. Less often a low platelet count (thrombocytopenia) may occur, which can cause serious bleeding or bruising; a new growth factor to stimulate platelet production is being introduced to address this problem. Anemia (low red blood count) can also occur but that rarely requires separate treatment during adjuvant chemotherapy for breast cancer. Blood counts are monitored before and frequently between courses of chemotherapy to ensure the safety of a regimen.

Uncommon toxicities of specific chemotherapeutic drugs include:

| Drug | Uncommon Complications |
| --- | --- |
| Cyclophosphamide | Bladder |
| Doxorubicin, cyclophosphamide, mitomycin-C, methotrexate | Pulmonary (lung) |
| Mitomycin-C | Renal (kidney) |
| Mitomycin-C, doxorubicin, vinorelbine | Skin ulcerations with extravasation |
| Methotrexate, mitomycin-C | Liver |
| Paclitaxel, docetaxel | Anaphylaxis (sudden collapse) |

Since many of the medications used can irritate the veins, great care must be exercised in starting an intravenous infusion for chemotherapy administration. A semipermanent venous access device can be implanted under the skin and attached to a catheter placed directly in a large vein. This infusion device, or port, can facilitate chemotherapy administration in selected patients and can often also be used for blood drawing, transfusion, or the administration of pain medications, if necessary.

## COMMON SIDE EFFECTS OF CHEMOTHERAPY DRUGS

| Drug | Hematologic | Nausea | Oral | Diarrhea | Cardiac | Neurologic | Skin | Hair Loss |
| --- | --- | --- | --- | --- | --- | --- | --- | --- |
| Cyclophosphamide (Cytoxan) | ++ | ++ | + | 0 | + | 0 | + | ++ |
| Methotrexate | ++ | + | ++ | + | 0 | + | ++ | + |
| 5-Fluorouracil (5-FU) | + | + | ++ | ++ | 0 | + | ++ | + |
| Doxorubicin (Adriamycin) | ++ | ++ | ++ | + | ++ | 0 | ++ | +++ |
| Vincristine (Oncovin) | + | + | 0 | 0 | 0 | ++ | + | + |
| Thiotepa (Thiopex) | ++ | ++ | 0 | 0 | 0 | 0 | + | + |
| Mitomycin-C | ++ | ++ | + | 0 | 0 | 0 | + | + |
| Mitoxantrone (Novantrone) | ++ | ++ | + | 0 | + | 0 | + | ++ |
| Paclitaxel (Taxol) | ++ | + | + | 0 | + | + | 0 | + |
| Docetaxil (Taxotere) | ++ | + | + | 0 | + | + | 0 | + |
| Vinorelbine (Navelbine) | + | + | + | 0 | 0 | + | 0 | 0 |

The specific symptoms of each chemotherapy program should be explained to the patient before treatment is initiated so that she is aware of the risks and practical steps to take to help herself. When chemotherapy is used to treat metastatic cancer, the goals of treatment should be clear to the patient and her family. Relief from the symptoms due to cancer is now the objective rather than preventing a recurrence or spread of cancer. We must be certain that the treatment actually provides a greater benefit to the patient compared to the toxicity. Regular assessment of symptoms and side effects is critical for adequate follow-up in women with metastatic breast cancer.

### Intensive Chemotherapy and Bone Marrow and Stem Cell Transplantation

Patients with large tumors and many positive nodes are treated with high doses of chemotherapy. Unfortunately, these high doses of chemotherapy are not only toxic to the cancer cells but are also toxic to normal cells, particularly the bone marrow cells, so much so that patient survival may be compromised without special procedures, such as bone marrow transplantation or peripheral stem cell transplantation to aid recovery of the bone marrow and the blood cells it produces. New developments have allowed the harvesting of stem cells (the origin of more mature bone marrow cells) from the blood using a cell separator machine after injections of growth factors. More intensive treatment can be given safely now than ever before in these very high-risk patients. Although high-dose therapy in breast cancer is still considered investigational, it is a consideration for selected patients with stage II and III breast cancers.

### Hormonal Therapy

By altering the patient's hormonal balance the physician can often control her breast cancer even when it has relapsed or spread. Estrogen and progesterone receptors should be documented in every patient with a new diagnosis of breast cancer. The test may help in predicting the risk of recurrence, but more important, it allows the selection of patients who might benefit from hormonal therapy. The detection of estrogen and progesterone receptors in the cancer tissue indicates whether the tumor is likely to be responsive to hormonal treatment. Approximately 50% of patients with positive estrogen receptors will respond to some hormonal treatment, especially anti-estrogen therapy, whereas less than 10% with negative receptors react favorably.

Hormonal therapy can take several forms. Today, the anti-estrogens tamoxifen (Nolvadex) and toremifene (Fareston) are the most widely used form of therapy in patients who have positive estrogen or progesterone receptors. The estrogen receptor assay along with other pathologic tests allows physicians to prescribe tamoxifen or toremifene as a preventive measure in those patients who might benefit. Tamoxifen or toremifene is now recommended in both postmenopausal and premenopausal patients who are at risk of recurrence of breast cancer after surgery and who have positive estrogen receptors measured in the cancer tissue. For women with receptor-positive tumors, 5 years of tamoxifen administration has been shown to lower the risk of recurrent cancer by 50%. This reduction is additive to any reduction from adjuvant chemotherapy.

Anti-estrogens usually produce few side effects. Hot flashes and vaginal dryness, symptoms similar to those many women experience during menopause, are the most common reaction. Patients who are on long-term tamoxifen or toremifene (over 2 years) should be screened for uterine cancer, although this is a very rare complication. Other unusual risks include thrombophlebitis (blood clots), vaginal bleeding or discharge, changes on specialized eye examinations without change in vision, low blood count, nausea, weight gain, skin rash, muscle cramps, and an elevated blood calcium level. Some patients may have an increase in bone pain or discomfort in an area of a metastasis after the start of anti-estrogen therapy, which usually abates with time. Contrary to many women's concerns, the use of anti-estrogens actually strengthens the bones in postmenopausal women and can lower serum cholesterol and other lipids.

The risk of breast cancer metastasis may be far greater than the toxicities listed here. In addition, there is evidence that there is a lower incidence of cancer of the opposite breast in patients who are taking tamoxifen. Chemotherapy Prevention Clinical Trials have shown the usefulness of tamoxifen in preventing breast cancer in the high-risk individual (see p. 95). Current anti-estrogen recommendations by the National Cancer Institute are that patients taking tamoxifen as an adjuvant or preventive treatment for stage I breast cancer should stop taking this anti-estrogen after 5 years of therapy.

A woman who is still having menstrual periods might benefit from an oophorectomy, an operation to remove her ovaries, the primary source of estrogen in her body. Oophorectomy has been used as a preventive measure after breast cancer surgery. Current data suggest that oophorectomy increases survival. This operation is now done with minimally invasive surgery (also called endoscopic-assisted surgery) through very short incisions. In the past the adrenal glands or pituitary gland was removed to eradicate other sources of estrogen; however, there are medications available today to accomplish this goal. Aminoglutethimide (Cytadren) blocks the production of adrenal hormones, including estrogens, and is used in selected cases. This anti-adrenal drug is difficult to use because of its side effects, including a severe skin rash, initial drowsiness, chemical imbalance, and nausea. A new group of drugs (luteinizing hormone–releasing hormone [LH-RH] agonists) that blocks some pituitary gland function has recently been approved for selected breast cancers.

Another type of "female" hormone that can be effective in controlling widespread breast cancer is a progestational hormone such as megestrol acetate (Megace) or medroxyprogesterone acetate (Provera). Progesterone has fewer side effects than estrogen, but an increase in appetite with subsequent weight gain is not uncommon. A new class of drugs, known as aromatase inhibitors, work to block estrogen metabolism with few if any side effects. Anastrozol (Arimidex) and letrozole (Femara) belong to this class of drugs and have been marketed for use after tamoxifen or toremifene. The use of male hormones such as androgens has been largely abandoned in breast cancer treatment since they are less effective and have many side effects.

## Drugs Commonly Used in Hormonal Therapy

Anti-estrogen
   Tamoxifen (Nolvadex)
   Toremifene (Fareston)
Progestational hormone
   Megestrol acetate (Megace)
Aromatase inhibitor
   Anastrozole (Arimidex)
   Letrozole (Femara)
Estrogen (dietheylstilbestrol)
Androgen (Halotestin)
Aminogluthemide (Cytadren)
Ketoconazole (Nizoral)
Luteinizing hormone–releasing hormone (LH-RH) agonist
   (leuprolide [Lupron] or goserelin [Zoladex])

## Monoclonal Antibodies

Another area of research is focusing on attacking tumors by using monoclonal antibodies (genetically engineered versions of natural human proteins that ordinarily seek out and destroy invading microbes). Monoclonal antibodies represent an exciting new approach to diagnosis and treatment of breast cancer patients. Some scientists are investigating the potential for injecting advanced cancer patients with monoclonal antibodies (immune system protein molecules); this experimental therapy has been found to shrink tumors in animal studies. A monoclonal antibody for non-Hodgkin's lymphoma therapy has recently been marketed. Herceptin, a monoclonal antibody being tested for breast cancer, has demonstrated promise in slowing the division of breast tumors. Initial tests of Hercepin in women with tumors that produce excessive growth-regulating proteins indicate that when combined with standard chemotherapy it has the potential to slow tumor progression, an improved response rate over standard chemotherapy alone. Herceptin may prove beneficial if given to women early in the course of the disease. Moreover, it has demonstrated few side effects beyond transient fever and chills and possible heart muscle damage if administered with anthracyclines. Although this therapy is still considered investigational and further studies are needed to establish its safety and efficacy requirements, the FDA has now designated Herceptin for speedy review, which means that availability could be expedited.

## Anti-Angiogenesis Agents

Anti-angiogenesis agents (angiogenesis inhibitors) are promising cancer drugs that hold the potential for shutting down blood vessel growth and stunting tumor growth. At least 11 of these agents have been identified and are being tested in humans and/or in animals and others are under development. This new therapy is based on the theory that a tumor needs a blood supply to grow. As long as a tumor generates vessels, it can grow indefinitely—and the bigger it gets, the more vessels it can generate. Unless a tumor can spawn a network of vessels to deliver nutrients and oxygen, it will grow to a small size and become dormant and harmless. However, if this small mass suddenly stimulates nearby blood vessels to send out new vessels and capillaries, this vascular flow, called angiogenesis, enables the tumors to grow uncontrollably, invading healthy tissues and spreading through the bloodstream. As long as a tumor generates vessels, it can grow indefinitely. Therefore anti-angiogenesis drugs seek to prevent new blood vessel formation. In research done on cancerous mice, treatment with two such vessel inhibitors (endostatin and angiostatin) has been shown to reduce the tumors to their original dormant state, often shrinking the tumor and preventing spread or metastases.

Other anti-angiogenesis agents have been reported to shrink tumors in human trials. Some pharmaceutical companies are synthesizing molecules that disrupt angiogenesis by binding with a particular growth factor or jamming a certain receptor. One company is studying an engineered antibody that blocks VEGF, one of the signaling molecules that tumors use to make blood vessels proliferate or grow. Others have developed several molecules that keep new vessel cells from picking up MMPs (the drill-bit enzymes). All of these antibodies and agents are still in investigational stages, with years of studies and trials needed to establish their safety and effectiveness.

## IF BREAST CANCER SPREADS . . .
GARY A. RATKIN, M.D.

If the local and systemic therapies are not totally effective in eradicating all disease, breast cancer can return and spread to other parts of the body. The unpredicted regrowth may occur within the first few years of the original breast cancer diagnosis or years later.

Once a metastasis has been found, an assessment of the patient's overall health and the degree of breast cancer spread is critical. Some metastases can be controlled with oral hormonal medications, others require local radiation therapy or surgery, and the most advanced might necessitate chemotherapy. The goal of treatment is to control the cancer so that the patient is able to live comfortably. Although a cure is not usually possible, once a recurrence is found, treatment can permit good-quality life for many years. Breast cancer, unlike many other forms of metastatic cancer, can be well controlled for long periods of time with the strategic use of medications. Recently, much progress has been made in the treatment of such widespread breast cancer.

Some of the most frequently used drugs in metastatic breast cancer are methotrexate, 5-fluorouracil, cyclophosphamide, doxorubicin, and mitoxantrone. New drugs used for breast cancer include paclitaxel, docetaxel, vinorelbine, and capecitabine. Paclitaxel (Taxol), a drug discovered from the bark of the slow-growing Pacific yew tree, has proved highly effective in treating women with advanced breast cancer. Recent studies have shown that adding Taxol to standard chemotherapy for breast cancer reduced the rate of recurrence by over 20% and decreased the number of deaths by approximately 25%. A newer synthetic form is called docetaxel (Taxotere). Typically, three or four drug combinations or sequences are given to obtain the best outcome. Side effects of chemotherapy for metastatic disease are similar to those described earlier in this chapter.

### Chemotherapy Drugs Commonly Used for Metastatic Disease

| | |
|---|---|
| Vinblastine (Velban) | Mitoxantrone (Novantrone) |
| Doxorubicin (Adriamycin) | Mitomycin-C (Mutamycin) |
| Cyclophosphamide (Cytoxan) | Paclitaxel (Taxol) |
| 5-Fluorouracil (5-FU) | Docetaxel (Taxotere) |
| Methotrexate | Vinorelbine (Navelbine) |
| Thiotepa (Thioplex) | Capecitabine (Xeloda) |

## FOLLOW-UP SURVEILLANCE AFTER BREAST CANCER TREATMENT

WILLIAM C. WOOD, M.D.

After completion of primary treatment of breast cancer, patients are routinely placed under follow-up surveillance to detect and treat any recurrence of the first cancer or to discover any new breast cancer in the opposite breast at the earliest possible stage. As mentioned previously, women who develop breast cancer have an increased risk of cancer in the other breast (see p. 56). For women over 50, this risk is about 4% for their remaining years; for those under 50, it is about 14%. Although the risk is not as great as many women imagine, careful evaluation is mandatory. It is essential that a cancer in the opposite breast be detected as early as possible to increase the likelihood of cure, as is the case with a primary tumor.

Detecting a new breast tumor in the opposite breast is accomplished by a familiar triad: monthly breast self-examination of the opposite breast, clinical examination by a physician or nurse practitioner every 6 to 12 months, and annual mammography. This combination provides the greatest assurance of early diagnosis. More frequent examinations have not been shown to be beneficial.

Surveillance for evidence of recurrence of the initial breast cancer is also a collaborative effort on the part of the patient and her surgeon, medical or radiation oncologist, and primary physician. The goal of self-examination of the chest wall or reconstructed breast (or the irradiated breast if breast-conserving therapy was performed), like examination of the normal breast, is to detect an area that feels different to the examining fingers or looks different in the mirror. Lumps, thickenings, or areas of different color can all be normal, but they should be checked by a woman's surgeon as soon as they are detected. Any new lump or swollen lymph gland that is discovered may arouse anxiety. If it persists for several weeks, the surgeon should check it to make a diagnosis and confirm whether there is reason for concern.

Initially, follow-up consists of a brief history and physical examination performed every 4 to 6 months. Physical examination focuses on parts of the body that are common sites of breast cancer spread. In time, this interval can be increased and a woman can return to her normal "whole person care" examination by her internal medicine physician, gynecologist, or family doctor.

The follow-up pattern of testing and its frequency are determined by a woman's physicians. Blood tests serve as screening tests for liver, bone, or bone marrow involvement. Chest x-ray films can screen for asymptomatic lung metastases, and mammograms can detect recurrences and screen for second (new) cancers of the breast. The great majority of recurrent cancers and second breast cancers are either detected by self-examination, by physical examination, or by mammography. Unless specific symptoms are present, there is little evidence to support additional laboratory studies such as chemistry studies, blood tumor markers, and even bone scans that are inconvenient for the patient, costly, and do not appear to improve survival. The value of these follow-up studies remains controversial. The American Society of Cancer Organizations (ASCO) has written a position paper discouraging the *routine* practice of follow-up laboratory studies as it does not change outcome (survival). Managed care companies also discourage this practice. On the other hand, any new symptom (e.g., ache or pain) or new finding (e.g., mass or lump) discovered on physical examination is a clear indication for specific studies. Because tumors that are faster growing recur sooner and more slowly growing tumors recur later, the interval between follow-up examinations can be increased over a period of years, but at no time should these examinations be discontinued.

Routine mammography of the reconstructed breast is not needed if a complete mastectomy has been done. Monthly self-examination of the rebuilt breast has proved the best method for detecting a recurrence. There is no evidence that reconstruction causes any significant delay in detecting the rare cases of recurrent disease behind or beneath the reconstructed breast.

## CLINICAL TRIALS: THEIR ROLE IN ASSESSING BREAST CANCER TREATMENT OPTIONS

ROGER S. FOSTER, Jr., M.D.

Before new treatments for breast cancer are accepted by the medical community for use on patients, they need to be compared to alternative treatments in carefully conducted scientific studies.

The clinical trial represents an excellent method for comparing and assessing different treatment approaches to breast cancer management. In these clinical trials, groups of doctors and their women patients agree to participate in studies in which the cancer treatment alternatives that these patients will ultimately receive may be decided by randomization. Randomization means that neither the patient nor her doctor chooses between the alternative treatments; instead, the treatments are chosen arbitrarily, or totally by chance, to avoid any bias creeping into the study. Randomized studies are particularly important when the differences between treatments being compared are likely to be either small or nonexistent.

Clinical trials in breast cancer have now involved many thousands of women whose medical data have been carefully collected to answer a variety of questions about breast cancer. Out of these trials has come an understanding that breast cancer is not one disease but many different diseases, or perhaps a disease with many variations. Increasingly, appropriate treatment requires understanding these many variations of breast cancer.

### Primary Treatment: Breast-Conserving Surgery vs. Total Mastectomy

The treatment of breast cancer by less than complete mastectomy has been studied in randomized clinical trials. Seven randomized trials in this area have contributed significantly to resolving questions that were unsatisfactorily answered previously. It has been shown that when carefully selected patients are treated by experienced surgeons and radiotherapists with breast-conserving operations, their survival at 10 to 15 years is comparable to the survival for women treated with operations that remove the entire breast. Some patients treated with breast-conserving surgery do, however, have a cancer recurrence in the remaining portion of their breast and require a total mastectomy at a later time. As further data develop from these studies, women and their physicians will have additional scientific information on which to base a decision regarding the alternatives of total mastectomy followed by reconstruction vs. breast-conserving surgery.

## Adjuvant Treatment

Adjuvant treatments are those treatments given in addition to surgical removal of the cancer. Alternative adjuvant management approaches for breast cancer have also been the subject of investigation. Scientifically valid studies have been conducted and demonstrate that the addition of radiation decreases recurrence in the treated area. We have learned that radiation treatment is also effective for those mastectomy patients in whom cancer recurs or for patients with more advanced cancers at the time of diagnosis.

Newer studies suggest that postoperative radiation to the chest wall may also have some survival benefit for women with several positive lymph nodes. This hypothesis is still under investigation. (See the discussion of postoperative radiation earlier in this chapter.)

Randomized studies have shown that irradiation after breast-conserving surgery greatly reduces the chance of recurrence of cancer in the breast, and therefore most of these patients are currently treated with radiotherapy. Other randomized clinical trials have investigated the question of alternative treatments for the axillary lymph nodes. These studies have shown that the axillary nodes can be treated by either surgery or radiation therapy with similar results. If the axillary nodes are not enlarged, they may simply be watched and treated only if they enlarge. These studies, which were conducted more than 15 years ago, proved that treating the axillary lymph nodes does not harm any immune response the patient's body may have triggered to fight cancer. Today, for most patients diagnosed with breast cancer under the age of 70, the axillary lymph nodes are routinely removed or sampled because up to 4 out of 10 patients will have microscopic spread of cancer into the lymph nodes, and that information is important in making decisions on additional treatments such as chemotherapy or hormonal therapy. Sentinel node biopsy (discussed earlier in this chapter) offers a new approach to node dissection that is currently under investigation.

Randomized clinical trials have been important in studying the effectiveness of combining systemic treatments (those affecting the entire body) with local and regional treatments of radiation and surgery. Over the past 20 years these randomized trials have been conducted to assess the effectiveness of systemic treatment with chemotherapy and/or hormonal therapy. The studies have clearly shown that it is possible to decrease the recurrence rates and improve survival for patients with some types of breast cancer by using these adjuvant treatments. Despite these advances there is still a need for better adjuvant treatments.

## Chemotherapy Induction Trials

Information has recently become available from a randomized clinical trial (conducted by the National Surgical Adjuvant Breast Project [NSABP]) comparing chemotherapy given before breast cancer surgery to the more common practice of giving chemotherapy after surgery. Chemotherapy given before surgery is sometimes called by names such as neoadjuvant chemotherapy or induction chemotherapy. According to one theory, the best time to give the chemotherapy is early in the course of treating any micrometastases outside the breast region when they are the smallest and have the least chance to develop resistant cells. This hypothesis suggested that it might be better to give chemotherapy before surgery. An alternative and competing theory argued for performing surgery to remove the primary cancer first to remove a potential source of cells that might spread to other parts of the body during the chemotherapy treatments. It turned out that neither theory prevails. The results of a large trial conducted by the NSABP have shown that recurrence and survival are similar when the adjuvant chemotherapy is given before rather than after surgery. There was an advantage to giving the chemotherapy first for some women when the breast cancer was relatively large in relation to the size of the breast. Giving the chemotherapy before surgery frequently made breast-conserving surgery possible when a mastectomy would otherwise have been required or made it possible to do a smaller lumpectomy. Chemotherapy is currently most commonly given after breast cancer surgery, but for more advanced cancers or when the size of the cancer in the breast might make breast-conserving surgery difficult or impossible, the option to give chemotherapy first is frequently considered.

## Breast Cancer Chemotherapy Prevention Trials

Observation of the beneficial effects that adjuvant (preventive) tamoxifen therapy has had in reducing the incidence of second primary breast cancer and cardiovascular deaths in breast cancer patients has led to the development of clinical trials to assess the value of tamoxifen in preventing breast cancer in women at high risk for its development. The U.S. trial conducted by the National Surgical Adjuvant Breast Project involved over 13,000 women: one half treated with tamoxifen and one half treated with a placebo. The trial has been closed, but follow-up continues. Since age is the most important risk factor for breast cancer, all women over the age of 60 were eligible. Women under the age of 60, down to the age of 35, were eligible if they had sufficient additional risk factors (including lobular carcinoma in situ, atypical hyperplasia, a family history of breast cancer, and were nulliparous, that is, not having borne children). A computer-generated assessment of breast cancer risk was used to determine a woman's eligibility. The younger the patient, the greater the degree of risk that was necessary for acceptance into the trial. Trial data seem to indicate that tamoxifen diminishes the risk of both invasive and in situ breast cancer but may increase the risk of two rare events, endometrial (uterus) cancer and deep vein clots and pulmonary embolism. Although the data on the benefits of tamoxifen in patients with breast cancer are compelling, the benefits must be proved in healthy women, with evidence that the benefits outweigh the side effects before tamoxifen is prescribed outside a clinical trial. (See p. 83 for information on side effects.)

Most breast cancer clinical trials require cooperation from physicians in many different medical centers. Numerous experts contribute to the design of each trial, thus providing "multiple second opinions." The National Cancer Institute reviews each trial design and commonly covers the expenses incurred in collecting the scientific data. In addition, each participating medical center has its own human investigation review committee that must approve the trial before it can begin at a medical center.

By participating in clinical trials, physicians are able to keep current with the most recent developments in cancer treatment, and patients can expect to receive either the best recognized treatment or a new treatment that a consensus of experts believes may represent an advance. In addition, information gained from the treatment will influence the future care of others.

The feelings of attachment a woman has about her breasts are profound and should not be lightly dismissed by the physician treating her. These feelings will influence a woman's decision to seek help initially and eventually will help determine the therapy she selects. Once the surprise of being stricken by a dreaded disease has passed, a woman desires and deserves honest information about her disease, her prognosis, and her options for treatment. In addition, she needs a physician who is sensitive to her psychological and aesthetic requirements. The physician who treats a woman afflicted with breast cancer must consider the effect of therapy not only on ultimate survival and rehabilitation but also on enhanced quality of life. Optimal patient care extends beyond medical management of the disease itself.

# What Your Doctors And Nurses Can Do For You

*It was frustrating. Each doctor wanted to do his part
but no one was coordinating the effort. I kept wondering where was
this team approach I've heard so much about?*

We live in an age of specialization. Nowhere is this phenomenon more obvious than in the field of medicine, where a single individual is no longer capable of staying current with the latest scientific data. Thus, when a woman has a breast problem, she may consult with several experts before she can decide on the appropriate course of action. Most likely she will begin by visiting her primary care doctor, who is familiar with her medical history and whom she has grown to trust for advice about her health care. This doctor may be her gynecologist, family practitioner, or internist, and he is the person she will first see for diagnosis of her problem and treatment advice. This doctor will refer her to other specialists if he feels that they can contribute to the diagnosis or treatment of her suspected problem. When her doctor sends her to another specialist, he is playing an important coordinating role by using his knowledge and taking advantage of recent developments in medicine to help her get the best specialty care possible.

A woman's needs, of course, will vary with her individual situation. Sometimes her breast problem will be diagnosed as fibrocystic change by her primary care physician, and he will monitor her breasts with regular checkups and mammograms. These mammograms will be interpreted by the diagnostic radiologist. If a lump or another suspicious area is discovered on physical examination or on a mammogram and warrants further investigation, possibly a biopsy (image-guided or surgical), she may be referred to a general surgeon for further examination and evaluation.

If a biopsy is indicated, a pathologist now becomes involved in the woman's health care. He analyzes the biopsy specimen and reports whether a cancer has been found, what kind it is, and whether it has spread to her lymph nodes. Even though the pathologist has no direct contact with the woman diagnosed with breast cancer or even with the woman whose biopsied lump proves benign, his report has a great influence on what happens to each of these women in the future. If the pathologist's report indicates cancer, the general surgeon explains her problem to the woman and outlines her treatment options (see Chapter 6). These options may include breast-conserving surgery and irradiation or mastectomy with possible breast reconstruction. If her tumor is large or her cancer has spread to the lymph nodes, adjunctive therapy also may be required, possibly before local surgical treatment. She may learn of chemotherapy, radiation therapy, and hormonal therapy. Depending on her individual situation and the therapy she ultimately selects, she may interact with a number of specialists associated with the breast management team; these experts include the radiologist, radiation oncologist, medical oncologist, general surgeon (surgical oncologist), and plastic surgeon.

The thought of facing more than one doctor is often frightening because we don't understand what each of these specialists does and who will coordinate care. It seems like an impersonal and expensive approach to health care. Women express confusion as to who is in charge. Furthermore, they don't always know what questions to ask these doctors or even how they can help them. To clear up some of the confusion and impersonality surrounding these medical specialists, we have asked experts we know and respect in each of the previously mentioned fields to write descriptions of what they do and how they can help you. The descriptions are organized according to the role these physicians play in a woman's health care and the stage at which she might consult with each expert. Therefore the gynecologist and internist are included under a heading entitled "Primary Care: Diagnosis, Management, and Referral" and the diagnostic radiologist, general surgeon, pathologist, radiation oncologist, medical oncologist, and plastic surgeon are listed under "The Breast Management Team: Diagnosis, Treatment, and Rehabilitation."

The nurse's role is also included in the discussion of "The Breast Management Team." When a woman has a breast problem, she is usually referred directly to a physician. Nurses, however, are active in all phases of the woman's breast care and play a valuable part in patient education, therapy, and rehabilitation. Therefore we have asked two nursing experts we know and admire, an oncology nurse and a plastic surgery nurse, to describe what they do and how they can assist you during this difficult time.

The final member of the team is the woman herself. As one of our readers reminded us, "A woman has an important role to play in this team effort. She needs to maintain a positive attitude, keep informed, and take responsibility for maintaining good basic health habits with attention to nutrition and exercise. In other words, the woman does not passively submit to treatments imposed by her doctors and other team members; rather, she is an active participant in her own treatment and recovery." We couldn't agree more. It is in a woman's best interest to play an active role in her own health care and to become an integral part of this team effort that contributes so significantly to her ultimate health and survival. (See Chapter 8 for more information on the woman's role.) The first step in this effort is learning what these health professionals do and how they can help you.

All of the physicians listed are board-certified members of their specialties. We feel that it is important for a woman to choose a physician who has met this standard. All physicians can practice medicine after medical school or residency, but board certification indicates that they have completed an approved training program and, after an initial period of clinical practice, have passed an examination that certifies that they meet the criteria for practice in the specialty.

## PRIMARY CARE: DIAGNOSIS, MANAGEMENT, AND REFERRAL

A yearly visit to the obstetrician-gynecologist or internist is routine for many women. If they develop a breast problem, they look to one of these doctors for advice and help.

### The Obstetrician-Gynecologist's Role in a Woman's Breast Care
JACOB KLEIN, M.D.

Specializing in the care of women and their reproductive organs, the obstetrician-gynecologist is in reality the primary care physician for most women and frequently is the only doctor that they see on a regular, ongoing basis. During a woman's annual or semiannual visits to her gynecologist he performs physical examinations that include a breast examination, pelvic examination, and Pap smear, which is a screening test for cervical cancer.

In the absence of breast disease the gynecologist is usually the physician who orders breast screening tests. It is his responsibility to be knowledgeable about the types of tests available, their advantages and disadvantages, and the frequency with which these examinations should be made. The newest developments in the area of breast screening must be part of every gynecologist's fund of knowledge.

The gynecologist is frequently the person most responsible for educating his patients about their bodies. This education includes information about the normal structure and function of their reproductive organs and what happens when these organs malfunction. In addition, the gynecologist stresses the value of regular gynecologic examinations and the importance of breast self-examination for early detection of breast cancer.

It is vital for the gynecologist to educate patients about the need for regular, monthly breast self-examination as well as the best timing for these inspections. Because a woman's hormonal cycle has a profound influence on her breast tissue, she needs to understand these cyclic changes in order to know when to examine her breasts. Women have numerous reasons for not performing this test, including fear of discovering a mass, ignorance of inspection techniques or the importance of early diagnosis, and lack of awareness of the prevalence of breast cancer. The gynecologist must be sensitive to a woman's concerns and aware of her reasons for procrastinating about initiating this health routine. With these reasons in mind, he should take responsibility for actually teaching his patients the appropriate techniques for breast self-inspection and then monitor a woman's performance to make sure that her inspections are adequate and to help her gain confidence in her ability to successfully practice self-examination. He also can assure her that she will gain proficiency with this inspection if she makes it a monthly routine.

When a woman discovers a questionable breast mass, the gynecologist is usually the first physician she contacts. The relationship that exists between a woman and her gynecologist is a unique and particularly trusting one. It allows the physician to deal with the physical and psychological aspects of a woman's breast disease. Therefore a gynecologist must sensitively respond to the patient's breast problem, from a total perspective, realizing that the discovery of a breast mass provokes unparalleled fear and anxiety in most women. The stress caused by the discovery of a breast lump must be dealt with as well as the treatment for the actual breast problem.

The process leading to definitive treatment of a suspected breast problem is initiated by the gynecologist after a routine breast examination. His findings will either reassure him that a disease state does not exist or prompt him to evaluate the breast mass further. The gynecologist will direct this evaluation by arranging for breast cyst aspiration, mammograms, or referral to a surgeon who is familiar with and sensitive to the issues involved with treating breast diseases. The patient will rely on her gynecologist for direction in her health care and will expect him to provide her with an explanation of the course of events that will likely follow. Once evaluation of her breast problem is complete and definitive treatment planned, a woman will frequently need to be reassured by her gynecologist that the other specialist's approach is medically sound. At this time the gynecologist plays an important role as a reliable source of information. He may also help in determining hormonal managment and whether hormonal replacement therapy is appropriate. He will continue the relationship with the patient concomitant with the care being provided to her by the surgeon, oncologist, radiotherapist, or plastic surgeon.

Prevention of breast disease and treatment of pathologic breast conditions when they do occur are an integral part of routine gynecologic care and should be expected and demanded by every patient.

## The Internist's Role in a Woman's Breast Care

BENJAMIN A. BOROWSKY, M.D.

In current medical practice the internist is the specialist responsible for the comprehensive medical care of his patients and the monitoring of their ongoing health care needs. His involvement in the treatment of a woman with a breast problem or breast cancer is continuous, beginning before the disease is detected and continuing after treatment is complete.

As part of health maintenance counseling, the internist will advise women on the need for self-examination and physician examination, appropriate use of mammograms, and effects of various drugs and hormones on her breasts. As more data become available on the influence of diet and environment on the incidence of breast cancer, he will discuss this information with her as well. In short, the internist's first duty is to educate the patient about practices that will prevent cancer when possible and lead to prompt detection if it does occur.

Once a breast mass has been discovered, the internist's first effort is to confirm its presence by examination. He must then choose from several options. If he feels certain that there is no indication of malignancy, he may decide not to proceed further. Repeat examination at a more suitable time in the menstrual cycle may be needed. In some cases the use of mammography is helpful. If he is uncertain about the diagnosis, he may wish to refer the patient to a surgeon for another opinion or for a biopsy and/or definitive surgery.

In selecting a general surgeon for patient referral the internist is guided by more than the surgeon's technical knowledge and skills. He must also consider how the individual woman will relate to a particular surgeon. Each person differs in the extent she desires to be informed about the many surgical options now available. Some women (and their families) wish to play an active role in planning treatment, whereas others prefer not to have to make a choice. It is important for the internist, who usually knows the patient best, to consider her preferences in recommending a surgeon. It is also his responsibility to advise the surgeon as to the woman's feelings. The surgeon usually will be the source of technical information regarding the woman's surgical options, but the internist can help her and her family understand these options and can offer his advice when a treatment choice is to be made.

During and immediately after surgery the internist manages any other coexisting conditions a patient may have. He also will participate in decisions regarding postoperative x-ray treatment or chemotherapy.

After the initial therapy is complete, follow-up is a coordinated effort between the surgeon, internist, and oncologist and/or radiation oncologist, when the latter are needed. It is usually the internist who is responsible for long-term follow-up and appropriate examinations to screen for signs of recurrent cancer. He also tailors his management of subsequent complaints based on the effect treatment may have on the woman's breast cancer.

The internist functions initially in the areas of prevention and detection. After cancer has been discovered, his relationship as principal medical advisor becomes most important. In this role he directs the patient to the proper specialists and advises her when treatment choices are necessary. Finally, he continues follow-up care of the patient indefinitely to ensure, if possible, the long-term success of treatment.

# THE BREAST MANAGEMENT TEAM:
# DIAGNOSIS, TREATMENT, AND REHABILITATION

Although the diagnostic radiologist is included here as a part of the breast management team, this specialist actually bridges the gap between the patient's primary care physicians and those members of the breast management team who will treat her breast problem. Screening or diagnostic mammograms may be ordered by any of these physicians, and the radiologist will confer with these specialists and with the woman herself to help screen for or diagnose any breast problems.

## The Diagnostic Radiologist's Role in the Detection and Diagnosis of Breast Disease

BARBARA S. MONSEES, M.D.

The diagnostic radiologist is a physician with special training in interpreting imaging studies such as mammograms, chest x-ray films, computed tomographic scans, ultrasonograms, and magnetic resonance imaging scans. Some diagnostic radiologists specialize in breast imaging and are called breast imagers.

Under most circumstances, the diagnostic radiologist functions as a consultant to physicians who order imaging studies to diagnose and evaluate their patient's problems. In the case of breast imaging, however, unlike other imaging tests, the imager assumes a more direct role, consulting with the patient herself and explaining the findings on her mammograms.

Although the radiologist does not position the patient for the mammogram and obtain the actual images (this is done by the radiologic technologist), he or she determines the number and quality of images obtained, maintains a standard of quality control, and interprets the examination itself.

When a woman has no signs or symptoms of breast problems, she is usually referred for a screening mammogram. Her breast images are then taken by the technologist and later interpreted by the radiologist. In this situation the patient has no contact with the radiologist.

If an abnormality is detected on a screening mammogram, however, the radiologist takes the lead in evaluating the problem because, lacking any signs or symptoms, it isn't observable on physical examination. Other mammographic views or ultrasound studies may then be suggested by the radiologist to fully evaluate the problem so that the radiologist can advise the referring physician as to whether an abnormality is present and whether it is likely to be benign or malignant. Often this information is also communicated directly to the woman herself by the radiologist so that she may seek consultation with a general surgeon who deals with breast problems. It is important for the radiologist to be sensitive to the patient's fears and to take the necessary time to explain what has been found on the mammogram and what that means for the patient.

When a woman or her physician finds a suspicious lump or thickening in the breast or a bloody nipple discharge, the woman should not be referred for a screening examination but for a diagnostic mammogram, which is performed under the direct supervision of the diagnostic radiologist. At that time the standard mammographic views will be taken, followed by any extra views necessary to better evaluate the suspicious area. The radiologist may also perform a clinical breast examination to correlate the mammograms with the physical findings. If an abnormality is suspected to be a cyst, ultrasonography (which is effective in distinguishing between a solid lump and a fluid-filled cyst) can be performed. If warranted, the cyst can be aspirated using ultrasound guidance. After all of the necessary images have been taken, the radiologist offers an opinion as to the type of follow-up needed, whether careful surveillance by the referring physician or surgical consultation. Frequently the radiologist will confer directly with the woman's primary care physician to expedite surgical consultation.

When a suspicious abnormality can be seen on the mammogram but cannot be felt, a biopsy is usually warranted. Until recently, it was standard procedure for the radiologist to place a small hookwire into the breast (breast needle localization) using mammography to ensure its accurate placement; this would then be followed by a surgical biopsy. With the recent advent of accurate equipment capable of placing a needle within even the tiniest lesion that can be seen on a mammogram, radiologists (as well as surgeons) have also begun to perform minimally invasive biopsies of suspicious areas seen only on mammography using either mammographic or ultrasound guidance. (See Chapter 5 for more information on these techniques.)

The breast imager plays a key role in detecting and diagnosing breast problems. This specialist not only interprets the breast x-ray films, but also consults with the woman and her referring physicians, offering solace when necessary and answering questions. The breast imager's role extends from detecting abnormalities that cannot be felt (through screening mammography) to characterization of detected abnormalities using diagnostic mammography, ultrasonography and other adjunctive techniques, and biopsy.

## The General Surgeon's Role in a Woman's Breast Care
KENNETH J. ARNOLD, M.D.

General surgeons are experienced in diseases of the breast, and this aspect of patient care represents a significant portion of many general surgery practices. When a woman or her primary care physician suspects a lump or abnormality, when a breast examination proves difficult, or when the mammographic results are questionable, it is usually the general surgeon who is consulted.

After examining the patient and reviewing her x-ray films, it is the surgeon who ultimately decides whether to recommend a breast biopsy. In arriving at that decision the patient's history, risk factors, and mammograms are all taken into consideration. In general, one of three conditions will result in a recommendation for breast biopsy: (1) a dominant lump, (2) a suspicious or indeterminate mammogram, or (3) bloody nipple discharge.

Frequently a mammogram will indicate a need for biopsy even though a palpable mass cannot be felt. In those cases a stereotactic needle biopsy or a needle-localized excisional biopsy is ordered rather than a surgical biopsy. The surgeon is in the best position to discuss those options with the patient and make recommendations as to which is most appropriate for her situation. When a lump is palpable, the surgeon often can place an ordinary hypodermic needle into the lump and gain valuable information quickly and with minimal discomfort. This usually can be done during the patient's office visit.

For the woman who requires a biopsy, the surgeon not only performs the biopsy, but provides the information and the emotional support that she requires. This means explaining the reason for the biopsy and the specifics involved in the procedure. It is important for the woman to know when she will receive a definitive report on the result of this procedure.

The surgeon can and should be more than an arbiter of treatment options. He should be a resource to the patient, knowledgeable about various conditions of the breast and their significance and able to answer the many questions that women have about their breasts. Many women do not require a biopsy, but they do need an expert to provide them with information about their breasts, to answer their questions, and to address their concerns. The general surgeon uses his expertise to reassure and educate these patients about benign breast conditions and breast cancer, the need for breast self-examination and physician breast examination, and the necessity for cancer screening. He must also make himself available to respond to the many questions today's informed women have about their breasts.

For the woman diagnosed with breast cancer, the general surgeon plays a key role in her care. The surgeon must be able to sensitively discuss with the woman and her family the many controversies surrounding the issue of breast cancer and the various choices available to her. Because the woman is faced with so much information and misinformation, it is important for the surgeon to take the time to help her sort through the plethora of fact and fantasy that confronts her.

In general, the surgeon will explain to the patient that there are two basic problems to be dealt with in breast cancer: local control of the disease within the breast itself and control of the disease within the rest of the body. Most women will have choices in these areas, and it is important that the surgeon adequately discuss these with the patient. It is also imperative that the patient, already distressed by her diagnosis, feel comfortable with her surgeon and be unafraid to ask even the most basic questions. Dealing with these issues is time consuming, but it is important for the patient to feel that she has been given sufficient information so that she can make the decisions that are required of her.

For the mastectomy patient, he will also inform the woman of the option of breast reconstruction. Then, if the woman is interested in this option, she and her surgeon can discuss the timing for reconstruction. If she desires immediate breast restoration during the same operation as her mastectomy, the general surgeon often will refer her to a plastic surgeon, either the one on his breast management team or one with whom he has worked before.

After fulfilling the role of teacher in educating the woman and her family about breast cancer, the surgeon must be able to make appropriate recommendations for treatment and then skillfully carry out the agreed upon surgical treatment, whether breast-conserving surgery or mastectomy, referring to other specialists as indicated. At this point the surgeon will often act as the coordinator of a team approach to the woman's breast cancer treatment, coordinating her care and referring her to various other specialists such as a radiation oncologist, medical oncologist, plastic surgeon, and support group personnel as they are needed.

Among the many questions a woman might consider asking her surgeon are the following:

- How should I examine myself? What time of the month is best and what am I looking for?
- When and how often should I see a physician?
- What are my risks of breast cancer and what can I do to lessen them?
- Is mammography necessary and will it increase my risk of developing cancer?

When a biopsy is necessary, she might ask:

- Should this procedure be done on an inpatient or outpatient basis and under local or general anesthesia?
- Can I have a fine-needle aspiration or a minimally invasive biopsy procedure?
- If I have a surgical biopsy, what type of scar will be left?
- Why is this biopsy necessary? Will the whole lump be gone or just a portion? When will the result be known with certainty?
- After biopsy, how long do I have to make up my mind on treatment if it reveals cancer?
- What happens if it is cancer? What are my treatment options? What are the associated benefits and risks associated with each option?
- What are the differences between breast-conserving surgery and mastectomy? Which is safer? Is survival the same? Is the recurrence rate the same?
- What are the aesthetic ramifications of treatment?
- Do I have to lose my breast?
- Can I have breast reconstruction if I need it?
- Will I need chemotherapy, hormonal therapy, or radiation therapy?

For the woman who ultimately develops breast cancer or for any woman conferring with a general surgeon, no question should be considered too trivial. She deserves a thoughtful answer to every inquiry. Above all, she must feel comfortable not only with the surgeon's ability, but also with his approachability since theirs is a relationship that will last through years of follow-up observation.

# The Pathologist's Role in the Diagnosis and Treatment of Breast Problems
JOHN S. MEYER, M.D.

A pathologist is a medical doctor specializing in the analysis and diagnosis of disease in the laboratory. He analyzes tissues obtained from biopsies or removal of organs and analyzes blood and other body fluids. He is an expert in cytology, which is the analysis of cells from tissues and fluids. In this role he will analyze Pap smears, smears of secretions from the nipple to detect malignant cells, and fine-needle aspirates from breast masses. To effectively diagnose breast cancer the pathologist must also have a thorough familiarity with the microscopic anatomy of the breast and various disease states that affect it.

Although the woman with a breast lump will talk to and be examined by her personal physician and surgeon, she is not likely to meet the pathologist who is responsible for diagnosing her condition if a biopsy is done. Ordinarily the specimen that the surgeon removes is sent to the laboratory, where the pathologist examines it in the light of the surgeon's findings, which are written on a form accompanying the specimen.

This examination involves two steps. First is the gross examination in which the pathologist uses his naked eye to scrutinize the specimen and select portions for microscopic study. After hardening and preserving these portions in formaldehyde or some other fluid, histotechnologists prepare microscopic slides on which very thin, transparent sections of the tissues are sliced and stained to make them visible under the microscope. Next, during microscopic examination of these slides, the pathologist analyzes the types of cells present and their relationship to each other.

In analyzing a biopsy specimen a pathologist does more than simply diagnose or rule out the presence of cancer. Breast cancer is actually not a single disease, but a classification containing many subtypes that have different implications for the patient and the doctors treating her. First, the pathologist decides whether the cancer is invasive (infiltrating) or intraductal (in situ). In situ cancer, either within the breast duct or lobule, does not metastasize and is virtually 100% curable by removal of the breast. If the cancer is invasive, it is classified as to the exact type. Certain invasive cancers are slow growing and usually do not metastasize. The great majority of women with these special types of breast cancer are cured by a mastectomy and axillary lymph node dissection without further treatment.

Most invasive breast cancers are not the slow-growing types mentioned above. The pathologist can classify these cancers further by noting the characteristics of their cells (whether well differentiated or poorly differentiated) and their patterns of growth in the breast tissues and axillary lymph nodes. If an axillary dissection has been done, he examines the lymph nodes microscopically to determine the presence or absence of carcinoma. The chances of having a recurrence of cancer or a metastasis depend strongly on the number of lymph nodes that contain cancer.

The pathologist may perform a battery of tests or assays to identify specific oncogenes (genes that play a role in producing cancers) and growth factors that predict breast carcinoma prognosis. One oncogene that he may look at is the oncogene *HER-2/neu* (also called *erb B-2/neu*), a protein present on the surface of breast cancer cells that is associated with a high probability of distant cancer spread (metastasis) when a patient has positive axillary lymph nodes. This gene is thought to be abnormal in up to 20% of women with breast cancer (particularly in women with a family history of breast cancer) and is capable of making tumors more aggressive and lethal. Tests are also conducted to measure the presence of epidermal growth factor receptors. Breast cancers with increased numbers of receptors for epidermal growth factor (a protein with growth-stimulating properties) have a relatively high likelihood of metastasis. The future role of these and similar tests is not yet clear.

The pathologist may also conduct tests to measure the enzymes that breast cancers secrete. These enzymes may attack surrounding tissues and help the carcinomas become invasive. One such enzyme that is related to breast cancer prognosis is cathepsin-D. Several studies have associated high levels of cathepsin-D with an unfavorable prognosis, but some questions remain about the utility of this test.

Much of the pathologist's attention focuses on growth rate measurements. Cancers with high rates of growth are more likely to produce recurrences within a few years of treatment than those with slow growth rates. Growth rates (S-phase fraction) may be measured by flow cytometry, which is an automated method for determining the ploidy (the amount of DNA in the cells). Tumors with abnormally high amounts of DNA are termed DNA-aneuploid and usually have a less favorable prognosis because they are faster growing than tumors with near-normal DNA content, which are called DNA-diploid. Labeling indexes and Ki-67 assays also are used to measure cell growth rate in tumors. Low labeling indexes are associated with a good prognosis and a smaller chance of tumor recurrence. Labeling index tests are technically difficult to perform, however, and are not available at all laboratories. Recent developments promise to increase the ease of performing these growth rate measurements.

Tests to measure the estrogen and progesterone receptors in cancer cells are an important means of determining the risk of cancer recurring, the subsequent need for further therapy (adjuvant chemotherapy, radiation therapy, or hormonal therapy), and which tumors are likely to respond to treatment with tamoxifen (an anti-estrogen) or other methods of hormonal therapy. Carcinomas that contain large amounts of estrogen and progesterone receptors, in general, are less likely to recur or metastasize within a few years of breast removal than are carcinomas with small amounts of these receptors or no detectable receptors. Thus information about the presence or absence of estrogen and progesterone receptors should be included in the pathologist's report.

The final report issued by the pathologist diagnoses the cancer and classifies it based on the various findings previously mentioned. This report is used by the general surgeon and other members of the breast management team in assessing the woman's risk of spread or possible recurrence of cancer and in determining the appropriate treatment and the need for any adjuvant therapies designed to prevent recurrence.

The identification of a breast cancer requires a woman to consult with still other members of the breast management team who will help with her treatment and rehabilitation.

## The Radiation Oncologist's Role in Treating a Woman With Breast Cancer

JOHN M. BEDWINEK, M.D.

A radiation oncologist is a physician who specializes in the study of cancer and its treatment with ionizing radiation—a potent killer of malignant cells. The radiation oncologist determines if and when radiation should be used and is a part of the cancer team (surgeon, radiation oncologist, and medical oncologist) that decides what is the optimum combination of the three cancer treatment modalities: surgery, irradiation, and chemotherapy. The radiation oncologist also decides how much and what type of radiation therapy should be used and is directly responsible for delivering the radiation dose effectively and safely.

The radiation oncologist must have a broad range of training. He must have a thorough understanding of all types of cancer and a familiarity with the capabilities, limitations, and side effects of the other two cancer treatment modalities: chemotherapy and surgery. He should be well versed in nuclear physics and the physics of ionizing radiation, understand the effects of radiation both on tumors and on normal human tissue, and know the latest techniques for precisely delivering the right amount of radiation to cancerous tissue while sparing normal tissue. In addition, he must be knowledgeable in general medicine so he can manage his patient's problems and know when to refer to other physicians if problems arise outside his area of expertise.

The radiation oncologist has a number of different responsibilities, beginning with the initial consultation, when he first sees the patient and studies all aspects of her condition. He reviews her current symptoms and past medical history, performs a physical examination, orders and evaluates all appropriate x-ray studies and blood tests, and reviews the biopsy specimen with the pathologist. Once the necessary data have been assessed, he confers with the surgeon and/or medical oncologist and they determine whether radiation is indicated or whether another form of treatment is more appropriate. Since he has conferred with the surgeon and/or medical oncologist, this decision carries the weight of a team approach.

Patient education is one of the radiation oncologist's most important functions. After deciding on the best mode of treatment he should be able to help the patient understand what that treatment is, why it is considered the best option, what are the anticipated side effects, and what is the expected outcome.

If radiation treatment is actually used, it is the radiation oncologist who determines how much radiation to give and what specific areas of the body should be targeted. For example, he must decide whether to treat the breast only or whether to treat the breast and the adjacent lymph node areas. The radiation treatment must be planned so that a precise and uniform radiation dose is delivered to all tumor-bearing tissue while minimizing the dose to normal tissues as much as possible. He may use high-technology equipment such as a simulator with fluoroscopy, a three-dimensional treatment planning computer, or computed tomography to assist him in this planning process.

Care of the patient during the course of and after completion of radiation therapy is also the responsibility of the radiation oncologist.

He must ensure that the daily radiation treatments are being given according to his plan and must monitor the effects of the radiation not only on the cancer, but also on the surrounding normal tissues. He must recognize which symptoms are side effects of the radiation dose and which symptoms are not and manage all side effects and problems that occur during the course of radiation therapy. Once radiation therapy has been completed, the radiation oncologist must assess the effectiveness of the treatment and monitor the patient at regular intervals to watch for radiation complications, regrowth of the cancer, and/or the development of new cancers.

Ongoing emotional support for the patient and her family pervades all stages of patient management. The patient needs to know that the radiation oncologist truly cares and will be there to answer all questions and to help with all problems.

A radiation oncologist must have compassion and sensitivity, qualities not easily taught in a formal training program. The patient who discovers that she has cancer has special psychological needs, and the radiation oncologist must be sensitive to these needs and be equipped to offer the necessary emotional support and understanding.

Of equal importance to compassion is the ability to communicate and teach effectively. It is crucial that the radiation oncologist provide clear and easily understandable answers to the following questions:

- What kind of cancer does the patient have, and how does it grow and spread?
- What are the treatment options for this particular kind of cancer? Will it be radiation therapy, surgery, chemotherapy, or a combination of these modalities?
- What is the specific purpose of each of the treatments?
- What are the potential side effects and complications of the proposed treatment, and what are the chances of these occurring?
- What are the consequences of the complications if they occur, and what is the treatment for the complications?
- Will the patient be able to engage in normal daily activities during the treatment? If not, what are the restrictions, and how soon can normal activity be resumed?

Are there any alternatives to the proposed treatment, and what are the chances of success and possible side effects of these alternatives? These issues are the bare minimum that must be explained clearly and simply without the patient having to ask. There will always be more questions, and the patient should be given ample opportunity to ask additional questions after she has had time to reflect.

The radiation oncologist must also make every effort to ensure that the patient fully understands what is said. Explanations and answers to questions should be given at least twice. It is the rare patient who can understand and fully grasp unfamiliar facts and concepts on the first explanation, particularly since she may still be in a state of shock and anxiety from recently being told that she has cancer. For this reason, the radiation oncologist should see the woman a second time a few days after the initial visit so that he can repeat earlier explanations and answer any questions that may have arisen since the first appointment. Also, it is helpful for the woman to have a close friend or family member present when explanations are given.

Being able to explain medical facts and concepts in an easily understandable fashion is, in part, a gift, but it is also a skill that can be acquired through patience, effort, and practice. The gift of communication is not possessed by all physicians and not all physicians take the time and effort to develop such skills. This is unfortunate since being able to help the patient understand all aspects of her disease and treatment will greatly diminish her fear. Patient education is one of the most important responsibilities of the radiation oncologist. It is, in fact, one of the most important responsibilities of any doctor. Most doctors, unfortunately, do not know that the origin of the title "doctor" comes from the Latin word *doceo,* which means "to teach" or "to explain." A doctor should first and foremost be a good teacher. If he is not, then the patient should find another doctor who is.

## The Medical Oncologist's Role in Treating a Woman With Breast Cancer

GARY A. RATKIN, M.D.

The medical oncologist's role in breast cancer managment has changed from treating metastatic cancer to the use of adjuvant chemotherapy to lower the chances of breast cancer spread or recurrence. Improvement in the use of systemic treatment, including chemotherapy, hormonal therapy, and supportive techniques have made consultation with an oncologist central to the managment of most patients with breast cancer.

A medical oncologist is a specialist in internal medicine who is knowledgeable in the management of malignancies (including breast cancer) and in the use of medications to treat cancer. A woman who has had primary treatment for breast cancer may consult a medical oncologist first when adjunctive therapy is being considered. She usually is referred to the medical oncologist by her surgeon or primary physician (internist, gynecologist, or family physician). Close communication with each of these physicians is key since the medical oncologist makes important recommendations to the patient based on the information he receives. If metastatic cancer develops, the medical oncologist may then manage the overall *palliative* treatment plan to relieve and reduce the severity of symptoms of the disease.

The oncologist reviews the original pathology report, hormone receptor and cell kinetic data (when available), and any clinical information such as x-ray films, laboratory tests, risk factors, symptoms, and physical findings. The medical oncologist can then advise the woman about the diagnosis, staging, and appropriate treatment.

Comprehensive knowledge of the latest drug therapies and experience in prescribing and administering chemotherapeutic drugs are required. When the patient requires chemotherapy or hormonal therapy, the medical oncologist is the one responsible for its administration. The common and unusual side effects of the drugs, how to prevent them, or how to treat them are addressed in the medical oncology consultation. In particular, the medical oncologist must have an in-depth knowledge of hematologic (blood) problems as well as broader experience in dealing with infectious diseases and lung, heart, or gastrointestinal problems. The oncologist must be aware of the many advances involving new chemotherapeutic drugs, new applications of hormones and chemotherapy, and current supportive techniques that allow the most effective and safest administration of these agents.

The oncologist must also be aware of and understand the many physical and emotional problems that confront the cancer patient. He should be able to sensitively address the patient's concerns to help her cope with the various aspects of her cancer and its treatment.

To meet the patient's individual needs the oncologist should be aware of the resources available to the patient in her community and nationally and be able to make the appropriate referrals and suggestions. She may need to consult with experts in radiation oncology, pathology, surgery, or plastic surgery. Knowledge of local nursing resources is critical, as is information on pharmacies and medical supply businesses that cater to the needs of cancer patients. Appropriate community service organizations, dieticians, psychologists, physical and occupational therapists, and social workers may be of great value to patients. Most communities and many hospitals have cancer information centers and support services available that may be of service.

Finally, the medical oncologist must be a scientist as well as a humanist. This means he must be able to scrutinize and critically evaluate medical reports in order to arrive at the best treatment plan. Many oncologists in the United States and Canada participate in clinical research on new treatment programs through local medical schools, hospitals, or national cooperative group efforts. Organized hospital cancer programs, tumor registries (organized by the American College of Surgeons), and the federally sponsored cooperative group efforts allow practicing physicians to contribute to the development of oncology as a science of cancer management.

A woman needs to understand the reason she is seeing an oncologist. Questions about the stage of her disease and the implications it has for her life or prognosis should be addressed to the medical oncologist. In addition, she should understand the goals of the suggested treatment. Further questions about the actual treatment program and how she can assess the effectiveness of treatment are very important. Some of the questions she might ask with anticipated answers include the following:

### Why are drugs used to treat cancer?

Cancer cells can escape from the original tumor and spread throughout the body. Chemotherapy or hormonal drugs can travel through the bloodstream to reach the cancer cells wherever they may be.

### How do you know which drugs to use?

Medical research has allowed physicians to compile experience with specific drugs to prove their effectiveness in controlling cancer. Once it is established which chemotherapy or hormonal agents work best, combinations are employed to increase their effectiveness. By combining drugs we hope to obtain additional therapeutic benefit and less toxicity. In general, drugs that work by different mechanisms are additive and produce a synergistic combination ($1 + 1 = 3$ or $4$).

### Why are there side effects of chemotherapy?

Chemotherapy drugs work to kill or damage cancer cells throughout the body. The cancer cells are thought to be more susceptible to this type of damage, whereas normal cells can heal themselves more easily. Side effects are the temporary effect of the chemotherapy on the normal tissue.

### What can be done to prevent side effects of chemotherapy?

Many side effects can be minimized by using drug combinations in more moderate doses. Certain side effects such as nausea can be prevented by using anti-nausea medications before or after treatment. Simple measures such as holding ice in the mouth while certain drugs are administered intravenously can prevent mouth sores. Patients who receive a drug such as cyclophosphamide that can irritate the bladder can prevent these symptoms by drinking adequate amounts of fluids.

### Why does my blood count have to be checked every time I go for chemotherapy?

Most chemotherapies can lower the red blood cell, white blood cell, or platelet count, which causes problems. If the white cell count is very low, the woman might be at high risk of serious infection. A low platelet count makes a person susceptible to bleeding or bruising. Anemia is the effect of a low red blood count and might require blood cell transfusions. The intensity of the chemotherapy regimen or the exact medications used determines how severely suppressed the count might be. Blood counts are usually allowed to recover before chemotherapy is safely administered again. Growth factors can be given in appropriate cases to stimulate normal white blood cell, platelet, or red cell production and recovery.

### Are there other generalized effects of which the patient needs to be aware?

Many patients who are being treated with chemotherapy will experience fatigue, which may be worst when the white or red blood cell count is lowest. Depression and anxiety are common symptoms when patients are undergoing cancer treatments. Even the end of a preventive chemotherapy program might cause anxiety.

### What are the most important side effects?

A suppressed blood count is usually the most serious aftermath of chemotherapy. If the white cell count is very low, the patient is at risk of bloodstream infection, which can be life threatening. A severely low platelet count may allow the patient to bleed internally, which could be critical or cause permanent damage to the body.

### What should you expect from cancer treatments?

The goal of a cancer treatment should be clear to the patient. Many patients receive adjunctive or preventive treatment with chemotherapy or hormonal medications (usually tamoxifen). The goal of treatment, therefore, is to eradicate the breast cancer. The intention is to improve the cure rate if possible. There is nothing specific to check except to look for the absence of symptoms or physical findings.

Women with metastatic cancer may have a more specific goal of treatment since there are symptoms that might be alleviated, x-ray findings or laboratory tests that could be measured, or even physical findings. Physicians hope to improve symptoms and lengthen survival, but cure is unlikely.

• • •

The patient also needs to understand the benefits and the potential ill-effects of the treatment. Common side effects of chemotherapy must be clearly outlined along with means of preventing or minimizing toxicities. The woman then may have specific questions about the drug therapy as it applies to her, its timing, and even its cost. She may also have questions about her activities, job, or exercise. Possible drug interactions should also be explained before chemotherapy or hormonal therapy is started. The oncologist may want to make use of literature designed for patients by the National Cancer Institute about breast cancer, chemotherapy programs, and specific drugs.

Although a woman may have a primary physician and/or surgeon caring for her before referral to a medical oncologist, the pattern of patient follow-up may be very different after that referral. The oncologist will make suggestions about the frequency of routine examinations, laboratory tests, and x-ray films. During the course of adjunctive chemotherapy the patient will be examined frequently by the medical oncologist. After preventive treatment, follow-up visits will be coordinated with all of her physicians. For the patient with metastatic disease, this pattern may be different, with the medical oncologist serving as a primary physician instead of her family physician or surgeon. The exact pattern of care is established by close communication between the woman and her doctors.

## The Oncology Nurse's Role in Caring for Breast Cancer Patients and Their Families
MARY ELLEN HAWF, R.N., O.C.N.

An oncology nurse is a professional registered nurse who is committed to providing optimal care to women diagnosed with breast cancer and their families. She is licensed in the state in which she practices and has completed educational training ranging from a diploma nursing program to a doctorate nursing program. He or she may also be certified in oncology nursing (O.C.N.), demonstrating a level of knowledge sufficient to perform the tasks necessary for competent practice. However, the level of education or degree should never be confused with one's level of competence. Frequently the oncology nurse has provided general nursing care prior to specializing in oncology. Much like physicians, nurses choose a particular area of expertise within the oncology field—surgery, gynecology, medicine, radiation, bone marrow transplantation, pediatrics, research, and hospice. The woman with breast cancer may encounter oncology nurses from several of these specialty areas throughout the course of her care.

Regardless of the nurse's specialty area, she must have extensive knowledge of the disease process, possible treatment modalities, and side effects of treatment and their management. She must also have a thorough understanding of the overall plan of care for each patient.

The nurse may be the woman's first contact when she arrives at the surgeon's office for consultation for a breast lump or for a breast biopsy. The woman is understandably anxious at this time, and the surgical oncology nurse can help alleviate this anxiety by explaining any planned procedures. After the consultation or biopsy, the nurse instructs the patient in care of the biopsy site or assists in coordinating additional tests such as mammography, ultrasonography, or surgery. Once pathology reports, surgical summaries, and x-ray/scan/laboratory reports are complete, more precise planning for definitive treatment will be recommended by the physician. Further discussion with the nurse regarding surgical options, expected recovery period, and postsurgical care is helpful for the woman and her family and permits them to freely express anxieties, fears, and concerns they may be experiencing during this difficult decision-making process. The surgical oncology nurse will focus on methods to minimize the impact of any subsequent surgery to facilitate a quick return to normal daily activity.

If radiation is recommended, the oncology nurse in the radiation oncology department will explain the plan of treatment (radiation therapy alone or in combination with other therapy), type of radiation therapy to be used, dates of treatment delivery, overall length of treatment, location of the planned radiation "field" on the body, types of markings used, possible side effects to expect, and testing to be done to monitor tolerance to the treatment (skin reaction, laboratory results, weight, etc.). The nurse will monitor the patient's skin daily for signs and symptoms of infection or skin breakdown, inquiring about the patient's level of comfort and her ability to manage the symptoms. Suggestions to help the patient maintain healthy skin and to promote comfort will be given as needed.

Referral to a medical oncologist might indicate the need for chemotherapy or hormonal therapy as a form of treatment. Once again, the oncology nurse will play a vital role. In-depth explanations of recommended drug therapy will be provided with ample opportunity before beginning therapy for the patient to ask questions and express concerns regarding expected side effects, scheduling of treatment, and anticipated lifestyle changes. Chemotherapy will be administered by a nurse who has been specifically trained to give chemotherapy drugs safely. This treatment may be given in an ambulatory care facility, hospital, the woman's home, or more frequently in the physician's office. The decision to administer treatment in one location or another is often determined by the intensity of the chemotherapy regimen prescribed, but it may also be determined by the physical surroundings and capabilities of the facility or insurance policy provider. The nurse, along with the physician, will monitor any toxicities and make recommendations or adjustments in the treatment regimen to safely administer therapy while still maintaining therapeutic efficacy.

The woman may encounter other oncology nurses who work within the hospital. Some hospitals have a designated floor or "unit" for oncology patients. The nurses who choose to work in these areas are specifically trained to care for patients with cancer and have the knowledge and experience to minister to their needs. This is not to say that the lack of such an oncology unit indicates less knowledgeable or trained personnel. But frequently a designated floor or unit allows for easier coordination of multiple services and more focused attention on the needs of the oncology patient. Women with breast cancer may be offered peripheral stem cell/bone marrow transplantation as a treatment option. The oncology nurse working on a unit where this treatment is given must possess additional intensive care nursing skills to accommodate the potentially acute needs of the person undergoing transplantation. (See Chapter 6 for more information on bone marrow transplantation.)

Oncology nurses working with a home care agency are available to meet the needs of the woman with breast cancer at various points in her therapy. Following surgery, assistance may be needed with dressing changes or drain care. Some chemotherapy regimens can be given at home instead of in the hospital or outpatient facility. Teaching the woman and/or her family members and loved ones the basics of self-care is invaluable to ensure that the necessary care can be safely provided in a home setting. Nurses may also make referrals to community agencies. If cancer is in the advanced stage, home health or hopice nurses are also available to meet the needs of the woman and her loved ones, assisting with long-term care issues, pain control, psychological support, and facilitating arrangements in the face of impending death.

Educating the woman and her family is a major responsibility of oncology nurses in all specialty areas. In addition to the details of a specific treatment modality, the oncology nurse will provide nutritional counseling with recommendations for follow-up care, including frequent physician examinations and breast examinations, as well as early detection methods recommended for the woman, her family, and caring others. Referrals to community agencies, prosthetic suppliers, support groups, and home care services are also initiated and coordinated by the oncology nurse.

In addition to providing "hands-on" care to these women, the oncology nurse frequently acts as the liaison between the physician and the woman with cancer. Women rely extensively on their nurses as a "sounding board" for their ideas, concerns, anger, grief, hopes, and fears. Given the predominance of females as nurses and males as physicians, a natural female bonding between patient and nurse frequently evolves. The nurse has the unique opportunity to become the patient's confidant.

Since multimodality therapy is commonplace in the treatment of breast cancer, coordination and timing of testing, surgery, treatment, and follow-up care can be quite a challenge for the woman. That challenge may be compounded by news that a newly diagnosed or recurrent breast cancer has been found, presenting a whole new set of decisions regarding treatment and care that needs to be made promptly. Although not intentional, it too frequently escapes the attention of medical professionals that this woman, regardless of her age, may also have a job that she enjoys (or financially needs), children that need car-pooling to and from school, an invalid spouse or relative dependent on her, or previously arranged engagements and commitments, to say nothing of the endless hopes and dreams she has for the rest of her life. The oncology nurse is uniquely aware of all of these pressures, and it is her responsibility to help coordinate a plan of treatment and care that is medically as well as emotionally therapeutic and accommodates a woman's needs and eases some of her tensions.

The role of the oncology nurse is a particularly rewarding one that enables her to establish lasting bonds with cancer patients that help these women cope with their disease and the problems it imposes. These women share with oncology nurses their joys and hopes, their idiosyncrasies, their family pictures and stories, their tears of sadness, as well as their tears of joy.

## The Plastic Surgeon's Role in the Rehabilitation of a Woman With Breast Cancer
JOHN BOSTWICK III, M.D.

Plastic surgeons treat patients with a wide range of problems and deformities. They perform aesthetic surgical procedures to counteract the effects of the aging process and reconstructive procedures to repair major body defects such as deformities resulting from birth defects, injuries and scars caused by accidents (including hand injuries and burns), and deformities resulting from cancer treatment.

Breast surgery is a major part of many plastic surgeons' practices. Women consult plastic surgeons for aesthetic breast operations to enlarge, reduce, or elevate their breasts and for reconstructive breast surgery to replace their missing breasts and nipple-areolae after mastectomy or reconstructing the defects after breast-conserving surgery. Recent developments in the field combined with the skills acquired from treating aesthetic breast problems enable plastic surgeons to create aesthetic breast reconstructions for patients with all types of mastectomy deformities.

A woman is referred to a plastic surgeon when she is interested in the option of reconstructive breast surgery either to replace a missing breast or to fill in a defect or correct an asymmetry after lumpectomy or quadrantectomy. This referral is often made by the general surgeon before the cancer operation. It also may be made by her family physician or by another member of the breast management team, of which the plastic surgeon is a member. Many women also come to the plastic surgeon after referral by other women who have been treated by him for similar problems.

When a woman consults with a plastic surgeon about breast reconstruction, he must consider her psychological state, the stage of her disease, and her need for additional therapy. Management of her tumor is a primary concern, and he will confer with the general surgeon and other members of the team to determine the best care for each woman and the best timing for reconstruction. Today, with the possibility of skin-sparing mastectomy, immediate breast reconstruction is becoming an option frequently selected by women desiring to avoid permanent breast loss and to achieve the most aesthetic reconstructive result. When immediate reconstruction is planned, the plastic surgeon works closely with the general surgeon to coordinate the mastectomy and reconstructive procedures.

The plastic surgeon is also aware of the ongoing concerns that a woman has about her cancer and must deal with her in a humane and sensitive fashion. A woman who is considering breast reconstruction has had to cope with the reality of breast cancer as well as that of partial or total breast loss. The emotional trauma that she has experienced should never be overlooked by the plastic surgeon in his dealings with her. He needs to provide support and understanding for the special problems and fears that she, as a cancer patient, is confronting.

The plastic surgeon also must be aware of some of the conflicts faced by the woman who inquires about reconstructive breast surgery. Although a woman may want to have her breast restored, she also may fear that reconstructive surgery will cause a recurrence of her cancer. The plastic surgeon needs to be sensitive to this fear and discuss it with his prospective patient. She also may worry that this elective surgery will be misconstrued as mere vanity on her part. The plastic surgeon's role is to reassure her that breast reconstruction is not merely a cosmetic procedure but a beneficial part of her total rehabilitation program.

The plastic surgeon's role in counseling patients is especially important. Today, this interaction often takes place before the mastectomy or lumpectomy. Consultations should be conducted in a private, quiet atmosphere to enable a woman to feel comfortable and free to speak frankly.

As a counselor, one of the plastic surgeon's chief obligations is to be a good listener as well as a teacher. If he does all of the talking, he will never really know what the woman's expectations are for treatment. He should ask open-ended questions that allow her to communicate her feelings and desires. He must understand what a woman expects so that he can plan an operation that most nearly produces her desired result. If her expectations cannot be met, he needs to explain the limitations of what surgery can accomplish.

The patient's medical history and the status and treatment of her breast cancer provide the plastic surgeon with important information in formulating a plan for breast reconstruction. He also will perform a physical examination to assess the options for reconstruction. These options will then be discussed with the woman, covering such topics as the pros and cons, expected results, anticipated hospital stay and recovery period, and risks of each approach. If a woman chooses an implant or expander reconstruction, this explanation will also include a full description of these devices and any problems or complications associated with them. In addition, the patient will be given an informed consent document that comprehensively describes the pros and cons of these devices and operations. The patient should read those documents and understand them before she signs them and agrees to this operation. Breast reconstruction is a very personal procedure, and the woman should understand that no one surgical technique is appropriate for all patients. She should be fully advised of all options. After these explanations, the plastic surgeon can formulate an operative plan that attempts to incorporate the patient's desires and expectations and is designed with her specific needs in mind. He should not assume, however, that a woman will naturally understand the details of her proposed surgery and should carefully review this plan with her.

The actual breast reconstruction is carried out by the plastic surgeon according to the preoperative plan that he and the patient have discussed and agreed on. After reconstruction, the woman returns to the plastic surgeon for periodic evaluations. On follow-up visits the plastic surgeon will continue to encourage his patient and to contribute to her rehabilitation from breast cancer.

## The Plastic Surgery Nurse's Role in Counseling and Caring for the Breast Reconstruction Patient

LYNNE A. McCAIN, B.S.N., R.N.

Plastic surgery nurses provide a variety of services for the woman undergoing breast reconstruction. Educating patients about their reconstructive options is an important part of the nurse's role. Nurses serve as a valuable resource for women, answering their questions and addressing their concerns. Once a reconstructive approach has been selected by the patient and the plastic surgeon, the nurse provides specific information on the details of the procedure and follow-up care.

In an educational session with the patient and her family the nurse provides information about tests to be taken, anticipated treatments, medicines that are safe to take and those to be avoided, blood donation requirements, diet and exercise recommendations before and after surgery, possible complications from surgery, expected pain and recovery, effect of smoking on healing, and clothing needed after surgery.

The nurse can show diagrams of the procedure followed by photographs depicting the before and after views of women who have had similar reconstructive procedures. Many women request the opportunity to speak with other patients who have had breast reconstruction performed by the plastic surgeon. These names are provided so that she may contact women who have already had the procedure that she is going to have. By talking to other reconstruction patients the woman will hear about the experiences of these other individuals and gain personal insights. Although pictures and diagrams are an important tool in educating patients about the different reconstructive techniques, nothing compares with the personal experience of speaking with another woman who has been there. It enables the woman contemplating breast reconstruction to realistically learn what to expect from this operation. It also gives her access to a networking system to share fears and worries and joys. Often women who have had reconstruction are willing to have a "show-and-tell" session with the new patient so that she may visualize and touch a reconstructed breast.

Before the patient meets with the physician, it is helpful to jot down questions on these subjects and others to ensure that nothing of importance is overlooked. Many patients have also found it helpful to write down the answers to their questions or to tape record their sessions with their physician and nurse so that this information is available for ready reference.

The nurse can also discuss insurance provider coverage with the patient. Seventeen states currently have laws mandating insurance coverage for breast reconstruction and for any surgery required for symmetry of the opposite breast. Most insurance providers will not cover surgery for the opposite breast, and the woman should be informed that she will be responsible for these expenses unless she resides in one of these states.

During the educational session the nurse may provide input about what clothing to pack to wear home from the hospital and what works best during the first few weeks after surgery. Many women who have had reconstructive surgery mention the importance of "loose, baggy" clothing. All agree that "the best" clothes are those that button down the front. These disguise the drains and dressings in the early postoperative phase.

During the reconstructive experience women encounter plastic surgery nurses from different specialties ranging from operating room and recovery room nurses to hospital and office based nurses. All contribute to the care and recovery of these women. The operating room nurses are probably the least familiar to the patient since preoperative medications may have been administered before the patient's encounter with these nurses in the operating room. These nurses are attired in hospital scrubs, caps, and masks; they greet the patient, introduce her to the operating room staff, and try to comfort her, often by tucking the woman in with warm blankets, holding her hand until the anesthesia has taken its effect, and answering questions or calming fears. Once the patient is under general anesthesia these highly skilled nurses provide assistance to the plastic surgeon, ensuring that all the surgical instruments are available and that the operation proceeds smoothly.

When the surgery is completed, the patient is transferred to the recovery room where the next team of specialty nurses assumes care of the patient. These recovery room nurses monitor the patient's vital signs, provide pain relief, and reassure the patient that all is well. The recovery room stay may last 1 to 2 hours, depending on the patient's ability to recuperate from the effects of the anesthesia. The nursing staff releases the patient once she is alert, awake, and oriented. Both the operating room and the recovery room nurses are the silent caregivers who provide invaluable assistance to ensure that the operation proceeds smoothly.

The last specialty nurse that the patient encounters during her hospitalization is the bedside nurse. This skilled professional cares for the patient during her time in the hospital and prepares her for discharge by teaching her how to monitor the surgical site(s), how to change dressings, how to empty a surgical drain, how to take prescribed medications, and what restrictions on physical activity are necessary until recovery is complete. These nurses provide teaching sessions throughout the patient's hospital stay to help facilitate her recuperation. In addition to these verbal instructions, the nurse also provides the patient with written instructions that restate the "how to" of home care and recovery.

Nurses are readily available and attentive to the patient 24 hours a day during the patient's hospitalization and are often the first to detect problems that may arise. These nurses are trained to detect even the subtle changes in vital signs, in the surgical site, or in urine output and to respond to these changes before they become problems. The nurse will alert the plastic surgeon to changes and implement necessary alterations in the care plan that are needed to ensure optimal care of the patient to facilitate a speedy recovery.

Nurses who care for breast cancer and breast reconstruction patients are in a unique position to serve as educators, confidants, and support personnel for these women. All of these nurses and the office-based nurses respond to the patient's physical and emotional needs. Nurses are attuned to the possible psychological responses their patients may have and are prepared to help the woman adjust. They recognize that the reconstructive process is not necessarily complete when the incisions are healed. Breast reconstruction after a mastectomy or lumpectomy begins a process of emotional healing. Losing a breast after mastectomy is an emotionally devastating experience. The patient finds herself overwhelmed by emotions ranging from anger, depression, isolation, sadness, and finally acceptance. Women newly diagnosed with breast cancer need to be aware that while the body may be physically healed enough to resume normal activities, the spirit or emotional self takes much longer. Often women say that in retrospect, they feel it takes nearly a full year to adjust to the emotional jolt of being diagnosed with breast cancer and the changes the body has undergone from chemotherapy, radiation, cancer surgery, and reconstructive surgery. Nurses are often the ones that women turn to for comfort as they try to cope. Many patients feel that they can open up to the nurse more readily because she has helped other women through the same experience and has worked closely with the woman through the reconstructive process.

Some plastic surgery nurses have become involved in organizing support groups for women undergoing breast reconstruction. These groups are often led by a nurse or social worker and they help women to educate themselves about what to expect from reconstructive surgery, to share feelings, and to know that they are not alone in this experience. During the meetings women discuss issues of self-image, the impact that mastectomy and reconstruction has on sexuality and body image, dating and relationship concerns for the single woman, and other personal concerns that they are hesitant to share with others who have not gone through the same experience. If available, women undergoing breast reconstruction are often encouraged to attend these meetings because they provide an accepting, supportive environment and a forum for sharing common experiences during the reconstructive process. The following poem, adapted from 1 Corinthians 15:44, is an example of the uplifting message and positive reinforcement often provided to women through these groups and through the support of nurses:

**What Cancer Can't Do**

Cancer is so limited
It cannot cripple love,
It cannot shatter hope,
It cannot corrode faith,
It cannot eat away peace,
It cannot destroy confidence,
It cannot kill friendship,
It cannot shut out memories,
It cannot silence courage,
It cannot invade the soul,
It cannot reduce eternal life,
It cannot quench the Spirit,
It cannot lessen the power of the resurrection.
Our greatest enemy is not disease,
     but despair.

Plastic surgery nurses are a major source of support to the woman undergoing breast reconstruction. They serve as educators, counselors, and caregivers, ministering to the physical and emotional needs of these women.

 *The Team Effort*

Many specialists are involved in the care of the woman with breast cancer. Most likely she has known her primary care doctors for years. She feels comfortable with them and trusts their judgment. Others, however, are specialists she sees for the first time on referral for treatment of her life-threatening illness. The thought of seeing strange doctors is often intimidating to an already stressed woman. Knowledge of what these doctors do and the positive benefit they can provide for the woman with breast cancer might alleviate some of her fears and help her to feel more in control of her own destiny so that she can regard herself as a participating member of the team rather than a passive recipient of care. In addition, knowledge of the support that nurses can provide throughout this ordeal may help in this coping process. This chapter has been designed to provide this information for women and to demonstrate how the team functions at its best and how individual doctors and nurses, regardless of specialty, can deal with their patients with caring and sensitivity.

# COMMUNICATING WITH YOUR DOCTORS

In society we place so much emphasis on "communication" that it is surprising that the doctor-patient relationship is so often marked by frustration and inability to convey thoughts and feelings effectively. This setting may be the stage for acting out the most significant of life's dramas yet communication is often halting and bewildering. When a woman develops breast cancer, the difficulties in communicating become magnified by the seriousness of the disease itself. Breast cancer attacks a woman's life as well as her femininity; that makes it a powerful silencer. Silence, however, is no solution and women need to be able to relate to their doctors about their health care concerns so that they can make reasonable, educated decisions.

Obviously communication problems are more easily confronted on paper than they are in real life. They are sufficiently important, however, to merit attention and active problem solving. In the previous chapter we explained ways in which specific doctors can help you and listed some of the questions that you might want to ask them. That is only half of the equation. No matter how frightened or intimidated a woman may be by the specter of her disease, she must bring something to the communication process for it to succeed. With that in mind, this chapter attempts to provide women with concrete suggestions for evaluating and selecting their doctors and with skills to facilitate the communication process. The goal is to ensure that women get the information that will empower them to cope with the decisions they have to make and the therapy they must undergo. As most women have emphasized in our surveys and interviews, the worst part of breast cancer is the feeling of loss of control and helplessness. The goal of this chapter is to enable a woman to reclaim some of that control.

First let's examine what you as a patient need from the doctor-patient relationship. Those needs are as various as the women who will be reading this book. Some women want the facts presented honestly and in as much detail as possible. They want to know what they have to deal with and then get on with it. Others need a softer, gentler approach, the diagnosis and prognosis presented in a *Reader's Digest* format, softened and accompanied by the appropriate handholding and solicitude. Still others don't want to hear what they term the "gory details" and prefer to trust their doctors to do "what is best for them." Obviously these are stereotypes, and many of us will find ourselves somewhere in between. None of these approaches is to be condemned as inappropriate, but it is beneficial for each woman to understand what her expectations of her doctors are and how much information she really wants. Only then can she establish a satisfactory doctor-patient relationship.

Once you have addressed these needs, some basic questions and considerations will help you select a doctor who will meet your expectations. Even though managed care may limit the pool of doctors a woman may choose from, she should always be aware that it does not eliminate choice.

## QUALIFICATIONS AND COMPETENCE
### What are your doctor's qualifications and training?

A woman has an obligation to herself to check her doctor out, to find out about his training and credentials, to ask for referrals, and to determine whether this is an area in which this physician has expertise. Information about a doctor's training is readily obtainable in the reference room of your local library in a book entitled *The Directory of Medical Specialists,* which lists only board-certified specialists (see Chapter 12). Board certification is an important credential. It means that after training and an initial period of practice, a doctor has passed a competence test showing that he meets the criteria for practice in the specialty. This book will list the doctor's year of birth, medical school, the year he was licensed to practice, the year of specialty certification, primary and secondary specialties, and type of practice. Other information on training and hospital and medical affiliations also is included. Doctors are listed geographically, making it easy to locate names of doctors in each community. The *American Medical*

*Directory* is another helpful reference, but unlike *The Directory of Medical Specialists,* it does not indicate whether a physician is board certified.

### Is your doctor on staff at a medical school–affiliated hospital? Does he have a teaching appointment with that hospital?

Association with a medical school suggests access to the latest techniques, technology, and developments in the field; knowledge of or participation in research efforts; and involvement in the education of residents. Breast cancer is a complex and life-threatening disease; you deserve the best care possible.

### What professional associations and societies does this doctor belong to?

He should belong to one or more professional societies, indicating that he has a specific interest in his specialty area and that he has access to the latest developments in his specialty.

### Does this physician specialize in breast cancer treatment?

It is not enough to just be a good doctor, the physician you choose, whatever his specialty, should have special expertise in treating breast cancer patients. You need to inquire what portion of his practice is devoted to treating breast cancer. How many breast cancer patients does he see in a year? How many has he treated this year? Last year? If you are consulting with a general surgeon, he should have experience with a variety of surgical techniques for treating breast cancer. You should ask if he performs lumpectomies and modified radical mastectomies and approximately how many of each in a typical year. You want a doctor who has the versatility to provide you with options for care. The same applies to a medical oncologist, radiation oncologist, or plastic surgeon. (More information on selecting a plastic surgeon is included in Chapter 12.)

You should also inquire whether the physician is a member of a breast management team. Comprehensive, coordinated treatment is provided by such a team effort. Members of a team are experienced in working with each other and pool their efforts to consult on your problems, to devise treatment plans that are individualized, and to ease some of the trauma involved in having to see various specialists. This team approach is common at major medical centers and will ensure that your doctors will have access to state-of-the-art technology and have the skills to use it. Ask what specialists are included on the team. At a minimum an effective team has a general surgeon, diagnostic radiologist/breast imager, pathologist, medical oncologist, radiation oncologist, and plastic surgeon.

## REPUTATION

### *What is this doctor's reputation within the medical community?*

Do you know any of his patients? Ask them about their level of satisfaction with this doctor's care. Patient referrals are an excellent way to find out about a doctor. Also, ask other physicians that you know and respect for their recommendations and their opinions of this particular physician. The local medical society will have a list of recommended physicians in your area, as will the specialty society for which he is board certified. Check all of these sources.

## PERSONALITY AND PROFESSIONAL MANNER

A doctor's presence and style may not be the most important consideration for some patients, but certain characteristics are basic to a sound doctor-patient relationship.

### *Is he courteous?*

Courteous treatment is a minimum standard of care that all patients have a right to expect.

### *Is he pleasant when he talks to you or examines you?*

Has he taken the time and effort to learn something about you? Does he make an honest effort to relate to you? Not all doctors can be "Mr. Personality," but it is important for a patient to feel that her doctor is humane and caring; this makes it easier for her to cope with her disease. After all, as one of the women we interviewed explained, "When a woman develops breast cancer, she goes steady with her doctors. She doesn't have to love them, but it is important that she like them because she is going to be spending a lot of time with them." How well you relate to your doctor has a bearing on your treatment program and how you respond. Therefore it is important that he has your respect and regards you as a person, not just a patient.

*Does he respect your sense of privacy and modesty?*

Obviously there will be times when your privacy will be invaded; physical examinations and preoperative and postoperative photographs are two cases in point. At those times it is difficult not to feel uncomfortable. But your physician can avoid creating situations that lead to an invasion of privacy and place you at a disadvantage. One such situation is when a doctor tells his patient her prognosis or explains her proposed treatment plan when she is still undressed in his examining room. No woman can think clearly when she is struggling to keep herself covered with a flimsy sheet or gown.

*Is he sensitive to your feelings? Does he allow you to express your emotions? Does he make light of your worries?*

No matter how insignificant your concerns may seem to someone else, they are important to you and your doctor should never downplay your feelings as trivial. Your emotions warrant similar consideration. Breast cancer is an emotional disease; at times women need to cry, to vent the feelings that tend to surface suddenly and sometimes unexpectedly. It is important to have a doctor who doesn't suppress or discourage these expressions of feelings. (It is also nice if he has a box of Kleenex conveniently located for those moments.)

## ADDITIONAL QUESTIONS

*Is he prompt or does he keep you waiting without an explanation? Is he tactful and diplomatic? Does he treat you like an adult? Does he address you by your first name, even though you have just been introduced? Does he seem brusque and hurried? Does he give you his undivided attention during your appointments? Does he refrain from taking phone calls during your examination and conference?*

Unfortunately, far too many physicians lack good bedside manners and are woefully unaware of this deficiency. Many of the women in our surveys complained about their doctors keeping them waiting, sometimes for hours, with no explanation and no apologies. Then when the doctor appeared, it was "business as usual" with no wasted time. Some even informed their patients that they were running behind "so let's get this over with." In response to just such a comment one women humorously wrote, "If he was in such a hurry, why couldn't he manage to get his butt in to see me 2 hours earlier when my appointment was scheduled?" Taking telephone calls from other patients during their consultations was another source of displeasure and frustration. Not only is this inconsiderate to the patient sitting in the doctor's office, but it is also a violation of privacy for the woman on the phone who thinks she is having a confidential conversation with her doctor.

Although the telephone provides an effective means of contact and communication between doctor and patient, it can be abused. Our surveys provided ample examples of this abuse, but two cited by Mimi Greenberg in her book *Invisible Scars* merit repeating. One concerns the gynecologist who invited the patient into his office, informed her that she had breast cancer, and before she could respond asked her to step into the waiting room while he answered a call. The other, and one we have heard frequently repeated in various versions, concerns the surgeon who telephoned the patient regarding her breast biopsy results. He cheerfully began, "I have good news and bad news. The bad news is you have breast cancer. The good news is yours is the best kind to get." Unless the patient is from out of town and a personal visit to the doctor would be an inconvenience, most women would appreciate and deserve the courtesy of receiving this highly charged, sensitive information in person.

• • •

There is a lesson to be learned from these vignettes. A diagnosis of breast cancer deserves and demands your doctor's full and undivided attention—in person (when possible) and without interruption. No patient should ever have to settle for anything less.

## COMMUNICATION SKILLS

### Are his explanations understandable?

Does he confuse you with medical jargon that you cannot understand? Are his explanations filled with statistics? Does he explain how these numbers actually relate to your prognosis?

### Does he take the time to inform you of all of your options?

A patient should demand to know her alternatives. It is unwise to make a decision based on partial information. That limits your alternatives right from the start. Learning all you can about your disease and the options means you can control the way your illness is handled.

*Does he ask you if you have any questions? Does he answer your questions to your satisfaction or just gloss over them?*

Frequently, particularly in an emotionally charged situation, a patient will not hear everything the doctor tells her during the first explanation. It is important to have a doctor who will take the time to repeat himself and to review his comments until the patient feels that she has a good grasp of what he is trying to tell her.

*Is he offended if you inquire about a second opinion?*

Second opinions are common in modern medical practice. Many insurance carriers insist on them before authorizing payment. A second opinion is an intelligent way to investigate options thoroughly. It is not meant as an insult. A doctor who implies that you are disloyal or says that he won't treat you if you get a second opinion is doing his patient a disservice.

*Is he honest with you?*

Your physician cannot always say what you want to hear, but you should expect honesty. He should tell you the truth and not circumvent the issue. A physician cannot promise a cure. What he can do, however, is bring honesty, integrity, and skill to bear on the problem. In all of our surveys with patients a perceived lack of honesty on the part of the doctor was judged to be the most damaging to the patient's well-being and was the main reason why many women said that they changed doctors. Fear of the unknown is far worse than fear of the worst known.

*Does your doctor respect your confidentiality?*

A patient has a right to expect confidentiality from her physician. It is her health problem, and no one else should be informed of it unless she agrees that this information can be divulged.

*Does he listen to you?*

Some of the most satisfied patients we have heard from are those who describe their doctors as good listeners. As one woman explained to us, "The best way a doctor can make you feel important is just to listen to you. Sometimes I just need to vent some of my frustrations or fears. I don't want someone to lecture to me; I just want someone to hear me. My doctor is very quiet, but he looks at me when I talk to him, he smiles and nods at the appropriate moments, and he makes me feel that he cares about me and about what I am saying. That makes all the difference to me; it also makes me more receptive to what he needs to tell me."

## ACCESSIBILITY

*How accessible is your doctor?*

Is it difficult to get in to see him or can you arrange appointments with relative ease? Does he have regular and convenient office hours. Is he genuinely interested in having you as a patient or do you have the feeling that he is overbooked and too busy to see you? Is his office within reasonable travel distance?

*Does he return your phone calls promptly? The same day? Does he set aside enough time for you to ask questions at the end of each visit?*

Does he encourage you to ask questions? Does he seem rushed when he is with you? Does he sit down to talk to you and establish eye contact or do you get the impression that he is in a hurry to get to his next patient? It is important to feel that your doctor is willing to invest the time that you need.

*When you have problems, is your doctor willing to accommodate you, to fit you into his schedule?*

It isn't reasonable to expect your doctor to spend hours with you every time you have an appointment, but if you need more time and you ask for it, your physician should be able to schedule it.

A woman should check to see if her doctor has designated someone in his office to assist patients when he is not available and should make an effort to meet this individual and talk with him or her.

• • •

The following list summarizes some of the fundamentals that you should look for and expect in your doctors:

- He should be willing to answer your questions.
- He should explain what you do not understand.
- He should spend a reasonable amount of time with you when you need it.
- He should treat you as an adult.
- He should not suppress your expressions of emotion.

- He should not discourage a second opinion.
- He should respect your confidentiality.
- He should always be honest with you.
- He should be sensitive to your feelings.
- He should treat you as a person as well as a patient.

Basically, you are looking for a doctor who is competent, caring, and informative. In turn, you as a patient also must bring something to this interaction. What can you do to facilitate communication? What is your responsibility?

## THE PATIENT'S RESPONSIBILITIES*

MIMI GREENBERG, Ph.D.

Let's take a look at the patient's responsibilities in the doctor-patient relationship. Following are some suggestions to help you improve the quality of this interaction:

Be prompt. If you want/expect your doctor to respect your time commitments, you must be willing to respect his.

Try not to cancel. Apart from the fact that cancellations, especially at the last minute, are usually annoying because they leave a big hole in the doctor's appointment schedule (and are not likely to increase your popularity with the nurses, technicians, and office staff), you may also wind up sabotaging your own treatment. Certain procedures are on timed schedules or doses (chemotherapy, radiation, and some surgical procedures), and you may be compromising your own prognosis and health. A good rule of thumb is this—don't cancel unless you are too sick to crawl out of bed. And frankly, if you are that sick, you need to be seen.

If you have several questions or wish extra time to speak with your doctor, tell the front desk when you set up the appointment. You will be given a time that is mutually convenient for both of you. Don't wait until the day of your appointment to request extra time. In all probability you won't get it because the schedule will be full. You will be disappointed and feel unnecessarily rejected.

Write down your questions ahead of time rather than trying to retrieve them from memory while you are talking with the doctor. If you don't, it's a cinch that you will forget them and then remember just as soon as you leave the doctor's office.

*Reprinted with permission from Greenberg M. Invisible Scars: A Guide to Coping With the Emotional Impact of Breast Cancer. New York: Walker & Co., 1988.

Take notes and write down the answers to your questions. This will save you many anxious hours and sleepless nights of wondering whether you are accurately remembering what was said.

Be direct in your communications. If you have a request, a problem, or a complaint, let your doctor know so that it can be resolved right away. Most physicians value your feedback and are genuinely interested in improving their services and meeting their patients' needs, but you have to let them know. Unfortunately, many of us insist on playing the role of the perfect patient who never complains and is always nice. This is not to suggest that you become nasty, but if you are unhappy with your doctor, his staff, the treatment, and/or anything else that is breast cancer related, you owe it to yourself and your emotional well-being to make your concerns heard.

Follow the doctor's instructions. Don't improvise. If the instructions seem unreasonable, check to make sure you understood them correctly and discuss the possibility of modification or change. For example, if you are told not to drive for 2 weeks following breast surgery and axillary node dissection but you feel up to driving within a week, get the medical okay before you take matters into your own hands. Without it you may be compromising your treatment and cosmetic results as well as irritating the doctor, who may see you as a difficult patient.

A difficult patient is one who creates unnecessary problems that complicate treatment and/or recovery and are time consuming to the physician and staff. Please be reassured that one misunderstanding will not earn you the reputation of being a difficult patient. But certainly habitual and chronic disregard for instructions will. For instance, if your doctor tells you it will take 6 to 8 weeks before you can safely return to work, it is pointless to call his office every few days to report that you feel fine and wonder if he has changed his mind. Why not use the time constructively to give yourself a special treat—like going to museums, art galleries, concerts, or catching up on your reading or movies you have missed? Physicians call it "patient compliance" and patients call it "following doctor's orders." One reason some women find it a problem is that they tend to feel so controlled by their doctors and/or breast cancer that they grasp (sometimes mistakenly) for any little bit of power that will prove to them and their doctors that they are not helpless. Rushing back to work and driving prematurely are two cases in point.

Be businesslike with your bill payments and with your health insurance refunds. If your company mistakenly sends the reimbursement check to you instead of your physician, present the check immediately to your doctor's office. Also, unless you have been advised to the contrary, you are expected to pay for whatever your insurance does not cover.

Your doctor is only human. Avoid placing him on a pedestal. Once there, the only place to go is down . . . and with a thud! The main problem with idealizing your doctor is that he cannot possibly live up to your expectations and fantasies. Once the bubble bursts, you are apt to feel disappointed, angry, and anxious to switch physicians. And if you do switch, you are likely to repeat the same pattern all over again.

Even in the best doctor-patient relationships there are awkward, embarrassing, and comical situations. One such awkward situation is the fear/belief that your doctor has made a mistake or isn't giving you the right treatment. This is a universal fear that each of us experiences at some point. This is not the initial reaction of "Not me . . . there must be some mistake." This is the wave of panic that washes over you at the moment you decide a serious and irreversible error has been made. When these panicky thoughts hit you, ask yourself two questions: (1) Why am I having these thoughts now? Usually you are upset at something or someone else, and without realizing it you seize the most convenient target. (2) What can I do to alleviate my panic? If you are certain you are not upset with someone else and are not transferring your feelings to your doctor or your treatment, then the healthiest and smartest course of action is to present your concerns to the doctor. This will give both of you a chance to examine the reality of the situation. There is no point in keeping your fears to yourself because it will only upset you and cause distance and mistrust in the doctor-patient relationship.

There is also no point in seeking a second opinion without first discussing the problem with the doctor who is treating you. Why? Because doctor No. 2 will need your records from doctor No. 1 to intelligently assess your diagnosis and treatment. In other words, doctor No. 1 is going to find out anyway, so why not give him the courtesy of finding out from you.

How does this affect the relationship? Most competent doctors will not try to talk you out of a second opinion. This is not to say that they love it, either. They don't. It's a big red flag that something is wrong in the relationship. Sometimes it isn't treatment competency at all, but rather the doctor's availability or bedside manner or a communication breakdown that is at the root of the problem.

In any case, you are not the first patient to feel that your doctor has made an error (or that you just feel more secure with another opinion), nor will you be the last. Doctors expect it. It comes with the territory. So take a deep breath, talk to doctor No. 1, and then for your own peace of mind talk to doctor No. 2 as well. You will sleep better for it. And if it turns out that it was all in your imagination, you needn't feel bad. . . .

## BUILDING A RELATIONSHIP

Much of what you feel about your disease depends on the kind of relationship you have with your doctors and their attitudes toward treatment and toward you. It is important to approach this relationship with realistic expectations and with a commitment to be an active partner with your doctors in your own care. Just as you will experience bad days, doctors will also, and they are as individual and various in their personalities as the patients that they minister to. Therefore it is important to keep in mind that your doctors will have off days. Furthermore, not all are good communicators. Some are quieter than others; some tend to overwhelm you with information; others only offer it if they are prompted. The patient has to bring something to the communication process. You have to help your doctors understand what you need. If your doctor is one of the reticent ones and you feel he is the doctor for you, then it is your responsibility to ask the questions and probe for information. If you don't know what to say, if you are stunned or upset by his diagnosis or plans for treatment, it is your responsibility to say so. It is okay to ask to have someone accompany you to your appointments if you want someone else to listen to what the doctor has to say as a backup. You may also want to take a list of questions with you for your visit so you don't waste time trying to remember what you wanted to ask. Some people suggest taking a tape recorder to the doctor's appointment to record what is said. Personally, we feel this would tend to create an artificial barrier between the patient and her doctor. And, considering the litigious environment we live in, it may even make your doctor hesitate to speak openly with you. Let your doctor know if you need more help and information. Ask for information on support groups and names of other patients with similar problems that you can talk to. One woman we talked to felt her doctor didn't spend enough time with her. She described him as "a butterfly, flitting in and out of the room before I had time to ask him what I wanted." Her solution was a simple one. During one appointment she placed her arm on his as he was exiting the room and asked if he could please sit down, slow down, and give her some more time. Surprisingly, he hadn't realized how rushed he had seemed. His response was to smile, sit down, and talk to her. From then on their relationship improved. The point is this relationship is one worth working on.

In the years that we have been interviewing women on this topic we have seen attitudes change. Women have become more assertive about their own health care needs, less passive and accepting, and more consumer oriented. This new attitude puts them more in control and positively contributes to their ability to cope with their treatment. They are demanding that their doctors consider the psychological as well as the physical aspects of their disease. They are asking questions and expecting answers. When they don't get them and they don't feel comfortable with their doctors, they are making the necessary changes. Sometimes this means changing doctors; other times it means concentrating their efforts to salvage and improve the situation. Similar to a marriage, the doctor-patient relationship requires mutual participation; it is an active partnership in which both members contribute and ultimately benefit.

# 9

# WHY WOMEN SEEK BREAST RECONSTRUCTION

*I was planting seedlings one day and my prosthesis fell out
while I was bending over. Crying, I picked it up out of the muddy
water. I called a plastic surgeon that same day.*

*I ached to once again be able to put on a beautiful
nightgown and fill it all out. I wanted to shop for pretty things
and feel feminine and sexy again.*

*My breast was an essential part of my femaleness (not femininity)
and I wanted to be breasted.*

*I began to feel good about life again. I decided that I was going to live
and beat cancer. I wanted to look as good as I felt.*

*I was only 17, an oddity for breast cancer patients. I had
a long life to live, and I wanted to live it whole.*

This chapter opens with just five of the many different responses that we received when we surveyed and interviewed women who had undergone breast reconstruction. Their motives for seeking reconstructive surgery were diverse, but all were touching manifestations of the sense of personal loss that these women had experienced after their mastectomies. For some women, the mastectomy was an experience that left them feeling "ugly" and "lopsided." Reconstruction therefore represented a means of regaining beauty and wholeness—harmony of body. For these women, femininity was a core issue, and they felt that their "mastectomy appearance" deprived them of feeling fully female. They loathed the very sight of their bodies and found the simple act of bathing to be repugnant. The mirror had become a fearsome presence in their homes. Furthermore, they avoided any situation in which they might have to disrobe in front of others— dressing rooms, locker rooms, the beach. For a good number of these women, dressing and undressing had become a strictly private act, conducted in closed bedrooms, closets, or bathrooms, until they had their breasts rebuilt and no longer felt the need to hide their bodies.

As one woman explained, "I am again a woman in my own mind. I don't look down anymore and cringe. I just know that something is there, and it has changed my whole life." Clearly, an improved self-image was one of the chief reasons for desiring breast reconstruction expressed by all of the women we surveyed. This elective plastic surgery allowed them to feel more relaxed and more positive about the future.

Relatively few of the women in our survey sought breast reconstruction because it would improve the quality of their sex lives or help to save their marriages or relationships. Motivation for reconstructive surgery was usually self-inspired. Breast reconstruction, however, often had a positive impact on a woman's ability to contribute to and feel good in a relationship. By making her feel better about herself this operation allowed the woman to relate to others, especially loved ones, with increased confidence and self-assurance.

Many women did allude to their children as a powerful motivating factor. Young women, in particular, worried that their small children would be frightened by their scarred chests, would ask uncomfortable questions, or would fear for themselves. They did not want their children to see them "deformed." They also wanted to set an example for their daughters if they, too, must face breast cancer one day—to give them hope for restitution. Other older women said they had breast reconstruction to encourage their daughters to consider the same option. As one woman explained, "My daughter had breast cancer at the age of 28. She and I had our breasts removed the same year, and I thought that if I had reconstruction she would follow."

A family history of breast cancer also figured into a woman's decision for breast reconstruction. It was sobering to see how many of the women who answered our surveys had mothers, sisters, grandmothers, and aunts who had breast cancer. They had witnessed their loved ones' struggles firsthand. They sought to avoid some of the traumas that their relatives had experienced. As one woman related, "I grew up seeing my mother with a radical mastectomy on one side and a modified on the other; I saw her struggle getting clothes so that she would look 'normal.' I did not want to spend the rest of my life going through the same thing that she did." Other women referred to the positive reconstructive experiences of close relatives. One woman's identical twin had breast reconstruction, and she laughingly related that "she needed reconstruction also to maintain the symmetry. After all, if she remained breastless, they would no longer be identical." For these women, reconstruction represented a positive way to confront their heritage.

The search for restitution and return to wholeness was a strong motivating factor for all of the women we interviewed, and this reason also pervaded the answers to our questionnaire. Even when the results of reconstruction were not perfect, the woman's dissatisfaction seemed to be minimal because the breast was now a part of her body and could again be incorporated into her self-image. As one woman said, "The reconstruction is not like a normal breast; there are some problems. It is too hard and it shifts around, but I wouldn't go back to the way I was for anything. I love my new breast, hardness and all. I am not embarrassed to undress in front of someone now. I don't feel like a freak anymore. I feel like a sexual person again. I am whole again."

Elimination of the need for an external prosthesis was another important reason why many women elected to have reconstructive surgery. Women seemed to feel constantly aware of the presence of a false breast, worrying that it would become dislodged and the lopsided chest would be exposed. In their attempts to hide their deformity some women even resorted to using surgical tape to solidly fix their false breasts to their chests.

Other women who were large-breasted objected to the size and weight of the prosthesis necessary for symmetry with their remaining breast. For these women, the weight of the prosthesis created a physical imbalance and they felt as if they were being pulled to one side. Furthermore, the heavier the prosthesis, the greater its tendency to pull away from the woman's body, resulting in her attempt to counterbalance this force by holding herself very straight. Some women actually said that they developed back problems and were unable to function without pain and disability. One woman, whose remaining breast was a bra size 41, had to be helped up from bed in the morning because the strain on her back had become so severe and debilitating.

The fit and coverage of the prosthesis was another area of concern and displeasure for women. Women with radical mastectomies consistently stated that the external prosthesis did not provide adequate coverage for their deformities. Their prostheses served primarily for filling out the form of their missing breasts; they did nothing to restore the anterior fold of the axilla or fill the upper chest area just under the collarbone.

Because a woman's prosthesis is fitted to provide breast symmetry when she is upright with her arms at her side, it does not move with her and is often unsuitable for the athletic woman who actively participates in sports. Accounts of prostheses that fell out on the tennis courts or slipped over to a woman's armpit during running or aerobic exercise were prevalent in our interviews and the source of much embarrassment to the women involved. With strenuous activity, this artificial breast was easily displaced or dislodged and could even float out of a bathing suit during swimming. It also could prevent the escape of heat from a woman's chest and cause skin irritation and skin rashes. Thus, for practical reasons of movement and comfort, many women felt that an external prosthesis was a nuisance and an inconvenience. "My prosthesis gets in my way. It interferes when I clean, exercise, or bend over." As one woman explained, "Prosthetic devices may be great in the beginning, but they are not totally comfortable. With breast reconstruction, one can feel whole again with no shifting of the prosthesis." The freedom afforded by reconstruction was emphasized by another woman who complained, "I enjoy being active; I am a swimmer and a golfer. My first prosthesis was large to match the existing breast, and it was cumbersome and floated when I dived."

For many women, one of the real bonuses of breast reconstruction was the increased variety of style and cut it allowed them in clothing. Reconstruction eliminated their need "to shop for clothes with higher necklines and specially designed swim wear." They now gained pleasure from the very act of shopping for clothing and once again felt excited about the possibility of purchasing lacy lingerie, pretty bras, and attractive blouses. Proud of their newfound ability to display a cleavage if they desired, they were also secure in the knowledge that when they were dressed there was absolutely no way that anyone could ever tell that their breasts had been reconstructed.

Before they had breast reconstruction none of these women regarded their prosthesis as a part of them or as a new breast. It was never incorporated into their body image, but instead was regarded as a necessity, a symbol of something missing and a constant reminder of the real breast. These women repeatedly emphasized their need to feel less obsessed with the cancer experience and a desire to rid themselves of their sense of deformity, which had resulted from having a mastectomy. Some felt that breast reconstruction relieved them of a cancer "stigma."

Interesting also was the reaction of older women we surveyed. Some of these individuals, in their late sixties and seventies, did not have reconstructive surgery because it was not a viable alternative when they had their mastectomies years earlier. They had lived so long without breasts they felt they were too old to bother with additional surgery. These women readily agreed, however, that if their daughters were to develop breast cancer and require mastectomies (and their daughters had an increased risk), they would urge them to have their breasts restored. Other women, in their seventies and eighties, had only recently developed breast cancer and their reaction was very different. They readily embraced the option of breast reconstruction, proclaiming that they had "lived this long with breasts and intended to live the rest of their lives with them as well." Age was not a deterrent, and these women expressed extreme satisfaction with their decision and were quick to recommend this option to their friends, who increasingly were being touched by this disease. For all of these women, breast reconstruction represented an exciting option and they felt that it would be "wonderful to have two breasts again."

In further examining motivations for seeking breast reconstruction, we noticed a definite correlation between age and marital status of a woman and her corresponding interest in reconstructive breast surgery.

Breast cancer is occurring with increasing frequency in young women. Moreover, breast cancer occurs with greater frequency in women who have never had children. Concomitantly, there are more childless women who are single than married. A mastectomy and the resultant deformity pose a number of especially uncomfortable and difficult questions for single women in the early stages of an intimate relationship.

How does one explain a missing breast to a potential lover? Some of the questions raised by women facing this situation follow:
- Do I tell my date I had a mastectomy?
- What is the right timing for this disclosure? Before or after discovery?
- Do I keep my body covered while we are having sex?
- Will I continue to be seen as desirable after I admit to a deformity?
- Can I feel sexy and good about myself with a deformity? Or is it easier to avoid sexual situations?

Many women choose the last option, preferring to steer clear of relationships that might lead to sexual intimacy. As one woman expressed it, "I could not face my life with just one breast. I was 42 years old and single when I had my mastectomy. I buried my sexuality for 13 months until I had the reconstruction."

Just as single and divorced women interested in meeting men and beginning new relationships often cite reconstruction as an attractive option, some widows reported feeling that breast surgery might be one step in a personal program of "starting over." Although many women who have had mastectomies after age 65 decide not to have additional elective surgery, age alone has no relationship to how women feel about themselves. Women at any age feel the sense of loss when they have a mastectomy. They still desire to return to wholeness. Many of the breast reconstruction patients we interviewed were over 50, and they felt that this surgery had renewed and invigorated them. In fact, some of the happiest and most satisfied women who have had breast reconstruction have been in these older age groups.

For many women, reconstruction is a symbol that they are completing the treatment and rehabilitation phase of their lives and are ready to get back to living. When the surgeon recommends reconstruction, he is saying that he feels good about the woman's chances for survival. In these cases, reconstruction represents a positive and reassuring statement from the general surgeon.

Reasons women seek reconstruction are as varied and individual as are the women themselves. Some women focus on the practical considerations of comfort and convenience, whereas others have psychological and aesthetic concerns; reconstruction bolsters their sense of femininity, self-confidence, and sexual attractiveness. Still other women seek peace of mind about the cancer experience, a realignment of their body image, and a return to wholeness. No one answer is better or more important than any other. The fact remains that after a woman's breast has been removed, a deformity exists and many women feel a deep sense of loss. The desire for restitution is a healthy reaction to this problem. It helps a woman to reconfirm her body image and bring her self-awareness back into harmony. For those women who feel the need to rebuild their bodies and replace their missing breast or breasts, reconstruction offers a positive source of hope for the future.

# QUESTIONS FREQUENTLY ASKED ABOUT BREAST RECONSTRUCTION

Over the past 15 years the approach to breast cancer treatment has undergone considerable change. Whereas once the emphasis was primarily on cancer removal, today treatment has a broader focus, including local tumor removal and quality of life issues such as breast preservation or breast restoration. Lumpectomy has withstood the test of time as a viable and effective primary treatment for breast cancer; women who choose this option can do so with confidence that survival rates are equivalent to those expected after mastectomy. As a consequence, lumpectomy and irradiation as well as immediate breast reconstruction following mastectomy have become the norm, enabling women to have the most effective cancer treatment while preserving their breasts. In this context the value of breast reconstruction, particularly immediate breast restoration with its considerable aesthetic and psychological benefits, is no longer questioned after mastectomy or after lumpectomy or partial mastectomy (when tumor removal will produce breast asymmetry or deformity). Women considering this option, however, continue to have numerous questions about the specifics and safety of breast reconstruction and whether they are appropriate candidates. Some worry that reconstruction can cause cancer or mask a recurrence; they may be concerned about the use of implants, which are foreign materials, and may be unaware of newer reconstructive techniques that allow women to have breast reconstruction using their own natural tissue. Others have anxieties about the appearance of the new breast, the prominence of breast scars, or the development of complications. Still others are concerned about the costs and the correct timing of surgery.

Some queries are so frequently posed to the doctor half of our writing team that we have compiled the following list of questions and answers to serve as a primer.

### Who is a candidate for breast restoration?

Today, most breast cancer patients can have their breasts rebuilt, and this option is increasingly being mentioned during the initial discussions concerning primary treatment so that women can avail themselves of an immediate procedure with skin-sparing mastectomy (provided there is no skin involvement) at the time of their mastectomy or lumpectomy. Age is not a factor in determining a woman's suitability nor is her type of mastectomy or the placement of her mastectomy scar. Women who have had radical mastectomies (removal of the breast and chest wall muscles), modified radical mastectomies (removal of the breast with chest wall muscles left intact), or partial mastectomies can now have satisfactory breast reconstructions. Partial reconstruction is best done prior to radiation therapy. Although breast reconstruction is increasingly being done at the time of the mastectomy, it does not matter how much time has elapsed since a woman's original cancer surgery. There is no statute of limitations for reconstruction and no disadvantage to waiting. Women have had successful reconstructive breast surgery 15 to 20 years after mastectomy.

### How does a person's age affect the success of reconstructive surgery? Are you ever too old?

A woman's age is not as important a factor in determining the ultimate success of her breast reconstruction as her motivation for the operation and her general health. Many women in their seventies have had successful reconstructive breast surgery and are very pleased with the results of this operation. A woman is never too old if she is in good health, is motivated to have breast reconstruction, and selects a type of reconstruction compatible with her general physical condition.

### Does the size and extent of a woman's cancer have any influence on whether she should have her breast reconstructed?

Women with small tumors have the best prognosis for survival, and breast reconstruction is most frequently performed for these women. Immediate breast reconstruction is a viable and appealing option for women who select a mastectomy and whose tumors have been discovered in the earlier stages. Women with larger tumors that have spread to the lymph nodes also may have their breasts restored, but the timing of their operation is influenced by the type and sequencing of the chemotherapy and radiation therapy they require.

### Are women with advanced disease eligible for this operation?

Occasionally a woman whose breast cancer has spread beyond her breast region requests this surgery. When this happens, the surgeon must reconcile the woman's present health status with her desire for "wholeness." Should he operate on a woman whose prognosis is poor and who may not live to enjoy her restored breast? Does this surgery justify the time, pain, and money it will cost when the potential time for enjoyment may be limited? For this woman, reconstruction must be discussed and performed in the context of improving the quality of her remaining life. Many women desire this procedure despite the presence of systemic disease. As one woman explained, "Even if I die tomorrow, it was worth it. I want to go out just like I came in." If the woman's motivation is strong and if she is fully informed about this surgery, then her psychological and emotional needs are an important consideration. Some surgeons feel that these women with advanced disease are among their most satisfied patients. The decision for breast reconstruction cannot be made in isolation and requires consultation and follow-up with the breast management team. The final decision must be made by a well-informed patient.

### Are there some women who are not suitable for breast reconstruction?

Yes, some women should not have breast reconstruction. Their emotional state, motivations, or personal circumstances may indicate that they cannot effectively cope with a major operation and recuperation. Women also may not be suitable candidates for this operation if their general health status is poor. For example, if a woman has advanced diabetes mellitus, a recent stroke or heart attack, severe chronic lung disease, or Alzheimer's disease, she should not be considered for this procedure.

### Are there any health considerations that would have a negative impact on the success of breast reconstruction?

The effects of smoking can have a detrimental effect on the success of any reconstructive procedure. This is primarily because of the effect on blood flow to the skin and underlying tissues. Skin and autologous tissues can fail to heal and infection is more common. Implants may have to be removed and flaps may fail to survive. All smokers are strongly advised to discontinue smoking before and after surgery.

Obesity is associated with an increased complication rate from anesthesia, blood clots from the legs, as well as pneumonia. Implant reconstructions are often unsatisfactory in the obese patient. There is also an increased risk of flap failure in these patients.

Autoimmune diseases that cause healing problems may impair potential reconstructive and radiation results. Women with these problems who decide to pursue breast reconstruction may want to avoid implants, but they should be aware that their condition will also make them more prone to possible flap failures. Consultation with their rheumatologist is important before considering any type of reconstructive surgery. Prior radiation therapy can affect the blood supply of the skin and underlying tissues and increase the possibility of poor healing or complications. Medications that affect blood clotting must also be discontinued.

### What are the timing options for breast reconstruction?

Reconstruction can be performed immediately, that is, right after the mastectomy or during the same hospital stay, or it can be performed on a delayed basis, that is, a few days, several months, or many years after the initial mastectomy. Many women had delayed breast reconstruction in the past, but immediate reconstruction is being requested and performed with much greater frequency today because it offers women a reprieve from the deforming effects of mastectomy and a reduction in the number of procedures they have to undergo. Today, most women who are considering mastectomy learn about breast reconstruction and the possibilities for immediate reconstruction from their general surgeons *before* they have their cancer surgery. Most medical centers now have breast management teams experienced in performing immediate breast reconstruction and able to offer this option to women who are having a mastectomy. Most women are pleased with the psychological and aesthetic results of immediate breast reconstruction. Frequently their surgeons will refer them to a plastic surgeon before the mastectomy so that they can investigate the option of breast reconstruction and the best timing for this operation. Although immediate breast reconstruction is now most frequently performed, the ultimate decision about the timing of reconstruction must be made by a fully informed patient in consultation and agreement with her cancer surgeon and her plastic surgeon to ensure the best treatment for her cancer. (See Chapter 13 for more detailed information on the advantages and disadvantages of immediate and delayed breast reconstruction.)

### Who are suitable candidates for immediate reconstruction?

Although immediate breast reconstruction is not appropriate for every patient, it is becoming a more frequently chosen approach for breast reconstruction, regardless of the stage of the disease. More breast cancers are being discovered at an early, more curable stage. Women with early breast cancer are the natural and obvious choices for immediate breast reconstruction should breast-conserving surgery not be selected; this would include women in general good health with small tumors (about 1 inch in diameter or less) and no involved axillary (armpit) lymph nodes (indicating less likelihood that the cancer has spread beyond their breast tissue). Of these early cancer patients, young women, women with a strong desire for breast preservation, women with small breasts, and women who require bilateral (both breasts) reconstruction are particularly appropriate for an immediate procedure.

### Who are suitable candidates for delayed reconstruction?

A woman who had a mastectomy before reconstructive procedures were offered or readily available is a natural candidate for delayed reconstruction. The woman with positive lymph nodes, indicating the disease has spread and additional therapy is necessary to treat her cancer, also is an appropriate candidate for a delayed procedure after chemotherapy and radiation therapy. Another candidate is the woman who needs time to evaluate whether she wants breast reconstruction. The delay between the mastectomy and the reconstruction gives her the opportunity to get acquainted with her plastic surgeon and decide on the best approach for her.

### Are the aesthetic results of immediate breast reconstruction as good as those that can be obtained with delayed reconstruction?

Experience with immediate reconstruction over the past 10 years indicates that results are as good as and usually better than those achieved with delayed reconstruction. With the newer mastectomy approaches aimed at skin conservation and preservation of the natural anatomic landmarks of the breast, immediate reconstruction often allows shorter mastectomy scars and more symmetrically shaped breasts. Breast sensation is usually better when more of the woman's own skin is spared rather than when an implant or flap procedure is done after traditional modified radical mastectomy with longer scars. To achieve the best possible aesthetic result some plastic surgeons prefer to perform immediate surgery because it is easier to match the remaining breast. Symmetry also is facilitated in women who are having both breasts removed. Women choosing immediate reconstruction need to understand, however, that the immediate operation is not the final operation. Similar to delayed reconstruction, additional procedures will be necessary to produce a symmetric, aesthetic breast appearance and nipple-areola reconstruction. (See the following questions for more information.)

A woman who desires an immediate breast reconstruction should inquire about how many immediate operations her reconstructive surgeon ordinarily performs (as compared to delayed procedures) and how the results he can obtain with an immediate breast reconstruction compare to those he can produce with a delayed procedure.

### What are the psychological benefits of breast reconstruction?

Each woman benefits from breast reconstruction in her own personal and individual manner. Patients having immediate breast reconstruction often say they appreciate not having to deal emotionally and physically with the mastectomy deformity. Many women who have had their breasts rebuilt have said that this operation made them "feel better about themselves . . . normal or whole again." Some women indicated that it relieved them of a constant reminder of the cancer and the mastectomy. Other women were pleased at the freedom it afforded them compared to wearing an external prosthesis. (See Chapters 9, 11, and 18 for more information.)

### How will a woman's breast reconstruction affect her relationship with her husband, family, friends, or loved ones?

Breast reconstruction usually does not change interpersonal relationships. It can, however, help a woman avoid having to deal with concerns about the physical deformity of a missing breast. It can also give the woman a boost in self-esteem, and as her feelings about herself improve, she can more thoroughly enjoy normal relationships and activities.

A woman will be disillusioned if she expects this surgery to remedy preexisting personal problems, repair a faltering relationship, or please another individual. To be worthwhile a woman's rebuilt chest must satisfy her personal, but reasonable expectations.

### How many operations are needed for breast reconstruction?

Aesthetically acceptable reconstructions usually can be completed in two operations. Immediate breast reconstruction allows the first operation to be done at the same time as the mastectomy or partial mastectomy. The first operation includes the reconstruction of the chest wall and breast mound and adjustments of the remaining breast (if indicated). Operation on the other breast would include enlargement, reduction, or uplifting to eventually achieve breasts of comparable size and position (see Chapter 14). (For the immediate breast reconstruction patient, these adjustments are often accomplished during a second procedure, although they can also be done at the time of the initial operation.) The second procedure is less extensive and includes nipple-areola reconstruction (see Chapter 16) and any additional operations that improve breast symmetry. When a temporary tissue expander is inserted initially, the permanent implant is placed during the second operation and nipple-areola reconstruction is usually delayed until a third operation, which can be performed on an outpatient basis. One-stage procedures (building both the breast and nipple-areola in one operation) have a higher incidence of malposition of the nipple-areola and breast asymmetries; these problems can be avoided with a two-stage procedure.

### How many doctor visits are necessary for each different reconstructive approach?

Before the operation the patient usually sees the reconstructive surgeon once or twice to discuss the details of the surgery and address questions. A follow-up visit is ordinarily scheduled approximately 1 week after the operation, with another visit planned about 6 weeks later. When tissue expansion is done, a woman may need to return for up to three or four additional visits so the saline volume in the tissue expander can be adjusted. No matter which reconstructive procedure has been used, the surgeon will want to see a woman yearly for follow-up visits after her breast reconstruction.

### Are blood transfusions necessary for breast reconstruction?

Although blood transfusions are occasionally necessary for flap procedures and microsurgical procedures and for some immediate breast reconstructions, newer surgical techniques tend to reduce blood loss and the need for transfusions. Simple implant or expander placement usually does not require transfusion. To alleviate patient concern about possible risks from blood-borne viruses, however, many surgeons request that patients donate 1 to 2 units of their own (autologous) blood for possible reinfusion in the operative and postoperative period. More blood will be needed for bilateral procedures and for mastectomies performed in conjunction with an immediate flap breast reconstruction. It is usually preferable to delay the operation for several weeks to allow enough time for the patient to donate her own blood. A few weeks' delay does not adversely affect the eventual treatment of the breast tumor, and it is best to prepare for the operation properly. Some patients prefer to obtain additional donor-directed blood (from relatives or friends) for transfusion when necessary. Use of blood from the general donor pool is almost never necessary for breast reconstruction patients.

### Will breast reconstruction cause cancer?

Breast reconstruction patients usually have already had a mastectomy in which the surgical oncologist removed as much breast tissue as possible. After mastectomy, sometimes a few cells from the breast tumor persist in the region of the mastectomy and later grow in this area (called a local recurrence). The likelihood of local recurrence is highest in women whose cancer has spread to the axillary lymph nodes. Radiation therapy and chemotherapy help reduce that risk. The rate of local recurrence after a mastectomy for early breast cancer is generally low.

There is no evidence of any kind, however, that breast reconstruction causes cancer to grow or increases the chance of recurrence. Many scientific studies have shown that the incidence of local recurrence after a mastectomy is not increased or the patient's survival affected by breast reconstruction, regardless of the technique used. Reconstruction with implant placement or the patient's own tissue does not increase the risk of local recurrence. It has also been noted that the type of tumors seen in local recurrences after breast reconstruction are the same as seen in patients who did not have breast reconstruction.

### Will the reconstruction hide the recurrence of cancer or prevent the detection of a new cancer?

The site of local recurrence of breast cancer is usually in the mastectomy scar, in the skin flaps, or in the axillary area. To monitor the woman's breast area for local recurrence after breast reconstruction with implants or expanders, the reconstructive surgeon places the breast implant behind the mastectomy area, usually beneath the underlying layer of muscle. When reconstructing the breast with a flap of the woman's own tissue, the tissue is placed behind the woman's chest skin. There is little difficulty in detecting an early local recurrence because the breast implant or the flap is beneath the skin and therefore does not obscure the most frequent sites of local recurrence. If a small area of recurrence is discovered in the mastectomy skin, this area is surgically removed (often as an outpatient procedure). The implant, expander, or flap does not need to be disturbed or removed. Additional therapy (radiation or chemotherapy) may be required, however, to protect against another recurrence or possible spread of the cancer to other parts of the body. (Detailed information on breast implants is provided in Chapter 11.)

### Will a woman be able to detect tumors as easily after reconstruction?

After reconstruction with an implant or expander placed beneath the muscle layer or with a flap* from the back (latissimus dorsi flap), the skin and scar are actually pushed forward and thus new tumors or local recurrences usually can be felt easily on breast self-examination (BSE). If the cancer recurs, it can be found by periodic checks of the skin to detect any new lumps. That is why it is equally as important for women to continue to perform BSE after a mastectomy whether they have had breast reconstruction or not.

Detection of tumors may be somewhat more difficult when a woman's breast has been reconstructed with the lower abdominal TRAM (transverse rectus abdominis musculocutaneous [muscle-skin] flap) or with the buttock (gluteus maximus) flap. Because this tissue is moved from a distant site and vascularity may be decreased, it sometimes develops firm, thickened areas of fat that may be confused with a local recurrence. These areas, however, are within the abdomi-

---

*A flap is a portion of tissue (with its blood supply) that is moved from one area of the body to another for reconstructive purposes such as breast reconstruction.

nal or buttock tissue and can be differentiated from a local recurrence. Sometimes mammography, ultrasonography, or a biopsy may be necessary for a definitive diagnosis. If a biopsy is needed, it can sometimes be done with a fine needle to avoid a surgical incision.

### Does breast reconstruction compromise a woman's immune system?

There is no medical evidence that breast reconstruction or general anesthesia compromises a woman's immune system. Some believe, however, that a woman who has breast cancer may already have a compromised immune system.

### What is the best placement of a mastectomy scar for the woman who desires breast reconstruction?

When skin-sparing mastectomy is to be done for immediate reconstruction, the best placement for this scar is usually around the areola with a 1- to 2-inch extension of the scar to the side or below the areola. For delayed reconstruction, the best placement of the mastectomy scar is in a low oblique position, extending from below the axilla to the inner lower breast area. Either of these scars is easily covered by a brassiere. For delayed reconstruction, frequently a portion of the scar can be reopened and an implant placed through it to avoid creating a new incision and thus a new scar. Sometimes, however, the primary cancer is located in an area of the breast that makes it impossible for the surgeon to leave an oblique scar, especially when it is high and medial in the breast area. When immediate breast reconstruction is done, the general surgeon and the reconstructive surgeon can plan the location of the incisions to ensure the best placement for the breast reconstruction. They may be able to minimize the incisions and preserve more skin, which improves the final breast appearance. Sometimes these incisions can resemble those used for a breast reduction in a woman with large, droopy breasts (see Chapter 14). Sometimes a separate, shorter incision is also made to remove the tumor in the upper breast region.

### What can be done if the mastectomy scar is in a bad location?

Breast reconstruction can be done with a mastectomy scar in any position. The scar position cannot be changed, but the reconstructive implant can be positioned through this scar and the scar revised to provide the best possible appearance.

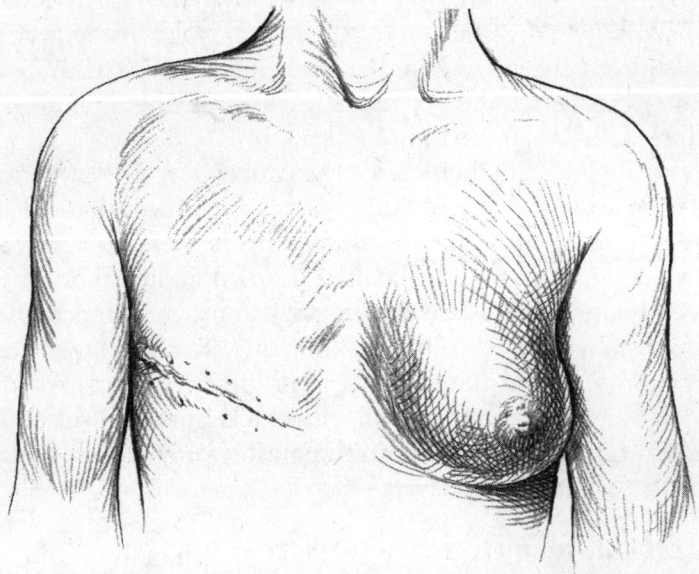

Modified radical mastectomy scar in oblique position

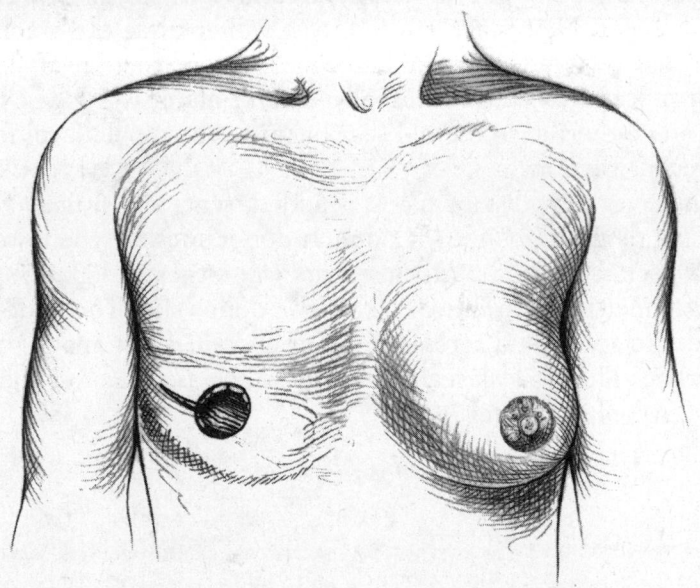

Skin-sparing mastectomy scar encircling areola with side extension

## Can the plastic surgeon totally remove the mastectomy scar when he restores the breast?

The scars from the mastectomy cannot be removed, although they sometimes can be reduced or made less obvious by a plastic surgery procedure called scar revision. A scar line will always be present where the original skin incision for the cancer surgery was performed. Initially the scars will be red and raised, a condition that will persist for several months after the operation. This redness (indicative of increased blood flow during the healing process) and thickness will subside over the next 1 or 2 years as the scars improve in appearance and become less obvious. Scars in fair-skinned women tend to remain red for a longer period of time. It takes less time for the scars of older women to fade. Some women heal with thick scars, and this tendency is obvious from the appearance of the mastectomy scar as well as any other scars that they may have.

## What type of new scars are created by reconstruction?

Reconstruction using the existing tissues or by expanding the existing tissues is most frequently accomplished through the mastectomy scar. No new scar is created. Sometimes, if additional skin is needed to reconstruct the breast, other scars will be created when this skin is inset into the breast. New scars on the breast will encircle the areola and extend into the underarm for immediate reconstruction after skin-sparing procedures and will usually extend along the lower breast crease and either up to the old scar or up to the nipple level for delayed reconstruction.

Whenever new distant tissue is added, scars will usually be left where the tissue is obtained. Common donor sites are the lower abdomen, back, side, and buttocks. Scars will either be left across the back or under the arm if the back is the donor site. The abdominal scar will usually extend across the lower abdomen just above the pubic hairline. The buttock scar will be in the crease or across the midportion of the buttock region.

## Types of Scars Created by Reconstruction

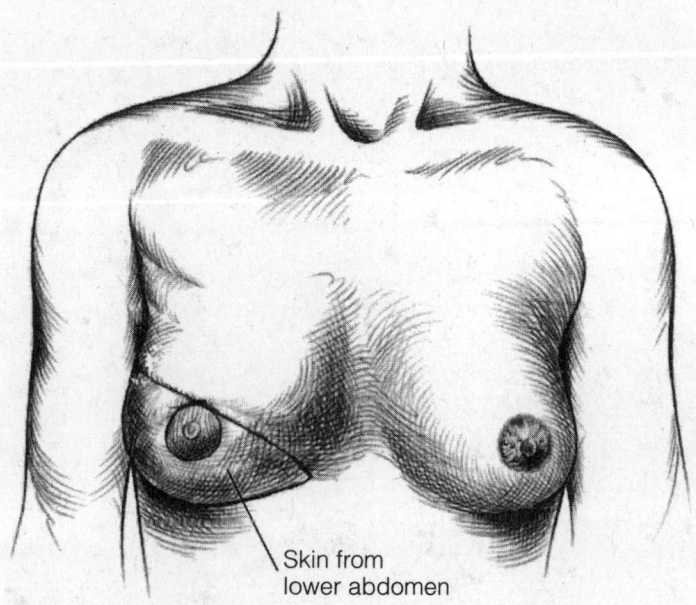

Skin from
lower abdomen

Breast reconstruction with a flap of tissue from the lower abdomen
(TRAM flap) after modified radical mastectomy

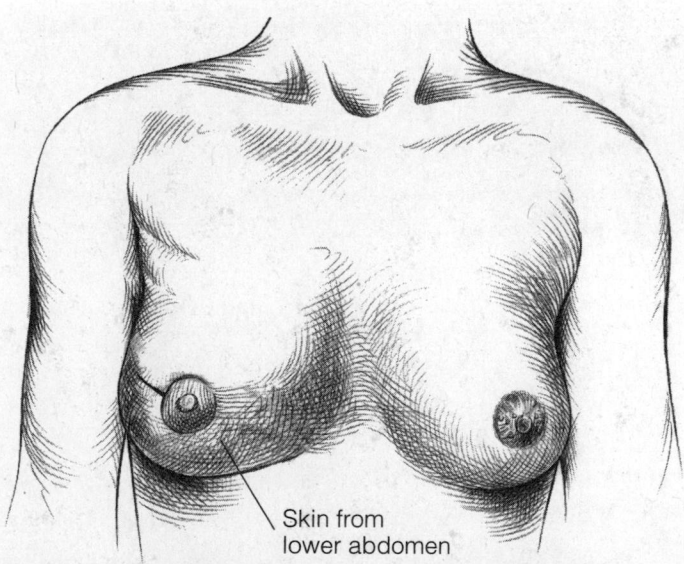

Skin from
lower abdomen

Immediate breast reconstruction with a flap of tissue from the lower abdomen
(TRAM flap) after skin-sparing mastectomy

## Types of Scars Created by Reconstruction—cont'd

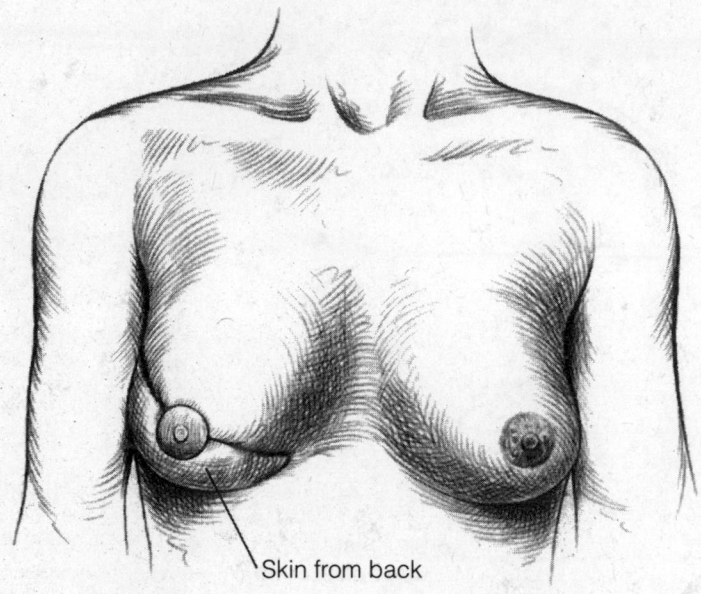

Skin from back

Breast reconstruction with a flap of tissue from the back
(latissimus dorsi) after modified radical mastectomy

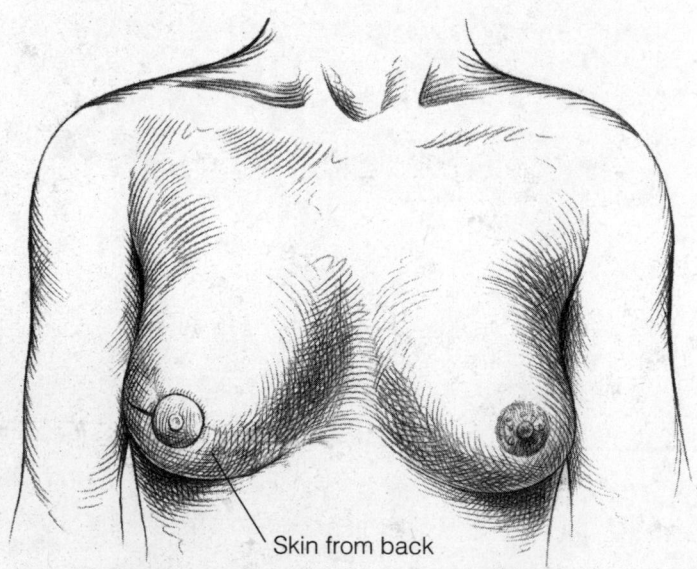

Skin from back

Immediate breast reconstruction with a flap of tissue from the back
(latissimus dorsi) after skin-sparing mastectomy

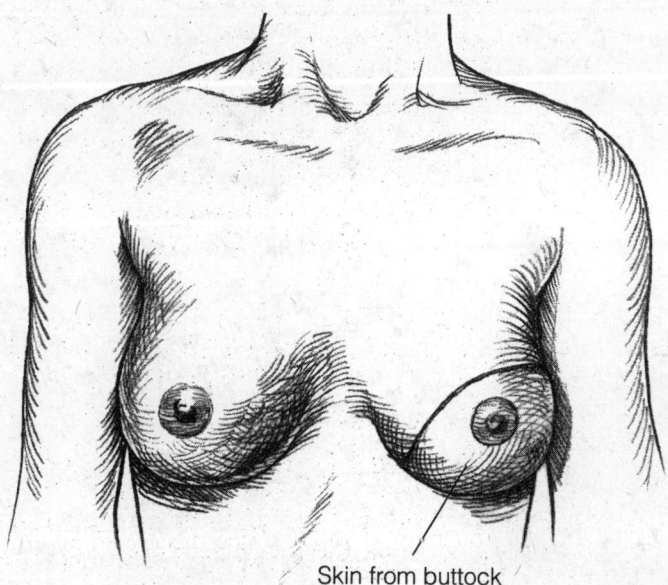

Skin from buttock

Breast reconstruction with a flap of tissue from the buttock
(gluteus maximus) after modified radical mastectomy

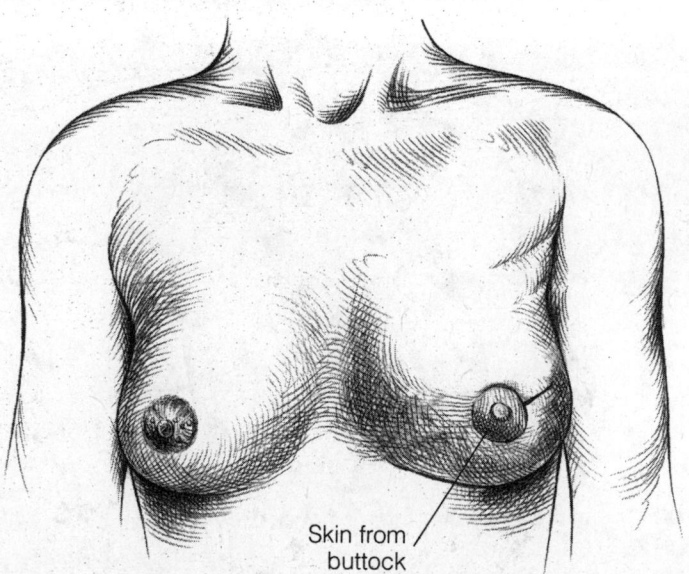

Skin from
buttock

Immediate breast reconstruction with a flap of tissue from the buttock
(gluteus maximus) after skin-sparing mastectomy

## Types of Scars Created by Reconstruction—cont'd

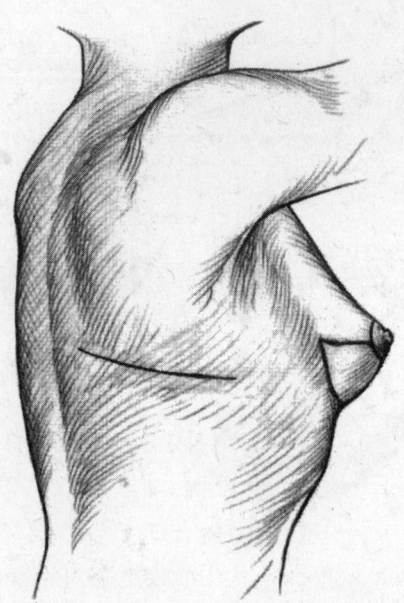

Donor scar left on back from latissimus dorsi reconstruction

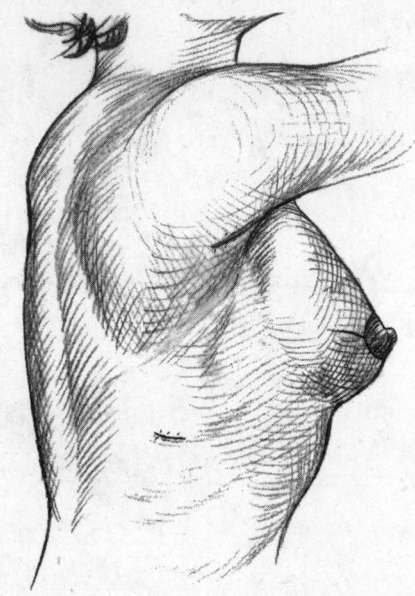

Donor scar left on back from immediate endoscopic latissimus dorsi reconstruction

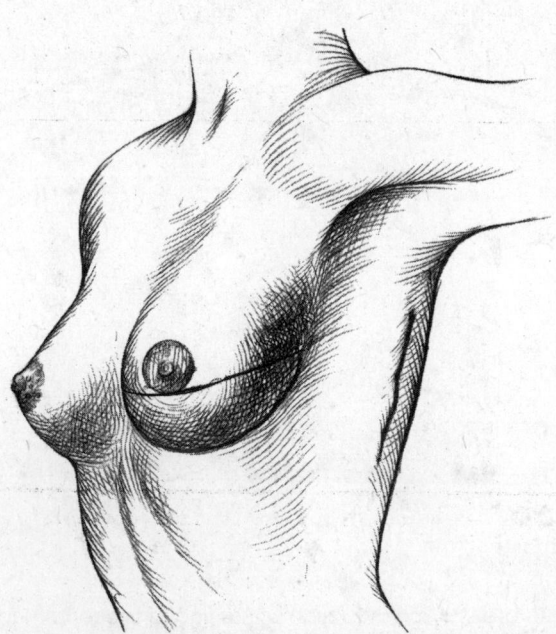

Alternate donor scar on side with a latissimus dorsi reconstruction

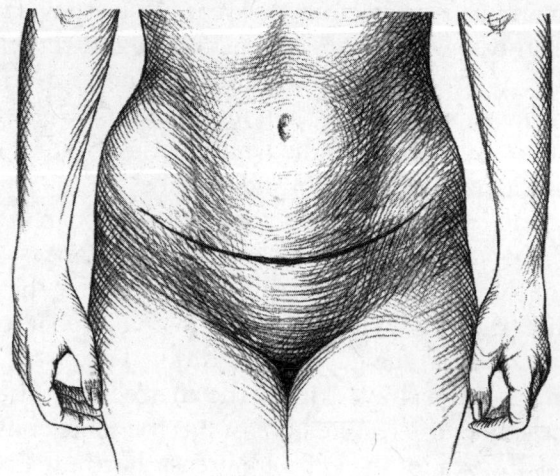

Donor scar on lower abdomen from
TRAM flap reconstruction

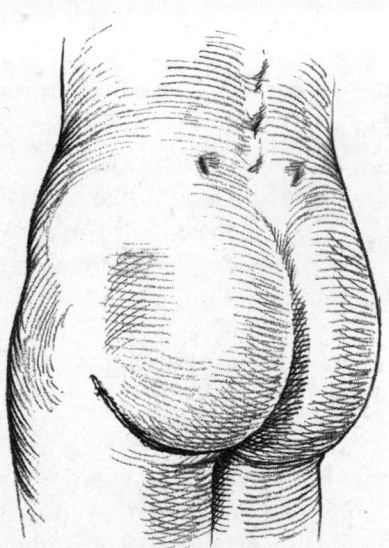

Donor scar left on buttock from
gluteus maximus reconstruction

### How much skin is removed during mastectomy and can you be sure enough can be preserved for breast reconstruction?

When a woman has a mastectomy to treat her breast cancer, the oncologic surgeon usually removes some skin around the biopsy site as well as the nipple-areola. Many surgeons can perform the operation through these incisions. The incision may need to be extended to the axillary region to gain access to the lymph nodes. Studies have shown that it is not necessary to remove additional skin from the breast region as was done in the past. Therefore more skin can be spared and preserved for breast reconstruction. In some instances, particularly when a flap of the patient's own tissue is available for the reconstruction, the skin at the biopsy site and area of nipple-areola removal is replaced with the skin on the flap. Any additional skin that is needed is supplied from the remaining skin at the mastectomy site. With this approach, the skin of the restored breast has the same consistency and appearance as the skin of the opposite breast. Furthermore, when less skin is removed initially, the mastectomy scars are shorter and the extra skin that is left is filled out by the transferred tissue or the breast implant or expander that is inserted.

Actually, a woman's breast can be reconstructed regardless of the amount of tissue remaining after the mastectomy. When the pectoralis major muscle and sufficient breast skin are present, a simple reconstruction with an implant or expander can usually be done. When much of the skin or pectoralis major muscle is missing and there is a significant skin deficiency, a flap, either from the back, lower abdomen, or buttock area, is usually necessary.

If a woman knows that she would like to have breast reconstruction before her mastectomy, her general surgeon should be informed so that he can confer with a plastic surgeon to ensure the best possible plan to facilitate the reconstruction.

### Is it necessary for a woman's normal breast to be modified to match the new one?

Many times a good match can be achieved with tissue expansion and implant placement without touching a woman's normal breast. Sometimes, to avoid altering the opposite breast, it may be necessary to reconstruct the missing breast using a flap procedure. When the normal breast is very large and sags or is very flat and small, the surgeon may not be able to match it and some modification might be required. (See Chapters 13 and 14 for additional information on this subject.)

### What areas can be reconstructed? Can large deformities and chest hollowness be filled in?

Predictably good restoration of the breast shape, contour, and size can now be achieved though breast reconstruction. It often improves the appearance of (but may not eliminate) scars, skin grafts, or radiation-damaged skin. For women who had a radical mastectomy many years ago, the upper chest and axillary deformity can be filled in and corrected. The infraclavicular area can be rebuilt, and the missing anterior axillary fold can be recreated. Restoration of these areas, however, requires the use of additional donor tissue from the back, lower abdomen, or buttocks and the subsequent creation of new scars in these areas.

### Can partial defects after lumpectomy and quadrantectomy be reconstructed?

After completion of the lumpectomy or quadrantectomy, the general or oncologic surgeon checks the margins of resection to ensure complete tumor removal. He also assesses the area of tumor excision to determine if it will leave an unsatisfactory breast shape or size after healing and/or radiation therapy. If this is the case, the volume of the breast may be restored with the latissimus dorsi back muscle and fat. The reconstructive surgeon uses an endoscopic technique to harvest a flap of latissimus muscle and its overlying fat through the incisions used for the primary local cancer treatment. This flap is then used to fill and contour the defect remaining after the breast-conserving procedure. This technique is also useful for secondary breast deformities that require some additional tissue.

### What are endoscopic techniques and how can they be used for breast reconstruction?

With the endoscopic technique for harvesting the latissimus dorsi back muscle and fat, the surgeon uses the incisions made at the time of primary cancer treatment, which are usually in the lateral breast region and in the underarm area (where the axillary lymph node dissection was done). A video camera is attached to the endoscope so the image can be viewed on the TV monitor by the surgeon while he operates using special long instruments that are inserted through the small incisions. The endoscope permits a video image of tissues beneath the skin to be projected on the video monitor via fiberoptic light. Sometimes separate incisions about an inch long are also needed in the middle to lower back. Through these small incisions the surgeon visualizes the area with the use of the endoscope, dissects the flap that contains the fat and muscle, preserves the blood supply to the tissue, and moves the flap through the underarm to the front of the chest for the breast reconstruction.

### Can the missing nipple-areola be reconstructed?

Both the central projecting nipple and the darker surrounding areola can be reconstructed. This procedure is usually done as a second operation after the proper breast shape and size have been obtained. Although there are several different methods for reconstructing the nipple, some of the most effective techniques use tissue available at the site of the new nipple. Earlier techniques primarily used tissues from other areas of the body. The areola can be reconstructed from a circular graft of excess skin near the mastectomy scar or from the abdominal scar if an abdominal (TRAM) flap has been used for the reconstruction. With increasing frequency, when extra skin is not available, a surgical tattoo can recreate the areola and the reconstructed nipple can be colored to the proper shade to match the opposite nipple. (See Chapter 16 for more detailed information on the different techniques for nipple-areola reconstruction.)

### What types of implants and expanders are available for breast reconstruction?

The different categories of implants and expanders and a detailed discussion of these devices and associated benefits and risks are presented in Chapters 11 and 13.

### How are breast implants and tissue expanders used for breast reconstruction?

A saline implant or expander is often inserted under a woman's skin or muscle to create a breast mound during breast reconstruction. For breast reconstruction with implants to be successful, the implant must provide volume, projection, and size that approximates that of the opposite breast. Just as the appearance of the normal female breast changes with age, breast implants may also need to be changed or adjusted over time to maintain the best results. The use of tissue expanders makes obtaining the proper size for the breast reconstruction more likely. The size of the expander can be adjusted if the fill valve is left in place.

### Can a woman's breast he huilt with her own natural tissue without the need for breast implants or expanders?

Reconstruction using flaps of the patient's own tissue (autologous breast reconstruction) is a viable and increasingly popular option for many women who wish to avoid breast implants but still have the most natural result possible. The consistency and feel of the reconstructed breast closely resemble a normal breast; this reconstructed breast ages similar to the opposite breast because it is the woman's own tissue and therefore is most likely to provide lasting symmetry. In many cases the reconstructed breast actually appears more natural over time. Sources of donor tissue are areas of excess tissue such as the lower abdomen, the back, the hips, or the buttocks. The donor scar can also be hidden so that a significant deformity is not created. Many women who have gained some weight over the years find this an excellent opportunity to accomplish two goals at one time: rebuilding a full and natural breast while contouring an area of abundant fatty tissue, usually in the lower abdomen. Most women have also noted some return of sensation to their breasts after they are rebuilt with their own tissue. The chance of sensory return is increased with the newer techniques that use shorter incisions and skin sparing at the time of the mastectomy.

When breasts are reconstructed with the patient's own tissue, breast implants are usually not necessary. One of the prime reasons that many women choose this approach is to avoid the insertion of a foreign material in the body. If a woman is very slender and lacks the excess fatty tissue necessary to build a breast without the need for a supplementary implant, particularly if she needs to have both of her breasts reconstructed (bilateral breast reconstruction), she may want to consider selecting a procedure involving implant or expander placement. (Autologous breast reconstruction techniques are discussed in detail in Chapter 13.)

### What is the TRAM flap? Is it the same as a "tummy tuck"?

The TRAM (transverse rectus abdominis musculocutaneous) flap is a method of breast reconstruction in which a woman's lower abdominal tissue is transferred to the breast region and reshaped to form a breast that is symmetric with her opposite breast. When this transverse ellipse of tissue is moved from the lower abdomen to the breast region, the blood supply is maintained because the tissue is left attached to strips or "pedicles" of the central abdominal muscle. The name

"TRAM flap" is derived in part from the muscle to which it is attached—the rectus abdominis muscle. This operation is often referred to as the "tummy tuck" procedure because the abdominal portion of the procedure in which the donor tissue is taken from the woman's abdomen is similar to the "tummy tuck" operation (abdominoplasty) to improve lower abdominal contour. In both procedures the excess lower abdominal tissue is removed, the abdominal area is closed and tightened, and the resulting scar extends across the lower abdomen.

### How are microsurgical techniques used for breast reconstruction?

One of the significant advances in plastic and reconstructive surgery over the past few years has been the development and refinement of microsurgical techniques for reconstructive surgery. These procedures are performed while visualizing the operative field through the magnification of an operating microscope, thereby permitting the repair and suture of tiny vessels and nerves. Microsurgical techniques are particularly helpful when tissue needs to be moved from a distant part of the body to an area to be reconstructed. These operations are called "free flaps" because the tissue is freed completely and separated from the donor area, moved to the reconstructive area, and reattached under the operating microscope. Donor sites for breast free flaps include the abdomen, buttocks, hips, and back. The buttocks were one of the first distant areas used for breast reconstruction via microsurgery. Since the blood supply cannot be preserved when moving buttock tissue this great a distance, a microvascular (involving the small blood vessels) technique is used to hook up the blood vessels of the buttocks to the blood vessels in the woman's breast region. The TRAM flap, described previously as a pedicle flap (one that is transferred while still attached to its blood supply), can also be transferred microsurgically as a free flap. The lateral hip flap (Rubens flap) is another possible donor site for breast reconstruction; this flap is transferred microsurgically.

### Is a breast implant or a woman's own tissues better for reconstruction?

This is difficult to answer because the specific method of reconstruction must be determined on an individual basis. Breasts reconstructed with implants or tissue expanders can look and feel quite natural. These operations can also be done without leaving additional scars. Sometimes, however, fibrous tissue develops around these implants (a condition called capsular contracture), causing them to feel firm and reducing the attractiveness of the breast. Placement of the implant under the muscle usually helps minimize any hardening. Implants with a textured surface have also proved effective in reducing the incidence of capsular formation around these implants and in keeping the breasts soft and natural. These textured implants have thicker envelopes, which can sometimes be seen as ripples or felt through thin skin.

Reconstruction with a woman's own tissue avoids the use of a foreign implant material and produces a soft, natural reconstructed breast that will not become firm. She pays a price for these advantages, however. When the lower abdominal or buttock tissue is transported to a woman's breast area, the surgeon must create additional scars on the breast, lower abdomen, or buttocks. These are the most involved procedures for breast reconstruction and can be associated with failure of some of the transferred tissue to survive, more pain, and a longer recovery. (This topic is discussed fully in Chapter 13.)

### *Does chest wall irradiation affect the success of breast reconstruction? Which techniques work best after radiation therapy?*

Radiation therapy can reduce the blood supply to the chest wall skin and muscle. It can also damage the skin, reducing its elasticity and healing potential. After radiation therapy to the chest wall, breast reconstruction with tissue expansion is often not as successful because the skin may be damaged and less resilient; this means that the potential for complications is greater. Radiation can also affect the success of a breast implant or flap reconstruction by causing fibrosis (or thickening), capsular contracture, and breast firmness. Therefore, if radiation is anticipated, breast reconstruction may be delayed until after this treatment is completed. The best and least complicated breast reconstructions after radiation are done with autologous tissue—the TRAM flap, latissimus dorsi flap, or gluteus maximus free flap.

### *How will a woman's breasts look over the long term, say 5 or 10 years after reconstruction? Which type of breast reconstruction produces the most aesthetic long-term results?*

Although it is impossible to predict with certainty how results will look in 5 to 10 years, generally some degree of capsular contracture will form after implant or expander reconstruction with each passing year. This usually results in some breast asymmetry as the reconstructed breast becomes elevated with time and the natural opposite breast droops subsequent to the aging process. With autologous reconstructions, the result is more lasting and less likely to change.

### If a person gains or loses a considerable amount of weight, how will that affect the results of breast reconstruction?

General weight losses or gains are reflected in some women's breasts; in others they are not. After an implant reconstruction, a major weight change will probably produce a change in the normal breast that will result in breast asymmetry. This asymmetry may require an implant change (an outpatient procedure). Such a change is often not needed with the expander implant because of its internal valve. This implant has the flexibility to permit future implant size adjustments to accommodate weight changes that have altered the woman's breast size. This may be the best solution for a woman who wants a breast reconstruction but plans on losing weight in the future. Similarly, if the woman gains additional weight, the breast can be enlarged to match the other larger, fuller breast.

Reconstructions with a woman's own lower abdominal or buttock tissues usually remain symmetric under these circumstances because of the major fatty components of both the normal and reconstructed breasts.

### What happens to breast symmetry as a woman's remaining unoperated breast ages?

Every woman's breasts age differently. Generally, however, there is gradual settling and lowering of the breast with time. Breast size also changes with aging; these changes are influenced by weight loss or gain, body fat content, and hormonal changes. When a woman's breast has been rebuilt with her own tissues, it tends to age more like her natural breast ages with better long-term symmetry. This symmetry is not as predictable over the long term with implant recontruction.

### What is the long-term appearance of a rebuilt nipple? Does it keep its projection?

If possible, the nipple built from a flap of chest wall skin is usually made longer than the remaining nipple to counter the tendency of nipple reconstructions to become shorter and flatter over time. When the nipple is built over a flap reconstruction, there is often more tissue available than when it is built over thin, expanded skin. Most of these chest wall flap nipple reconstructions can be expected to lose about one half of their initial projection over time. When built with a graft from the other nipple, symmetry is usually easier to maintain.

### Can another person tell if a woman has had breast reconstruction?

A woman who has had breast reconstruction can dress normally without anyone realizing that her breast has been rebuilt. Unless she is naked, her scars will not be noticeable to anyone. (The newer skin-sparing techniques minimize the scars from reconstruction.) When she is clothed, her breasts will appear the same as any other woman's.

### If a woman has reconstruction, will she be able to wear V necklines and ordinary clothing without high necks?

A woman who has had a modified radical mastectomy with a scar that falls under her brassiere will be able to wear V necklines again. If she has had a radical mastectomy in which the pectoralis major muscle has been removed, reconstruction (which requires flap tissue) can still permit her to wear V-neck clothing unless the mastectomy scar extends into this central area of the chest and she is concerned about it showing.

Sports clothes also can be worn, but sometimes the style might have to accommodate any unusually positioned mastectomy scar or a donor flap scar on her back, underarm, lower abdomen, or buttocks.

### How do the results of breast reconstruction compare with a woman's expectations? Do her breasts look and feel normal?

It is important for a woman to carefully define her expectations before she has this operation to make sure that the plastic surgeon knows what she wants and can tell her if it is possible. She also needs to understand the limitations of the operation. Breast reconstruction can fill in and rebuild the deformities resulting from mastectomy. A woman may be disappointed, however, if she expects her new breast to be the same as the one it is meant to replace. Her new breast with an implant will often be cooler, firmer, and more rounded than her remaining one. It will not move as naturally with changes in position or posture. Firmness is often associated with the use of implants. Also, the lower portion of the breast implant can sometimes be felt through the breast skin; this is not bothersome to most women and is considered a natural accompaniment of breast reconstruction with implants.

When the skin and overlying tissue cover is thin or irradiated, any irregularities or ripples in the breast implant can show through the skin. This rippling can give an unattractive contour to the reconstructed breast and can be reduced by placing the implant under autologous tissue or a layer of latissimus dorsi back muscle. A more normal breast "feel" and flow can usually be obtained by using the patient's own tissue from the lower abdomen, back, or buttocks.

### In what ways will a woman's rebuilt breast differ from her original breast?

It will be less mobile and have less sensation. It cannot produce milk. There are scars from the mastectomy and reconstruction. Furthermore, the nipple-areola does not totally match the other natural one and does not respond to stimuli.

### What are the chances for breast symmetry?

The chances for acceptable breast symmetry are good. Each reconstruction must be individualized. Preoperatively the surgeon must determine if symmetry can be achieved with or without modification of the other breast. Bilateral reconstructions are often the most symmetric.

### Will the reconstructed breast have projection?

The reconstructed breast often has a similar projection to the opposite normal breast. However, reconstructed breasts can be flatter and thus have less projection than natural breasts. Occasionally an implant is used to optimize projection after a flap reconstruction. Sometimes, when an implant breast reconstruction develops capsular contracture, the breast becomes rounder and firmer and the projection can actually increase.

### Is the reconstructed breast sensitive to touch and to sexual stimulation?

Because sensation or feeling in the chest wall area is lost during the mastectomy, the reconstructed breast can feel numb or at least have less sensation than the normal side. The skin-sparing mastectomy tends to result in more residual sensitivity to touch. The underarm may also be numb and feel strange to the touch. Some women say that shaving their underarms becomes a rather unpleasant, uncomfortable experience. The underside of the upper arm is usually also numb; however, surgeons often attempt to preserve the sensation to this area. Sometimes, as some of these nerves grow back after the mastectomy, the woman may notice some radiating, "shooting," or "tingling" pains in the area where these nerves are located, particularly in her underarm region or in the breast area.

This lack of sensation is more common when an implant has been used for breast reconstruction. Many of the women whose breasts are reconstructed with their own tissue (autologous tissue) from the lower abdomen will develop some sensation to touch in the region of their reconstructed breasts. Their chances for developing additional breast sensation are further enhanced when the reconstruction with autologous tissue is performed immediately after a skin-sparing mastectomy. The patient can maximize return of sensation by reeducating the involved area of numbness with daily massage.

The special, pleasant sensation associated with the nipple-areola area with its responsiveness to sexual stimulation is usually lost and does not return.

### If a woman has breast reconstruction with implants, will her breast be warm like a normal breast?

Usually the temperature of a reconstructed breast is determined by the thickness of the skin cover and adequacy of the blood supply. When the cover is thin and the ambient air is cold, a cooler temperature of the implant will be noticeable and the breast can feel cold. Flap reconstructions usually are not affected in this manner because they are nourished and warmed by their own blood supply.

### Will there be nerve loss?

No additional nerve loss is to be expected after breast reconstruction with implants. With a TRAM flap reconstruction, the area just above the abdominal wall donor site scar is usually numb for a few months. With a latissimus dorsi flap, it is below the back incision; and with a gluteus maximus flap, down the back of the leg.

### What is the expected hospitalization for the different reconstructive procedures?

The usual hospital stay for simple implant placement or tissue expansion is 1 to 2 days, although many women can have these operations as outpatient procedures. For the latissimus dorsi (back) flap, hospitalization is 1 to 4 days; for the TRAM (lower abdominal) flap, 4 to 8 days, and for a microsurgical buttock, hip, or TRAM flap procedure, 4 to 8 days.

### What is the anticipated pain and recovery time?

After breast reconstruction a woman will experience pain in her chest area as well as in any donor sites where additional tissue was taken to build her new breast. The degree of pain and length of the recuperative period will vary with the individual patient, the extent of her defect, and the operative procedure chosen. The postoperative pain comes from the effects of the cut nerves in the breast region. As these nerves grow back, they can often be reeducated by massage of the skin a few weeks after the operation. (Specific information on these matters is provided in Chapter 13.)

An advance in pain control after an operation, the PCA (patient-controlled analgesia) unit, is now available to alleviate some of the patient's pain and discomfort during her hospital stay. This device enables the patient to press a button when she needs pain relief. The machine then delivers a predetermined amount of pain medication. In the past it was necessary for a nurse to give an injection to relieve the pain every 2 to 4 hours. Current thinking indicates that better pain relief may be possible if pain medication is administered as the patient needs it. This approach allows the patient to be in control of her pain relief medication.

Some women do not handle pain medication well, even the relatively small doses delivered by the PCA. A potentially distressing side effect for these women is nausea and vomiting from the effects of the anesthesia and the medication given immediately after surgery. This can be alleviated by reducing the dosage of the pain relief medication to the absolute minimum that the patient needs and can tolerate or by changing the medication. A patient who does not tolerate medication well should alert the anesthesiologist and surgeon of this problem preoperatively so that some accommodation can be made to avoid nausea following the operation. Alternatively, an epidural spinal catheter can be inserted to administer medication to control pain.

### Is it painful when the tissue expander is inflated? How does it feel?

Most women describe a "full, tight feeling" during tissue expansion. For a minority of patients, expansion can be painful. To relieve the discomfort for these individuals the expansion process is paced more slowly, which means more frequent visits and lower volume expansion. In some cases some of the saline solution may even be removed temporarily until the patient feels more comfortable. When expansion is begun soon after the mastectomy, there is less pain because the nerves have not grown back yet.

### What aftereffects and adjustments should a woman expect after breast reconstruction?

Following breast reconstruction a woman's breast may be swollen and bruised. These are expected and natural responses to healing and the patient should not be alarmed; the swelling will subside in a few days and the bruising will fade and disappear over a period of weeks, leaving her breast with a far more acceptable appearance. Her breast may also appear smaller or larger than expected and may not be completely symmetric with the opposite breast. Some asymmetries will lessen with time. If they persist, the breast usually can be adjusted a few months later during a second procedure and at the time of the nipple-areola reconstruction.

When an expander is used, the reconstructed breast will look smaller and flatter at first. It will become enlarged after several postoperative visits as additional saline solution is added to the expander.

### If muscles are used for reconstruction, how will it affect movement and physical strength in the future?

The muscles and portions of muscles used for breast reconstruction are considered functionally expendable; other muscle groups usually take over when one of these muscles has been transferred. Therefore muscle flap reconstructions normally do not impose functional restrictions on a woman after the healing period is over. A postoperative exercise program can contribute to rebuilding strength. Practically all patients can expect to return to their normal preoperative activities after the healing process.

### What limitations or weaknesses does a woman experience after a musculocutaneous flap reconstruction?

Most of the activities of daily living, including sports activities, are not affected by breast reconstruction with a muscle or muscle and skin flap. However, a woman's ability to perform sit-ups may be reduced after a TRAM flap. This problem can be more noticeable if both rectus abdominis muscles (bipedicle or bilateral) are used. Some activities that rely heavily on upper extremity strength, such as cross-country skiing, may also be more difficult after a latissimus dorsi flap procedure.

### Will a woman have full use of her arm after breast reconstruction?

Breast reconstruction will not impose any permanent restrictions on arm mobility or strength. Because some free flap breast reconstructions and the latissimus dorsi flap require surgery in the arm area, a woman will be instructed to limit arm activity for a few weeks after surgery to avoid complications.

### If a muscle is used for reconstruction, will it still function when it has been transferred?

When the latissimus dorsi back muscle is used, some patients notice that certain movements of the arm cause the transferred muscle to contract, thereby causing the reconstructed breast to move. This can be disconcerting. If this proves a major problem for a woman, it can be remedied during a later procedure that divides the nerve to the muscle. The muscles moved from the abdomen are not functional after they are moved.

### When can a woman resume an exercise program after breast reconstruction? Will any activities be permanently restricted?

Although each patient recovers at a different rate, most women who have implant reconstruction can resume normal upper extremity activity after 3 to 4 weeks. After a flap procedure, activity can be resumed in 6 to 8 weeks.

### Is any depression experienced after this operation?

Some women go through a limited but normal period of depression after breast reconstruction. The operation, general anesthesia, postoperative pain, and medications may combine to produce these feelings. Because this operation represents a major step for a woman, there is an emotional buildup to prepare for it as well as heightened expectations for a lovely result. Therefore a woman may feel a letdown once the operation is over because the postoperative appearance will not reflect the final result. Instead, her breast may look bruised and possibly flat, far removed from the result she expected. This depression usually subsides in a few days as the patient recovers and the appearance of her breast improves.

### What are possible complications from breast reconstruction? When do they occur and why?

Complications of breast reconstruction appear either immediately after the operation or develop later. The type and degree of complications relate to the method of reconstruction used.

When an implant or expander is used to reconstruct the breast with existing tissues, a blood collection (hematoma) can develop around the implant; this problem usually requires drainage, often in the operating room. When the skin is thin or irradiated, actual exposure of the implant can occur because of the poor cover; the implant must be removed, the wound allowed to heal, and reconstruction restarted a few months later. Infection and delayed healing also may occur. The implant or expander can deflate. Capsular contracture is the most frequent late problem associated with implant and expander reconstruction; this topic is addressed in Chapters 11 and 13.

Complications are more likely after flap reconstructions, particularly after the more complex microsurgical procedures. Hematoma may occur in both the site of the reconstruction and in the donor site. If the flap tissue that is moved does not have an adequate blood supply, a portion or occasionally the entire flap may be lost. With microsurgical reconstruction, sometimes the microanastomosis (where the blood vessels are connected) develops a blood clot and the patient may need to return to the operating room immediately for a second procedure to remove the clot and resuture the blood vessels. (A more detailed discussion of the potential complications associated with the different breast reconstruction operations is included in Chapter 13.)

### Is infection a serious problem after breast reconstruction?

Infection is an infrequent problem after breast reconstruction. It is more likely to occur after an immediate implant or expander reconstruction (a 2% to 10% chance). If infection occurs, the implant or expander usually must be removed to control the infection. Reconstruction can begin again a few months later. Infection after a flap procedure may result in partial flap loss, which would require revision of the flap during another procedure.

### Do flaps used in breast reconstruction ever die or fail? If so, what can be done to complete the reconstruction?

Flaps are an essential component of some reconstructions. A flap is a portion of tissue that is moved from one area of the body to another. For the flap to be successful, transferred tissue must have a plentiful blood supply. If this blood supply is marginal or partially insufficient, a portion of the flap can die· this portion of the flap is therefore lost as a source of tissue for reconstruction.

Reconstruction usually can be completed after partial flap loss. Rarely is the blood supply to the flap so impaired that the entire flap is lost. Potential flap loss usually can be identified during the operation and appropriate measures taken by the surgeon to avoid this problem. Certain general health conditions can impair blood supply to flaps and result in flap loss; for instance, if a woman has diabetes, has received radiation to the flap vessels, has an autoimmune disease, or is a cigarette smoker, blood flow may be reduced.

### What is a worst case scenario for each of the different reconstructive procedures?

Implants and expanders can become exposed and infected, requiring removal. In this instance reconstruction must begin again at a later date. The implant can be reinserted or a flap procedure may be needed. Flaps can fail because of partial or total loss of the blood supply. When a flap fails, another reconstructive technique, either a different flap or an implant procedure, usually will be necessary to complete the reconstruction. More serious complications such as deep vein thrombosis (blood clots in the leg veins or pelvic veins) and pulmonary embolus (blood clots to the lungs) can develop, usually after longer operations; these are rare occurrences, but they are life threatening (see Chapter 13).

### Can a woman die from breast reconstruction?

The risks to life from breast reconstruction are very low. One obvious risk is from anesthetic complications; however, administration of anesthetics is safe in the hands of well-trained anesthesiologists. Reconstruction with implants is also safe. Flap reconstructions, especially with the lower abdominal flap and buttock flap, carry somewhat more risk because of the length of these operations and the risk of blood loss and the development of venous blood clots in the woman's legs. It is possible for these clots to go from the legs (deep vein thrombosis) to the blood vessels of the lungs (pulmonary embolus), a potentially life-threatening condition. The development of blood clots is linked to the length of the operative procedure; these clots are more likely to occur when the operation lasts more than 4 or 5 hours. The use of compression stockings enhances the blood flow and venous return from the legs during the procedure and in the postoperative period and thus decreases the possibility that this problem will develop. The surgeon may also decide to use an anticoagulant in a low dosage to reduce the possibility of a blood clot.

## What are the costs of breast reconstruction?

The costs of breast reconstruction depend on the extent of surgical repair needed, the type of reconstructive operation a woman selects, whether this surgery is performed as an immediate or a delayed procedure, and the number of operations required. Insertion of an implant costs less than a procedure requiring a flap of additional tissue supplied from the back, buttocks, or abdomen. Creating a nipple-areola further increases the price. These decisions affect the length of hospitalization, the length of the operation, and the anesthesia that is required. Costs include the plastic surgeon's fees and the hospital charges. In addition, costs may vary depending on the region of the country. The cost of surgery, as with the cost of living, seems to be higher on the East or West Coast than in other areas of the country.

Immediate breast reconstruction usually costs less. The patient is already hospitalized for a mastectomy and is only anesthetized one time. She recovers from the mastectomy and reconstruction simultaneously. A surgeon's fee for immediate reconstruction without a flap and with the tissues remaining after the mastectomy usually begins at $2500 and goes up from there. Flap operations start at $5000; microsurgical flap procedures are even higher, starting at $8000. It is important to note, however, that some plastic surgeons prefer not to do a flap reconstruction as an immediate procedure because the complexity requires a longer operating time and a greater chance of complications.

If the breast reconstruction is delayed, costs are usually greater. Thus charges for reconstruction with available tissues and implants and expanders may start at $3000, reconstruction with the latissimus dorsi (back muscle) flap at $6000, reconstruction with the TRAM (abdominal) flap at $8000, and microsurgical reconstruction with the gluteus maximus (buttock muscle) flap at $10,000. A second procedure to restore a woman's nipple-areola usually costs upward from $1500 and can be done on an outpatient basis. Reconstruction with available tissues or tissue expansion, if performed as a delayed procedure, also can be done on an outpatient basis, thus lowering the costs. The cost for the implant is additional and now ranges from $1500 to $3500. Costs for managed care contracts, preferred provider organizations, and Medicare are predetermined by contracts and by insurance policies.

These costs are approximate and reflect a range seen in the country today. They are offered merely to give women an idea of the expenses to be anticipated when considering breast reconstruction. Your reconstructive surgeon will tell you the specific costs.

## Will the insurance carrier, HMO, or Medicare cover the costs of breast reconstruction?

Most major medical carriers cover the costs of breast reconstruction after mastectomy based on the restrictions specified in their individual policies. This surgery is not considered cosmetic, but rather reconstructive, and many states have passed laws to ensure coverage by any company delivering health insurance within the state. Coverage varies, however, from state to state. It is wise to check with your insurance carrier before you have breast reconstruction to be sure that part or all of your expenses will be reimbursed. Persistence and assertiveness will sometimes be necessary to get the information that you need. If only a portion of the cost is covered, you need to inquire what percentage is covered and if this coverage is based on the actual cost of the surgery or on a preassigned payment schedule that identifies the "usual and customary fee" for a particular operation as determined by the insurance company. If there is a "usual and customary fee," you need to know what that fee is and how much of your anticipated bill will not be covered so that you can plan accordingly.

Dealing with the medical carrier can be a frustrating experience. It may require additional letters and phone calls, but you should not become discouraged. This is a legitimate reconstructive procedure that qualifies for coverage. It is your right to insist on information and specifically to know the extent of coverage before the operation. A letter from your doctor to the third-party provider may be needed to explain your condition and the need for surgery. Although some carriers still do not cover rehabilitation of any kind, fortunately they are the exception, not the rule. Some insurance carriers may, however, not be familiar with some of the more recently developed breast reconstruction techniques, and you may have to help educate them about the technique that you have selected. Your plastic surgeon can also assist you in this process with a telephone call to the insurance provider and a follow-up letter.

Before a woman decides on reconstructive breast surgery, she should carefully read her health care policy. Some policies stipulate that either a prosthesis or breast reconstruction will be covered but not both. If a woman receives reimbursement for the cost of her prosthesis, the cost of her reconstruction will thus not be covered later. It is necessary for her to be aware of these stipulations so that her eligibility for reimbursement for the costs of reconstruction, which are far greater than the cost of a prosthesis, will not be jeopardized.

In deciding whether she can afford breast reconstruction a woman needs to assess all aspects of her reconstructive surgery. What type of procedure does she plan to have done? Is it going to be done on an immediate or delayed basis? Is her other breast going to be modified? What is her insurance coverage? Does it cover both a prosthesis and reconstruction or does it cover one or the other? Does it cover modification of the other breast? Many policies will cover prophylactic (risk-reducing) mastectomies (the removal of breast tissue as a preventive therapy against the development of cancer in the future), but they will not cover what they consider to be aesthetic changes such as augmentation (enlargement), mastopexy (tightening and lifting of the breast), and reduction (reducing the size of the breast).

If a woman has implants from a former cosmetic breast procedure, she should check to ensure that this will not affect her insurance coverage. Some insurance carriers have withdrawn coverage for women with implants.

For women with no health care coverage and/or limited assets, breast reconstruction is often available through the plastic surgery divisions of university teaching hospitals.

### If considering breast surgery, how should a woman become informed?

When a woman is considering an operation to restructure or reconstruct her breasts, she needs to obtain as much information as possible about the proposed procedure and to consult with a board-certified plastic surgeon with special expertise in breast surgery. (See Chapter 12 for more information on selecting a plastic surgeon.) During the consultation the plastic surgeon should review the patient's condition, discuss her options, and answer any questions she may have. If breast implants and tissue expanders are being considered, the plastic surgeon should describe these devices, detail all potential benefits and risks, and answer questions concerning them or the implant surgery itself. He should also provide the patient with the manufacturer's informed consent documents (these are also approved by the FDA) and have the patient read these documents carefully and ask questions. The plastic surgeon can often provide reading materials to explain the different procedures. A woman should also discuss the operation with her other physicians, and if additional questions need addressing, a second opinion is in order. A woman should make her decision only after all her questions are answered and she understands all of the possible risks and benefits.

### *How does breast reconstruction affect survival rates from breast cancer?*

Many breast cancer experts believe that knowledge about breast reconstruction will save thousands of women's lives. Some women will come for treatment earlier on discovering a mass in their breast if they are aware of the chance for reconstruction after mastectomy. As one expert explains, "This procedure could conceivably have an immense impact upon the entire problem of early detection and treatment of breast cancer."

As breast reconstruction techniques become increasingly sophisticated and widely accepted, more women are seeking information about them. Before deciding for or against breast reconstruction, a woman needs to be apprised of the essential facts concerning this surgery. Her questions should be answered and her doubts should be addressed. This chapter has attempted to provide some of these answers.

# WHAT WOMEN WANT TO KNOW ABOUT BREAST IMPLANTS

Breast implants have been an integral part of breast surgery for almost 35 years. They have been successfully used to restore breast shape and contour after mastectomy, correct breast and chest wall deformities and asymmetries, augment small breasts, and lift sagging ones. Although the efficacy of these devices is widely recognized and acknowledged, in recent years major concerns have arisen about their safety. The intense media coverage of the so-called implant controversy and the Food and Drug Administration (FDA) restrictions on implant availability pending further research heightened public concern. Emotions often triumphed over logic. Today, however, with the passage of time and after numerous scientific studies, this topic can be approached with a fresh perspective. Questions about safety are being fully addressed, the hysteria has largely dissipated, and the breast implant story is no longer front-page news. The scientific facts can stand on their own merit. Recent clinical studies have assuaged earlier fears, allowing these devices to be judged impartially based on the scientific data accumulated.

The following discussion attempts to address women's questions and concerns, to present the facts, to review the latest scientific studies, and to put this topic into perspective so that women can judge for themselves. The majority of this discussion is devoted to questions that women want answered. These queries are those posed by women in personal interviews and surveys. The answers are based on published medical studies and reports, data supplied by experts, and current documented scientific evidence. Unlike the anecdotal reports of individual patients often featured in the media, these scientifically controlled studies compare women with and without implants. The latter group of women, called a *control group*, serves to determine whether health problems in those with implants are occurring more frequently than might be expected in the general population.

We begin by discussing the benefits and risks of these devices.

### What is the value of breast implants?

Breast implants were originally developed in the early 1960s for women who desired breast enhancement. Some of these women's breasts became smaller after pregnancy, and they wanted their breasts to be fuller once again; others thought their breasts were too small, poorly formed, or out of proportion to their total body shape. Implants offered a viable and effective solution to their problems. Building on patient satisfaction with implant surgery for breast enlargement, surgeons soon recognized that these devices were also well suited for restoring breast shape and contour after mastectomy for breast cancer and for correcting breast and chest wall asymmetries and congenital chest wall deformities.

Since the introduction of implants almost 35 years ago, approximately 1 million women in the United States have had breast implant surgery. Implants have made a difference to these women. They have offered a return to normalcy for women with breast cancer and an opportunity to put the cancer experience behind them and get on with their lives. Breast reconstruction has helped these women to feel whole again; they have reported feeling good about themselves once again, with renewed self-confidence and a new zest for life. Still others say that implants have provided them with a more normal body image, a more flattering breast form, or an improved self-image. The benefits of breast implants have been both physical and psychological, and their value for women's health has become more obvious with time. Many cancer specialists believe and our experience would suggest that knowing that breast reconstruction is an option will save many women's lives because they will not procrastinate in seeking care for breast problems for fear of breast loss.

### What are the psychological benefits of breast implants?

Since breast implants are used to enhance small breasts and reconstruct breasts after mastectomy, the benefit is primarily psychological. Women who have had breast implants report that their self-esteem is enhanced—that they feel more attractive, less self-conscious, more feminine, and more self-confident. Women who have had implants for breast reconstruction report that they no longer feel deformed as they did following mastectomy; they feel more normal and less depressed over their appearance. Most describe a restored sense of well-being and relief at not having a "constant reminder of their cancer and mortality."

### What are the physical benefits of implants?

Implants can be used to correct breast or chest wall asymmetries associated with developmental conditions or trauma. They are also used for breast reconstruction after mastectomy. Many women who have had mastectomies report that the implant helps restore a feeling of balance. For women with a large opposite breast, it may also alleviate back and shoulder pain and postural problems caused by attempts to disguise the uneven chest with a heavy external prosthesis. The implant can provide cover for the exposed chest wall, which may be sensitive after breast removal. It can also be used to replace an external prosthesis, thereby affording a woman greater freedom in selecting clothing styles and avoiding the discomfort and skin irritation that sometime accompany use of an external breast prosthesis.

### What is the reported satisfaction rate of women who have had implant surgery?

A number of studies have been done to assess the satisfaction rate after breast implant operations. These studies have shown that over 60% and sometimes as many as 80% to 90% of the women who have had implant surgery for augmentation are pleased with the results of the procedure. Approximately 94% of these women reported that the results of augmentation met their expectations. A 1997 study involving 504 patients at 11 different centers adds further credence to these statistics, reporting overall patient satisfaction at 94.2% after surgery with saline-filled implants (usually for breast augmentation). Similar satisfaction rates have been reported with implant surgery for breast reconstruction; however, because skin may be thinner at the mastectomy site, the possibility of complications is higher for reconstructive procedures than for breast augmentation. Despite problems, most women say, and our surveys confirm, that they would choose to have implant surgery again.

### What kind of breast implants are currently available? What type of fillings are used in them?

Basically there are two broad categories of implants: fixed-volume breast implants and implants in which the volume can be changed after they are implanted (tissue expanders). All of the currently available implants have an outer layer or envelope of silicone that is in contact with the body tissues. These implants are usually filled with saline (saltwater) solution. Silicone gel–filled implants are also available but only on a relatively limited basis in the United States.

Alternate filling materials for the implant envelopes are under investigation to determine if these materials are radiolucent, as opposed to opaque, and easily eliminated or removed by the body if they leak. These fillings will provide possible alternatives to those currently in use. Some of the fillings being investigated include water-based gels; gel-like solutions consisting of water, salts, and organic polymers; and purified soybean oil. Currently no breast implants with alternative fillings are commercially available in the United States. An implant that has a silicone shell filled with a purified soybean oil is presently being studied to determine whether mammograms can more effectively detect breast masses with this type of implant than with a silicone gel–filled or a saline-filled implant.

Implants are also available with smooth and with textured silicone surfaces. Many surgeons believe that these textured surfaces have helped to reduce the incidence of breast hardness (capsular contracture) after implant surgery. However, in some patients these textured-surface implants are more visible and may exhibit a rippled appearance through the skin.

### How do the aesthetic results of operations with saline-filled implants compare to those achieved with silicone gel–filled implants?

Certain characteristics of silicone gel–filled breast implants make them preferable to saline-filled implants. The gel has a more natural consistency than saltwater and feels and flows more like a natural breast. These implants also offer flexibility in designing different breast shapes—some wider, some with additional projection to allow for individualization. Saline-filled implants are more limited in their shape; they are also slightly heavier than silicone gel–filled implants and when overfilled are firm, almost spherical, and therefore feel and look unnatural. When underfilled they can be soft, and their envelopes, which are generally thicker than those containing silicone gel, can develop noticeable and palpable folds and ripples, particularly through thin skin at the mastectomy site. Some of the newer models of saline implants have "shaped" contours that seem to help minimize wrinkling problems and improve the contour of the reconstructed breast.

### Is one brand or type of breast implant better or safer than another?

Although some surgeons have expressed "a higher level of comfort" with the safety of saline-filled implants and others prefer a particular type of implant because they have experienced more success with it, for example, in avoiding certain adverse effects such as capsular contracture, it will not be known for certain whether one brand or model is more effective than another until the FDA evaluates the safety and effectiveness of all breast implants. Ongoing clinical trials are underway to evaluate silicone gel–filled implants. The formal review of the safety and effectiveness of saline-filled implants began in 1993. The information gathered by two U.S. manufacturers has already been submitted to the FDA for evaluation. All preclinical data as well as the deflation and complication rates will be submitted toward the end of 1998.

### Is silicone safe to use in humans?

Silicone, a commonly used substance for various implantable devices, is considered by many to be one of the least reactive biomaterials. Initially introduced for evaluation in medical applications in the 1940s, silicone is used for artificial joints, implantable pumps, shunts, drains, ocular implants, and other devices that require a material that is relatively nonreactive, nonallergenic, and easily tolerated by the body. Implantable silicone devices include pacemakers, hydrocephalus shunts, breast implants, penile implants, and testicular implants. Anyone who has ever taken a capsule has probably ingested silicone, for it is used to coat many capsules to make them more easily swallowed. Silicone is also present in processed foods, in cosmetics, and in many drugs (especially antacids). Silicone is used to lubricate syringes, in intravenous tubing, and in shunts used for chemotherapy. Anyone who has had blood drawn or been given an injection has had some silicone introduced into his or her body. Many infant pacifiers are made of silicone. As Dr. James Potchen, a radiologist at the University of Michigan explains, "Some systemic levels of silicone will be found in every patient with an implant. The fact is that a very low level of silicone is present in everyone. The relationship between use of insulin syringes by diabetics and systemic levels of silicone is just as impressive as that in patients with implants that bleed." If silicone represents a serious chemical hazard to the human body, this should already be apparent because of this chemical's widespread use. The fact is it doesn't. Nevertheless, studies continue to rule out the possibility of currently unrecognized and rare problems. New silicone devices are routinely receiving FDA approval. For example, silicone oil, a new product for reattaching the retina in complicated cases of retinal detachment, has received FDA authorization to be marketed.

### What problems are associated with implants and how often do they occur?

As with all devices, implants are not without problems. They are subject to local complications such as rupture, possible leakage, deflation, displacement, deformation, and capsular contracture, the latter being the most common problem. They also may interfere with mammograms and cause calcium deposits to accumulate in the capsule tissue that forms around implants. Breast implant surgery may cause changes in breast and nipple sensation. These problems are not life threatening, however, and are usually correctable.

One of our most accurate sources on the frequency of local complications is the unaudited 4-year results of the Mentor Adjunct Study (a cooperative effort between Mentor Corporation and the FDA). This study reports the incidence of capsular contracture and the occurrence of complications in 15,544 patients receiving silicone gel–filled breast implants. In this 5-year study the researchers reported capsular contracture rates as follows: 8.8% of patients experienced minimal contracture, 3.7% moderate, and 1.1% severe. The three most frequently cited complications were breast pain, implant wrinkling, and breast asymmetry. Interestingly, only a small percentage of patients (less than 1%) chose to have secondary surgery to have these problems corrected.

### How do the risks associated with saline-filled implants compare to those associated with silicone gel–filled implants?

Shrinkage of the scar tissue (capsular contracture) and calcium deposit formation occur with both saline-filled and silicone gel–filled implants. Deflation of the implant may be more likely with the saline-filled type. When a saline-filled implant develops a leak, it is likely to deflate over a period of hours to days or even weeks, requiring surgical replacement within a month or two or when the implant has lost most of its volume and become flat. Some saline-filled implants will deflate spontaneously, losing all the saline solution at once and requiring re-operation for implant replacement.

### Is there a special risk for women with polyurethane-coated implants?

In about 11% of women who had silicone gel–filled breast implants a type of implant coated with polyurethane foam was used. The coating was designed to reduce the incidence of capsular contracture. These implants are no longer available in the United States because the company manufacturing them has discontinued production.

The polyurethane coating can be chemically broken down under specific laboratory conditions to release tiny amounts of a substance called toluene diamine (TDA), which has been found to cause cancer in laboratory mice. It is not known whether the foam breaks down to TDA in the body; however, the FDA has determined that "it is unlikely that even one of the estimated 110,000 women who got polyurethane foam–covered implants will get cancer as a result of exposure to TDA." Studies using the latest tests to detect minute levels of TDA were conducted under FDA guidance and showed a slight increase in levels of TDA but no indication of an increased risk. According to the FDA, a woman's lifetime cancer risk, if any, is likely to be miniscule, about one in a million over a lifetime.

### What is capsular contracture? Does this pose a serious risk for women who have implant surgery?

A capsule is firm, fibrous scar tissue that forms around a breast implant. This is a characteristic response of the body to isolate any foreign substance; similar scar formation can be observed around most other implants, regardless of whether they contain silicone, including hip implants, artificial joints, hydrocephalus shunts, heart valves, and pacemakers. For unknown reasons, in some cases, the scar tissue capsule may become thick and constrict a soft implant. This phenomenon is referred to as capsular contracture. This condition can make the breast feel harder and firmer than desirable, producing a rounded or spherical breast appearance; sometimes it can also cause pain. The severity of this problem varies with each individual. Ideally, the capsular layer surrounding the implant does not contract and affect the shape of the breast. In some women it manifests itself as a slight breast firmness. Mild contracture requires no treatment. Most women find this minimal firmness acceptable and are not motivated to undergo further adjustments of their reconstructed or augmented breasts. In more severe cases of capsular contracture, however, a woman may experience significant discomfort and elect to have an operation to release some or all of the scar tissue (capsulotomy) or to remove it (capsulectomy). During this secondary operation the surgeon may reposition the implant under the pectoralis major muscle if previously placed over the muscle or he may replace it with a textured-surface implant after releasing or removing the capsule. These textured-surface implants appear to have a lower incidence of capsular contracture. It is usually necessary to remove the scar capsule around the smooth implant before replacing it with the textured-surface implant. Patients who continue to experience problems after surgical correction may decide to have their implants removed. After implant removal (explantation), an aesthetic correction such as a breast lift (mastopexy) may be necessary to achieve an optimal breast appearance. A woman should be informed of this possibility. Some women with firm breasts decide to have the implant and scar tissue removed and replaced or covered with fatty and muscle flap tissue from the back, lower abdomen, or buttocks.

Although capsular contracture may be uncomfortable and produce breast distortion and asymmetry, it is not a health hazard. Rarely this contracture may result in the implant being exposed through thin breast skin. It does not, however, threaten a woman's life or health, and most women who experience this problem can have satisfactory surgical correction. With the newer textured breast implants, capsular contracture is estimated to occur in approximately 2% to 4% of cases in some studies and in as many as 4% to 9% of cases in others. These implants have been on the market for 10 years now, and contracture rates with these devices seem to have remained at this level over time.

### What can be done to avoid capsular contracture? Will exercises help?

The incidence of capsular contracture is lower when the implant is placed behind the pectoral muscle. Using implants with a textured covering also seems to reduce the likelihood of capsular contracture; it is thought that the rough surface prevents a smooth, uniform scar from forming and constricting the implant. When smooth-surface implants are used, some surgeons recommend breast massage of the implant throughout the breast pocket in an effort to prevent or reduce the incidence and severity of fibrous capsule formation around the implant. There is no scientific evidence, however, that breast massage is helpful in preventing contracture, and some surgeons have stopped recommending massage to patients with smooth implants. Massage is not necessary for implants with a textured surface.

### What are calcium deposits? Can they be mistaken for the calcifications associated with breast cancer?

Sometimes calcium forms in the capsule around the breast implant after it has been implanted for many years. These deposits may increase the hardening; however, they have a characteristic appearance on mammography and can be differentiated from calcifications associated with breast cancer. Breast surgery, including breast reduction, breast lift (mastopexy), and breast reconstruction with a woman's own tissues (autologous), can also cause calcifications visible on mammography.

### What effects will breast implant surgery have on breast sensation?

Women having implant surgery for augmentation may experience changes in breast and nipple-areola sensation. Most of these changes are temporary, but in some cases they prove permanent. Women having breast reconstruction with or without implants already have diminished sensation because of the nerves severed during the mastectomy.

### Does a woman who has an implant breast reconstruction still need to have mammograms?

Mammograms are usually not necessary after a mastectomy and breast reconstruction. However, if an implant is placed in the opposite breast for symmetry or balance, this breast still needs to be monitored. Women should inform the breast imager that they have a breast implant or expander so that additional displacement views can be taken to help visualize the extent of the breast tissue.

### Will breast implants interfere with mammograms?

Both saline-filled and silicone gel–filled implants can pose some imaging problems. Silicone gel–filled implants are opaque to x-rays; saline-filled implants are less so; therefore any breast tissue overlying or underlying the implant may be masked by the implant on the breast films. Women who have implants in place should make sure that they inform the breast imager so that the automatic equipment can be properly adjusted and special displacement views can be taken (in addition to the "standard" or routine mammography compression views) to better visualize the breast tissue. Many physicians recommend that patients with implants should have two additional displacement views. The displacement technique (also known as the Eklund or "pinch" technique) was introduced to allow more breast tissue to be visualized in women with breast implants. With these special views and in the absence of significant capsular contracture, satisfactory breast images can be obtained in most women and their breasts can be effectively monitored for possible breast problems. Both compression and displacement views provide better visualization if the implant has been placed under rather than over the chest wall muscle. The new implant fill materials being studied appear to be more radiolucent and may permit better visualization of breast tissue when an implant is in place.

### Should women with implants have more frequent mammograms?

According to Dr. Potchen, "The use of screening mammography in a patient with an implant should be no different than in any other patient. At Michigan State University we currently adhere to the American Cancer Society's guidelines [that recommend yearly mammography for all women 40 years of age and older]. We do not see a need for additional mammographic examinations in individuals who have an implant, and we would not advocate doing mammograms in younger patients." The FDA Update of March 1996 further states that "women with breast implants who are in an age group where routine mammograms are recommended should be sure to have these exams at the recommended intervals."

### What is the proper way to examine the breasts if a woman has implants?

Like all women, those with breast implants should perform regular breast self-examination (BSE) and have regular physician examinations. These examinations take on added significance for women with breast implants because they can also help to reveal any problems that may develop with their implants.

### Can implants slip, shift, or become displaced?

During the initial operation the plastic surgeon places the implant in the best position to provide the desired breast appearance. During the process of healing, with the development of capsular contracture, and over time the implants can shift or become displaced. This can occur because of the pull of gravity on a smooth implant or subsequent to a capsular contracture, which can elevate the implant. This problem occurs less frequently when a textured breast implant has been used because the rough surface usually adheres to the surrounding tissue, thereby minimizing the chance of displacement.

### Can the implant be rejected by a woman's body?

"Rejection" means an allergic or immune response that causes the body to literally reject a foreign substance. In this sense implants are not rejected. However, the overlying breast skin may become thinned, infection can develop, or healing may be incomplete, leading to exposure and necessitating removal of the implant. Although these are complications, they are not tantamount to rejection.

### Can an implant be removed?

Yes. When an implant is not performing the function for which it was intended, or if the woman feels that she would be better off without the implant, it can be removed. In most cases this is a relatively minor operation, that can often be performed on an outpatient basis. She should ask her plastic surgeon if the capsule should also be removed. The procedure for capsule removal is called capsulectomy. The patient should decide, in consultation with the plastic surgeon, if additional aesthetic corrections will be necessary after removal.

### Should women diagnosed with rheumatic diseases have their implants removed?

This is not necessary, according to noted rhematologists, Drs. John Sergent, Howard Fuchs, and John Johnson. "We do not recommend that women with implants who acquire rheumatic diseases have intact implants removed. It has been recommended for some time that ruptured implants be removed, although this, too, is somewhat controversial if the rupture is contained within the fibrous capsule. If contractures are painful and tender, the decision to remove the implant must be balanced against the expected cosmetic result and the operative risks. . . . It is sometimes appropriate to have the implant and associated capsule removed in these patients."

### Should women who have polyurethane-coated breast implants consider having them removed?

According to the FDA, "There is insufficient evidence at present to support having polyurethane-coated breast implants surgically removed because of concerns about cancer. The risks of the operation itself to remove or replace the implants are far higher than the risks of keeping the implants."

### If a woman needs to have her implants removed because of a problem, or chooses to have them removed because she is concerned about them, will this procedure be reimbursed?

Some insurance carriers will cover implant removal for certain types of problems. The financial arrangements for implant removal should be discussed with your surgeon and your insurance carrier before any decision is made.

### What are the manufacturers' replacement policies for saline-filled implants in case of leakage or deflation?

Both McGhan Medical (Inamed) Corporation and Mentor Corporation, the two companies supplying the bulk of saline-filled implants in the United States, offer patients full lifetime replacement in the event of deflation due to loss of shell or valve integrity.

### How long do breast implants last?

The silicone breast implant has been available for use in patients since 1964, and many of the original devices are still in place. Just as human and artificial organs can fail and require transplantation, breast implants also may have to be replaced.

No precise figures on the life span of silicone gel–filled or saline-filled implants are available at present. The ongoing clinical studies and product research should help clarify this. It is known that implants can last from a very short time to many years, depending on the surgical technique used, the patient, and her implant. In any case, breast implants should not be considered "lifetime" devices. Women should be followed up by their physicians over the long term so their breasts can be monitored for possible problems as a part of their general health care regimen.

### How strong are implants? Will they break on impact? Can they be broken during mammography?

Breast implants are manufactured to specific standards requiring that they resist breast compression as well as multiple and long-term physical stress. These devices, however, are not indestructible. Although the outer shell of the implant is quite sturdy, it can break if subjected to severe physical trauma. A sharp or blunt injury to the chest wall and breast, such as pressure from a seat belt during a car accident, can cause this problem. The envelope can also tear if it is inadvertently cut or nicked by instruments during surgery. Compression views taken during mammography are calibrated to avoid undue pressure that could rupture a breast implant. According to Dr. Potchen, "There is no evidence that compression or displacement mammography has caused implant rupture."

### What factors increase the chance that an implant will rupture?

The chance for rupture may increase with the length of time the implant has been in the body and with normal wear and tear. The incidence of rupture is increased when the implant develops folds or rippling on the outer surface. Trauma or injury to the breast also increases the chance of rupture, as may closed capsulotomy (a technique to correct capsular contracture in which strong pressure is applied to the breast to break up the scar tissue around the implant). This technique is less frequently used today and is not recommended by the manufacturers.

### What percentage of implants rupture?

Results from recently released clinical studies revealed a low rupture rate of 0.06% for silicone gel–filled implants. Researchers at Mallinckrodt Institute of Radiology and Washington University Medical School in St. Louis have detected a 5% to 6% rate of implant rupture or leakage among the women with implants they studied. Researchers at the Mayo Clinic found a similar rupture incidence of 5.7%. Other reports from Scotland and California revealed even lower rates of rupture.

Earlier model implants, made with thinner envelopes and containing a different gel configuration, are thought to have a higher rate of rupture and leakage. These thin-walled implants, produced in the mid-1970s to the mid-1980s, are no longer being made. Some have suggested that the envelope failure rate seems to increase after 10

years of implantation. Since the mid-1980s a low-bleed implant envelope has been used and is more resistant to rupture.

### How can a woman tell if she has a ruptured or deflated implant?

Any noticeable change in the shape, size, feel, or comfort of the breast
could signal implant rupture. For women with saline-filled implants,
this change in breast size and shape is often more noticeable when
leakage and absorption of the saltwater solution by the surrounding
tissues causes implant deflation. When such symptoms occur, a patient should see her plastic surgeon for evaluation. According to the
FDA, "It is possible for a woman to experience rupture of the implant
without symptoms, but women should not have routine mammograms
(x-rays of the breasts) just to detect these 'silent' ruptures if they are
not experiencing any symptoms."

### What happens if a saline-filled implant deflates?

There is a possibility of deflation with saline-filled implants if a leak
develops in the implant covering and will require possible reoperation
with implant replacement. Currently available saline-filled inflatable
implants have a relatively low deflation rate. One-year cumulative
results from the clinical trials conducted by the two remaining U.S.
implant manufacturers reveal deflation rates ranging from 1.7% by
one of the companies to 3.7% by the other. A study conducted at the
University of Minnesota of 504 patients receiving saline-filled implants reported a 5.5% deflation rate. As with silicone gel–filled implants, saline-filled implants should not be considered lifetime devices.

### What happens if a silicone gel–filled implant leaks?

When the cover of a silicone gel–filled implant is pierced or ruptures,
the gel usually remains within the fibrous capsule or membrane that
develops naturally around the implant and does not travel to other
parts of the body. Significant trauma can cause tears in the surrounding capsule, and the gel can migrate into the breast and possibly beyond the breast to form lumps (granulomas) nearby. Some of this silicone can cause enlarged lymph nodes in the armpit area (lym-
phadenopathy). When silicone escapes to other parts of the body,
such as the arm or upper abdomen, removal can be difficult. Gel
migration outside the capsule rarely occurs, however, and, if it does,

the viscosity (or thickness) of the gel seems to reduce its ability to migrate.

### What is silicone bleed?

Silicone bleed refers to microscopic amounts of silicone fluid that seep through the implant's envelope. Although most of this is trapped within the implant pocket or the surrounding scar tissue, minute amounts of silicone could possibly migrate through the capsule. The majority of implants manufactured after 1985 have a low-bleed design that reduces leakage.

### Can ultrasound, magnetic resonance imaging, or mammography be used to detect implant leakage or rupture?

Ultrasonography is an adjunct to mammography that can be useful in detecting implant rupture. Computed tomography (CT) scans have also been used but require a relatively high dose of radiation compared with mammography. Magnetic resonance imaging (MRI) is not recommended for routine screening, but it is a useful adjunct to mammography for evaluation of implant integrity for possible leakage as well as the actual breast for masses and cancer. Dr. Potchen reports that "MRI is currently the most accurate way of determining whether an implant has ruptured. It is an expensive and perhaps unnecessary approach depending on whether the rupture produces symptoms or is likely to create subsequent problems. It also depends on whether it is a *capsulated* [italics ours] rupture [in which the gel is contained in the capsule that surrounds the implant] or whether silicone has leaked into other tissues. Generally a crude estimate of rupture can be pretty well determined on a mammogram. Even at that, I would not recommend using mammography in patients younger than 30. One advantage of ultrasonography or MRI is that there is no ionizing radiation."

### Is there a test to detect silicone in the body or determine whether a woman is sensitive to silicone?

No. According to the FDA, "There is no FDA-approved, standard test to detect silicone in the body. . . . Even if simple techniques for silicone detection were available, they might not be useful in detecting a rupture, because small amounts of silicone ordinarily 'bleed' even from intact implants." Furthermore, since silicone is found in food and many other products, including commonly used medicines and cosmetics, individuals have quantities of silicone in their bodies regardless of whether they have breast implants. Therefore, "the tests would not easily determine whether the silicone came from the implant or another source."

As the FDA has indicated, "Determining that silicon or silicone is present in body fluids does not indicate whether a person is sensitive to these substances or at risk for any specific disease. There is presently no test to determine if a person is sensitive to silicone or silicon."

### Do ruptured implants and leakage of silicone gel pose a major health hazard?

Not according to Drs. John E. Woods and Phillip G. Arnold, two plastic surgeons from the Mayo Clinic. In an article in *The Wall Street Journal* they explain that "over the years, we have removed many ruptured implants, not because the patient has complained of any symptoms but simply in the process of releasing capsules or exchanging the implants. We have not seen any serious consequences in patients with ruptured implants. Silicone gel is readily removed from the pocket and has only extremely rarely been associated with postoperative problems. We believe that when ruptures are known to exist, it is appropriate to remove the implants. In most patients, however, the presence of ruptured implants is not detectable, is asymptomatic, and is not likely to cause problems."

A more recent Mayo Clinic study conducted by Drs. John E. Woods and Michael Duffy concluded that their 30-year clinical experience with silicone gel breast implants for augmentation mammaplasty and breast reconstruction "failed to demonstrate that clinically evident adverse health problems are incurred by those women who subsequently experience a silicone gel breast implant failure."

These data do not suggest that women with breast implants are not subject to the usual health problems that affect the population at large. Breast cancer, heart disease, and arthritis, to name a few, are common health problems confronted by all women.

### What are the risks if a saline-filled implant ruptures?

Although the safety of saline-filled implants is being evaluated by the FDA, leakage or deflation of these implants results in release of saline solution (saltwater), which is not foreign to the body, thus avoiding some of the concerns associated with silicone gel. (The saltwater is absorbed after it leaks out, resulting in deflation of the implant.) Because saline-filled implants do not contain silicone gel, fewer questions have been raised about their safety; they are still available without restriction for both augmentation and reconstruction. But since both types of implants have an outer silicone elastomer envelope, the long-term safety of which is being studied, the saline-filled implants may not be entirely without risk and are being reviewed by the FDA.

### What should be done if an implant ruptures?

If a woman suspects possible implant rupture, she should see her doctor. Many experts recommend that removal of a ruptured implant be considered. Frequently the capsule surrounding the implant or a portion of it may have to be removed at this time. If the implant rupture is confined to the capsule, many women have chosen to avoid an operation, to leave the contained leaking implant in place, and to take a "wait and watch" approach under medical supervision.

### What should women with implants do to minimize possible problems?

Women with implants should take the time to inform themselves about their implants. This means finding out specifically what type of implants they have, the date of implantation, the manufacturer, and the model number. They can obtain a copy of the package insert (instructions accompanying the implant and providing information on possible risks and complications for that device model). It is also crucial for all breast cancer patients and for women with implants to practice monthly BSE, to have regular physician examinations, and to report any problems, changes, or concerns to their doctors. They should keep in close contact with their doctors for adequate follow-up. Finally, joining a breast implant registry through the implant manufacturer will help to ensure that women are kept informed about safety issues for these devices. Tracking of breast implants is mandated by the FDA.

### Can silicone gel–filled or saline-filled implants cause cancer?

Silicone breast implants have been available for almost 35 years and during that time have been studied extensively by plastic surgeons, implant manufacturers, scientists, and government regulatory agencies such as the FDA. In all of that time no scientific studies have documented an increased risk of breast cancer attributable to breast implants nor is there any evidence that these devices have adversely affected the course of breast cancer when they are used for breast reconstruction. Large population studies from California, Denmark, Sweden, France, and Canada have all indicated that the incidence of breast cancer in women with silicone breast implants is the same or possibly lower than in women who have not had implants. Interestingly, several studies (such as the one conducted in Los Angeles) reported a lower incidence of cancer occurring in women with implants. The FDA's current informed consent document serves to underscore these findings. It states, "There is presently no scientific evidence that links either silicone gel–filled or saline-filled breast implants with cancer."

### Is there any scientific evidence to prove that silicone gel–filled implants pose potential dangers to a woman's health?

After studying the information about silicone gel–filled breast implants provided by its consultants, the FDA stated that more data are needed about these devices, but there is no evidence that they cause breast cancer or autoimmune diseases.

### What do cancer specialists say about the dangers of breast implants? Is there a risk of cancer from breast implants?

The research from cancer experts and institutions throughout the world seems to indicate a general consensus that breast implants do not increase a woman's risk of developing breast cancer. Studies conducted by researchers from the U.S. National Cancer Institute, the International Epidemiology Institute and the Karolinska Institute in Sweden, the Danish Cancer Registry, the Fred Hutchinson Cancer Research Center, the Institut Gustave Roussy in France, the Alberta Canada Cancer Board, and the U.S. Centers for Disease Control and Prevention, among others, have all found that there was no greater incidence of breast cancer among women with implants than in the general population. Large population studies seem to confirm this finding, such as the one conducted at the University of Southern California School of Medicine, which concluded "that there is no increase in breast cancer incidence following augmentation mammaplasty." Additional studies are under way to study implants and their long-term impact on a woman's health.

### What are connective tissue disorders? What symptoms are associated with these diseases?

These are rare disorders such as lupus erythematosus, dermatomyositis, scleroderma, and rheumatoid arthritis in which the body reacts to its own tissue as though it were a foreign material. A combination of symptoms may characterize these disorders, including the generalized symptoms of joint pain and swelling; tight, red, or swollen skin; swollen glands and lymph nodes; extreme fatigue; local symptoms of swelling of the hands and feet; skin rashes; and unusual hair loss.

The FDA advises a woman who experiences these symptoms to "see her regular doctor if the symptoms do not subside, because these complaints could be indicators of a variety of health problems, not just immune-related disorders."

### Can implants cause connective tissue or autoimmune disease in healthy women?

There have been allegations that implants can cause or exacerbate immune-related or connective tissue disorders (also referred to as collagen vascular diseases or incorrectly as human adjuvant disease). This possibility has been carefully evaluated by respected immunologists and rheumatologists in numerous national and international scientific studies. The consensus after extensive scientific investigation seems to be that there is no conclusive scientific evidence to indicate that there is an increased incidence of such diseases in patients with breast implants. Although these conditions may exist concurrently, there is no evidence that a silicone implant has caused or contributed to autoimmune disease. Even the FDA's own *Epidemiological Review* published in 1996 concurs that "current research has tended to rule out large increases in risk for connective tissue disease caused by breast implants." Following is an overview of some of the studies that address this question.

Scientific studies conducted at the Mayo Clinic, Harvard Medical School, University of Michigan School of Public Health, Emory University, University of Kansas Arthritis Center, University of Texas M.D. Anderson Cancer Center, University of Washington Fred Hutchinson Cancer Research Center, University of Toronto, University of Maryland, University of Pittsburgh, University of California, San Diego, and Johns Hopkins University Schools of Medicine have revealed no association between silicone gel breast implants and connective tissue disease. The 1996 Women's Health Cohort Study conducted at Brigham & Women's Hospital, Harvard Medical School, evaluated 10,380 women with silicone breast implants and a control group of 384,713 women without implants. After considering all available evidence, this large study concluded that "women with breast implants should be reassured that there is no large risk of connective tissue disease."

In a *New England Journal of Medicine* article published in 1995 Dr. Jorge Sánchez-Guerrero and his colleagues analyzed the data from 14 years of follow-up of a National Institutes of Health (NIH)–funded study from Brigham & Women's Hospital, Harvard Medical School. This study examined the incidence of connective tissue disease and 41 signs, symptoms, or laboratory findings of connective tissue disease among a group of 87,500 registered nurses between the ages of 30 and 55. The authors concluded that "there was no evidence of an association between silicone breast implants and connective-tissue diseases defined according to a variety of standardized criteria or signs and symptoms of these diseases."

International studies have come to the same overall conclusions. Research conducted in Australia, Canada, Denmark, and Sweden also failed to find "a causal relationship between the implantation and the development of connective tissue disease."

An article published in *Arthritis and Rheumatism* summarizes recent research by investigators from Brigham & Women's Hospital, Harvard Medical School, Robert B. Brigham Multipurpose Arthritis Center, Saint Thomas Hospital, and Vanderbilt University School of Medicine. This article reports that the clinical, immunologic, and epidemiologic evidence to date "suggests little or no association between silicone breast implants and CTD [connective tissue disease] or a unique arthralgia/myalgia/fibromyalgia syndrome."

This lack of causal relationship is given additional support and credibility by the American College of Rhematology's Revised Statement on Silicone Breast Implants published in the *Journal of the American Medical Association* in 1996. The College concludes that current large studies "provide compelling evidence that silicone implants expose patients to no demonstrable additional risk for connective tissue or rheumatic disease. Anecdotal evidence should no longer be used to support this relationship in the courts or by the FDA."

### What advice should rheumatologists and immunologists give to patients contemplating implant surgery?

Dr. John Sergent, a respected rheumatologist, advises informing patients that "a few reports have indicated a relationship between implants and various rheumatic diseases. The number of patients reported is small, and considering the total number of implants, it may not even be a valid observation. If there is a causal relationship, it is clearly a rare event."

### Should women diagnosed with connective tissue diseases or autoimmune diseases have reconstruction with breast implants?

These diseases are rare, and scientific studies are under way to define and better understand these conditions. As a precaution, however, if a woman has any of these conditions or has a family history of these conditions, she should probably not have silicone gel–filled or saline-filled implants until the results of current population studies and other information are available. As Dr. John Sergent explains, "My recommendation for patients with scleroderma is to minimize trauma of any kind. That would include all cosmetic surgery, not just implants. Many patients with scleroderma request cosmetic surgery to correct the perioral wrinkles they all have, and I strongly discourage them. Most of them do well with surgery; the skin heals quite well. However, there are some patients who have an exuberant fibrotic reaction. My across-the-board recommendation for patients with scleroderma is that all elective surgery should be avoided—implants or anything else." Women with these problems are also poor candidates for radiation therapy and musculocutaneous flaps.

### Can implants cause neurologic disease in healthy women?

According to the American Academy of Neurology, "there really is no evidence from what has been published that breast implants are associated with or cause neurologic disease." Dr. John Ferguson, chairman of the Academy's Therapeutics and Technology Assessment Subcommittee, speculates that the reason many people think breast implants cause health problems is because the FDA took implants off the market in 1992. "That made women think, 'Maybe there's something wrong and maybe this ache or that pain is caused by this device.' I think the women who have complaints are suffering, but I think there's no good evidence from what I can see regarding either autoimmune disease or certainly not in neurologic disease that that's the cause of their problems."

### Is it possible to be allergic to silicone implants or to the silicone gel within them?

As mentioned earlier, silicone has been used in medical devices and oral and parenteral medications for over 40 years, and there is no scientific evidence that individuals can develop allergies to these devices. It may be possible, however, to develop antibodies to the silicone. The mere presence of antibodies, however, does not indicate the presence of disease. The body's normal process of dealing with foreign bodies is an immune response with subsequent development of antibodies. Further studies will need to be conducted to determine if there are actually any allergic reactions.

### What possible complications can occur with implant surgery?

As with any surgical procedure, there is the potential for complications, including reactions to anesthesia as well as infection, hematoma, bleeding, seroma, and delayed wound healing with possible implant exposure requiring removal.

### Are there any recorded deaths from breast implants?

There are no reports in the medical literature of breast implants being responsible for a single death. There is an inherent risk of serious complications and even death from any operation, but this is usually related to the risk of anesthesia for a period of time. This risk is somewhat higher for longer operations, particularly if the operation lasts for more than 4 hours. However, the risk is still considered very small.

### How does the incidence of complications from implant surgery compare to the incidence of complications from other common operations such as appendectomies, mastectomies, and hysterectomies?

The rate of complications experienced after breast implantation is comparable to and sometimes lower than the rate of complications from other commonly performed operations. A study by Dr. Sherine Gabriel and colleagues published in the *New England Journal of Medicine* in 1997 examined the rate of local complications requiring reoperation in women with breast implants. The researchers found that approximately 24% of the women studied experienced at least one surgically treated complication over the period of follow-up. According to Dr. Gabriel, "These rates are about the same as the rates reported for breast reconstruction without implants and are comparable to reports from other centers." Patients having breast implant surgery generally have a lower incidence of conditions such as infection, hematoma, pulmonary emboli, and deep vein thrombosis. However, reoperation because of capsular contracture or to achieve a better final breast appearance is necessary in a significant number of cases.

**Why don't women just have reconstruction with their own natural tissue from their abdomen, buttock, or back instead of incurring the risks of a foreign material?**

Many women want an operation that can be done either as an outpatient procedure or with minimal down time, expense, and inconvenience. For them, implant reconstruction is the best choice because it affords the convenience, short recovery period, and reduced cost they desire. This is also the procedure of choice for a woman who does not want any additional scars, a necessary consequence of most flap procedures. Implant surgery is a good choice for a slender woman who may not have enough fatty tissue for a flap procedure or for a woman with a medical condition that places her at increased risk if she has a more complex operation such as a TRAM (abdominal) flap, latissimus dorsi (back) flap, or a free flap. Furthermore, many surgeons experienced in breast reconstruction techniques with implants and expanders prefer these operations for most patients over the more involved flap procedures.

**What are the risks involved with flap surgery? How do these risks compare to those encountered in implant surgery?**

The decision to have breast reconstruction with a flap or with a breast implant involves an analysis of the risks and benefits of the two approaches. Flap operations take longer, which means increased risks of major surgical complications such as deep vein thrombosis, pulmonary complications, and fluid retention. The success of flap procedures depends on the blood supply of the flaps; if this is compromised, part or all of the flap can be lost. Fortunately, this is a rare occurrence. The shaping of the flap tissue into a breast form also requires more skill and artistry on the part of the surgeon than that required for placement of a breast implant or expander. The obvious benefit of autologous flap reconstruction is that it creates a lasting, more natural breast symmetry that is usually maintained for a lifetime and uses the woman's own tissues, generally without the need for an implant.

The perioperative risks of implant reconstruction are less serious and pose a lower chance of major complications. The benefits of breast reconstruction with breast implants are also significant for the patient who can have a successful procedure with minimal inconvenience and cost. The drawback of this approach is that a deflation or rupture can occur or a capsular contracture can develop around the breast implant and may require additional procedures in the future. Additionally, implants are not considered lifetime devices and may have to be replaced at some point in the future.

## What is the FDA's role in testing and evaluating implants and expanders?

The FDA has been charged with regulating all medical devices since 1976 and is involved in an ongoing evaluation of the safety and efficacy of breast implants. The FDA designates these devices as class III, which means that they must have premarket approval of their safety and efficacy. During the early 1990s the FDA conducted hearings on polyurethane-covered implants and silicone gel–filled implants. Saline-filled implants are currently in the final phases of FDA review. It is anticipated that the final clinical study documentation along with the premarket approval application will be required to be submitted to the FDA on all saline products before the close of 1998.

## Why has the FDA evaluated breast implants if they are not dangerous?

The FDA investigation into the safety of silicone breast implants is merely an example of a government agency performing its legally mandated regulatory function. When the FDA was granted authority to regulate medical devices in 1976, 100,000 devices being distributed were required to be registered with the FDA and were permitted to remain on the market pending later review. Breast implants were included on the FDA's list for review, but devices such as heart valves and intrauterine devices (IUDs) were scrutinized first. It took from 1976 until 1988 (when the review process was completed for some of these other devices) before the FDA turned its attention to breast implants and officially placed them into a class III category, a designation assigned to most other permanently implantable medical devices. This classification requires manufacturers to submit comprehensive safety and effectiveness data in order to secure premarket approval. FDA hearings and mandated clinical trials are part of this ongoing review process as silicone gel–filled and saline-filled implants are scrutinized to ensure that they meet certain safety and effectiveness standards.

### What is the current ruling concerning silicone gel–filled breast implant availability?

All women desiring silicone gel–filled breast implants are required to enter clinical trials sponsored by the implant manufacturer and approved by the FDA. Any woman who needs an implant for breast reconstruction is permitted access to these trials or studies, including women who have had breast cancer surgery, women with traumatic breast injuries, and women with severe breast or chest wall deformities or asymmetries. Also eligible are women with an existing breast implant that needs to be replaced for medical reasons. Only a very limited number of women are able to receive silicone gel–filled breast implants for reoperative breast augmentation (as a secondary procedure never as a primary procedure), and these women must enroll in strictly controlled clinical studies referred to as adjunct studies. Participants in all of these studies must read and sign a detailed informed consent form, be closely followed by their doctors after their operation, and have periodic checkups for 5 years after implantation. Women in these studies are enrolled in a patient registry established by the manufacturers.

### What is a clinical trial?

A clinical trial is basically a controlled study of patients who are receiving a prescribed treatment or combination of treatments. Clinical trials may be used to determine the usefulness of operations, drugs, devices, or treatments as well as their safety and effectiveness and risks and benefits. Each study is designed to answer scientific questions and to find new and better ways to help patients. Clinical trials have long been used in breast cancer research for evaluating new treatments. Often one or more treatments are compared. Currently clinical trials have been designed to study the safety and effectiveness of breast implants. Many of these studies have been completed.

*Are women who want these implants for breast augmentation
allowed to get them in the United States if they are not participating
in the clinical studies?*

No. Although silicone gel–filled implants are still manufactured by
two companies in the United States, their distribution and use in the
United States is restricted to these studies. However, they are widely
available in many other countries through their respective National
Health Services. In the United States saline implants continue to be
widely available for reconstruction and the only alternative for augmentation.

*What actions are other countries taking concerning silicone
gel–filled breast implants?*

Other countries have also investigated the allegations concerning
breast implants and their possible link to systemic disease. The British
government has concluded that there is "no evidence of any association between breast implants and connective tissue disease and therefore no reason to alter practice or policy in the United Kingdom." The
Australian Medical Association issued a statement that said, "Despite
legal interest and media publicity, scientific evidence for silicone-asso-
ciated diseases is lacking." A similar conclusion was reached by a
Swedish study of 10,000 women published in the *British Medical Journal* in February 1998. This study found that women who receive
breast implants have no increased risk of developing connective tissue
disorders.

The European Committee on Quality Assurance and Medical
Devices (EQUAM) in Plastic Surgery has issued a consensus declara-
tion stating that "there is conclusive scientific, clinical, immunologi-
cal, and epidemiological proof that silicone breast implants do not
cause identified and recognized autoimmune diseases nor connective
tissue diseases. At present there is no scientifically identified 'new disease' caused by silicone implants . . . [and] . . . no such thing as silicone allergy, nor silicone [associated] disease nor intoxication. There
is an immune reaction to every foreign body, but this is not identical
with immune disease."

*Why are women who want implants for augmentation restricted
in their access whereas women who want them for reconstruction
are not subject to the same restrictions?*

The rationale for this distinction seems to go beyond the scientific evidence available. Scientific studies have revealed no evidence to link

these devices with cancer or autoimmune conditions. Even so, access to silicone gel–filled breast implants is restricted to all women who need them for breast reconstruction for "compassionate use" but only to a limited number of women desiring them for secondary breast augmentation operations, never for primary augmentation. All women receiving implants must participate in controlled clinical trials. Many physicians and breast cancer patients have questioned the logic of these restrictions. Why are implants not safe for healthy women but okay for women with breast cancer whose immune systems may already be compromised by their bout with cancer?

### Why were women with intact older model silicone gel–filled implants told not to have them removed whereas access to the newer models was restricted?

To gather more information on silicone gel–filled breast implants, the FDA requires all women receiving them to enter controlled clinical trials. However, since the scientific information from numerous clinical studies seems to indicate that these devices do not pose a serious health risk (i.e., cause cancer or autoimmune problems), the FDA has advised patients not to have them removed as long as they have not ruptured and continue to give the patient some benefit. The FDA and physicians believe that the risk of an operation, with the attendant anesthetic and operative risks, is far greater than leaving the devices intact. Why have a potentially risky operation to change something that is performing well and is not broken?

### Why are silicone implants subject to such stringent regulation when other silicone products are not subject to similar regulations?

Governmental agencies such as the FDA are bound by specific laws and directives in carrying out their regulatory duties. They are also susceptible to political pressures, the press, and individual interest groups. The individuals interested in this product made their positions known and lobbied the FDA to ban silicone gel–filled implants. The agency responded accordingly. Other silicone devices, however, will be reviewed in the future, but lobbying efforts against these silicone products have not been as intense or attracted as much media attention.

### What should women who already have silicone gel–filled implants do about their implants?

It is important to bear in mind that most women do not experience serious problems with their implants. Women who are not experiencing any problems with their breast implants should monitor their breasts just as if they did not have implants. This includes careful, monthly BSE, regular physician examination, and breast imaging as recommended. They should also schedule periodical follow-up visits to their plastic surgeon.

### What is the status of saline-filled breast implants and tissue expanders?

Saline-filled breast implants, which contain saltwater rather than silicone gel, are currently on the market and available to all patients. In 1993 the FDA directed the two manufacturers of saline-filled implants (Mentor and McGhan Medical) to conduct clinical trials to prove the safety and effectiveness of these products. These studies focus on frequency of problems such as rupture/deflation, capsular contracture, infection, and short-term complications. Quality-of-life issues are also being examined. Mentor and McGhan Medical have now completed all preclinical testing as well as clinical retrospective and prospective studies. It is anticipated that the FDA will call for all remaining data by the end of 1998.

### With silicone gel–filled implants available only to women enrolled in clinical trials, will women who need them for reconstruction be reimbursed as before?

Reimbursement policies of health insurance companies or other health care providers are not determined by government agencies. However, since the legal status of implants used for breast reconstruction has not changed and they are not considered "investigational," there appears to be no reason why reimbursement policies should change. To be certain about payment issues, however, a woman should always check with her insurance company or health care provider before she schedules an operation.

### How have the regulations on breast implants affected insurance coverage for women who have already had implant surgery? Is their insurance coverage jeopardized?

This, of course, has been a major concern for individuals with silicone breast implants. Coverage varies with the different companies and group policies and with different health maintenance organizations and managed health care organizations. There is evidence that individual insurance companies with individual policies have sometimes excluded coverage for future breast problems for women with silicone breast implants (even when the problems are not related to their implants). A number of lawsuits have been filed against insurance companies concerning this issue. Now with the accumulating scientific data to support women's claims for coverage, the pendulum seems to be swinging back in their favor.

### *If a woman wants to have breast implants for reconstruction, what should she do to make sure they are covered by insurance?*

Most insurance companies do not cover "cosmetic" surgery; however, they do reimburse breast cancer patients for the costs of breast reconstruction after mastectomy, including the cost of breast implants. Seventeen states now mandate coverage for breast reconstruction, ranging from covering just the mastectomy breast to covering a procedure on the opposite breast (augmentation, reduction, or breast lift) for symmetry or risk prevention (prophylactic mastectomy). Currently, federal legislation is under consideration to mandate breast reconstruction with the option of an opposite breast implant for symmetry. As a precaution, it is best to contact your insurance company before any anticipated operation. Your physician can often provide essential information to give to the insurance company related to the specific medical diagnosis, the specifics of the procedure, and the computer code numbers necessary for predetermination of coverage and an explanation of your benefits under the policy.

In addition, the FDA advises women to get written answers from their insurance company to the following questions:
- Does my policy cover the costs of the implant surgery, the implant, the anesthesia, and other related hospital costs?
- Does it cover treatments for medical problems that may be caused by either the implant or the reconstruction?
- Does it cover removal of the implants if this becomes necessary?

### *What types of information are we attempting to gather about silicone gel–filled breast implants from the clinical trials and other studies that are being conducted?*

The studies are seeking answers to the following questions:
- What is the expected life of implants?
- How often do implants leak or rupture?

- What happens to gel that escapes into the body?
- How do you measure silicone in the body?
- How do you measure sensitivity to silicone?
- How often do women with implants suffer problems?
- Do implants cause or increase the risk of cancer?
- Do implants cause or exacerbate connective tissue disorders?

### What types of information are the saline-filled implant clinical trials trying to gather?

The trials are seeking answers to the following questions:
- How often do saline-filled implants leak/deflate?
- What is the incidence of capsular contracture after saline-filled implant surgery?
- How often do infections occur before, during, or after saline-filled implant surgery?
- How often do women with saline-filled implants suffer with short-term complications?
- How does breast implant surgery affect a patient's quality of life?

### What is an IDE?

An Investigational Device Exemption (IDE) is a permit that allows a physician to use a device that has not been approved if it is part of a closely controlled clinical study. Participation in an IDE study requires the investigator to supply additional information concerning the safety and effectiveness of the devices. Classification of the study under an IDE ensures that the clinical trials will be structured to gather this information under strictly controlled circumstances. Currently, silicone gel–filled implants used for reconstruction are not included under an IDE, but are monitored under a study referred to as an Adjunct Study.

### What does informed consent really mean?

"Informed consent" is a legal term that means that the individual contemplating a certain treatment be fully informed of all of the goals and specifics of the treatment as well as its possible consequences. To be truly "informed" this patient must be provided with this information in verbal and in written form and in terms that are clear and understandable. Risks and benefits of the procedure as well as possible complications and their consequences must be fully described and explained.

### What type of informed consent is required for a woman getting silicone gel–filled or saline-filled breast implants?

Informed consent documents for silicone gel–filled and saline-filled implants have been developed by the implant manufacturers in cooperation with the FDA.

### What is an implant registry? What is its purpose? Why should a woman participate?

An implant registry is a (FDA-mandated) central computerized data bank established by manufacturers in the implant business. (Former manufacturers do not have registries.) The registry contains pertinent information on patients and their implants. The woman's name, address, and other personal data are kept on file. It also contains information concerning her saline- or silicone-filled breast implant. For the registry to function optimally, this information should be updated periodically. The purpose of the registry is to provide ready access to women who are enrolled so that they can be contacted if there is new information concerning their implants. Information recorded in the registry can also be used to provide data to direct further study of the device. The implant registry is confidential. The FDA is the only group, other than the manufacturers themselves, that has access to this data.

### How can a woman find out how to join a registry? Is there a fee?

Each of the two U.S. implant manufacturers still in the implant business provides a registry for women using that company's implants. This type of registry is funded and organized by the manufacturer and there is no fee for participation. A patient can sign up for the prospective (for new patients) or retrospective (for previous patients) registry sponsored by the manufacturer through her doctor. As a member of the registry a patient agrees to inform the registry via change-of-address cards or by calling a toll-free number if her name or address has changed and/or if her implant has been removed or replaced subsequent to implant surgery.

### If a woman already has implants, is she still eligible to join an implant registry? Or if she didn't sign up for the manufacturer registry, can she still do so?

Yes. The manufacturers offer both a retrospective registry and a prospective registry. Contact the company that manufactured the implants you have to enroll.

### How can a woman find out what type of implants she has?

Women who already have implants can find out what implant was used from their surgeons or from hospital records, if available. Those planning on having implants can ask their surgeons for a photocopy of the "sticker" that identifies the implant by brand name, type, product number, manufacturer, and date of implant. The manufacturers also provide copies of a "Patient Card" that describes the specifics of the device being implanted. Women who had their implant surgery over 15 years ago may have more difficulty locating records of implant specifications for their implants.

### How can a woman report problems with her implants?

If a woman develops problems with her implants, she should first contact the doctor who performed her implant surgery. She can also report problems to the company that manufactured the implants. Manufacturers are required by law to report all problems associated with these devices to the FDA. Problems can also be reported directly to the FDA through the MedWatch voluntary reporting system (1-800-FDA-1088), although the FDA recommends physician reporting as the preferred method.

### How can a woman sort through the media reports about implants to discover the truth about their safety and efficacy?

That is a difficult question. In our judgment the media is not the place to turn for objective scientific information. Rather, a woman seeking more information about implants or about any medical concern should look to the scientific literature and to respected medical professionals for guidance. She may want to ask her physician to assist her by recommending articles, books, and videotapes on this topic. In addition, the information presented here is culled from the scientific literature and from acknowledged experts. We have included an extensive bibliography to assist the reader in securing more information. The FDA has a toll-free telephone line for consumers (1-800-532-4440); by calling this number women can receive up-to-date, accurate information on silicone breast implants and their regulatory status.

### What is the American Cancer Society's position on silicone gel–filled breast implants?

According to the American Cancer Society's position statement, "The American Cancer Society believes that breast implants should continue to be made available as an option in cancer rehabilitation. Any decision regarding breast reconstruction should be discussed by the woman and her physician to determine the individual's benefits and risks. The American Cancer Society supports further research into long-term safety issues related to breast implants."

## What are the latest American Medical Association's recommendations concerning silicone breast implants?

In an article published in the *Journal of the American Medical Association* in December 1993 the AMA noted that the FDA hearings were "characterized by excessive emphasis on evidence based on anecdotal opinion rather than . . . scientifically proved data. This imbalance likely facilitated the inappropriate media coverage that produced undue anxiety in women with implants." The AMA recommended (1) establishment of a registry of all patients with breast implants to regularly review and report health outcome data; (2) support for the position that women have the "right to choose silicone gel–filled or saline-filled breast implants for both augmentation and reconstruction after being fully informed about the risks and benefits"; (3) physicians be informed of current scientific data available to address the public anxiety over the safety of breast implants ("an anxiety not warranted based on current scientific evidence"); (4) "continued availability of silicone gel implants for both augmentation and reconstruction provided that there is appropriate data collection and follow-up . . . and that clinical trials as proposed by the FDA do not limit a woman's right to choose"; (5) "the AMA monitor the decision-making process of the FDA on the use of not only silicone gel breast implants, but also all silicone-based devices, with particular attention to use of expert medical judgment and to issues of conflict of interest"; and (6) "the AMA request that specific FDA policies regarding the process of device evaluation be developed and publicized to the medical profession and the public and that the process be sensitive to the emotional impact on the patient."

## Why have some manufacturers gotten out of the implant business?

In view of the negative publicity generated by the scrutiny of implants in the national media and the subsequent litigation surrounding this controversy, most implant manufacturers decided that the best business decision was to withdraw from the market in the early 1990s. Many of these were large multinational companies, and for them the breast implant business represented a small contribution to their bottom line.

### What companies still sell implants? How have these companies been affected by the FDA rulings? What steps have they taken to ensure the safety of implants?

Currently, there are only two companies in the United States that continue to make breast implants, McGhan Medical and Mentor, and two international companies, PIP and Hutchinson. The two U.S. companies are carefully monitored by the FDA and must meet rigorous criteria for manufacture. They are required to establish registries, participate in ongoing clinical trials, and conduct far-reaching product testing to ensure the continued safety and effectiveness of their products. These companies have completed or are completing numerous tests to evaluate the safety and effectiveness of these devices. They are also involved in research to develop and test new and improved devices. These studies have been ongoing for many years; in addition, new studies are now mandated by the FDA. It is not clear whether PIP and Hutchinson must adhere to similar rigorous standards for their products. They have, however, submitted an application for marketing saline-filled implants in the United States, claiming equivalency to the McGhan Medical and Mentor saline implants.

### What part do these companies play in the clinical trials?

The companies play a pivotal role in the clinical trials. In the current studies the companies are required to work with specific doctors and centers around the country who agree to use their implants and to comply with the rules of the study. The companies must provide an FDA-approved protocol to doctors as well as the necessary forms to be completed on each patient. In addition, they must establish and support a patient registry and monitor each participating surgeon for compliance to the protocol. On request from the FDA these companies are also required to collect and organize data on each patient for possible FDA evaluation.

### How have FDA regulations affected the price of implants?

The two U.S. companies that continue to manufacture silicone gel–filled breast implants must contend with a smaller market, decreased consumer demand, higher costs associated with implementing FDA regulations and financing registries, the expense of clinical

trials and studies, and substantial legal costs. These additional financial and workload burdens have understandably increased their cost
of doing business. To remain in business they must pass this cost on to
the consumer. Consequently, the cost of breast implants has risen approximately 300% and most likely will continue to rise as new tech-
nologies are introduced.

### Will implant manufacturers discontinue manufacturing silicone gel? What alternate fillings are being suggested?

Both remaining U.S. manufacturers are committed to the silicone gel
market. Their clinical studies will be presented to the FDA for approval. Various new substances that promise to be radiolucent and
easily absorbed by the body are under development. It is hoped that
these fillings can be evaluated under the current clinical trials so that
they can receive FDA approval and be used as alternative fills.

### What role have the manufacturers played in the silicone implant debate?

The manufacturers have played a key role in the breast implant debate, and these companies have been the subject of intense scrutiny
and publicity. Some plastic surgeons believe that they relied too heavily on the companies for supportive data, and now question the accuracy of some of the information that they received. All parties acknowledge that over the years these companies have invested enormous resources in developing, testing, and improving their products
and in conducting ongoing research. Critics think that the companies
were initially lax in conducting the specific studies needed to assess
the long-term efficacy and safety of these devices and to meet FDA
standards for premarket approval. Perhaps they should have taken the
lead in coordinating follow-up with plastic surgeons to assess the rate
and severity of complications. If they had established a better dialogue
with the FDA, misunderstandings may have been avoided. However,
some of the responsibility clearly lies with the FDA. It was not until
1991 that these companies were given any formal guidance as to the
specific testing that the FDA wanted performed. The companies
therefore could not be certain what the FDA wanted until just before
the results of their product research were to be submitted for review. If
this guidance had been provided earlier, with better communication
on both sides, the manufacturers' dollars and research efforts could
have been directed with those goals in mind, providing ready answers

to questions about safety and efficacy and avoiding much of the controversy that has surrounded these devices.

Most would agree, including the independent investigators, that there were no deliberate cover-ups or wrongdoing. None of the information that has been disclosed indicates that these mistakes resulted in increased risk to the health and safety of women with implants. Furthermore, once the FDA informed the manufacturers of what testing requirements they were expected to meet, these companies cooperated with the FDA to provide full disclosure, to set up the additional studies that the FDA requested, and to produce the information that the FDA demanded. It is unfortunate that this information was not requested and gathered years earlier so that it would have been available to answer the FDA's queries and to prevent the concerns and fears that resulted.

The manufacturers are also continuing to fund research to address potential complications and to investigate whether breast implants are associated with systemic disease.

### What role have lawyers played in the silicone implant debate?

Reports in the press and media have pointed out the close relationship of the plaintiff's bar and the consumer advocacy groups that have been vocal in pressing the FDA to ban breast implants. Prior to the escalation of the breast implant debate, lawyers' groups set up special committees and organizations to solicit women as potential plaintiffs in lawsuits against the implant companies. The plaintiff lawyers' trade group, the Association of Trial Lawyers of America, set up a special Breast Implant Litigation Group. Numerous ads were placed in newspapers and on television encouraging women to contact these attorneys to report problems with implants.

The plaintiff's bar requires continuous product liability activity to thrive. Contingency-fee lawyers get approximately one third or more of the money awarded in such cases. The banning of these implants would provide them with a virtual gold mine in potential lawsuits to be filed against the implant manufacturers. As *The Wall Street Journal* reports, "The business of the contingency-fee lawyers . . . is speculating in litigation, hoping to hit deep pockets with big awards, of which they pocket a third or more." Numerous lawsuits have been filed against implant companies and individual physicians. And, as reported in the *Boston Globe* in a story headline that read "Lawyers Fight Over Limits of Implant Trials," these lawyers were also locked in battle with each other over the perceived rewards.

### Have the courts decided on the safety of silicone breast implants?

Early in the implant debate, a panel of federal judges consolidated supervision of the silicone implant cases nationwide and assigned it to U.S. District Judge Sam C. Pointer, Jr., in federal court in Birmingham, Alabama. Judge Pointer has played a major role in negotiating the various settlements and in adjudicating this issue and assessing the scientific evidence presented in these cases.

### What steps have been taken by judges to ensure that decisions about implant safety are based on reliable scientific evidence?

Judge Pointer has convened a scientific panel of four doctors (a rheumatologist, a toxicologist, an immunologist, and an epidemiologist) to hear scholarly presentations from scientists on both sides of this issue to evaluate current evidence of whether silicone may cause human immune system illnesses. Extensive documents, including studies and reports, have been submitted to the panel for their review and consideration. The establishment of a national science panel has been widely applauded by the medical community and the manufacturers who have pushed to have decisions on implant safety based on sound scientific evidence from well-defined studies and not on what has widely been termed "junk science" whereby so-called hired experts provide anecdotal (personal) stories and opinions that are not verifiable.

Another landmark judicial decision in support of sound science in the courtroom was made by Judge Robert E. Jones, of the U.S. District Court for the District of Oregon on December 27, 1996. Judge Jones ruled that plaintiff's evidence supporting a link between silicone breast implants and serious systemic disease did not meet the standard for scientific proof and therefore was inadmissible in court and should not be presented to juries under the Supreme Court's test in *Daubert v. Merrill Dow Pharmaceuticals, Inc.* (The Supreme Court instructed trial courts to make better use of their gatekeeping authority to keep unproved scientific evidence out of the courtroom and to aggressively screen out ill-founded or speculative theories.)

### How have recent court decisions been affected by reliance on the Daubert standards for evaluating scientific evidence in silicone implant cases?

Rulings from judges are beginning to match the judgments of the scientific community finding insufficient evidence to support claims that silicone implants cause disease. For example, in February 1997, in

*Pick v. American Medical Systems, Inc.*, Judge Ginger Berrigan of the U.S. District Court for the Eastern District of Louisiana issued a Daubert decision granting a summary judgment excluding the testimony of 13 plaintiffs' disease causation experts. In *Kelly v. American Heyer-Schulte* in January 1997, Judge Edward Prado of the U.S. District Court for the Western District of Texas ruled in favor of Baxter HealthCare Corporation in a case in which the plaintiff claimed that silicone implants caused her systemic disease. Citing the Daubert case, Judge Prado excluded testimony from the plaintiffs' disease causation experts.

### What is the current status of implant settlement talks? Have any settlements been reached? What are the provisions of these settlements?

The breast implant controversy that arose in 1992 resulted in a virtual onslaught of litigation and court cases. Plaintiffs' attorneys sought to recover damages from the manufacturers for possible systemic diseases and other local complications that their clients claimed had been caused by silicone gel implants. To stem the flood of litigation and resolve this issue, the manufacturers began discussing plans for a settlement.

In 1993 a proposed settlement for Mentor was approved by the court. It established a $24 million fund to cover patients who received Mentor silicone gel–filled or saline-filled implants between April 1, 1984, and June 1, 1993. This settlement has proceeded as planned, and Mentor payments or dispersements have already been made to claimants. Three types of payments were provided with this settlement. They included payments for patients who (1) only had Mentor implants, (2) had Mentor or Bioplasty implants, and (3) had Mentor implants and implants from one other manufacturer.

In 1994 a number of the other implant manufacturers proposed a "no liability" $4.25 billion Global Class Settlement (in response to a class action lawsuit filed in federal district court in Birmingham, Alabama). The settlement granted compensation to women who claimed that breast implants manufactured by any of these companies caused a variety of diseases and afflictions. The Global Settlement Plan was dissolved after Dow Corning Corporation filed for Chapter 11 bankruptcy protection. Subsequently, a Revised Settlement Program, which provides for a smaller class action settlement, was proposed.

### What are the terms of the Revised Settlement Program and who does it cover?

The Revised Settlement Program involves Baxter HealthCare, Bristol-Meyers Squibb, 3M (Minnesota Mining and Manufacturing), and McGhan Medical Corporation. The court approved this plan in 1995. The Revised Settlement Program provides a fund to compensate women who have health complaints associated with breast implants manufactured by these companies. It is divided into two categories: Current Claimants and Other Registrants who satisfy certain disease and severity criteria. The benefits for Current Claimants range from $10,000 to $50,000. The benefits for Other Registrants range from a minimum of $75,000 to a maximum of $250,000, depending on the disease and severity level.

The Revised Settlement Program covers U.S. women with silicone breast implants, saline-filled breast implants, and breast implants with polyurethane coverings manufactured by one of the participating companies. Current and future claims for a 15-year period will be reimbursed for medical diagnosis and evaluation, removal of breast implants and implant rupture, as well as specific diseases such as immune system, rheumatologic, or neurologic disorders. Women who wanted to preserve their right to file a claim during the 15-year time period were required to register a claim with the court. The opt-out period has now expired for most registrants. This settlement has proceeded as planned and payments or dispersements are being made to claimants.

The Dow Corning Corporation Chapter 11 bankruptcy is a completely independent court proceeding from the Revised Settlement Program. Women who became members of the class in the Revised Settlement Program must sign up separately by filing a bankruptcy Proof of Claim Form with the Bankruptcy Docketing Agent if they also wish to assert claims against Dow Corning Corporation.

### How were women notified about the Revised Settlement Program?

Women were notified of settlement details and requirements for participation through worldwide advertisements and announcements. Fairness hearings were also held by Judge Sam C. Pointer. A toll-free hotline number(1-800-887-6828) was established to provide information on the Revised Settlement Plan. Information could also be obtained on the Internet on Judge Pointer's home page.

Women did not need an attorney to participate in the settlement.

They could register with the court if they had no current problem and had recourse for the next 15 years should problems develop. They also did not need to prove that their illness was caused by breast implants to become part of the settlement. They only had to meet the court's criteria for the various funds. This latter point was particularly important in light of the results of numerous studies that are now available and show no link between breast implants and disease.

### Why did Dow Corning declare bankruptcy? What impact will this have on claims that have been filed against the company?

Dow Corning filed for protection under Chapter 11 of the U.S. Bankruptcy Code on May 15, 1995, due to extensive litigation and lack of support from their insurers. The company had been a named defendant in an extensive class action lawsuit against several silicone breast implant manufacturers in which a tentative Global Settlement was reached. However, thousands of implant recipients opted out of the Global Settlement and filed individual lawsuits against Dow Corning. By mid-1995 the company was facing dozens of trials each month in locations throughout the United States involving hundreds of plaintiffs. The company then filed for Chapter 11 bankruptcy protection to reorganize its affairs under the supervision of the Bankruptcy Court.

Filing for bankruptcy was not an admission of the validity of the claims filed against the company, but rather a process by which such claims could be resolved. According to Richard Hazleton, Chairman and CEO of Dow Corning, "the time had come to resolve this situation in everyone's best interest."

### Where does Dow Corning's Chapter 11 case currently stand?

In February 1998 Dow Corning filed an amended Plan of Reorganization to settle breast implant claims. The Bankruptcy Court must first approve the documents related to this proposed plan before Dow Corning can send it out to claimants for a vote. In addition, the Tort Committee, composed primarily of lawyers representing women with breast implant claims, has filed a motion to withdraw Dow Corning's exclusive right to send its plan out for a vote. A hearing on these matters is scheduled for April 1998.

### When will women be able to vote on a plan?

Voting on a plan is a court-supervised process. When the court approves sending a plan out for a vote, claimants will begin receiving information and a ballot. Whenever the voting period begins, women will have several weeks to make a decision and will not need to take any action until they fully understand the plan. Anyone who has filed a claim in Dow Corning's case will receive the required information for voting through the mail.

### What are the proposed terms of Dow Corning's most recent plan?

Dow Corning's $4.4 billion Revised Settlement Plan targets $3 billion primarily for resolving breast implant claims. The balance of those funds would satisfy commercial claims. The new plan offers women more than 15 different settlement choices with payments ranging from $1000 to $200,000—or more for women who have uninsured medical bills that exceed their settlement payments. The plan is designed to provide a range of choices so that women can select the best option to meet their individual circumstances. Settlement options are available over the 16 years of the plan so that women who may want to file claims in the future have a reasonable safety net.

### How does Dow Corning's plan address rupture claims or explantation surgery?

The plan offers expanded payments for women whose implants were found ruptured following removal surgery. Payments for those claims range from $15,000 to $50,000, depending on the severity of the rupture. Women who may want to have their implants removed in the future would have access to a Medical Procedures Program to cover the costs related to removal and reconstruction (if that is their choice) as well as a $1000 payment to cover personal expenses.

### How does Dow Corning's plan address medical conditions?

Dow Corning's plan offers payments for medical conditions or symptoms ranging from $5000 to $200,000, depending on the level of severity and disability. Women who have uninsured medical bills that exceed their settlement can also file for additional payments.

### What if a woman doesn't have anything wrong now, but she filed a claim in case her condition changes? How does Dow Corning's plan address claims filed in the future?

Dow Corning's plan provides a 16-year period to file claims. Women can file a claim for a qualified medical condition at any time during that period and be eligible for the same payments as women who file claims immediately. Furthermore, if a woman settles a claim for a medical condition with a payment of less than $50,000 and her condition later changes, she can refile a claim for an additional payment up to $50,000. Women also will have access to a Medical Procedures Program that will operate over the 16-year period. This program covers the costs involved with removing an implant and reconstruction if a woman so chooses.

### Does the manufacturer's willingness to settle suggest that silicone breast implants are linked to serious disease?

The willingness of the manufacturers "to settle" does not signify that silicone implants are harmful. In fact, a growing number of scientific studies conducted by independent researchers at prestigious institutions such as the Mayo Clinic, Johns Hopkins Medical School, and the University of Texas M.D. Anderson Cancer Center have shown that women with implants have no greater incidence of systemic disease than women without implants and that there is no link with cancer. These settlements have been proposed by the manufacturers to provide reasonable and timely options for women to resolve their claims and as a more sensible financial alternative than litigating each case independently, which would likely result in bankruptcy for some companies as it has for Dow Corning. It is estimated that the manufacturers were paying in excess of $1 million per litigated case in legal fees with none of this money going to patients. A settlement seemed the logical solution for all involved. The companies believe that protracted litigation will not be in the best interests of women or the manufacturers. The goal is to resolve this controversy, address claims, and return to normal business operations.

### Why did so many different consumer groups present themselves as spokesmen for women in the implant debate? Which groups truly represent women's interests?

It is often difficult to distinguish among the many consumer and support groups that speak for women's interests. Many women have complained that these groups misrepresent themselves as impartial support groups for women seeking information, whereas in reality they represent a specific bias. Women have complained that these groups do not provide them the balanced information they desire.

Potential conflict-of-interest allegations raised against the most vocal of these consumer groups, the Public Citizen Health Research Group, focused on the group's possible ties to the American Trial Lawyers Association. Some have suggested that this group can profit from the banning of these devices and that this organization is indebted to plaintiffs' attorneys for some of its funding. In an article in *Forbes*, several plaintiffs' attorneys were quoted as openly admitting to supporting the organization "overtly, covertly, in every possible way." Additionally, *The Wall Street Journal* reported that "the Public Citizen Health Research Group has prepared how-to kits on suing implant manufacturers; plaintiffs' lawyers pay the group $750 per kit."

To determine if a group will provide the unbiased scientific information you seek we suggest that you start by asking your physician about the names of groups that may be helpful. Many hospitals have support groups set up to aid breast cancer patients and their families. You might also check with the local chapter of the American Cancer Society for names of groups in your area. In addition, Y-ME, the largest national support organization for breast cancer patients, and NABCO, the National Association of Breast Cancer Organizations, are excellent, reliable sources of balanced information.

### What experts should a woman consult about the advisability of breast implants for breast reconstruction or cosmetic breast surgery?

The woman considering breast surgery that involves breast implants should obtain detailed information about these devices before deciding if they are for her. Plastic surgeons are well informed about breast implants and can give detailed information. If questions remain, she should consult with her individual physician or surgeon. Information is also available from the FDA, the manufacturers, the American Society of Plastic and Reconstructive Surgeons (1-800-636-0635), and Internet sites of respected medical groups and associations.

## PUTTING THE ISSUE INTO PERSPECTIVE

Now that the media hype has subsided and the scientific studies have been completed, what does it all mean? What are the ramifications for women desiring implant surgery? Are the dangers real or have they been distorted? What is the impact on women, their choices, their health care, and ultimately their peace of mind?

### Evaluating the Risks

The growing preponderance of available scientific evidence suggests and many credible experts agree that there are no lurking dangers that should unduly alarm us. Most women are not in any serious danger from silicone gel–filled or saline-filled implants or expanders. As the FDA itself has concluded, "These devices do not present a health hazard." As is true of all surgical procedures and all implantable devices, benefits must be weighed against associated problems, risks, and complications, and women need to be alert to these dangers and fully informed about them.

Most women, however, do not experience serious complications from breast implants. Ongoing surveys of women who have had breast implant surgery continue to indicate a high satisfaction level. When queried, most women indicate that they would choose to have implant surgery again. These devices have been used for almost 35 years, and if they had been linked to serious, debilitating health problems, surely we would have heard about it by now, not only in association with implants but in connection with the numerous devices, medications, and products that contain silicone and are widely ingested, injected, or implanted. Silicone is a commonly used material; there are few people in our society who do not have minute quantities of silicone in their bodies as a result of normal activities of daily life.

## Defining the Problems: The Scientific Process

What of the women who have experienced serious health problems after implant surgery? Their concerns and anguish are not to be minimized, but the source of their problems needs to be scrutinized more closely. Are these conditions a result of the operation itself, are they associated with the implants, or are they coincidental? This investigation should be conducted not by lawyers in a courtroom, not by expert witnesses receiving payment for their testimony, not by the media in the headlines and on the talk shows, not by self-proclaimed consumer groups receiving funding from malpractice attorneys, but by skilled scientists with expertise in this area who have no special interests beyond the quest for answers to these women's problems. We need to examine the source of these problems to determine why they occurred and how they can be prevented or alleviated. It is a disservice to women to attribute particular symptoms to implants when in fact these problems may have another cause that could be effectively treated if correctly diagnosed.

Peer review and randomized studies are the raw materials that have long supported the scientific process. These well-respected scientific methods were largely ignored as the FDA hearings became politicized and sensationalized. Recent judicial decisions, however, have served to reverse the trend to junk science in the courtroom and to confirm the need for valid scientific evidence as a basis for judicial decision making. It is time to redirect our efforts in the interest of women and of scientific progress.

## FDA Ruling: Positives and Negatives

Although some may disagree with the FDA handling of the breast implant evaluation process and with the specifics of its ruling, most would concur that the goal of obtaining reliable scientific information to answer the question of implant safety and effectiveness is admirable and worth pursuing. The FDA sought more information about possible health problems related to the use of these devices. The ruling called for additional detailed scientific studies while allowing the use of silicone gel–filled breast implants under certain limited provisions. Similar studies were also required for saline-filled breast implants; the results of these studies are now becoming available.

These clinical trials have provided positive benefits. They ensure comprehensive informed consent and follow-up for all women having silicone gel–filled implants for breast surgery as well as for those having saline-filled implants. They are designed to provide a means for discovering the true incidence of problems experienced by women who have had these devices implanted, such as the rate of rupture, deflation, infection, and contracture. Additionally, they can look for possible links between these devices and other health conditions.

In the United States access to the clinical trials and to silicone gel–filled implants is available to all women seeking breast reconstruction after mastectomy or for other breast deformities but is strictly limited to a small number of women requesting reoperative breast augmentation. The distinction between breast reconstruction patients and augmentation patients seems to interject a moral judgment in what should be a scientific investigation. The trials should study the safety of these devices, not whether some women have a "better" or more "pressing" need for them. Access to saline-filled implants is not similarly restricted to a specific group of patients; they are used for both augmentation and reconstructive purposes.

## Impact of Breast Implant Controversy on the Doctor-Patient Relationship

The implant controversy called into question the competence and motives of medical professionals. They became targets of much media criticism; malpractice attorneys sought to isolate them, along with the implant manufacturers, as villains in the implant debate, even though implants, the object of these attacks, were satisfactory to the vast majority of patients and had never been proved unsafe. As a result, women's confidence in their doctors (particularly in plastic surgeons since they perform implant surgery) was eroded. This was unfortunate. The ties that bind patients to their doctors are crucial to patient well-being. Women facing breast cancer need to have a positive attitude and faith that their doctors will recommend the best treatment and provide the best care possible. They need to know that their doctors are on their team and are committed to helping them.

Few will benefit from this erosion of confidence, certainly not women or the doctors who care for them. If plastic surgeons erred in this scenario, it was by acts of omission, not acts of commission. They could have taken the lead years earlier in establishing registries for better patient follow-up and designing and implementing clinical and research studies on the long-term safety and viability of these devices. They could have worked with the manufacturers to provide a comprehensive, understandable informed consent document to be used for all patients contemplating implant surgery. Most likely they were lulled into complacency by the high level of patient satisfaction and low incidence of complications that they saw after implant surgery. If these measures had been taken, the hysteria generated over the safety of breast implants may have been averted. The much-needed supporting studies and data would have been available to address questions raised.

The female half of this writing team has spent the past 21 years observing and working with doctors and has generally been impressed with their genuine desire to provide optimal health care. Some are indeed more skilled than others, some are better communicators than others, and some are more devoted to their patients than others, but this is true of all people, all professionals. The ongoing FDA scrutiny of breast implants should not reflect on the motives of all caregivers who used them, often in response to patient desires. This is not to excuse those individuals who may not have acted in the best interest of their patients, particularly those physicians who were not qualified to perform implant surgery. But a few bad actors should not cast doubt on the total performance. It would be unfortunate if the implant debate served to permanently undermine the doctor-patient relationship. When a woman is diagnosed with breast cancer, she needs to have confidence that her doctors will help her survive and overcome this life-threatening disease.

## Impact of Breast Implant Controversy on Women

For breast cancer patients who have had reconstruction with implants, the breast implant controversy was anxiety provoking. Some of these women were led to believe that their reconstructive implants posed as serious a threat as the cancer they survived. Some were made to feel that they had "time bombs" implanted in their breasts; others were hounded by guilt for having wanted to restore their missing breasts. An atmosphere of fear was generated in the name of women, but not in their interest.

The restriction of silicone gel–filled breast implants primarily to breast reconstruction patients has unfairly penalized and stigmatized women who seek to enhance their self-image. Furthermore, it served to negate some of the positive psychological benefits of reconstructive surgery, sending a message to breast cancer patients that implants are not safe for healthy women. For many breast cancer patients, the doctor's recommendation for breast reconstruction is a sign that their prognosis is good and he considers them candidates for the same type of breast surgery as normal, healthy women. Now this positive reinforcement has been blunted. This may not have been the message that the FDA intended to send, but it was the message that the process delivered.

Healthy women have also been affected by this decision. Many cancer experts believe that breast reconstruction is a lifesaving option for many women who would delay seeking care for breast problems for fear of breast loss. (Implant reconstruction represents the least expensive, least complicated, least time consuming, and therefore one of the most frequently selected methods of breast restoration.) If women are aware that such rehabilitation is available, the hope is that they will be encouraged to practice BSE, to get regular physical examinations, and to go for regular mammograms. Thus, if a cancer is found, it will be in an earlier, more curable stage. Unfortunately, many women will now continue to regard implants, all implants, as hazardous despite the results of subsequent studies. Our surveys and interviews with women over the past 15 years confirm that some will choose to avoid or delay seeking treatment for a breast lump because of their overwhelming fear of breast mutilation. According to some reports, only 50% of the women who discover a breast lump see a doctor within 1 month, and 20% wait a year or more before seeing a physician. Delay in seeking treatment could be a serious blow to the progress that has been made in the early detection of breast cancer.

## A Woman's Decision

Women's rights continue to be assailed from many quarters. The FDA in its ruling regarding silicone gel breast implants limited a woman's right to make an informed decision in consultation with her doctor about her own health care. This is a personal decision, but the FDA inserted itself between a woman and her doctor. As Peter Huber, author of *Galileo's Revenge: Junk Science in the Courtroom,* aptly points out in an article in *Forbes,* "If the state can regulate whether or not a woman can put a bag of silicone into her chest, it obviously can also regulate whether she can put an aspirator into her uterus or a contraceptive pill into her mouth. . . . Given all the recent publicity, no one can even plausibly claim that a woman who now opts in favor of a silicone implant has not been fully informed of the risks. If anything, she has been overinformed. The choice should now be hers. . . . When you compromise on the principle of personal autonomy—of freedom of individual choice—you are soon left with all compromise and no principle. . . . A breast implant, safe or dangerous, intact or ruptured, is still just a bag of plastic. When a woman stands in her doctor's office discussing a breast implant, there's only one body and one life involved: her own."

●　●　●

The decision of the FDA and the sensational stories of the media that surfaced in 1992 portrayed women as pawns and second-class citizens. According to Peter Huber, the entire debate "revolved around a vision of vain, foolish, helpless women—women at the mercy of manipulative doctors and conspiring chemical companies, women more like children than adults, women incapable of making intelligent, individual choices for themselves." Those of us who know and work with women with breast cancer know that this is not the case. Women can only gain control over this devastating disease if they have the necessary information and knowledge, and most women who investigate breast cancer treatment and breast reconstruction do so with great intelligence and diligence.

*Getting the Priorities Straight*

Breast cancer is an overriding threat for all women. It is the most common malignancy in American women, with approximately 180,000 new cases diagnosed each year. It is also the second most common cause of cancer death in women; this year alone over 45,000 women will die from this disease. It seems somehow frivolous for the media and the government to focus so much time and money on breast implants when the real culprit remains virtually ignored.

The breast implant debate has now subsided, the scientific evidence is in, and women can now feel relieved and reassured that their fears about possible serious health concerns tied to breast implants have proved unfounded. As time passes, many women reading this material will be unaware of the controversy that raged and will not be faced with the same issues and concerns. Breast implants are not perfect, but they are not the public enemy that they have been portrayed, and they probably did not warrant all of the attention that they received. The positive psychological, aesthetic, and physical benefits they confer have been all but overlooked in a media blitz of unparalleled proportions. If these devices had not been implanted in women's breasts but rather in some other area of the body, they probably would not have received such widespread attention.

This discussion has attempted to examine the issues and controversies surrounding silicone gel and saline implants based on logic and scientific evidence. We now know a lot more about these devices, and the good news is that they do not pose any serious threat to a woman's health. The scientific evidence is convincing and, hopefully, the media that made the implant controversy front-page news can now give science its fair share of coverage. We hope that this discussion will provide women with the information they need to alleviate some of the anxiety that has been generated and allow them to direct their attention to a far more ominous threat that confronts them. Breast cancer is the enemy, and women need to be fully empowered to face this serious challenge.

# SELECTING AND COMMUNICATING WITH A PLASTIC SURGEON

Having made a decision to seek breast reconstruction, a woman needs to choose her plastic surgeon carefully. Although newspapers, the *Yellow Pages*, and magazines on the newsstand feature ads for plastic surgery, these are not discriminating and therefore are not the best means for selecting a plastic surgeon to perform breast reconstruction or any procedure for that matter. Furthermore, in many cases a woman's degree of freedom in making a choice is limited by her circumstances. If she is already under the care of a general surgeon who is a member of a breast team, he will likely recommend one of the plastic surgeons he works with regularly. This is particularly true when immediate breast reconstruction is planned and the general surgeon and plastic surgeon must work together closely. Her choice also may be directly affected by her insurance provider's list of approved physicians. If she is under a managed care program, she will have to select from that list or there may be an additional copayment if she selects someone who is not on the approved list.

When selecting a plastic surgeon, a prospective patient should consider the guidelines described below.

## TRAINING

The physician a woman selects should be trained in plastic surgery and have met the qualifications of the American Board of Plastic Surgery, which grants board certification in this specialty. To be able to take the board examination a surgeon must have 3 to 5 years of training in general surgery or in a surgical subspecialty and an additional 2 to 3 years of specialized training in the broad aspects of plastic surgery. Furthermore, he must demonstrate competence by completing an approved residency training program; this means the doctor's peers have approved his moral and ethical qualifications as well as his knowledge, training, and experience in the field. Approximately 1 to 2 years after residency training is completed, he is eligible to take board examinations and once again subject himself to the scrutiny of peers in order to obtain board certification. Once certified, he may apply for membership in the American Society of Plastic and Reconstructive Surgeons (ASPRS).

## EXPERIENCE

The plastic surgeon a woman chooses should have a special interest in breast reconstruction and should regularly operate with general surgeons as a part of the breast team. In addition, he should be experienced with the different techniques appropriate for breast reconstruction and have a record of successful operations. If he has a teaching appointment at a medical school–affiliated hospital, this association suggests access to the latest surgical techniques, involvement in the education of residents, and awareness of recent developments in the field. It is not enough just to be a well-trained plastic surgeon. A good doctor must know about the specific procedures that apply to the patient's problem if he is to render optimal care.

## HOW DO YOU INVESTIGATE A DOCTOR'S CREDENTIALS?

Getting information about a doctor's training is easy to do and worth the effort. This information is available in the reference room at the local library. It can be found in a book entitled *The Directory of Medical Specialists,* which lists only board-certified specialists. It will list the doctor's year of birth, medical school, the year he was licensed to practice, the year of specialty certification, primary and secondary specialties, and type of practice. Other information on training and hospital and medical affiliations also is included. Doctors in this book are listed geographically, so it is easy to locate the names of doctors in each community. The *American Medical Directory* is another helpful reference, but, unlike *The Directory of Medical Specialists,* it does not indicate if a physician is board certified. Doctors who are on the staff of hospitals accredited by the JCAH (Joint Commission on Accreditation of Hospitals) in a specific specialty have had their credentials approved by their peers representing the hospital and meet their criteria to practice the specialty.

## FINDING A PLASTIC SURGEON

How do you find out whose surgical competence is highly regarded? How do you know who is experienced in breast reconstruction? Most people do not know where to go for reliable information. This information, however, can be obtained from numerous sources. One of the best sources of referral is another physician in the community or another member of the breast management team. The general surgeon is a knowledgeable person to ask; frequently he works with a plastic surgeon as part of a breast team and feels comfortable with this expert's skill and in his ability to work with the other team members to achieve the best result for the patient. He also may have patients who have had breast reconstruction and are willing to discuss this topic and recommend their doctors. Other women who have had breast reconstruction provide an excellent source of information and reliable recommendations about their plastic surgeons; they have firsthand knowledge of this surgery and can personally relate to the surgeon's skill and bedside manner. A woman's gynecologist or family physician also may know the names of plastic surgeons who have performed successful breast reconstructions.

The American Society of Plastic and Reconstructive Surgeons (444 E. Algonquin Rd., Arlington Heights, IL 60051; 708-228-9900) provides information on breast reconstruction; it also will supply a list of board-certified plastic surgeons performing reconstructive breast surgery in different communities throughout the United States. The American Cancer Society, through its Reach to Recovery Program, is now providing information on breast reconstruction. By contacting this organization through the local chapter of the American Cancer Society, the woman desiring information on breast reconstruction will be placed in touch with a woman who has had her breast reconstructed and will share her experiences. Breast cancer and breast reconstruction support groups also provide valuable information and access to other women of similar age and background who have had breast reconstruction. Many times these support groups are affiliated with local hospitals. The local medical society is another source of information; it often has lists of specialists in the community and their areas of interest. (See Appendix A for more information on this topic.)

# FINDING THE RIGHT PLASTIC SURGEON

Locating a qualified plastic surgeon does not necessarily mean a woman has found the right surgeon for her. She needs to determine if this physician will meet both her physical and emotional needs. Breast reconstruction is a very emotional experience; a woman's breasts have far greater psychological implications than their anatomy and physiology would suggest. A woman needs a doctor who listens, who treats her as an individual, and who has time to deal with her concerns.

Remember, as with any anticipated surgery, a woman should consider a second opinion before finally selecting a surgeon. Some women, however, hesitate to request another opinion for fear it will offend their doctors. They are intimidated by their doctors and are reluctant to question their statements and seek more information. Time spent in finding the right plastic surgeon is well invested, however. Unfortunately, most people do not devote the necessary effort in making this important choice. As one woman in our survey so aptly explained, "Most women devote more attention to buying a vacuum cleaner than they do to selecting a doctor."

# QUESTIONS TO ASK A PLASTIC SURGEON

Before selecting a plastic surgeon a woman needs to know that he is receptive to her questions and concerns. To assist in making a satisfactory choice of a plastic surgeon, we have included some questions a woman might ask during her consultation.*

- How many breast reconstructions have you done and what type of results have you achieved?
- May I talk with several of your patients who have had this surgery?
- What are the different options for breast reconstruction?
- What is the best timing for reconstructive surgery? Can I have immediate breast reconstruction at the time of my cancer surgery?
- What are the benefits and risks associated with the different reconstructive techniques?
- What are the benefits and risks associated with breast implants? With tissue expanders?

---

*Chapters 9 through 13 and 18 are totally devoted to answering women's frequently asked questions about breast reconstruction.

- Is it possible to have reconstruction with my own tissue and without an implant?
- Is it possible to have endoscopic-assisted breast reconstruction?
- Which reconstructive approach is appropriate for me and why?
- What is involved in this surgery?
- What type of anesthesia will be used: local or general?
- How many different procedures and hospitalizations will be needed? How long will I be in surgery for each operation?
- What type of scars will I have and exactly where will they be placed?
- What are the expected results of surgery? Can I expect good long-term results?
- Will my breasts be symmetric?
- How long will it take me to recuperate?
- What are the anticipated costs of surgery?
- Will you help me file for insurance coverage?
- What are possible complications from this surgery?

Most plastic surgeons will have photographs of breast reconstruction patients. These might help the patient understand the results that can be achieved for a deformity such as hers.

## QUESTIONS TO ASK YOURSELF BEFORE YOU SCHEDULE SURGERY

- Is this the plastic surgeon I want to do my breast reconstruction?
- Is he properly trained and qualified?
- Does this surgeon seem to understand how I feel and is he sensitive to my needs?
- Has he taken the time to understand what I want done?
- Has he provided me with enough information so that I can make an informed decision?
- Is he going to spend the necessary time with me to answer my questions and deal with my concerns?
- Does he have the necessary skill to perform this surgery?
- Has he explained what he plans to do in terms that I can understand?
- Does he treat me as a responsible adult?
- Does his plan for surgery agree with my expectations for what I would like done?
- If there is a problem, do I feel comfortable with this surgeon handling it?

# COMMUNICATING WITH A PLASTIC SURGEON

Good communication not only helps the patient find the best plastic surgeon to perform her breast restoration, but also enables her to work with him to achieve the result she desires. Preoperative consultations provide the patient and surgeon with an ideal setting for discussing their thoughts and exploring their expectations for a final result.

A typical consultation with a plastic surgeon about breast reconstruction should begin with an explanation of the woman's concerns and expectations for this operation and a complete review of her medical and surgical history. It is in a woman's best interest to have a plastic surgeon who is well informed about all aspects of her health and tumor care so that he can consider these factors in discussing reconstructive options with her. It is helpful if he has copies of the general surgeon's operative report and the pathologist's report or has communicated directly with the other physicians. He also needs to be aware of the radiation and chemotherapy that she has received, the status of her opposite breast, and her feelings about it.

After this initial discussion the plastic surgeon will need to physically examine the woman's chest, back, and abdomen to determine the reconstructive approaches that are appropriate for her physical situation.

Preoperative photographs are taken during this initial examination by a plastic surgeon, and a woman should expect to be photographed during her visit. If she visits more than one doctor, she usually will have photographs taken by each doctor. Although these photographs do not show the patient's face, sometimes this picture-taking process is unsettling for the woman. These photographs are important, however, because the plastic surgeon will use them for evaluating her condition and planning her operation. They also provide a record of her treatment. He may eventually use them (with the woman's permission) for educational purposes to demonstrate the results of this surgery to other patients and physicians and for publication in the professional literature.

Once this examination has been concluded, the woman can again meet with the doctor to review the different options for breast reconstruction. Final determination of the operative plan must often wait until the plastic surgeon has consulted with the other members of the breast management team.

If a woman has a husband or significant other in her life, it is often helpful for this person to accompany her on her preoperative visits with the plastic surgeon. Mutual expectations can then be aired and discussed, and the influence of the man's feelings on the woman can be observed and evaluated. Even though the man and woman share in the learning process, the final decision about surgery must be made by the woman herself. At no time should a woman feel pressured into this surgery by a relative, friend, husband, or even the plastic surgeon with whom she is consulting.

If a woman has a consultation with her plastic surgeon before her cancer surgery, they should discuss the correct timing of reconstructive surgery, whether immediate or delayed. If she desires an immediate reconstruction, the general surgeon and plastic surgeon need to confer and agree on the suitability of this approach for her. Before an immediate breast reconstruction is done, the details of timing, operative care, and team cooperation must be carefully planned.

The woman who consults with a plastic surgeon after her mastectomy or lumpectomy should remember that reconstructive breast surgery is never an emergency procedure. In the interest of good communication she may require several visits to her plastic surgeon to answer all of her questions, to clearly explain her expectations for reconstruction, and to work with him to define a specific surgical plan appropriate for her. There are many methods for reconstructing breasts today, and a well-trained plastic surgeon will probably be knowledgeable in a number of different procedures. It is important, however, that the type of reconstruction a woman selects be the simplest and safest procedure yet still be the most likely to meet her expectations for a good result.

# SURGICAL OPTIONS FOR BREAST RECONSTRUCTION

As recently as 25 years ago a woman who had a mastectomy had few options if she desired breast restoration. Breast reconstruction techniques had not been perfected, and the most a woman could expect was the creation of a breast mound that bore little resemblance to her remaining breast. Most breast reconstructions were done months to years after the mastectomy. Without reconstructive surgery she faced the prospect of living with a lopsided chest or wearing a breast prosthesis to hide her deformity. A prosthesis, however, was not always the solution to her problem. Sometimes it made a woman feel increasingly self-conscious because she worried that her artificial breast would become dislodged and be obvious to others. Betty Rollins' humorous yet poignant account of her attempt to find a suitable external prosthesis after her mastectomy reveals the frustration felt by many women in trying to appear whole again.

Today, with the development and refinement of techniques to satisfy the requests of women seeking breast restoration, the results of reconstructive surgery have improved dramatically. The focus now is on breast preservation and avoidance of a mastectomy deformity. Skin-sparing mastectomy, tissue expansion, endoscopic techniques, and autologous tissue refinements have enhanced the results of immediate reconstruction, which is now often the preferred timing for breast reconstruction. Women who require or choose a mastectomy or women who choose a lumpectomy but require reconstructive surgery to prevent breast asymmetry or contour defects can now select from a number of reliable procedures that meet their psychological and aesthetic expectations for breast restoration. Breasts can be rebuilt using implants or expanders and the tissue remaining after the mastectomy or with flaps of muscle or muscle and skin (musculocutaneous) obtained from the abdomen, back, hips, or buttocks and then transferred to the chest wall. The choice of reconstructive method depends on the amount and quality of the tissue remaining after the mastectomy, the surgeon's experience with each technique, and the patient's preferences and expectations. In addition to these basic operations, the patient may request additional procedures to enhance appearance and symmetry.

In deciding which surgical option is appropriate for her a woman first must resolve her feelings about her remaining breast. Does she like the way it looks and want the rebuilt breast to match it? (With the new reconstructive techniques available, it is often possible to achieve breast symmetry without altering the opposite breast.) Is she willing to consider an operation on her normal breast if this will make both breasts appear symmetric? If her remaining breast is large and full and she does not want it modified, will she agree to a flap procedure that will provide sufficient tissue to match her large breast but will also result in an abdominal or back scar? (Most women have strong feelings about preserving their remaining breast intact.) Her feelings about her remaining breast will affect the type of procedure chosen and the ultimate success of the reconstructive effort.

This chapter is designed to serve as a woman's guide to the different techniques available for breast restoration, their indications for use, and their advantages and disadvantages. In addition, the various types of implants and expanders and their applications are described. The optimal timing of breast reconstruction is also considered, with a full discussion of the benefits and risks of immediate and delayed breast reconstruction. No one procedure is advocated above any other. The particular approach must be selected with the individual woman's needs and her deformity in mind.

## TIMING OF BREAST RECONSTRUCTION

Once a woman has decided that she wants breast reconstruction, timing becomes an important consideration. When should this operation be performed? Should she have breast reconstruction immediately at the time of the mastectomy or wait until some time after the mastectomy for a delayed breast reconstruction. For some women, the decision is made by circumstance because they are unaware that reconstruction is possible until long after the mastectomy has been performed. For others, the delay is practical reality to allow them to recover from the systemic therapy that is necessary to treat their cancer. For most women, however, immediate breast reconstruction performed at the same time as mastectomy is an exciting and appealing option. Today, with increased emphasis on informed consent, many women learn of the option of immediate reconstruction from their general surgeons or other doctors before they have their cancer surgery and have the opportunity to contact a plastic surgeon to discuss reconstructive surgery as a component of the total treatment plan.

The past 25 years have witnessed important changes in breast cancer detection and management. Today, the diagnosis of breast cancer does not mean that a woman must experience permanent breast loss after breast cancer treatment. Increasing experience with conservative surgery and radiation therapy and mastectomy and immediate breast reconstruction have demonstrated the validity, efficacy, and safety of these approaches in providing women with optimal treatment of their cancer with minimal deformity. Furthermore, many breast cancers are being detected at an early, more curable stage, breast reconstruction techniques have improved, and cooperation between reconstructive surgeons and general surgeons or surgical oncologists (surgeons who specialize in cancer surgery) have increased. With experience gained over time and refinements in technique, immediate breast reconstruction is now being requested and performed with much greater frequency and with better results. For most breast cancer patients who desire breast preservation and are not candidates for conservative surgery, general surgeons and surgical oncologists have come to accept that immediate breast reconstruction is a viable and appealing option. In fact, when combined with new skin-sparing techniques, it is often the preferred timing because it produces a superior, natural aesthetic breast that closely resembles the normal opposite breast.

Before the decision for immediate breast reconstruction can be made, the foremost consideration of the general surgeon and the patient is the proper management of the breast cancer. No aspect of treatment should be compromised. The possible need for adjunctive treatment, either radiation therapy or chemotherapy, and the best timing for this therapy are key factors in planning the scheduling of mastectomy and breast reconstruction. For some women with large tumors, preoperative chemotherapy (also called induction or neoadjuvant chemotherapy) will be administered in an effort to shrink the tumor before surgical removal. When this approach is used, the patient is sometimes able to have less extensive cancer surgery because the tumor is substantially diminished in size. In this instance surgery and reconstruction should be delayed for at least 1 month and more typically for 2 or 3 months until the patient's blood count has returned to normal. If postoperative chemotherapy is planned, breast reconstruction should not delay its administration, which generally should begin within 2 months. Consideration is also given to delaying breast reconstruction until after radiation therapy has been completed. However, this is not always necessary for autologous tissue reconstructions since they seem to tolerate radiation well. The potential for achieving the most aesthetic breast appearance is also an important consideration. To help the patient make the best decision the reconstructive surgeon should let her know which approach he thinks will produce the optimal result.

The choice between immediate reconstruction or a delayed procedure several months later makes the decisions a woman must make before her breast cancer treatment even more complex. Not only must she decide on the appropriate tumor management, but she also has to select the best reconstructive technique, the correct timing for her breast reconstruction, and the plastic surgeon to perform it. A sense of urgency pervades her decision making if she is not to delay or compromise the treatment of her cancer. She has much additional information to process and more specialists to consult. All of this can be overwhelming for some women, and they understandably choose not to respond promptly but to face treatment one step at a time. Most opt for an immediate procedure to avoid experiencing breast loss and the pain and added time and cost of yet another major surgical procedure. Fortunately, access to information and care is now more readily available to women interested in immediate reconstruction. With increasing experience, many breast management teams and breast centers have now fully incorporated immediate breast reconstruction into the choices presented to the patient during her initial discussions about tumor management. The plastic surgeon is often part of these initial discussions, and the scheduling of appointments and the actual operation can be streamlined through this type of teamwork. Ultimately, however, the decision to have immediate or delayed reconstruction is a personal one influenced by the patient's individual needs, the stage of her cancer, and the recommendations of her general surgeon and plastic surgeon. She makes this decision after she has had full opportunity to weigh the advantages and disadvantages of each approach and choose the one that is best for her.

## What Are the Advantages of Immediate Reconstruction?

Immediate reconstruction, or reconstructive surgery performed at the same time as the mastectomy, has a definite psychological appeal for many women and offers major advantages for obtaining an optimal result. Dealing with a life-threatening disease and simultaneously coping with the loss of a breast are devastating to most women. Some women even delay seeking medical help because they fear losing a breast. Others will not consider a mastectomy unless they can have immediate breast reconstruction to avoid the mastectomy deformity. In recent interviews with young women in their twenties and thirties who had chosen mastectomy and immediate breast reconstruction, many explained that they felt that immediate reconstruction was a compelling necessity for them in order to adjust to their diagnosis and to continue to conduct normal social lives. The desire to be seen as "normal" among their peers and to be able to interact comfortably with the opposite sex was crucially important to them.

Obvious psychological and aesthetic advantages are associated with an immediate procedure; the patient who requests it is usually pleased with her decision. The breast management team is sending her a message that her prognosis is positive enough to justify beginning her rehabilitation without delay. The patient feels that her doctors are addressing not only her tumor but also her overall concerns and well-being.

Cooperation between the oncologic surgeon and plastic surgeon has led to major advances in technique and to more attractive reconstructed breasts, usually with less scarring than was previously the case. Improvements in immediate breast reconstruction have led many plastic surgeons to believe that the results they achieve with immediate reconstruction are usually as good or even better than those attained with delayed reconstruction. Often immediate reconstruction can permit the surgeon to remove less breast skin than would ordinarily be removed for a mastectomy alone, thus reducing or shortening the breast scar. This technique is called skin-sparing mastectomy and is only appropriate if there is no tumor involvement in the skin. With this approach, the surgeon removes the nipple-areola and only as much skin as is needed for ideal tumor treatment. The reduced scar is even less conspicuous later when most of it is covered by the nipple-areola reconstruction. The preserved skin used to cover the new breast reduces the need for skin expansion and requires less skin to be transferred from the abdomen or back if autologous breast reconstruction has been selected. The surgeon can also help preserve the natural landmarks of the breast such as the inframammary fold (where the breast meets the chest wall), medial cleavage, and lateral, outer limits of the breast. These boundaries can then be used to more accurately define breast shape when rebuilding the woman's breast. The result is a reconstructed breast that often has optimal symmetry with the remaining breast.

Studies by Schain et al. and Noone et al. reveal that immediate reconstruction has positive psychological benefits for women who wish to avoid breast loss and rid themselves of their preoccupation with cancer. Furthermore, these women are, for the most part, satisfied with the results of their immediate surgery. The study by Schain et al. indicates that women having immediate breast reconstruction experience less overall psychological trauma and have less recall of the pain associated with their mastectomy. Their new breasts are incorporated more quickly into a redefined body image and they exhibit a lower level of distress, probably because they awaken from the mastectomy with a breast contour intact and thus do not see the mastectomy deformity and experience the sense of mutilation that so often accompanies breast amputation. They also do not feel the anxiety, disappointment, and embarassment sometimes associated with camouflaging the defect or having the external prosthesis become dislodged. These women are particularly grateful that they did not have to live without their breast or breasts for any period of time. These studies and others have also shown that the survival rate of immediate breast reconstruction patients is comparable to that of patients who have not had reconstructive surgery and that the local recurrence rate is no higher in this group.

Essentially the same techniques are used for immediate breast reconstruction as for delayed breast reconstruction, but newer modifications such as skin-sparing mastectomy (discussed previously) and the increasing use of autologous tissues (the patient's natural tissue) have substantially improved the aesthetic results expected from immediate breast restoration and decreased the residual scarring. The primary procedures used include implant or tissue expander reconstruction with the available tissues left at the mastectomy site or breast reconstruction with autologous tissue usually taken from the lower abdomen or back and less frequently from the buttocks or hip. Immediate breast reconstruction also provides for a quicker resolution of the mastectomy deformity and reduces the number of operations the woman has to undergo without significantly lengthening her hospitalization. She benefits from the reduced cost of having one operation under general anesthesia performed during one hospitalization. She can recover from the mastectomy and the breast reconstruction at the same time without the need to schedule additional time for another operation for the reconstruction later.

## What Are the Disadvantages of an Immediate Procedure?

The major disadvantage is that there are many decisions to be made at once and the time constraints of an immediate procedure may place the woman under even greater stress. She will also have to undergo more surgery at the time of the initial primary cancer treatment, which will increase her hospitalization, recovery time, and initial cost.

The added complexity of the operation means that there is a higher complication rate from skin loss, hematoma, and infection with immediate reconstruction. For implant and expander reconstruction, fluid accumulation (seroma) in the mastectomy wound and low-grade infection add to the potential for fibrous formation around an implant, possibly resulting in capsular contracture or hardening of the reconstructed breast. Infection can pose a problem if a tissue expander is in place; the expander may have to be removed to allow time for the tissues to heal before once again attempting reconstruction, this time on a delayed basis. The reconstructive surgeon may suggest that a portion of the latissimus dorsi muscle be transferred from the back to enhance implant cover and lower the chance of infection or implant exposure.

Immediate breast reconstruction with an implant or expander typically requires about the same amount of time as the mastectomy. When a TRAM flap is done, it usually takes twice as long as the mastectomy. Free flaps (transferred by microsurgery) can take even longer. The woman who elects immediate reconstruction must have realistic expectations about her breast appearance after immediate reconstruction. Even though modern skin-sparing techniques permit remarkably natural reconstructions, there are differences. A woman's rebuilt breast will not be an exact replica of the breast that she lost. Sensation will be diminished and initially absent and lactation will not be possible. Furthermore, the breast reconstruction will not be complete with this one operation. A second and sometimes a third procedure is necessary to complete the process, depending on the type of breast reconstruction selected, the individual healing process, and the expectations and preferences of the surgeon and the patient.

Some plastic surgeons fear that a less than perfect reconstruction could cause further emotional distress for an already stressed patient. Since the patient has not seen the mastectomy deformity, she measures the reconstruction against her normal breast. Some plastic surgeons and women who have had a delayed reconstruction feel that the mastectomy experience is traumatic enough without adding reconstruction to it. Since reconstruction is for a lifetime, the woman should have the best possible result, which additional time may help the surgeon to achieve in some cases. Today, however, most immediate breast reconstructions, especially those done after skin-sparing mastectomy, have better results with shorter scars and improved contour.

Close teamwork between the general surgeon and the plastic surgeon is required for this surgical approach. The general surgeon should be supportive of the decision for immediate breast reconstruction, and he must work with the plastic surgeon to plan and perform this operation.

There are obvious benefits and risks to be considered in immediate reconstruction. They are summarized as follows:

| Benefits | Risks |
| --- | --- |
| Probable improved aesthetic result | More complex procedure |
| Reduction of psychologic trauma attending the mastectomy | Less time for woman to cope with cancer diagnosis and evaluate her experience options |
| Reduced overall cost and hospitalization | Higher complication rate |
| Reduced overall operative, anesthetic, and recovery time | Longer initial operative, anesthesia, and recovery time |
| Shorter mastectomy scar and improved sensation | |

## What Are the Advantages of Delayed Reconstruction?

Delayed reconstruction can be performed from a few days to years after the mastectomy. For patients with early-stage disease who do not require chemotherapy or radiation therapy, some plastic surgeons prefer reconstruction 3 to 6 months after mastectomy.

Delayed surgery affords the woman time to cope with her initial cancer. In recent interviews, 14 women who had delayed reconstruction were asked if they would have preferred their reconstruction done immediately. Although four admitted that they could have had the procedure earlier than they did (after 11-, 9-, 6-, and 3-year delays, respectively), they all felt that a waiting period allowed them to "cope with their cancer, get their emotional lives in order, and separate the negative cancer experience from the very positive reconstruction." In addition, these patients also felt delaying their surgery gave them more time to investigate reconstructive surgery, and thus they had more realistic expectations of the results that could be achieved.

By delaying her reconstructive surgery a woman has time to fully evaluate her decision to have her breast rebuilt; some women change their minds after a waiting period and decide not to pursue this option. This time also allows a woman to recover from any additional therapy that might be required and to fully explore the topic of reconstruction, find the right plastic surgeon, get to know him, and decide on the correct reconstructive approach.

For the plastic surgeon, delay offers the psychological benefit of a patient committed to this procedure. In addition, for health considerations, the plastic surgeon and general surgeon often prefer to assess and to help the patient understand the full extent of her disease and the anticipated treatment before she embarks on further surgery.

Delayed reconstruction allows the breast tissues time to heal, soften, and settle. There is less chance of infection, seroma, and implant extrusion. For the woman having breast reconstruction with her own tissues, she can plan the timing, select the surgeon, and donate her own blood prior to a more extensive procedure, which involves a longer recovery period. The surgeon has more time to plan his surgery to achieve breast symmetry and accurate placement of the nipple-areola (if it is to be reconstructed). The plastic surgeon may feel he has better control of the variables than when a new operation is initiated at the end of a mastectomy operation.

## What Are the Disadvantages of a Delayed Procedure?

One of the primary disadvantages of a delayed procedure is the period of time that a woman must live without her breast and the associated psychological and emotional trauma she will experience. Because more skin is removed during a delayed reconstruction, the scars are often longer and the results may not be as good as those achieved with immediate breast reconstruction. A second operation also involves another hospitalization with the associated risks of general anesthesia and additional pain, recuperation time, and cost. Some women who do not have this procedure at the time of their mastectomy may not have the opportunity for breast reconstruction again.

Again, there are risks and benefits of a delayed procedure:

| Benefits | Risks |
| --- | --- |
| Time to recover from mastectomy | Time to dwell on cancer and on the deformity |
| Time to recover from adjunctive therapy | Patient may experience depression from mastectomy status |
| Time to get acquainted with plastic surgeon | Patient may never "get around" to having reconstruction |
| Time to make an informed decision | Additional cost of two surgeries (both financial and time) |
| | Additional potential for problems from two surgeries and two anesthetics |
| | Probably more skin removal with longer scars from initial mastectomy |

## What Is the Correct Timing for Breast Reconstruction if the Patient Requires Chemotherapy or Radiation Therapy?

Most patients with positive lymph nodes have chemotherapy, hormonal therapy, or radiation therapy after the mastectomy and axillary lymph node dissection. Most adjunctive chemotherapy now lasts for 6 months. Chemotherapy can impair the body's ability to resist infection by lowering the white blood cell count; therefore it is important to delay breast reconstruction for at least 1 month and preferably 2 to 3 months after the completion of chemotherapy to be sure that the patient's blood count has returned to normal. Because radiation therapy causes some changes in the skin and underlying subcutaneous and fatty tissues, the reconstructive surgeon also will recommend that the patient wait at least 6 weeks after radiation therapy to reduce the possibility of healing problems after the operation. Many women do not want to wait until the adjunctive therapy has been completed and opt to have immediate reconstruction and then radiation treatment and/or chemotherapy. Implant reconstructions do not perform well after irradiation or when the implants are placed into irradiated breast tissue. There is a high incidence of capsular contracture, firmness, and breast distortion. When postoperative radiation is planned, an autologous tissue flap reconstruction should be a strong consideration to reduce the possibility of implant problems.

## What Timing Is Suggested for Patients With Advanced Disease?

Once the woman with advanced disease and her surgeon decide to proceed with reconstructive breast surgery, they need to determine the correct timing for this procedure. On one hand, these women have a less favorable prognosis than if they did not require chemotherapy; thus they often prefer to go ahead with reconstruction without delay. On the other hand, they also have a greater risk of developing local recurrences, and chemotherapy can affect their blood count and modify the wound-healing potential. Most surgeons prefer to delay breast reconstruction until after mastectomy and chemotherapy and/or radiation therapy. Because some patients with advanced disease have earlier recurrences or relapses after cessation of chemotherapy, some oncologists suggest that reconstructive surgery be delayed 1 to 2 years after chemotherapy. However, the blood count and other variables that can affect wound healing usually return to normal by 1 month. Each case is individual and the reconstructive surgeon and medical oncologist should confer concerning the proper interval after chemotherapy. Patients with larger tumors who are receiving preoperative chemotherapy (also called induction and neoadjuvant therapy) can complete this therapy and then have a mastectomy and immediate breast reconstruction with autologous tissue followed by radiation therapy. This approach has not been associated with compromise of local control or general disease control in the first few years it has been studied.

## Results With Immediate Breast Reconstruction

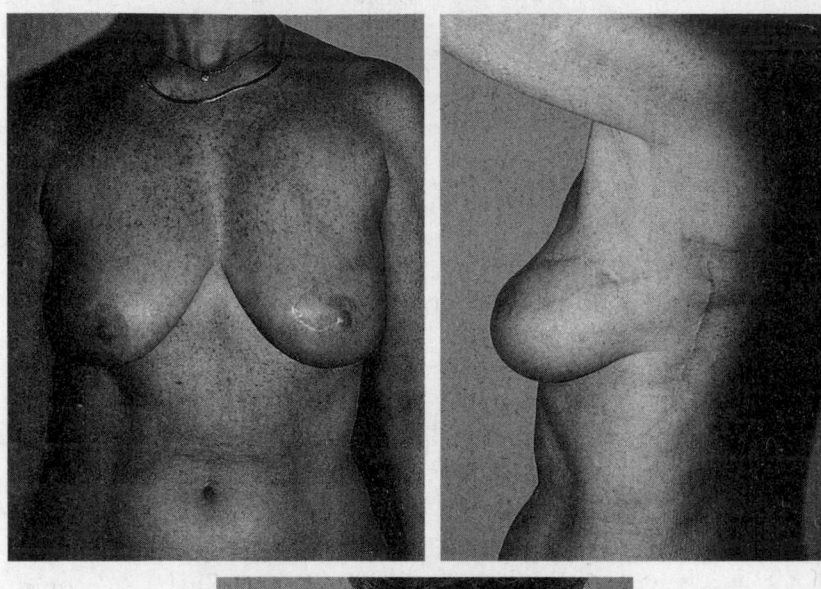

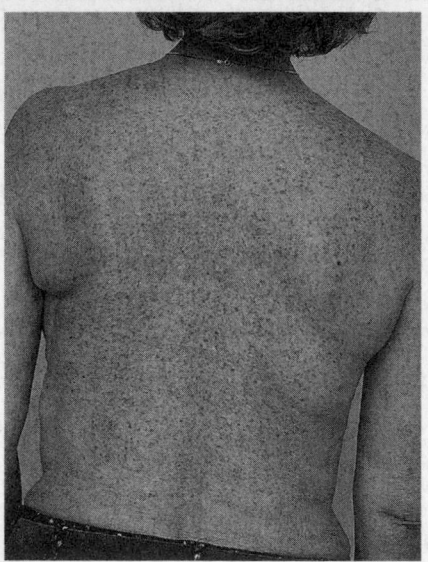

This 45-year-old woman, whose natural breasts were reasonably symmetric, had a skin-sparing mastectomy of her left breast and immediate breast reconstruction with a laterally based latissimus dorsi musculocutaneous flap and an implant. She did not want her opposite breast modified. She is shown 4 years after breast reconstruction. She considered her back and side incisions acceptable trade-offs for a symmetric breast reconstruction without the need to alter her other breast. Her nipple-areola was reconstructed with a local flap and a tattoo.

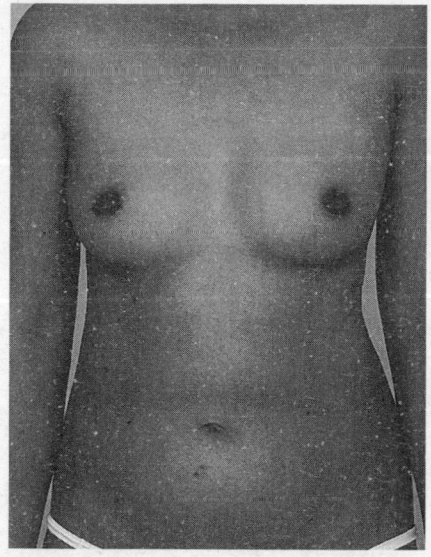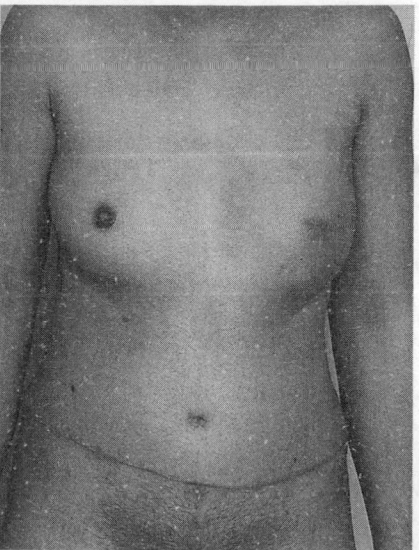

After breast cancer developed in her left breast, this 29-year-old woman had a modified radical mastectomy using a skin-sparing technique and reduced incisions. She is shown 6 months after immediate breast reconstruction with a TRAM flap. Because of the small diameter of the nipple, it was closed as a small round scar, simulating a nipple-areola.

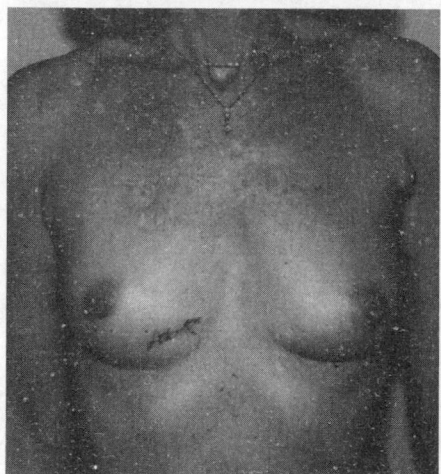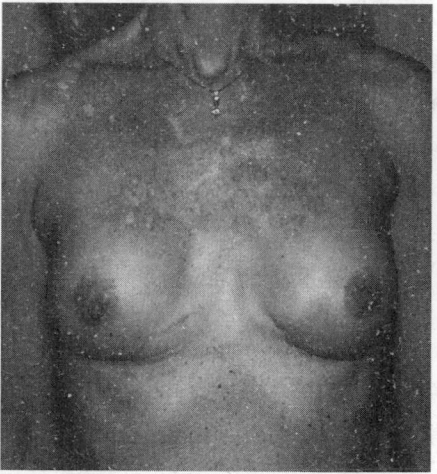

Lumpectomy and axillary lymph node dissection were used to treat cancer of the left breast in this 40-year-old woman. An extensive intraductal component and positive tumor margins were found on pathologic examination. Bilateral total mastectomies and immediate breast reconstruction were performed with breast implants placed beneath the muscle. No new scars were created and her nipple-areolae were spared. She is shown 2 years after breast reconstruction.

## Results With Immediate Breast Reconstruction—cont'd

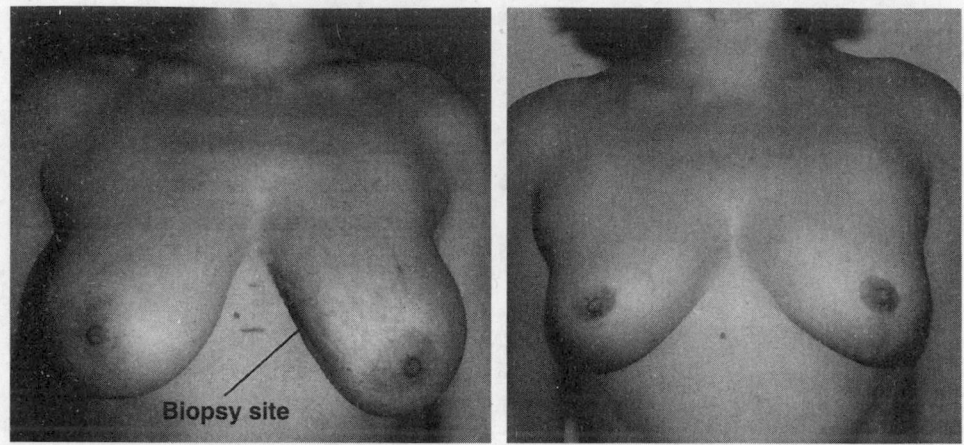

This 28-year-old woman requested lumpectomy to treat cancer of her left beast. Since she wanted smaller breasts, lumpectomy was combined with reduction of both breasts. The result is shown 3 years after breast reconstruction.

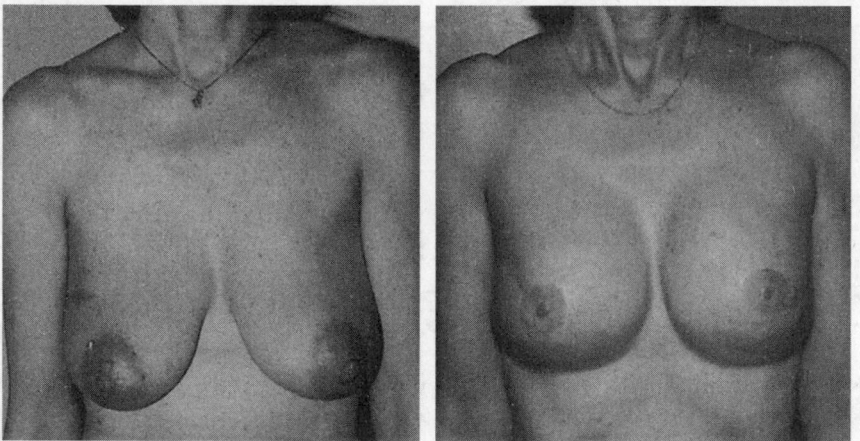

This 44-year-old woman had bilateral prophylactic mastectomies and immediate reconstruction with tissue expansion. She is shown 2 years after nipple-areola reconstruction.

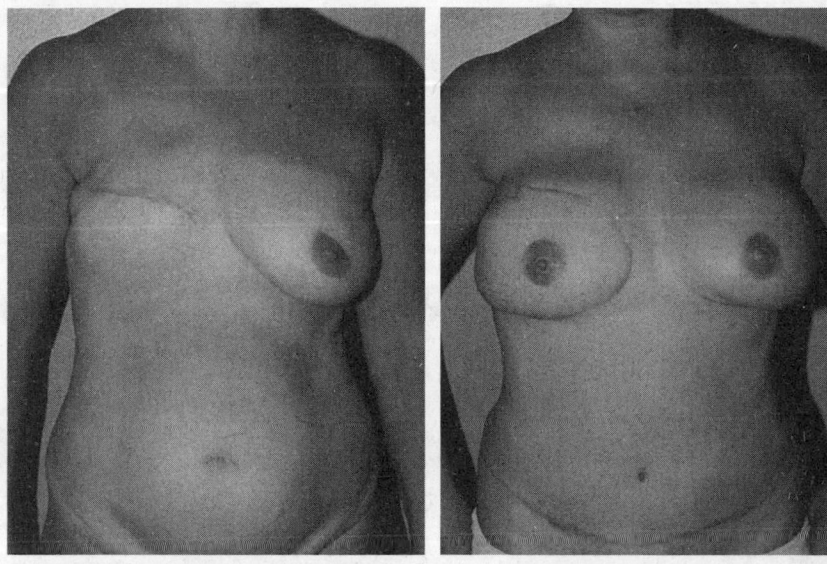

This 44-year-old woman, who previously had a modified radical mastectomy of her right breast, elected to have a left prophylactic mastectomy and immediate TRAM reconstruction and a delayed TRAM reconstruction of her right breast. Skin-sparing incisions were used around the areola and in the inframammary fold. This patient, shown 1 year later, illustrates how the length of incisions can be reduced when immediate breast reconstruction is performed.

## RECONSTRUCTION WITH AVAILABLE TISSUE

Despite their desire for breast restoration after treatment for breast cancer, many women will forego reconstructive surgery if it means a lengthy or complicated operation, convalescence, and rehabilitation. Constraints of time and money or psychological needs often limit their choices to a simple procedure or to no procedure at all. Women who choose these simpler procedures do not object to the use of a foreign material in their bodies and do not express overriding concerns about breast implants. Their chief goal is the simplest and most convenient method of breast restoration. For these women, implant or expander reconstruction provides the perfect solution. Unlike the more complex flap techniques, the operative variables are not increased, new scars are not created, and the potential for perioperative complications is minimized. Furthermore, these procedures do not rule out other procedures, especially flap operations, should they become necessary in the future. The patient who chooses implant reconstruction should be aware, however, that this reconstructive approach usually is not a one-stage procedure. A second operation will be required to reconstruct the nipple-areola and if necessary to make appropriate adjustments in implant size, shape, and position or to release scar tissue (capsular contracture release). Similarly, tissue expansion will require additional office visits to inflate the expander and for implant placement or adjustment and nipple-areola reconstruction. Under most circumstances these secondary procedures can be performed on an outpatient basis.

Before we discuss implant and expander reconstruction techniques and the anticipated postoperative care and recuperation, a brief review of the available implants and tissue expanders is appropriate.

## Types of Implants and Expanders

Basically, there are two broad categories of implants: fixed-volume breast implants and implants in which the volume can be changed after they are implanted (the latter are called tissue expanders). All current implants have a silicone elastomer layer or envelope that contains the filling (which is now usually saline solution); this covering is the outer material in contact with the body tissues.

Of the fixed-volume implants available, the ones most commonly used today are those that can be inflated with saline solution. (In the United States silicone gel can only be used if a woman is enrolled in clinical trials.) Alternative implant fill materials that are radiolucent on mammography, compatible with the surrounding tissues, and absorbed by the body if a leak occurs are under development. The radiolucence of implant fill materials is not as great an issue when these implants are used for breast reconstruction after mastectomy because this operation removes the majority of breast tissue, and subsequent mammography of the reconstructed breast is usually not necessary.

Although concerns about silicone gel leakage are avoided by implants that contain only saline solution, they may not, however, have the natural feel that implants containing some gel do. When saline-filled implants are soft and have good cover, they can feel natural. When there is thin tissue over these implants, a margin of the implant may be felt or the breast may have a rippled appearance. If leakage develops, they will deflate, requiring another procedure to replace the implant. Although leakage and deflation were problems associated with earlier saline implants, today's saline inflatable implants have a much lower incidence of deflation. Shaped or anatomic saline implants also provide more versatile options for achieving breast symmetry and more natural contour. They are often designed to use in conjunction with anatomic expanders.

Tissue expanders are adjustable implants that can be inflated with saltwater (saline solution) to stretch the tissues at the mastectomy site. These tissue expanders have a textured silicone shell that is filled with saline solution and adjusted after their placement. The saline solution is injected through the skin and into a valve leading to the implant. This fill valve is either a separate valve connected with tubing to the device near the breast reconstruction site or most commonly it is attached to the front of the implant. This temporary expander is left in place until the breast has been expanded and adjusted to the optimal volume and shape; the expander is then exchanged for a permanent fixed-volume implant, usually after 4 to 6 months or longer.

There are two basic designs of tissue expander valves through which the saltwater is injected to inflate the expander and stretch the tissues. One type of valve is connected to the tissue expander through

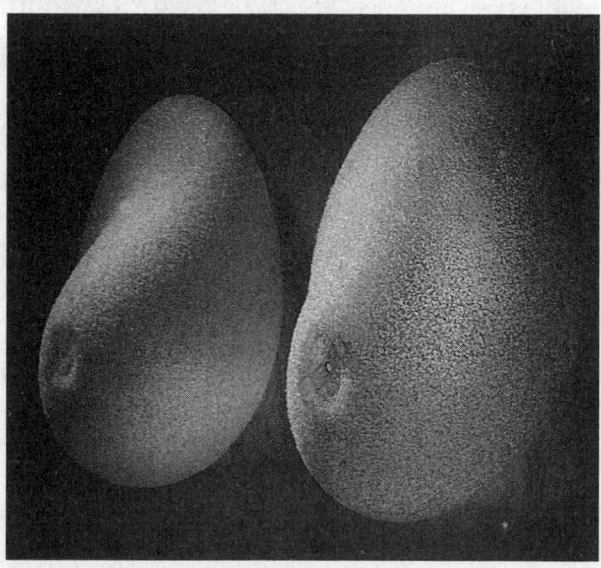

Anatomic-shaped, textured-surface saline-filled implants

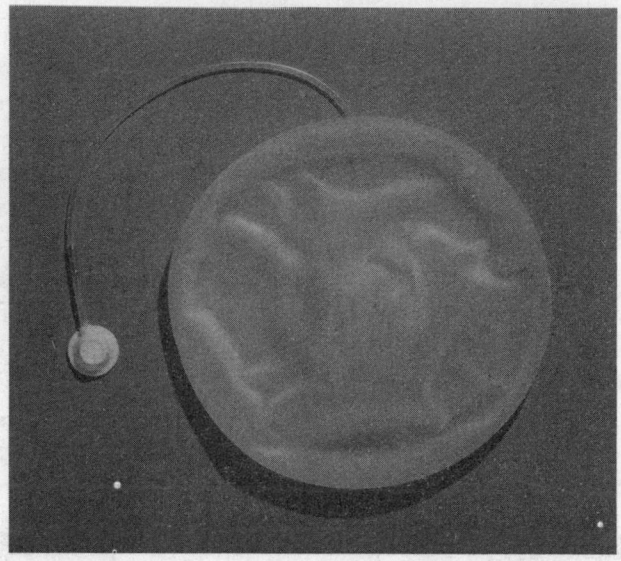

Textured-surface permanent expander implant with remote fill port

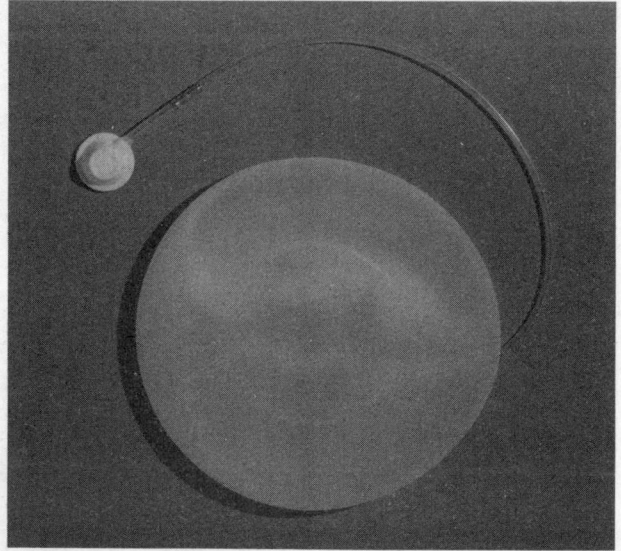

Postoperatively adjustable saline-filled, textured-surface
implant with remote valve

silicone tubing. This valve may be removed or in the case of the smaller valves (less than ½ inch in diameter) it can be left in for an extended period of time to permit future adjustments in breast size. Another type of valve is an integral part of the tissue expander. A metal disk is incorporated in the back of this integral valve, and a magnetic finder is then used to locate the site for injection of the saline solution. This valve is often palpable and can sometimes be felt through thin skin cover.

The postoperatively adjustable implant is an alternative to the temporary expander. This device permits postoperative adjustments in breast size over a relatively narrow range of volumes. The postoperatively adjustable implant contains only saline solution; it is basically a saline implant that has separate tubing connecting it to a small fill valve, usually located in the underarm area. With this model of adjustable implant, the small, separate fill valve can remain in place for months or even years so that breast size can be altered over a long period of time, or it can be removed when breast volume is judged ideal. Most women tolerate the small valve without a problem and appreciate the option of changing their breast size and volume should it be necessary or desirable. Once the valve has been removed, this device becomes a permanent fixed-volume implant.

Another alternative for tissue expansion is the permanent expander implant. This device has an outer lumen that contains a thin layer of silicone gel, an inner expander that is injected with saline solution, and a separate valve. Similar to the postoperatively adjustable implant, the permanent expander implant has separate tubing connecting the implant to a small valve placed under the skin, usually at the side of the breast, below the breast, or in the axilla. This valve can remain in place for an extended period of time to permit alterations in breast size.

All silicone implants and expanders once had a smooth outer envelope. Today, the surfaces of these devices may also be textured as a possible means of reducing the incidence of firmness produced from scar formation (capsular contracture). Textured tissue expanders seem to have less capsular contracture and produce softer breasts. Currently, breast expanders are available only with a textured surface. Textured implants do not perform as well when overlying skin cover is thin and may be unnaturally palpable or may exhibit visible wrinkling through the skin. The smooth-surface saline implant may produce less visible rippling when the skin cover is thin.

## Implant Reconstruction

Implant reconstruction using the available tissue remaining after the mastectomy is often the choice for the woman who has sufficient healthy tissue at the mastectomy site to adequately cover a breast implant or a postoperatively adjustable implant. This method is appropriate for the woman who has had a total mastectomy in which her breast is removed but her chest muscles are preserved. Skin-sparing mastectomy increases the probability that the skin remaining at the mastectomy site will not be tightly stretched. For delayed implant reconstruction, the surgeon should be able to move the skin over the muscle, which indicates the presence of tissue beneath the skin that can be used to provide a smooth contour for a pleasing breast shape. Reconstruction with this technique is particularly suitable for obtaining a symmetric appearance in a woman whose remaining breast is of normal size, has a somewhat rounded shape, and does not sag. It is also suitable for bilateral reconstructions; in fact, the best symmetry is often possible when both breasts are reconstructed simultaneously with the same technique.

When immediate reconstruction is planned, the same general indications apply, but the preferred candidate's breasts should be somewhat smaller. There are limitations to the size of the breast implant that can be placed at the time of the mastectomy to avoid complications and not compromise healing. These size limitations make tissue expansion, which permits more flexibility, accuracy, and safety in sizing the reconstructed breast for larger reconstructions, an appealing option for an immediate operation.

### Surgical Procedure and Postoperative Appearance

Breast restoration using the tissue remaining after the mastectomy is the simplest technique available today. This operation normally takes 1 to 2 hours to perform. If the remaining breast is to be altered, this modification can be made during the same operation, and any further adjustments on the reconstructed breast can be made during a second operation to rebuild the nipple-areola. Either a general (the most common) or local anesthetic can be used with adequate sedation. This operation may be done on an outpatient or inpatient basis.

The plastic surgeon places a breast implant beneath the patient's skin and upper chest muscles to produce a breast shape. To avoid creating new breast scars the surgeon will frequently reopen a portion of the mastectomy scar and insert the implant through it. Endoscopic surgery (often referred to as video surgery or minimally invasive surgery) can be helpful in this situation. This technique allows the surgeon to operate through short incisions using special long instruments. The operative cavity is visualized through small video cameras attached to the endoscope; these cameras project a video image of the tissues beneath the skin on the video monitor via fiberoptic light. This endoscopic approach helps minimize the length of the scar and the patient's postoperative pain.

If an immediate reconstruction is being performed, the implant can be placed through the mastectomy incision. The plastic surgeon may even remove the entire mastectomy scar and resuture it to produce a thinner scar line. When the mastectomy scar is not in the best location, a small incision can be made near the new inframammary crease (where the lower part of the breast joins the chest wall). The implant is then placed through this new incision. Because this inframammary scar falls in a crease, it is barely noticeable.

The technique for immediate breast reconstruction is similar to that just described. However, with the introduction of skin-sparing mastectomy, it is now possible to shorten the length of the scars. After the general surgeon removes the breast and the pathologist examines it, the plastic surgeon begins the breast reconstruction. He elevates the layer of muscular tissue just under the breast, selects a breast implant or expander, and positions it to obtain the best symmetry with the other breast. He then closes the muscle layer and sutures the skin incision. If the surgeon predicts preoperatively that there will not be sufficient cover for the implant or expander, sometimes a strip of latissimus dorsi muscle is obtained through the mastectomy incision to provide better cover for the lower portion of the implant and reduce postoperative complications. This portion of the latissimus dorsi (back) muscle can be harvested with endoscopic techniques to reduce any additional scarring.

Although this approach is designed to produce a reconstructed breast of the correct volume and shape at the initial procedure, in practice, this goal is not always attainable in one operation, especially if the breast is to appear as natural and symmetric as possible. It is frequently necessary to adjust or change the implant during a second

## Breast Reconstruction With Implants

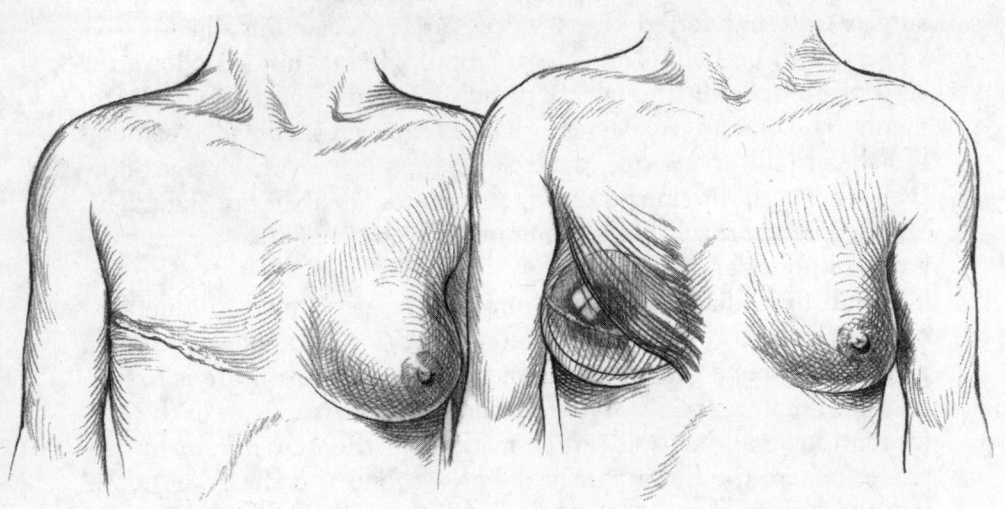

Modified radical mastectomy

Implant placed under muscle
and through existing scar

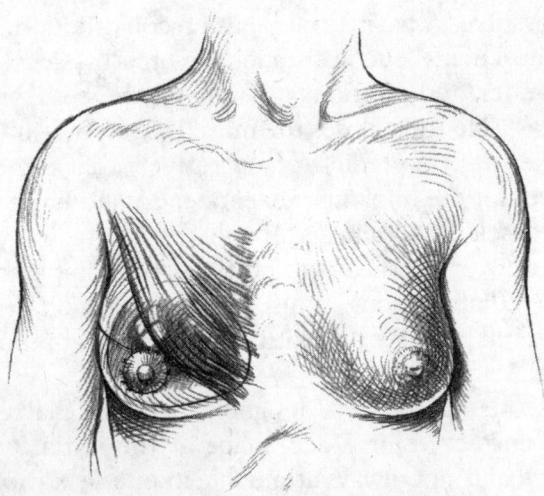

Nipple-areola reconstructed several months later

procedure. If the adjustments are minor, nipple-areola reconstruction is done during the same operation; otherwise it is best to wait until a third operation to ensure proper positioning.

The newly restored breast often appears flattened immediately after reconstruction with available tissue (immediate or delayed). This flatness results from the implant being positioned behind tissues that are relatively tight, restricting normal projection. These tissues stretch and soften over the next few weeks and months to provide better breast projection and shape. When a permanent expander implant or postoperatively adjustable implant is used, further adjustments can be made later to improve projection and give the patient some control over final breast size.

### Postoperative Care

A suction drain is often inserted into the reconstructed breast after surgery and left for 1 to 3 days to remove any excess fluid from the operative sites. The drain may need to be in place longer if there is increased drainage from the removal of axillary lymph nodes. The postoperative dressing selected should provide the best support for the new breast. A brassiere is chosen if the implant needs to be guided upward; an elastic "tube top" or light dressing is selected if it is to be maintained in place or allowed to move downward. If nonabsorbable stitches are used, they are removed approximately 1 week after surgery. This is usually not painful because the skin in that area is numb and relatively insensitive. Today, however, most reconstructive surgeons use absorbable sutures that do not require removal.

Because the breast has decreased sensitivity, the patient should not use a heating pad at the site of the operation to relieve breast discomfort; this area will be numb and she could accidently burn herself. After the stitches have dissolved or are removed, the surgeon may suggest that the patient massage and move her new breast around to keep it as soft and natural as possible. Massage is not needed, however, if textured implants have been used for reconstruction.

In a few weeks the scars will become red; this is a natural healing response and should not alarm the patient. This redness will fade with time. When the woman has fair, translucent skin, the increased blood flow into the healing scars will make them appear red for a longer period of time, sometimes for several years. Some patients naturally tend to heal with thick, raised scars. (A woman can get some idea of how she will heal by checking the appearance of any other scars she may have.) There are various recommendations for improving the appearance of these thickened scars, even though time is often the best solution; they will often fade and soften naturally over a period of months to years. Some surgeons recommend that surgical tapes be placed over the scars for several weeks or months to support the scar and to reduce the likelihood that they will widen and thicken. These scars may also be treated by injecting a cortisone solution into them or using silicone sheeting over them to provide gentle pressure to flatten and help fade them. In more severe cases the surgeon may re-excise, revise, and resuture the scars. When the scars are tight, they can be lengthened by a technique called a Z-plasty. With this technique, the skin is cut in the shape of a Z and then reshifted and sutured to relieve some of the skin tightness.

After reconstruction the patient's breast skin may be dry because of contact with the dressings. A nonallergenic skin moisturizer can help relieve dryness. In addition, if there are no drainage problems, some surgeons may suggest the use of vitamin E oil or cocoa butter; the patient can lightly massage this oil into her scars to help them soften and fade. Prolonged use of vitamin E oil can cause a rash, and if this condition develops, it should be discontinued.

### Complications

Implant reconstruction with available tissue has a low rate of complications. Complications are somewhat more common with immediate breast reconstruction. The most troublesome problem is excessive formation of hard fibrous tissue around the implant—the body's normal reaction to all foreign material. This reaction is called capsular contracture. There is some scar formation around all implants, and most reconstructed breasts feel firmer than normal breasts. To reduce breast firmness some surgeons use implants that have a textured surface. Surgeons recommend placement of smooth-surface implants under the chest wall muscle to help avoid this problem; in this location the implant is covered and protected by a layer of muscle. Although textured implants work equally well to reduce breast firmness in either location (above or below the muscle), most surgeons feel that they are best placed under thicker cover so that their texture and ripples are not visible under thin skin. When a smooth-surface implant is placed, many surgeons suggest that the woman massage her breasts on a regular basis to keep them soft and natural in appearance. Massage is not necessary for women with textured-surface implants; in fact, it may disturb the tissue adherence that the texturing promotes and that serves as a deterrent to fibrous scar formation. Sometimes a smooth-surface permanent saline implant is used to replace a textured expander or implant if the first device produces rippling.

In some cases this fibrous formation around the implant becomes tight, the implant becomes hard, and the breast appears deformed. Placement of an implant into an irradiated mastectomy site or subsequent radiation of an implant after reconstructive surgery often causes capsular contracture to develop. This problem is often managed by a capsulectomy, a procedure in which the thickened capsule and implant are surgically removed and the implant repositioned or replaced (for example, a smooth-surface implant may be exchanged for an implant with a textured surface). Alternatively, a layer of latissimus dorsi muscle may be inserted between the breast skin and implant to cover and cushion the implant. For some patients, the implant is removed, a flap of autologous tissue from the abdomen or buttocks is substituted for the implant, and the breast is thereby reconstructed entirely with the woman's own tissues.

Problems with implant leakage and displacement may also occur and are usually treated by removing the implant and replacing it during an outpatient procedure. Patients should be advised that implants are not lifetime devices; their life spans vary and they may have to be exchanged or replaced at some later date. (See Chapter 11 for more information on implants and possible complications.)

Bleeding and infection are rarely encountered after this operation. If the patient has had radiation therapy or her breast skin is thin or taut, infection may develop, or in an immediate breast reconstruction some of the skin may die because of poor blood supply, thereby exposing the implant. This complication is managed by removing the implant temporarily and transferring additional tissue to cover the implant or occasionally by resuturing the wound. Breast reconstruction is then started over a few months later; the technique selected at this time is dependent on the individual's situation.

Women who are cigarette smokers can have more difficulty with healing of the mastectomy skin flaps and experience a higher incidence of infection and exposure of the breast implant or tissue expander at the time of immediate breast reconstruction. In fact, smoking is a detriment to any surgical or reconstructive procedure. It reduces blood flow to the tissues, impairs healing, is associated with increased coughing, lung complications, and infections, and may severely compromise the result of any reconstructive attempt. *All smokers are strongly advised to discontinue smoking for at least 3 weeks and preferably several months before and after surgery. They should also not be around other cigarette smokers to avoid being exposed to second-hand smoke.*

### Pain and Recuperation

Most women who select implant reconstruction with available tissue say that it is not as painful or debilitating as the original mastectomy. The breast area is somewhat numb after the operation, but this lack of sensation is a residual effect from the mastectomy. The reconstruction avoids the armpit area, so pain in this region and shoulder stiffness are not concerns as they were after the mastectomy.

This operation may be done on an outpatient basis or during a brief hospitalization of 1 to 2 days. Women recover quickly from this procedure and are usually out of bed the afternoon of the surgery or the next day and may return to work or normal activity within a week. The patient may take a tub bath the day after the operation, but the incision should be kept dry and the dressing intact. Showers may be resumed 1 to 3 days after the operation if all is going well. Some surgeons place waterproof surgical tapes over the incisions to protect them and allow the patient to shower the day after the operation. One to two days after surgery the patient may lift her arms enough to comb her hair. It is possible to drive a car after 1 to 2 weeks, but the patient should not take any pain medications or sleeping pills that could impair her alertness and reflexes. Before driving, the woman should attempt turning the wheel while the car is still parked in the garage or driveway to see if this causes discomfort. It is best to wait 4 to 6 weeks before gradually resuming upper extremity exercise and sports activities. Although the woman may be feeling fine, she has been inactive for a period of time and even the muscles not affected by the operation need to be gradually retrained and stretched to regain their suppleness and strength.

## Results With Implant Reconstruction

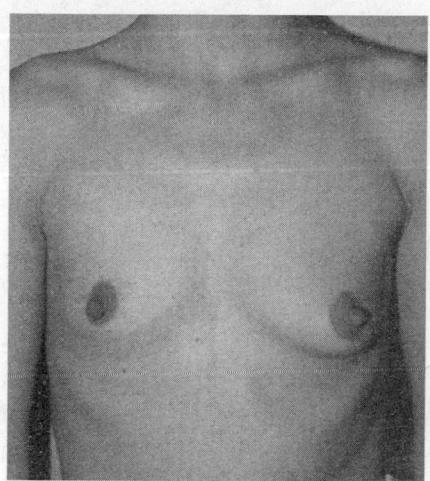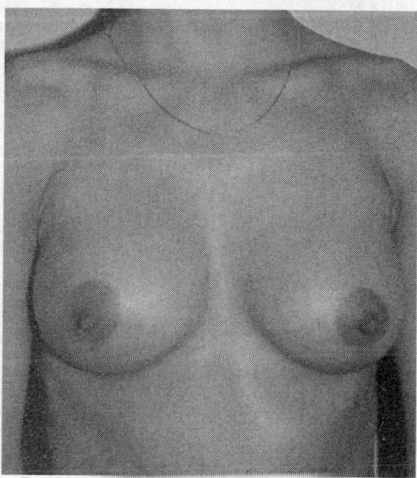

This 26-year-old woman wanted fuller breasts with minimal incisions and requested immediate breast reconstruction after a partial mastectomy. Implants were placed under the muscle in both breasts to achieve symmetry.

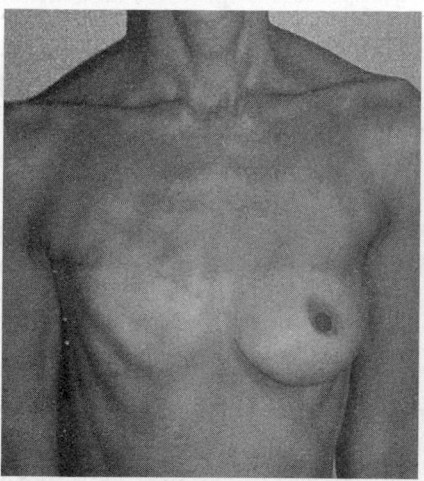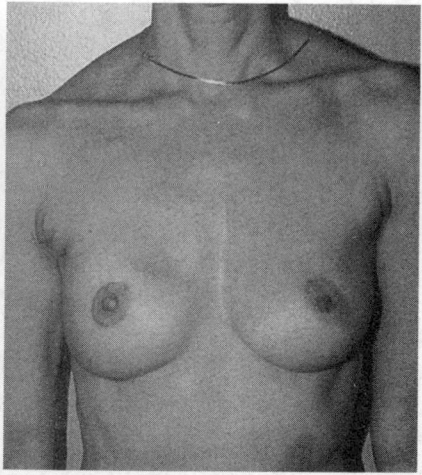

This 52-year-old woman had a modified radical mastectomy. Her breast was reconstructed using intraoperative tissue expansion and immediate implant placement. Her opposite breast was not modified. She is shown 1 year after breast reconstruction.

## Results With Implant Reconstruction—cont'd

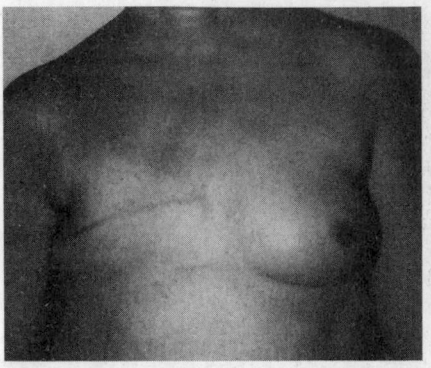 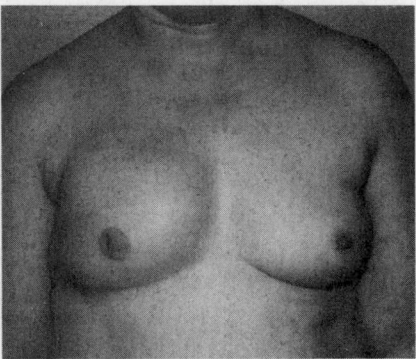

This 42-year-old woman had a right modified radical mastectomy. Her right breast was reconstructed with a breast implant placed beneath the muscle and her nipple-areola was reconstructed 3 months later. No opposite breast modification or additional breast scars were required. She is shown 2 years after breast reconstruction.

## Tissue Expansion

Despite tight skin at their mastectomy site, some women prefer to have simple reconstruction with available tissues rather than a more compli-cated flap procedure. For these women, the tissue expansion method is a good alternative. This type of breast reconstruction is frequently cho-sen by women who desire a simpler reconstructive approach that af-fords some flexibility in breast size. With this approach, the taut skin in the area of the mastectomy is stretched and expanded, thus avoiding a more complex flap operation and permitting placement of a perma-nent breast implant of suitable size and shape. Although this operation is similar to the approach described in the previous section, it differs in the type of implant used and the postoperative management.

Tissue expansion has a number of advantages for the patient and the reconstructive surgeon. The reconstruction can usually be accom-plished without additional breast scars, and the patient can help make the final determination of the volume and size of her reconstructed breast. She has input into decisions about final breast symmetry and the timing of inflation and second-stage breast reconstruction. This approach is particularly applicable for bilateral breast reconstruction because it permits the woman to determine final breast volume with-out the tissue restrictions she might encounter if she were depending on donor tissue from a flap from her abdomen, back, or buttocks, which could be insufficient to build two breasts.

Breast reconstruction with tissue expansion has its drawbacks; it is time intensive, and the woman who is looking for the quickest approach should understand that usually two or even three procedures may be required. Although the length of hospitalization necessary for the initial placement of the device is not great and even can be done as an outpatient procedure in many cases, the patient requires a number of additional postoperative visits for the actual stretching of the tissues. These office visits and procedures can be inconvenient, require traveling long distances, and interfere with the demands of family and work. The procedure takes longer than breast reconstruction with other techniques, often a matter of months. Even though the desired breast volume is usually attained within a few weeks, additional time is required to complete the reconstruction. For the best results, the breast tissue should be overexpanded, the expanded reconstructed breast allowed time to heal, and the breast evaluated for any further adjustments prior to second-stage breast reconstruction when the tissue expander is exchanged for a breast implant or the expander implant is converted to a permanent implant by removing its valves. These valves can be small and some women choose to keep them in case they require later volume adjustments.

Today, most patients having immediate breast reconstruction with available tissue have a temporary expander or a postoperatively adjustable implant placed rather than a fixed-volume implant. These expandable devices permit a larger breast to be built and adjusted as it is inflated, avoiding the problem of placing an implant that is not symmetric or is initially too large for the tissues and could complicate the healing process. When a fixed-volume implant is placed, it is usually either too large or too small. The expander enables the surgeon to fine-tune this volume for each individual. When tissue expansion is used after skin-sparing mastectomy for immediate breast reconstruction, it also has the advantage of avoiding skin tension over an implant while accurately achieving symmetry with the opposite breast.

### Surgical Procedure and Postoperative Appearance

Tissue expansion usually requires two operations. The first operation normally takes 1 to 2 hours to perform. It may be done under local or general (the most common) anesthesia and may be done on an inpatient or outpatient basis. During the first procedure the surgeon inserts a temporary expander or a postoperatively adjustable implant through the mastectomy incision or an inframammary incision, similar to implant placement (as described on p. 258). The upper part of the expander is usually positioned below the chest wall muscle, with the low-

## Breast Reconstruction With Tissue Expansion

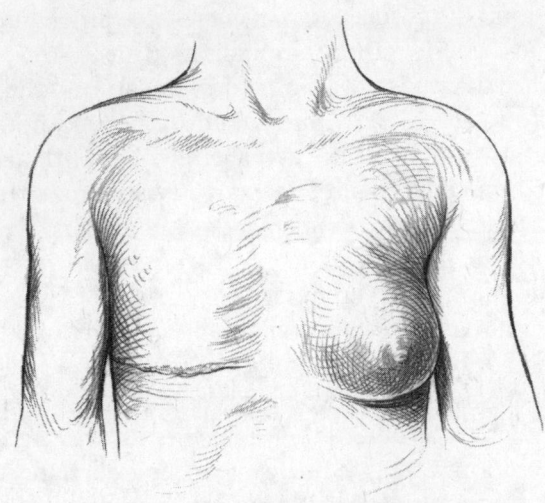

Modified radical mastectomy

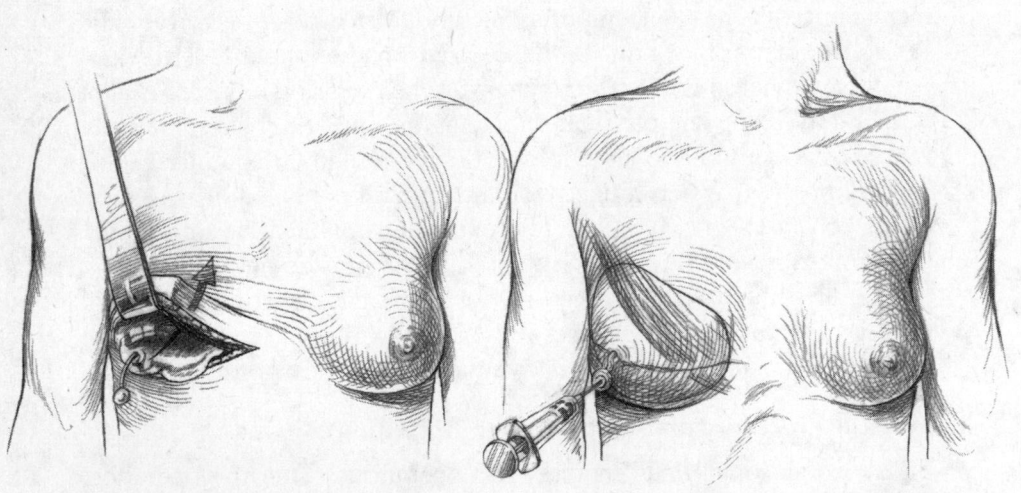

Tissue expander inserted
under skin muscle

Expander inflated with saline solution
during postoperative visits

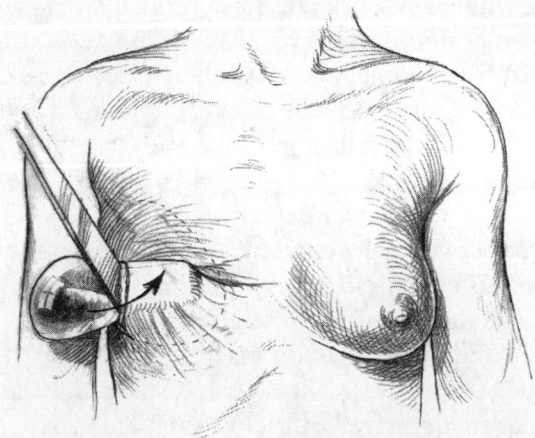

Expander removed and permanent implant inserted
in stretched pocket (with the permanent expander implant
only the fill tube and valve are removed)

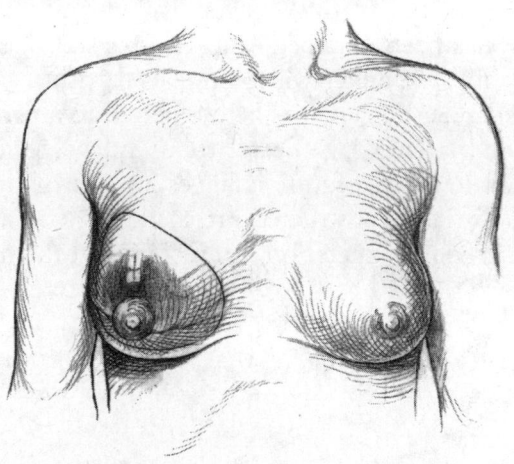

Nipple-areola reconstructed several months later

er part just under skin. The surgeon often manually stretches the breast skin during this initial operation to permit more rapid expansion later or may use some volume expansion to stretch the overlying skin intraoperatively. He then positions the valve to allow injection of saline solution for enlargement of the implant. In this early postoperative period the breast skin is still tight and the reconstructed breast appears flattened and smaller than the remaining breast on the opposite side.

Once this implant is in place and the valve is positioned under the skin for easy access, the woman schedules visits to the plastic surgeon to have her expander gradually inflated. A typical expansion session lasts from 5 to 15 minutes. The saltwater solution is usually injected through the skin into the valve, which is often on the upper front surface of the expander and is found by palpation or by using a magnet. The rate of inflation is influenced by the quality of the healing and the tightness and discomfort being experienced by the patient. This gradual enlargement of the implant produces pressure on the woman's skin, causing it to become tense, stretch, and eventually expand to a larger area. Much the same phenomenon occurs when the abdominal skin stretches during pregnancy. This process can be painful for some women, and the volume and timing of the injection and fill process must be individualized. After the breast skin has been distended sufficiently, which is somewhat larger than the other breast (this is called overexpansion), and the optimal breast size has been obtained, during a second outpatient procedure the temporary expander will be replaced with a permanent implant or the expander implant will be converted to a permanent fixed-volume implant by removing the fill tube and valve. (Alternatively, these can be left in place if future changes are anticipated.) After this second operation the reconstructed breast usually has a more natural appearance and the final operation can reconstruct the nipple-areola.

### Postoperative Care

Postoperative care is the same as that described for implant reconstruction on p. 261.

### Complications

Capsular contracture, device failure, expander exposure (requiring removal), and implant displacement are all potential problems associated with tissue expanders. The use of textured-surface expanders that adhere to the surrounding tissue has significantly reduced the incidence of breast firmness and implant displacement. The incidence of device failure and leakage is greater with tissue expanders than it is with implants because of valve problems, displacement of a remote fill port, inadvertent puncture of the tissue expander during saline inflation, and possible introduction of bacteria that can lead to infection. If this occurs, the device or the fill port may need to be removed and the wound allowed to heal before it is replaced.

Tissue expansion can lead to thinning of the stretched skin. If the skin at the mastectomy site is already thin, healing problems may occur. To lower the chance of tissue expander exposure through this thin skin necessitating removal, the reconstructive surgeon may decide to place the tissue expander under the muscle and fascial layer. As an alternative, he can shift a layer of muscle from the latissimus dorsi (back) muscle to the lower portion of the reconstructed breast at the time of the mastectomy (the pectoralis major [chest wall] muscle is used to cover the upper part of the expander); this muscle cushion seems to reduce the incidence of complications from implant exposure, is especially useful for immediate breast reconstruction, and provides better skin cover over the lower portion of the reconstructed breast. This technique can be performed without additional incisions or scars and without significant functional impairment. (This technique is discussed later in this chapter.)

As with implant reconstruction, women who are cigarette smokers can experience an increased incidence of healing problems after tissue expansion. This potential complication is discussed on p. 263 under complications after implant surgery.

### Pain and Recuperation

The pain associated with tissue expansion is similar to that described previously for implant reconstruction. When tissue expansion is done at the time of mastectomy, the patient experiences additional pain from the stretching of healing tissues, which are undergoing wound contraction. Patients often describe a tight, pulling sensation following inflation. Usually this pain is not severe. If it is, the tissue expansion is terminated temporarily to allow the tissues to heal for a week or two and then resumed. If it is too tight, some saline solution can be removed for a few days. The site for the fill valve is usually in an area where some nerves were removed during the mastectomy and thus is relatively numb.

This operation may be done on an outpatient basis or during a brief hospital stay. If done in the hospital, the usual stay is 1 to 2 days. Recovery from this operation is reasonably quick. The patient can usually return to nonstrenuous activity in 2 to 3 weeks and resume sports in 6 to 8 weeks. All other aspects of recovery are the same as those described earlier on p. 264.

## Results With Tissue Expansion

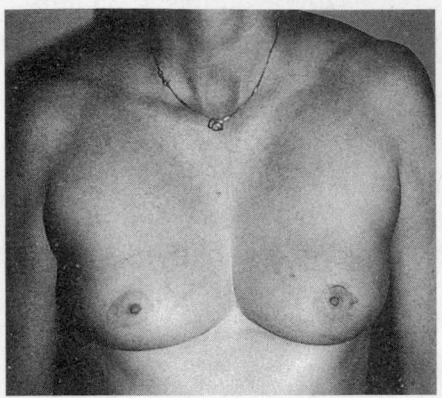 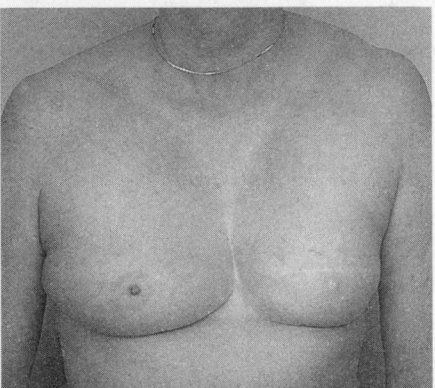

This 52-year-old woman with cancer of the left breast had a modified radical mastectomy and immediate breast reconstruction. She decided to have reconstruction with placement of a tissue expander. This was followed by placement of a permanent breast implant, which made it possible to match her opposite breast. She is shown 1 year after breast reconstruction. Her nipple-areola was reconstructed with a local flap and a tattoo.

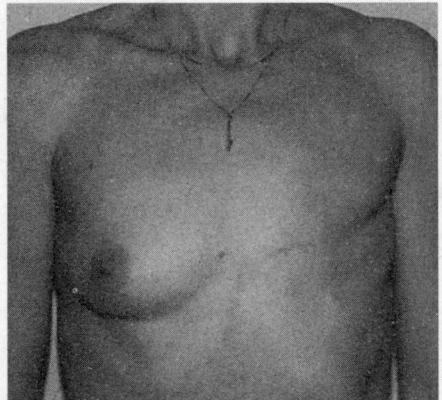 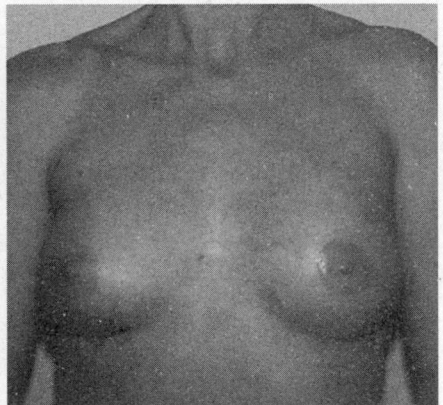

This 35-year-old woman had a left modified radical mastectomy that left tight local tissue. She requested breast reconstruction with tissue expanders and a right breast augmentation. She did not want to have a TRAM flap procedure. She is shown 2 years following breast reconstruction.

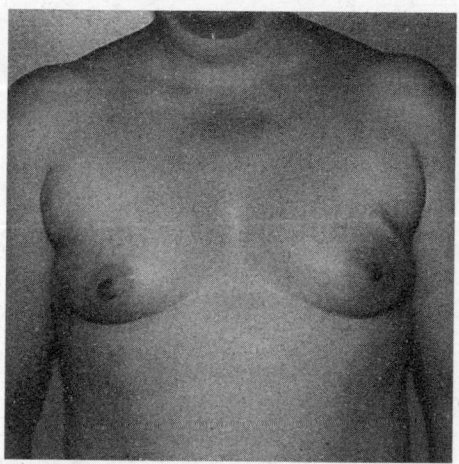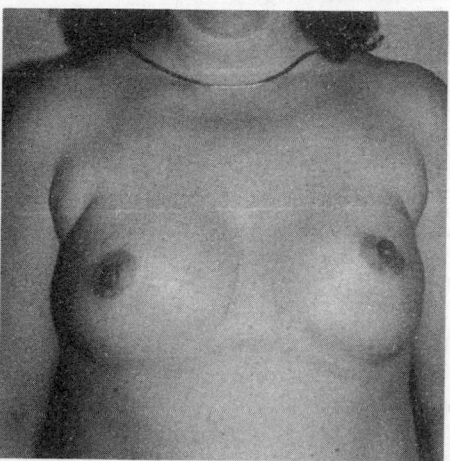

This 38-year-old woman had bilateral mastectomies and immediate breast reconstruction with tissue expander implants placed under the muscle. She is shown 15 months following breast reconstruction.

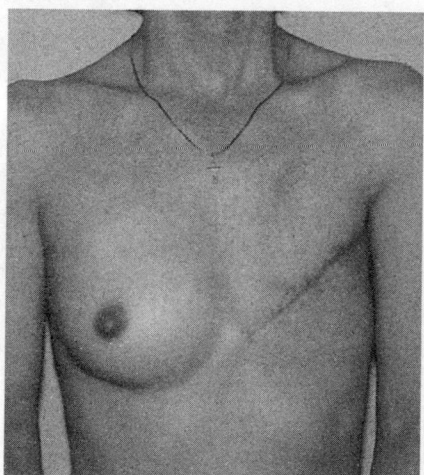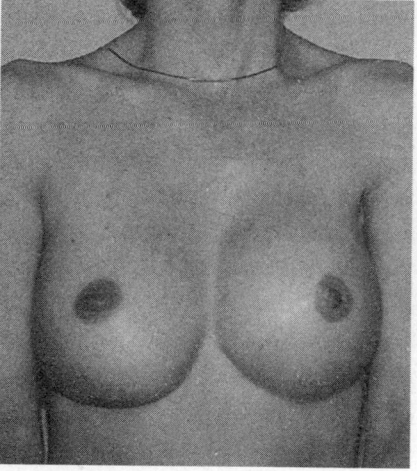

This 34-year-old woman had breast reconstruction after a modified radical mastectomy. Permanent expander implants were used for reconstruction and augmentation mammaplasty. She is shown 12 months following breast reconstruction.

## *Results With Tissue Expansion—cont'd*

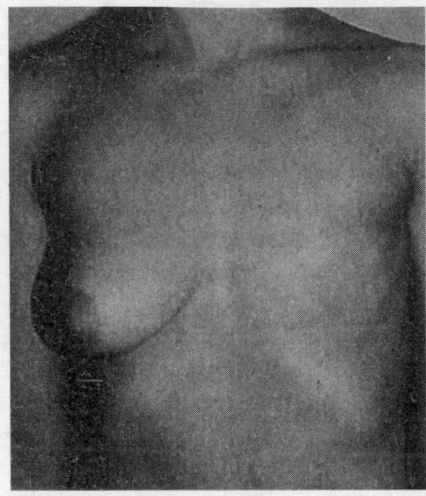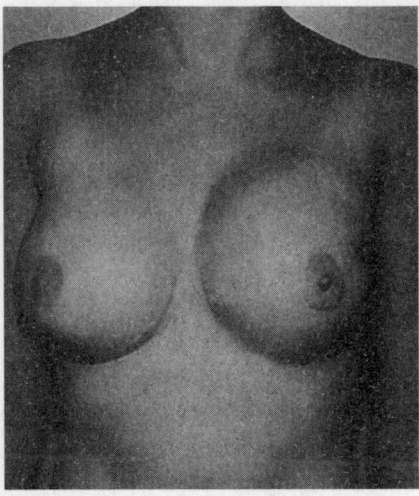

This 28-year-old woman had a modified radical mastectomy of her left breast. When she was referred for prophylactic mastectomy of the opposite breast, she requested bilateral breast reconstruction at the time of her mastectomy. Since she wanted to avoid back or abdominal scars, a flap procedure was not selected. She is shown 3 years after bilateral breast reconstruction with tissue expanders.

## When Available Tissue Reconstruction Is Not the Right Choice

Because reconstruction with available tissues and implants or tissue expanders is the simplest of breast reconstruction techniques and offers excellent results, you would assume that these techniques would be the best choice for every patient. Some circumstances, however, prompt a woman to consider other reconstructive options. For instance, when her remaining breast is large and she does not want it changed, reconstruction with these methods will produce breasts of an unequal size because there will not be enough tissue present to build a large breast. Although she might be satisfied with the newly reconstructed breast initially, eventually she will feel lopsided and will probably still need to wear a prosthesis to make her breasts appear equal in size. Consequently, unless the normal large breast is reduced to match the rebuilt breast, reconstruction with the available tissue may not be a permanent solution for this patient because it will not produce symmetric breasts. The experienced surgeon can predict in advance if the other breast will need to be modified or if a flap is needed.

Although breast implants and tissue expanders have a good track record when used for aesthetic and reconstructive breast surgery, some women prefer not to have a foreign material permanently placed in their reconstructed breast. For them, breast reconstruction with their own tissue is the only logical choice.

Nor is reconstruction with available tissue or tissue expansion appropriate for a woman with a radical mastectomy deformity because it does not satisfactorily restore the missing chest wall muscle (pectoralis major muscle), the hollow under the collarbone (infraclavicular hollow), and the fold produced by the arm and breast in the armpit area (anterior axillary fold). Additional tissue must be brought in to reconstruct these areas. For some patients, a combination of additional tissue from the back or the lower abdomen and an implant or expander will offer the most symmetric breast reconstruction.

If a patient has tight, thin, irradiated, or grafted skin, she also may have limited or unsatisfactory results because the skin remaining at the mastectomy site, even with tissue expansion, is insufficient to cover the implant and to provide her with a breast that looks and feels natural. A flap reconstruction technique is a more logical choice for the patient with major skin, muscle, and contour deficiencies. If a woman has had conservative surgery followed by radiation therapy (also called lumpectomy with irradiation) and for some reason has to have a completion mastectomy, in all but rare circumstances a flap of the patient's own tissue from the lower abdomen or back is necessary to obtain a satisfactory breast reconstruction. Implants and expanders usually do not provide satisfactory results if the breast has been irradiated.

Sometimes an implant or expander must be used in conjunction with a flap. This may be necessary when a woman needs both breasts rebuilt and has insufficient flap tissue or to permit the design of a smaller but necessary flap with a shorter donor scar. For example, a TRAM flap or latissimus dorsi flap may be combined with a tissue expander. The flap can then provide muscle or skin and muscle for the reconstruction, and the tissue expander can be used to create a new breast of the correct size. When the latissimus dorsi muscle is being used for immediate breast reconstruction, it can be obtained through the mastectomy incision using endoscopic techniques. ( See p. 259 for a fuller discussion of endoscopic techniques.) This approach allows the surgeon to harvest the flap tissue with shorter scars, often improving the result and also causing less pain. A flap of tissue is also used to provide good cover for the breast implant or tissue expander. Sometimes the TRAM flap reconstruction is enhanced by placing an implant or expander. The newer devices, particularly those which are inflatable and have textured surfaces, are made with thicker outer envelopes; these cause wrinkles and are easily seen and felt through thin skin. If the skin is thin, the result is better if a flap of the patient's own tissue is interposed to provide better cover for the implant.

## FLAP RECONSTRUCTION

The use of flaps of muscle or skin and muscle (musculocutaneous) to supplement the tissue remaining after a mastectomy represents a major advance in breast reconstruction. With the newest flap techniques, most women's breasts can now be rebuilt with their own tissue and usually without a breast implant. Furthermore, because the donor sites are often areas of tissue excess such as the lower abdomen or buttocks, these women can expect a full and natural breast that closely resembles the size and shape of their opposite breast. As a benefit, the area from which the donor tissue is taken can sometimes be contoured to produce a more aesthetic appearance. Now even women with radical mastectomy deformities, radiation injuries, or recurrences after lumpectomy with irradiation requiring a mastectomy can have their deformities filled in and rebuilt. The patient's own tissue is preferred in these situations.

The two most common sources of tissue for breast reconstruction with the patient's own tissue (autologous) are the lower abdominal wall and the back. The buttock or lateral hip areas can also be used as donor sites, although some women and surgeons find the hip scars objectionable. When the tissue from the abdominal wall or back is used, it is left attached to the blood supply of the muscle beneath it (a musculocutaneous flap). When buttock or lateral hip tissue is used, microsurgery techniques are necessary to restore the blood supply of the flap by reattaching the vessels supplying this tissue to those in the breast region. Microsurgery can also be used to move a flap of abdominal wall tissue (TRAM flap). The surgeon uses an operating microscope and special fine instruments and sutures to disconnect the tissue and vessels from the donor area and reattach them to tiny vessels in the region of the breast, usually in the axilla and occasionionally in the inner breast area. Many surgeons prefer to reserve the use of microsurgery for TRAM flap operations for those patients with abdominal scars that preclude the usual TRAM flap and for patients with risk factors that make the free TRAM flap safer. Some surgeons feel that this abdominal tissue can be moved more reliably and expeditiously when it remains attached to its muscle and blood supply. Others, however, who are skilled microsurgeons, prefer to transfer this tissue microsurgically. This is a highly versatile flap for breast reconstruction, and whether it is transferred as a pedicle flap or via microsurgery often depends on the surgeon's expertise and the patient's preference.

All of these flap procedures are associated with more blood loss than breast reconstruction with local tissues and implants or expanders. For this reason, the reconstructive surgeon may discuss the possibility of blood transfusions with the patient and recommend that the patient donate her own (autologous) blood before the operation. Her blood is then stored in the blood bank until it is needed. Usually this blood is donated during the month before the operation. For immediate breast reconstruction with a flap, it is usually recommended that 1 to 2 units of the patient's blood be available. This can sometimes necessitate scheduling the operation a few weeks later; this short delay will not lessen the patient's chance of a cure from the breast cancer treatment and can reduce the patient's concern about the possibility of receiving a blood transfusion from the general donor pool.

## Reconstruction With the Lower Abdominal (TRAM) Flap

Creation of the breast with a flap of lower abdominal skin and fat over a strip of muscle (rectus abdominis) is a major contribution to breast reconstruction. This operation, developed in the early 1980s, is now the most frequently used flap procedure and provides some of the most attractive and realistic breast reconstructions. This technique allows the surgeon to restore a woman's breast with her own tissues, usually without the need for a silicone breast implant, and at the same time give her a slimmer abdomen. With this approach, the surgeon uses excess abdominal tissue to rebuild the breast after a total mastectomy, modified radical mastectomy, or even radical mastectomy.

The transverse rectus abdominis musculocutaneous flap, also known as the TRAM flap, is recommended for the woman who requires the extra tissue supplied by a flap reconstruction. She prefers a breast reconstruction without a breast implant and is pleased or will accept the prospect of having a "tummy tuck" as a bonus. Sometimes the patient's lower abdominal tissue is insufficient to create a breast of satisfactory volume. This most often occurs with bilateral reconstruction. The patient should discuss her preferences and thoughts with the reconstructive surgeon and get his opinion of whether implants will be needed. As with the other flap operations, this is major surgery and the woman who selects this operation should be in good health. Her tissue is moved a long distance (from the lower abdomen to the chest), and its blood supply must be healthy and sufficient to nourish the new tissue for breast reconstruction.

It has been found that the TRAM flap blood supply is particularly sensitive and precarious in the overweight woman, the hypertensive woman, the woman who has had radiation therapy, the woman with certain types of abdominal scars, and the woman who is a cigarette smoker. Because cigarette smoking can constrict and narrow blood vessels and precipitate flap failure, the plastic surgeon will insist that the patient avoid cigarettes before and after the operation. Additionally, the surgeon might suggest an exercise program consisting of sit-ups and modified sit-ups for several weeks before surgery to increase blood flow and strengthen her abdominal area. If there is evidence that the blood supply may be impaired from many years of cigarette smoking, another method of breast reconstruction should be selected, either tissue expansion or the latissimus dorsi flap. Microsurgical TRAM flap reconstruction and TRAM flap delay are other strategies to increase blood flow to the TRAM flap tissues. (The TRAM flap delay is discussed in the next section.)

The TRAM flap is not appropriate for every patient. When the woman's abdominal wall is very thin or she does not want scars in this region, another procedure should be considered. Women who are cigarette smokers, women who are significantly overweight, women over 65 years of age, women with medical problems such as diabetes mellitus or heart disease, and women who have had abdominal irradiation or who have abdominal scars, or women who have had liposuction, particularly across their upper abdomen, should strongly consider other techniques, for these conditions can increase the complication rate of the TRAM flap.

An immediate TRAM flap reconstruction offers a number of advantages. By combining the mastectomy and the breast reconstruction during one operation, the general surgeon is able to limit the amount of skin removed to only that which is necessary to properly treat the breast cancer. The removed skin is then replaced with the abdominal skin supplied by the TRAM flap. When the nipple-areola has a small diameter, the entire TRAM flap can be buried, thus further reducing the breast scars. By preserving the remaining breast skin and by restoring the important landmarks of the breast such as the inframammary fold and the lateral breast, immediate breast reconstruction with the TRAM flap creates a natural, well-contoured breast with minimal breast scars. Of course, an abdominal wall procedure is necessary to obtain the TRAM flap.

The TRAM flap is now frequently used for immediate breast reconstruction with skin-sparing mastectomy when there is no tumor involvement in the skin. The skin-sparing mastectomy saves most of the breast skin and its peripheral landmarks, thus permitting a better shaped breast with fewer scars.

When immediate breast reconstruction with the TRAM flap is planned, close cooperation between the general surgeon and the reconstructive surgeon is essential and the patient needs to be fully informed about the specifics of the procedure, possible complications, and the expected recuperation. Usually it is necessary for the patient to donate her own blood so it is available if needed during the procedure or in the postoperative period.

### Surgical Procedure and Postoperative Appearance

TRAM flap breast reconstruction is major surgery and usually takes approximately 3 to 6 hours in the operating room compared to the 1 to 2 hours required for implant or expander reconstruction. This procedure is done under general anesthesia and requires a hospital stay of 4 to 8 days. This operation can only be done once, and the patient should be advised that if the need arises in the future for another breast reconstruction, another technique will have to be used.

Using this reconstructive method the surgeon designs a transverse flap of skin and fat on the middle to lower abdomen. The tissue for the new breast is surgically freed from the abdomen but left attached to a strip of the vertical abdominal wall muscle (the rectus abdominis). Sometimes strips of both rectus abdominus muscles (bipedicle TRAM flap) are used to ensure a better blood supply to the flap. The donor site is closed by bringing the remaining muscles together and tightening the entire central abdomen to restore abdominal wall strength. The scar that is left on the abdomen is similar but may not be quite as low and inconspicuous as the horizontal scar left from an abdominoplasty (tummy tuck), which removes excess abdominal tissue for aesthetic reasons. The flap is then ready for transfer to the chest. In preparation for transfer the plastic surgeon removes the mastectomy scar (if it is in an inconspicuous position) or he creates a new incision that will allow for a more aesthetic reconstruction. The flap is then elevated and transferred to the chest wall area through a tunnel under the upper abdominal skin and extending to the new incision in the breast area. The upper part of the flap is sutured into position to give the best contour for the upper breast area, and the lower portion of the flap is positioned, folded under, and contoured to form a breast mound. The breasts are then checked for symmetry and form with the patient positioned upright, and the flap is carefully stitched in place. If the patient has sufficient excess abdominal fat, there ordinarily is no need for a breast implant.

If the surgeon is concerned preoperatively about the adequacy of the blood supply of the abdominal flap, usually in patients with a combination of findings such as obesity, cigarette smoking, previous abdominal scars, or chest wall irradiation, he may decide on an operative delay. In this approach the operation is sequenced into two procedures. One to two weeks before the definitive flap operation the patient has a minor operation during which the surgeon divides some of the blood vessels going into the lower portion of the TRAM flap. He does this through two short incisions placed in the lower abdomen along the lower line of the planned TRAM flap. Later, during the major operation, these short incisions will be incorporated into the TRAM flap incisions. This so-called delay of the vessels serves to redirect and increase the flap's blood flow and venous drainage and is designed to improve its blood supply and therefore help ensure flap survival.

Several months after the TRAM flap procedure the plastic surgeon restores the nipple-areola in a second or third procedure (if a TRAM flap delay has been used) under local anesthesia followed later by a tattoo if additional pigmentation is desirable. Frequently the flap shape is altered and the abdominal wall is contoured with liposuction or ultrasound-assisted liposuction during a second operation. When ultrasound energy is applied, it cavitates, emulsifies, and loosens the fat before it is suctioned out.

The procedure for immediate TRAM flap reconstruction is similar to that described for the delayed approach, but it does not take as long because the surgeon's mastectomy has prepared the recipient area and more breast skin can be preserved to help shape the new breast and shorten the mastectomy scar. Results of immediate surgery with this technique have improved dramatically over the past several years. Often a woman's breasts are closely matched after the initial procedure and there is less need to adjust the opposite breast later. However, the woman who decides on an immediate procedure needs to be fully prepared for the donor deformity and scar and the additional breast scars required for placing the TRAM flap. Sometimes the mastectomy and immediate TRAM flap breast reconstruction are delayed for several weeks to enable the woman to have time to donate her blood for future transfusions during the breast reconstruction. The oncologic surgeon should have input in this timing decision. Most oncologic surgeons feel that this short delay has no adverse effect on the patient's outcome.

After this operation, if the breast reconstruction is to be delayed, the new breast usually has an elliptic pattern of stitches running along the lower breast crease and up toward the nipple area. When an immediate reconstruction is planned, the skin patch can be smaller and just extend around the area of the areola and sometimes laterally toward the axilla or there is only a short breast scar after the skin-sparing mastectomy. A donor scar extends across the lower abdomen between the pubic area and umbilicus. In addition, there is often some fullness on the inner portion of the new breast because of the addition of the rectus abdominis muscle, which supplies nourishment to the flap. This fullness usually subsides in the first 2 to 3 months after the operation as the transferred, unexercised muscle becomes thinner. If this fullness persists, if the reconstructed breast is larger than the opposite breast, or if there are other areas of fat accumulation in the lateral or lower abdomen, these areas can be contoured later using liposuction or ultrasound-assisted liposuction to suction out the excess fat.

## Breast Reconstruction With TRAM Flap

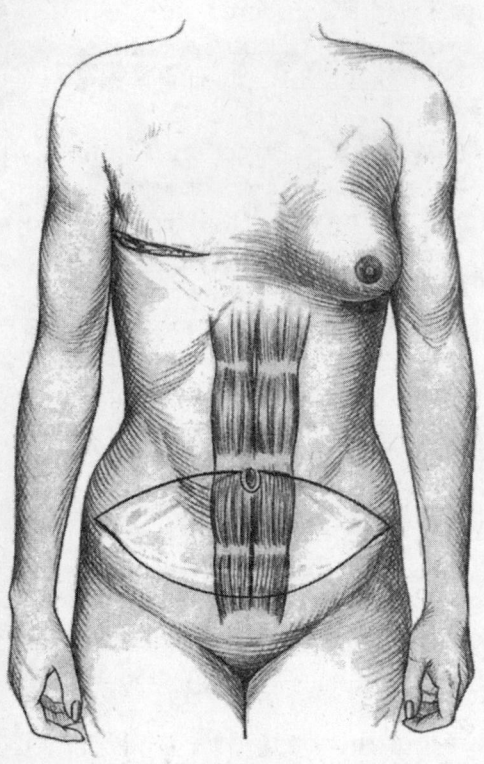

TRAM flap designed on lower abdomen

Abdominal tissue transferred to breast area while still attached to abdominal muscle (rectus abdominis)

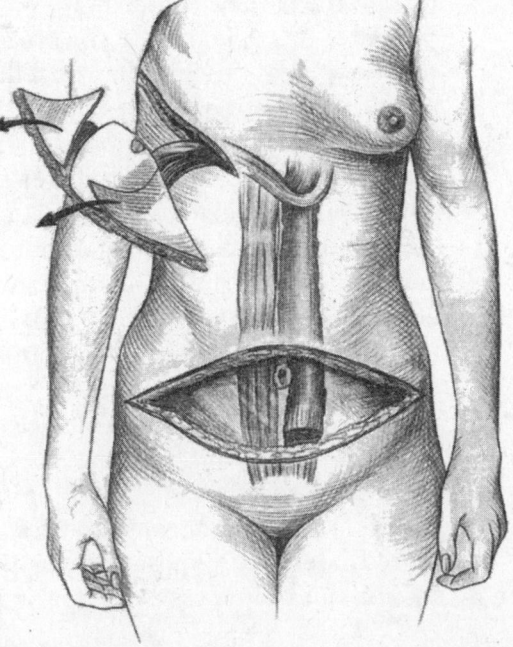

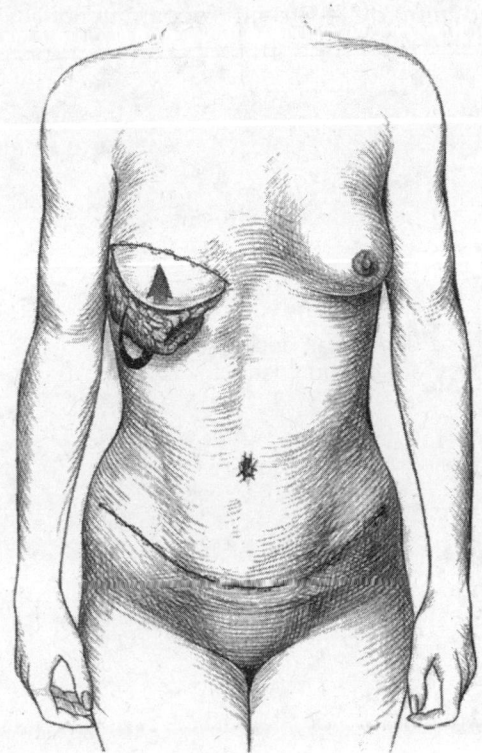

Abdominal tissue fashioned into breast and lower abdomen closed as transverse (tummy tuck) scar

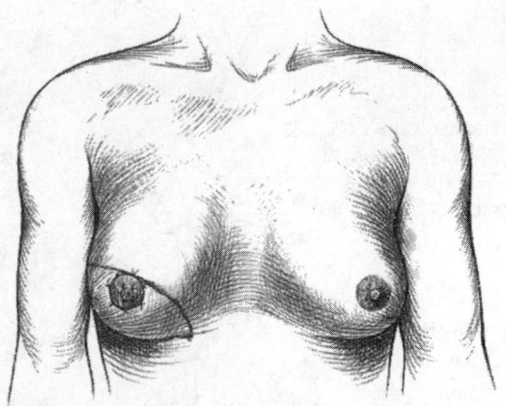

Nipple-areola reconstructed several months later

## Skin-Sparing Mastectomy and Immediate Breast Reconstruction With TRAM Flap

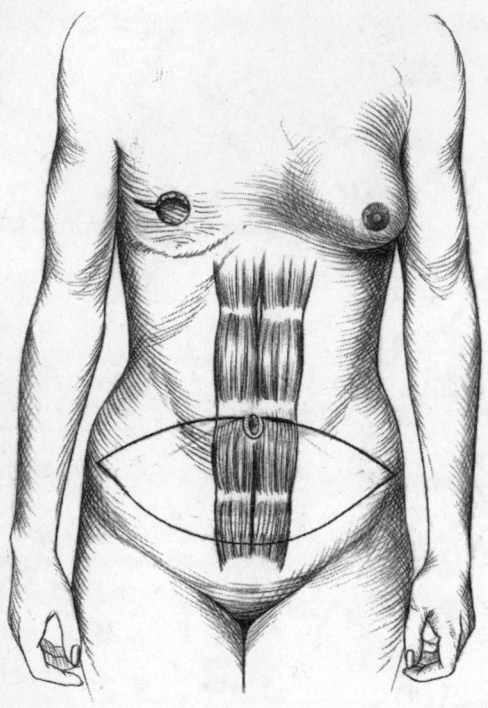

TRAM flap designed on lower abdomen

Abdominal tissue transferred to breast area while still attached to abdominal muscle (rectus abdominis)

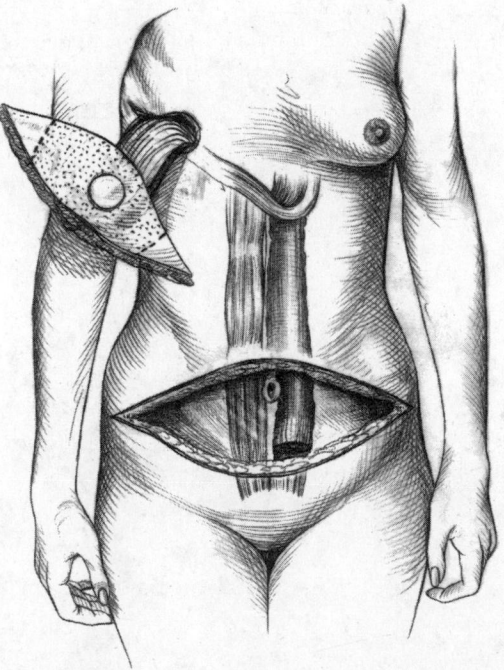

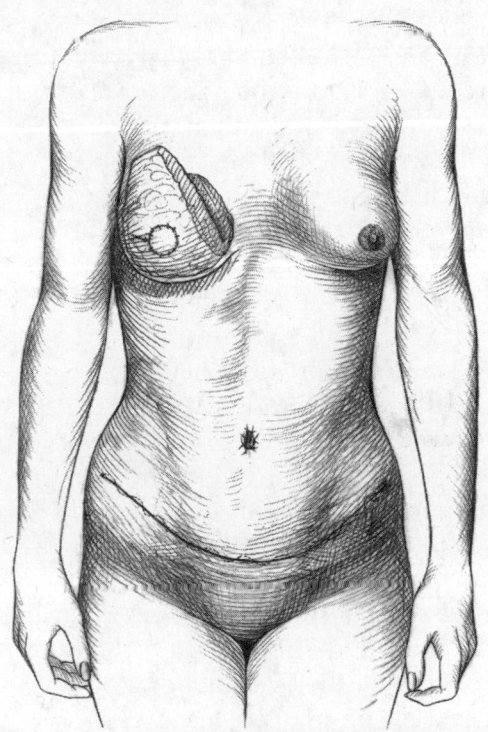

Abdominal tissue fashioned
into a breast and lower abdomen
closed as transverse scar

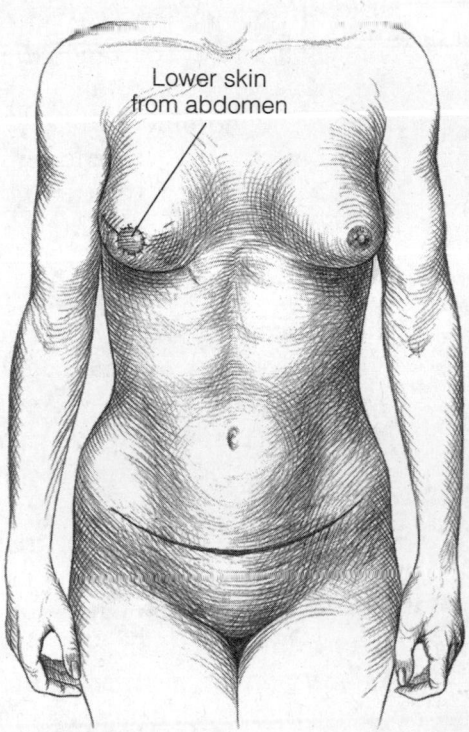

Lower skin
from abdomen

Breast reconstructed and
short incision (encircling areola
with side extension) closed

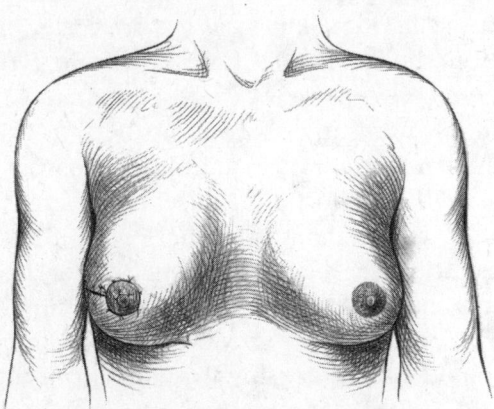

Nipple-areola reconstructed several months later

## Postoperative Care

Surgical drains are placed in the breast and abdomen for 3 to 4 days after the operation but are usually removed before the patient goes home. The hospital bed is flexed to relieve abdominal tension caused by the removal of lower abdominal tissue and muscle during the operation. The patient is usually asked to get out of bed the next day and walk. Even though her abdomen may be tight, it is important for a safe recovery. Activity enhances the blood flow throughout the body and can lower the chance of developing blood clots in the legs, which could travel to the lungs. The reconstructive surgeon may ask the patient to wear support hose before the operation and for the first few days after the operation to use sequentially compressive stockings or wear support hose to further enhance the blood return from the legs and lessen the chance of deep vein thrombosis. When the patient first gets out of bed, she may be unable to stand up straight; this is to be expected. It often takes days to weeks for the patient to stand erect, depending on the tightness of the abdomen. This tightness may also make her feel full after eating only a small amount of food and she may find that smaller, more frequent meals are better. The other specifics of postoperative care are described in the section on implant reconstruction on p. 261.

## Complications

Because this is major surgery, there are more possibilities for complications. About 1 in 10 patients experiences some healing problems, resulting in an area of skin loss, fat drainage, or firmness of the fatty tissue on the flap. This hard, thickened tissue can be frightening to a woman because of its resemblance to her original tumor. It sometimes softens in 6 to 18 months. This thickening can be differentiated from a tumor by examination, mammography, and sometimes fine-needle aspiration. These thick areas can be removed surgically or with standard liposuction or ultrasound-assisted liposuction techniques. Delayed healing or even loss of some or rarely all of the flap because of insufficient blood supply is a potential complication. Sometimes a portion of the skin edge or fat will have a reduced blood supply, causing drainage from the new breast for a few weeks. To avoid this drainage the surgeon may want to remove this strip of tissue as a minor outpatient procedure. If fluid accumulates beneath the abdominal skin, it may need to be aspirated or a small drain placed through the incision to allow this liquid to be removed.

Other less frequently occurring complications include bleeding (hematoma) and infection. If blood accumulates at the operative or donor site, a brief trip to the operating room is necessary to drain the hematoma. Antibiotics are frequently used to minimize the problem of infection. The development of venous clots in the legs or pelvic region is a rare but serious complication. These clots can potentially travel to the lungs (pulmonary embolus). If clots develop, the woman will be placed on anticoagulants (blood thinners). In addition, the patient should be encouraged to resume some activity right away, actively exercising her leg muscles when she is in bed and getting out of bed and attempting to walk the day after surgery. While she is inactive in bed, compression stockings are recommended.

Since the TRAM flap is obtained from the abdominal wall, there is some chance of a hernia developing. As a preventive measure to strengthen the abdominal wall and reduce the possibility of hernia, the reconstructive surgeon may place a sheet of mesh over the site where the strip of abdominal muscle is removed. This complication is now reported to occur in less than 2% of patients having this operation. If a hernia develops, mesh may also be used to repair it, and this can be done at the time of the nipple reconstruction.

### Pain and Recuperation

The TRAM flap operation is potentially more painful and uncomfortable than any of the other methods of breast reconstruction, especially in the abdominal area. Because the surgeon removes a strip of lower abdominal tissue during surgery, the abdomen is tighter and the woman feels a distinct pull. It may be difficult for the patient to stand upright until the muscle is stretched out again. A day or two after the operation when she is ready to eat, she may notice that she gets full quickly because the abdomen is tighter. However, as with most operations, each patient has a different tolerance level for pain; some patients take very little if any pain medication, whereas others may experience a great deal of pain and require analgesics for several weeks.

The discomfort involved in a TRAM flap has been compared by patients to the pain experienced after an abdominal hysterectomy or a cesarean section. During the first week after surgery most patients report soreness and pain in the abdominal area; movement is difficult and quite uncomfortable.

The PCA (patient-controlled analgesia) unit is now used to alleviate patient discomfort during hospitalization. This device represents a real advance in the management of pain in the postoperative period. It is safe, provides excellent pain relief, and the patient is in control. The PCA unit is connected to the patient's intravenous tubing, the proper pain-relieving drug and dosage are determined, and the machine is set so that the patient can press a button and administer the pain-relieving medication as she needs it. With this device, the pain medication can also be given much more often than when a nurse administers shots to the patient. In 2 to 3 days the patient's pain is usually controlled with analgesics taken by mouth.

The TRAM flap procedure requires a hospital stay of 4 to 8 days. The patient usually can gets out of bed the first day after the operation, but it takes another 1 to 2 weeks before she can stand upright. Recuperation is somewhat slower with this operation than with the implant procedures discussed earlier. Most women find that they can gradually resume normal basic activities within the first 4 weeks after returning home but that it takes 4 to 8 weeks before they are ready to return to work. Usually they are able to participate in sporting activities within 3 to 6 months.

Few functional problems exist after transfer of the rectus abdominis muscle. Most patients can return to the same level of activity as before the operation. They can also usually perform athletic activities at the same level and intensity as before. A preoperative and postoperative exercise program helps strengthen the abdominal wall muscles and makes recovery less difficult. Although sit-ups sometimes may be difficult and women may have to push up when rising from the reclining position, most athletic activities can be continued without difficulty, and many women have returned to tennis, golf, and jogging.

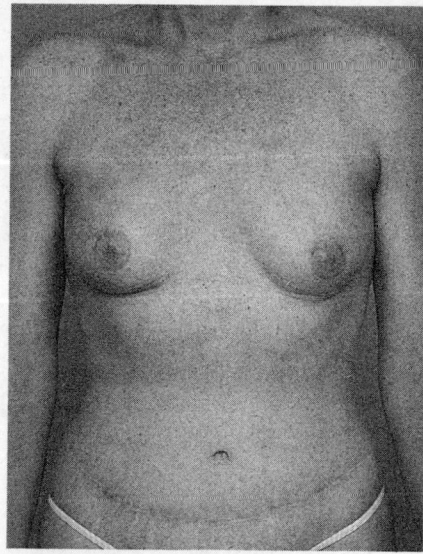

After being diagnosed with bilateral breast cancer, this 38-year-old woman had modified radical mastectomies using skin-sparing techniques and immediate breast reconstruction with TRAM flaps. She is shown 1 years later. Her reconstructed breasts are similar in size to her natural breasts. Her nipple-areolae were reconstructed with local flaps and then tattooed.

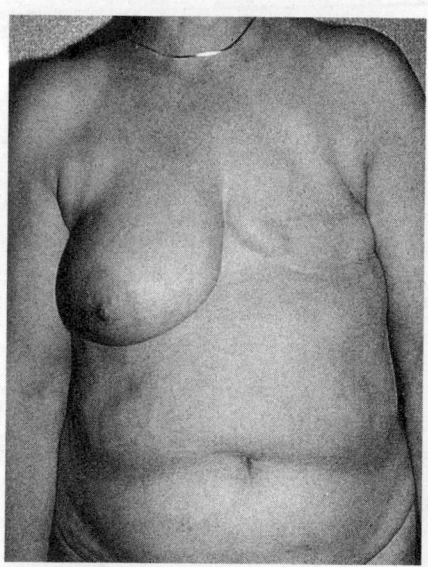 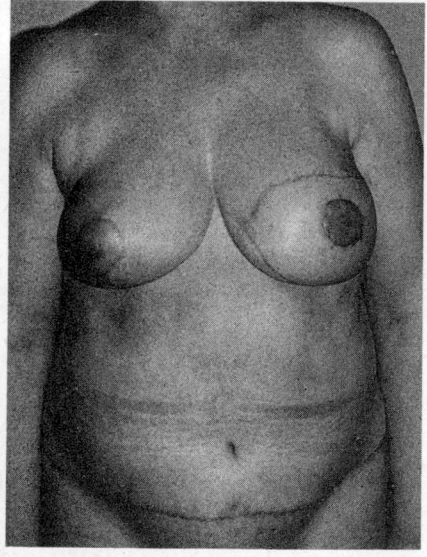

When cancer of the left breast was diagnosed, this 54-year-old woman chose to have a modified radical mastectomy and delayed breast reconstruction with a TRAM flap. Because her opposite breast was ptotic and heavy, she also had a small reduction mammaplasty of her opposite breast. She is shown 1 year later. Her nipple-areola was reconstructed with a local flap and a tattoo.

## *Results With the TRAM Flap—cont'd*

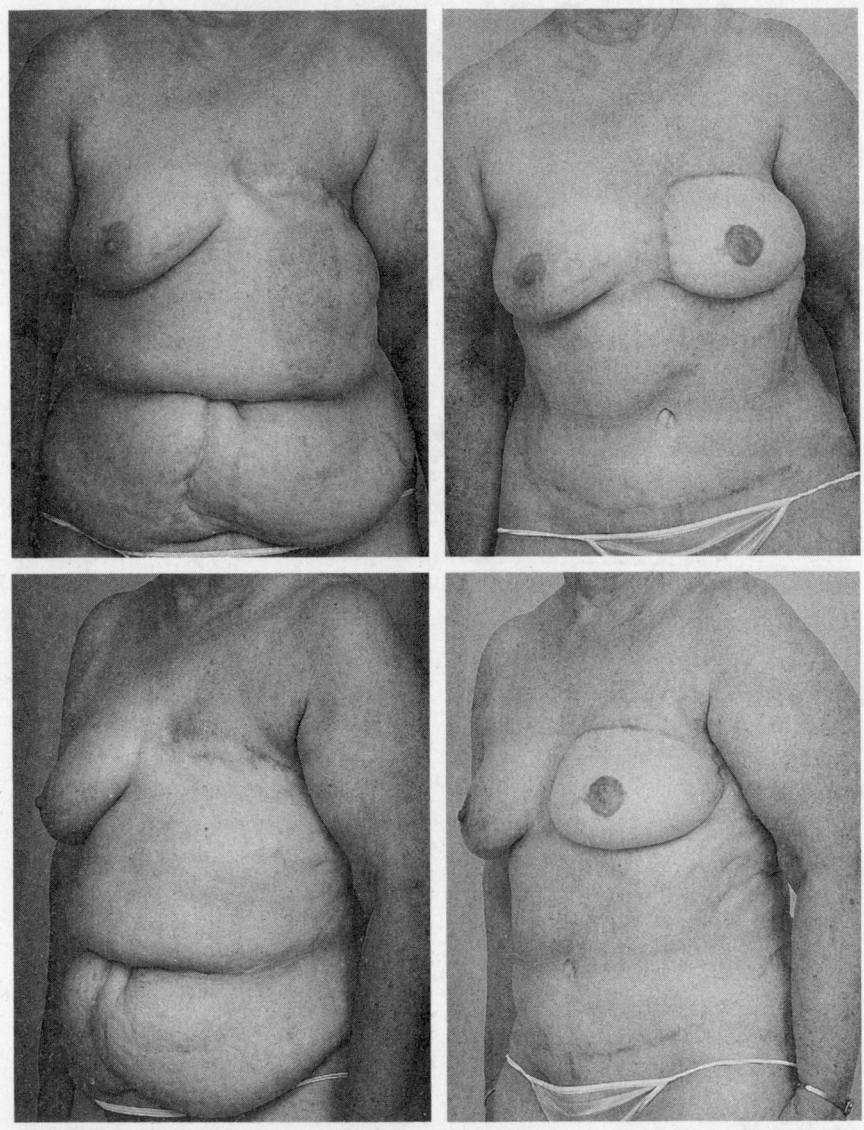

This 62-year-old woman had cancer of the left breast. She had a modified radical mastectomy and decided to have a delayed breast reconstruction. Her opposite breast was ptotic and heavy; however, she wanted the breast reconstruction to match it. She also desired treatment of her heavy and scarred abdominal wall. She is shown 1 year after breast reconstruction with a TRAM flap. Her nipple-areola was reconstructed with a local flap and a tattoo.

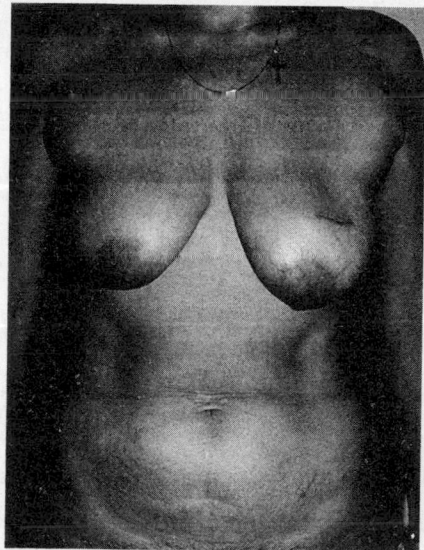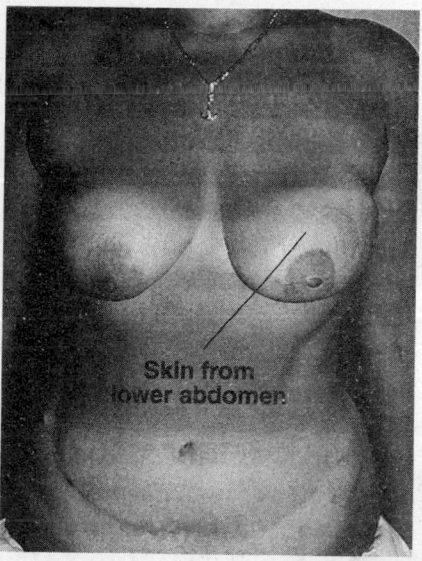

This 42-year-old woman had cancer of the left breast. She had a modified radical mastectomy with skin-sparing incisions and immediate reconstruction with a TRAM flap. Her opposite breast was ptotic; however, it was possible to match it using the TRAM flap. She is shown 1 year after breast reconstruction. Her nipple-areola was reconstructed with a local flap and a tattoo.

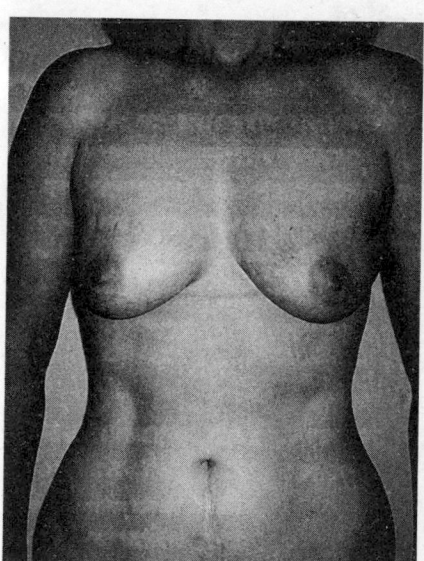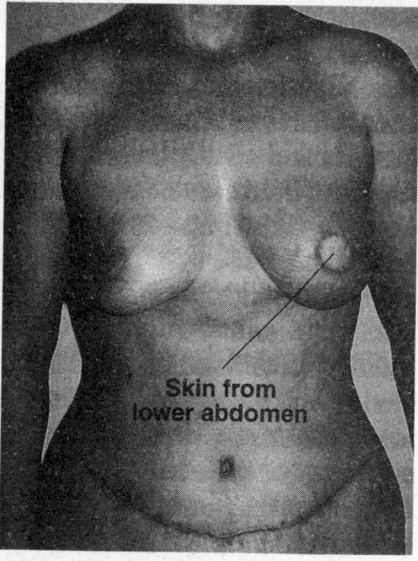

After cancer of the left breast was diagnosed, this 37-year-old woman had a skin-sparing mastectomy with shorter incisions and immediate breast reconstruction with a TRAM flap. The tissue from the abdomen was used to replace the breast tissue and a round piece of the abdominal wall skin was used to fill the defect left after the nipple-areola was removed. She is shown 6 months after breast reconstruction before her nipple-areola reconstruction was performed.

## Results With the TRAM Flap—cont'd

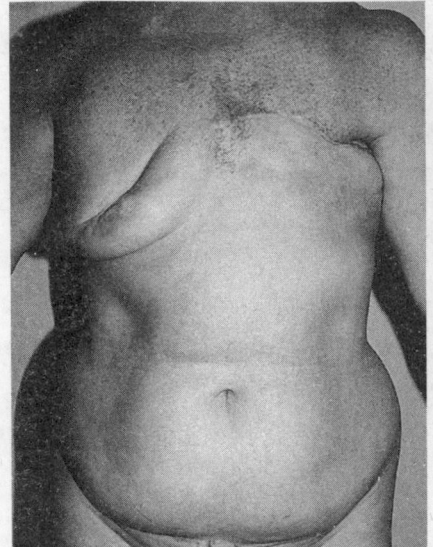
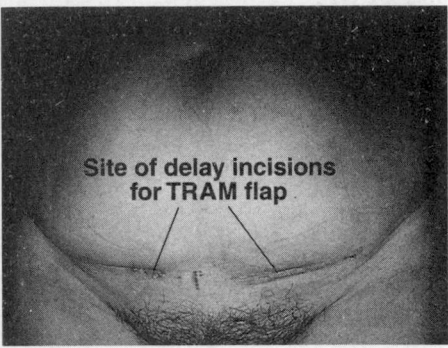

Site of delay incisions
for TRAM flap

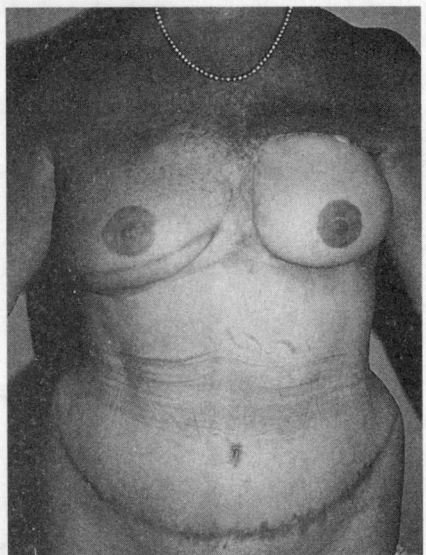

This 58-year-old woman had a modified radical mastectomy and postoperative radiation therapy for cancer of the left breast. She had a history of cigarette smoking and was somewhat overweight. Subsequently, a second breast cancer developed and she had a left modified radical mastectomy. She decided to have delayed breast reconstruction. Because of her risk factors, she had a TRAM flap vascular delay in which two lower abdominal wall incisions were made 1 week before the main TRAM flap breast reconstruction. She is shown 1 year after bilateral reconstruction. Her nipple-areolae were reconstructed with local flaps and tattoos.

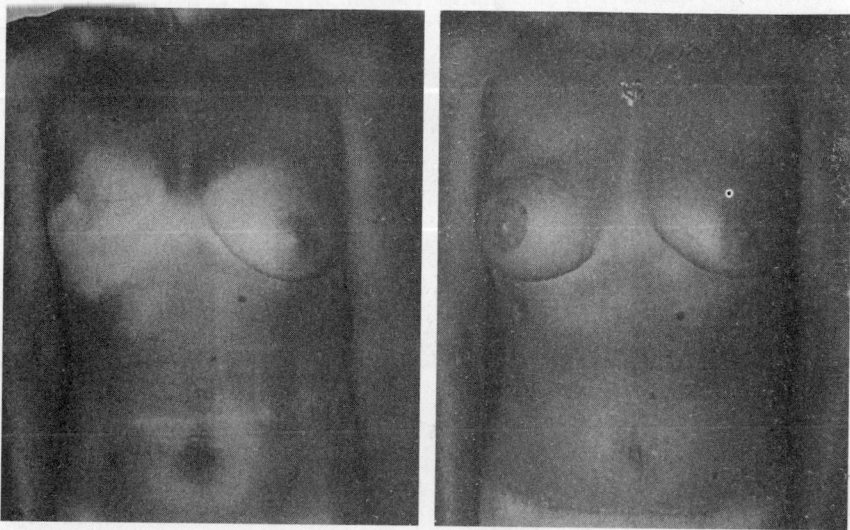

This 43 year-old woman, who had a modified radical mastectomy, requested breast reconstruction with her own tissues. Her right breast was reconstructed with a TRAM flap to match her remaining breast. She is shown 1 year after breast reconstruction.

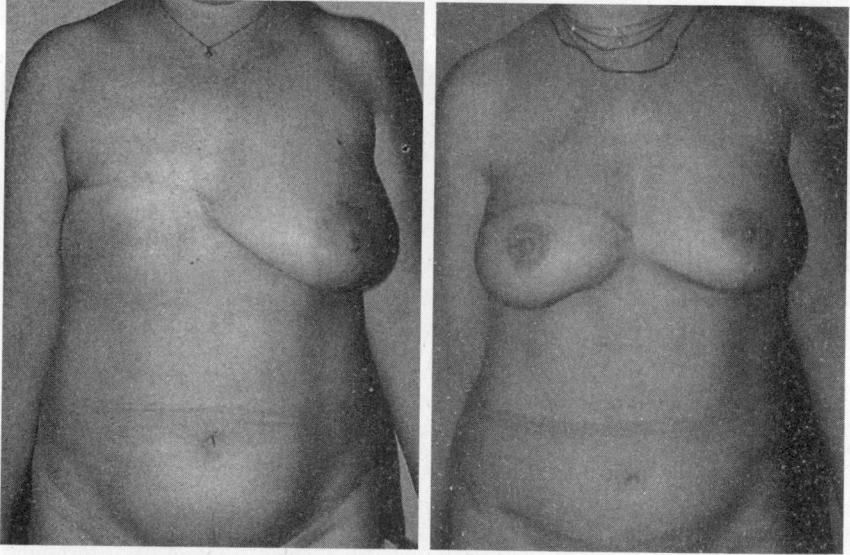

This 55-year-old woman had a right modified radical mastectomy. Her left breast was heavy and her abdomen was flabby. A TRAM flap was used for her right breast reconstruction and a small reduction mammaplasty was performed on her left breast. The patient is shown 2 years later.

*Results With the TRAM Flap—cont'd*

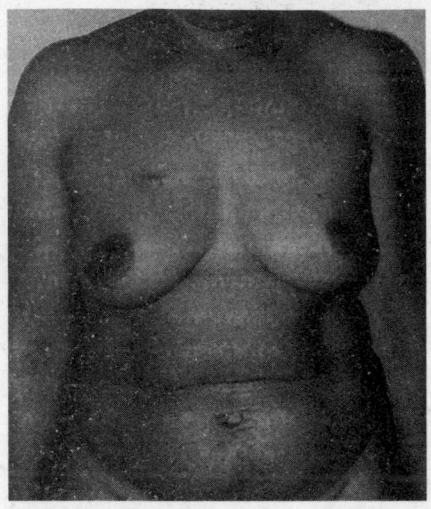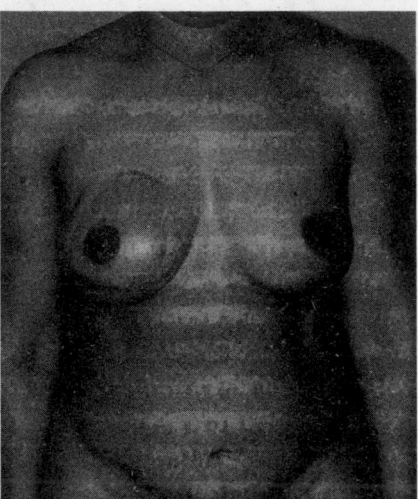

This 48-year-old woman had a modified radical mastectomy of her right breast followed by immediate TRAM breast reconstruction. Three months later liposuction was used to contour her upper abdomen and breast. Her nipple-areola was also reconstructed and later tattooed. She is shown 2 years after breast reconstruction.

## Reconstruction With the Latissimus Dorsi (Back) Flap After Mastectomy and After Breast-Conserving Surgery

A latissimus dorsi flap technique is selected when additional tissue is needed to rebuild mastectomy defects. This is a safe, reliable flap with a good blood supply, and endoscopic surgery offers the advantage of leaving minimal scars. The latissimus dorsi flap is most often used when the reconstructed breast needs to be large or ptotic to match the opposite one, the patient does not want a TRAM flap, or a TRAM flap would pose too much risk and prolonged recovery. Because it has a long track record for safety and predictability, many surgeons feel more comfortable recommending it than the other flaps.

With this procedure, skin and muscle or sometimes only muscle is transferred from a woman's back around to the breast area to replace the skin and chest muscle that were removed during a mastectomy or a partial mastectomy. The latissimus dorsi flap provides functioning, healthy muscle tissue for covering an implant or expander, for filling the hollow areas beneath the collarbone left by removal of the pectoralis major muscle (a standard part of the radical mastectomy procedure), and for recreating the anterior axillary fold.

Adding additional skin to the chest wall area also permits the formation of a more naturally shaped, fuller, larger breast than could be created by simple implant placement or tissue expansion. The healthy skin added is often thicker and of better quality than the thin expanded skin. This muscle and skin (musculocutaneous) flap is also useful for patients who have skin grafts or very tight or irradiated skin, although the TRAM flap is often the flap of first choice for the woman who has had a mastectomy after radiation therapy. The latissimus dorsi muscle and skin flap can be used after a modified radical mastectomy to eliminate the need to alter the patient's remaining breast if it is too large to match by expanding the existing tissue. Many women prefer a donor scar on their back or side to a scar on their remaining breast, which would be necessary to adjust it to match the expanded breast reconstruction. In addition, the use of flap tissue provides additional cover and a measure of protection for the breast implant or expander. This is often the case when a woman has immediate breast reconstruction. A strip of the latissimus dorsi muscle can be elevated and brought through the mastectomy incision to provide better cover and safety for the breast implant or tissue expander and to reduce its visibility and palpability. No additional incisions are required.

Sometimes a woman's breast can be reconstructed entirely with the back tissue without a breast implant. This autologous latissimus dorsi flap reconstruction is used when the woman has excess back tissue, especially in her midback, or if she does not have a particularly large breast. In this instance the skin, muscle, and fatty tissue of the back can be brought around to the front and shaped into a breast. Usually this can be done with a single scar across the midback. When there is fullness of the lateral chest wall area, additional skin can be harvested. One of the drawbacks of this approach is that when a large amount of skin and fat are removed from the back, there can be delayed healing, the resulting scar can be unattractive, and the back area from which the flap was taken can appear flatter than the opposite side of the back.

The latissimus dorsi muscle alone can be used for immediate breast reconstruction to enhance implant cover or transferred with some additional skin to replace missing skin. The introduction of endoscopic surgery (described earlier) allows the surgeon to transfer the latissimus dorsi muscle from the back through the mastectomy site either without additional scars or with minimal scars on the back and in the axilla.

Latissimus dorsi fat and muscle flaps are now being used to fill localized defects within the breast after lumpectomy and quadrantectomy. This reconstructive procedure extends the application of breast preservation to women who require larger breast areas removed during breast-conserving surgery. After the lumpectomy or quandrantectomy is done, the general or oncologic surgeon checks the margins of resection to ensure complete tumor removal. He also assesses the area of tumor excision to determine if it will leave an unsatisfactory breast shape or size after healing and/or radiation therapy. If this is the case, the volume of the breast may be restored with the latissimus dorsi back tissues. In this situation the reconstructive surgeon uses an endoscopic technique to harvest a flap of latissimus muscle and its overlying fat through the incisions used for the primary local cancer treatment. This flap is then used to fill and contour the defect remaining after the breast-conserving procedure. This technique is also useful for secondary breast deformities that require some additional tissue.

### Surgical Procedure and Postoperative Appearance

Reconstruction with the latissimus dorsi flap is a longer, more complex procedure than techniques using local tissue or tissue expansion. This operation takes between 2 to 4 hours to perform. Since the operation is longer and there is additional back pain, it is done under general anesthesia and hospitalization is required.

When using the latissimus dorsi flap for breast replacement, the plastic surgeon separates the latissimus dorsi muscle from its deep attachments and frees it with its attached skin from the back. This muscle-skin flap is left attached to its nourishing vessel, a main artery in the armpit area that the surgical oncologist saves during the mastectomy. The flap is now ready to be transferred to the chest area. In preparation for this transfer the mastectomy scar is excised or removed (if it is located in an inconspicuous position) or a new, better placed incision is made along the lower outer area where the new breast will be reconstructed. Next the flap is rotated to the front of the chest and passed through a tunnel created high in the underarm so that it extends through to the new incision or to the opening left by the removal of the mastectomy scar. The back donor incision is then closed. The flap is adjusted for the most aesthetic appearance and sutured to the front of the chest; the latissimus dorsi muscle is stitched to the pectoralis major muscle, and back skin is stitched to breast skin to supplement deficient tissue in this area. When an axillary fold is needed, some of the outer layer of skin and a portion of the latissimus dorsi muscle are brought around and stitched out onto the upper arm. This tissue will span from the arm to the chest, thus simulating a new anterior axillary fold. An opening is left in the outer part of the incision for the insertion of a breast implant or tissue expander to provide a breast shape symmetric with the opposite remaining breast. The surgeon positions the expander under the muscle, which provides good cover and permits a more natural reconstruction; he then closes the incision. The nipple-areola is created during a later operation under local anesthesia.

For immediate breast reconstruction, the upper part of the expander is placed under the chest wall muscle (pectoralis major) above and the lower part is covered by the back muscle (latissimus dorsi). When skin is needed, it replaces the skin removed at the time of mastectomy. If necessary, an expander implant is placed to permit accurate postoperative sizing.

With the endoscopic technique for harvesting latissimus dorsi back muscle and fat, the surgeon uses the incisions made at the time of primary cancer treatment, which are usually in the lateral breast region and in the underarm area (where the axillary lymph node dissection was done). A video camera is attached to the endoscope and the image is displayed on the TV monitor for the surgeon to see while he operates using special long instruments that are inserted through the small incisions. The endoscope permits a video image of tissues beneath the skin to be projected on the video monitor via fiberoptic light. Separate incisions about an inch long may also be needed in the mid to lower back. Through these small incisions the surgeon visualizes the area with the use of the endoscope, dissects the flap which contains the fat and muscle, preserves the blood supply to the tissue, and moves the flap through the underarm to the front of the chest for the breast reconstruction.

The latissimus dorsi reconstruction leaves a donor scar on the patient's back (under her bra line) or on her side (in a diagonal under her upper arm) and additional scars on her breast when the flap is placed into the breast area. The reconstructed breast can be somewhat rounder and firmer than the normal breast. In addition, the woman may have a slight bulge under her arm where the latissimus dorsi flap was tunneled through to her chest area. This bulge will shrink with time as the muscle atrophies with inactivity, but it will not completely disappear. This fullness is usually positioned in the axillary region to reduce the hollowness after axillary lymph node removal.

## Delayed Breast Reconstruction With Latissimus Dorsi Flap and Tissue Expansion

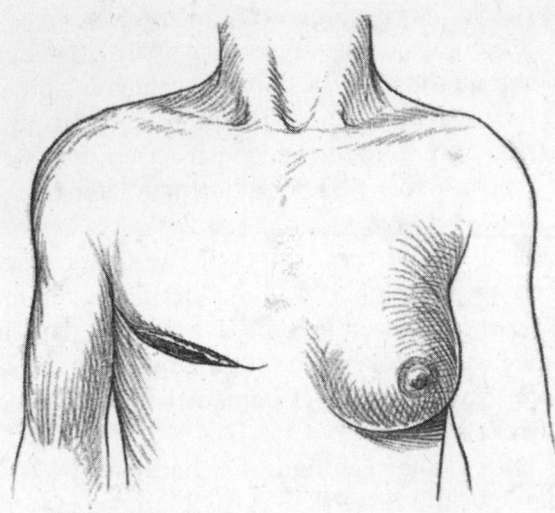

Modified radical mastectomy scar opened

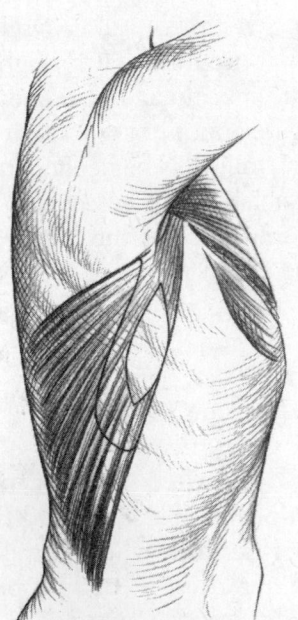

Latissimus dorsi flap
designed on side

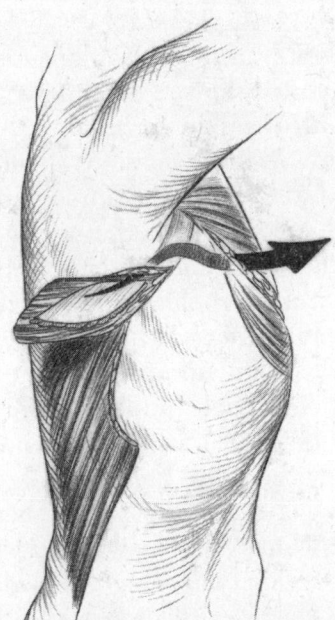

Skin and strip of latissimus dorsi
muscle elevated on side of chest

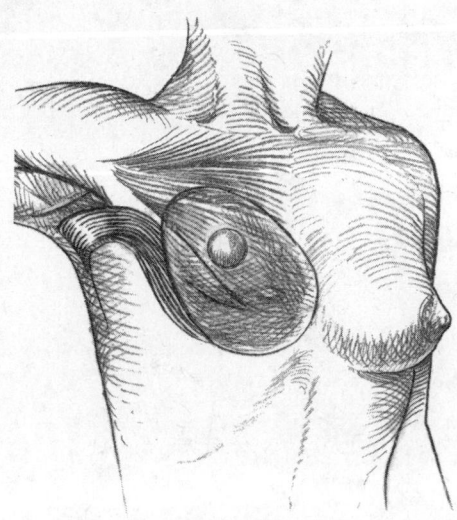

Latissimus dorsi muscle
covering a textured anatomic-shaped
expander

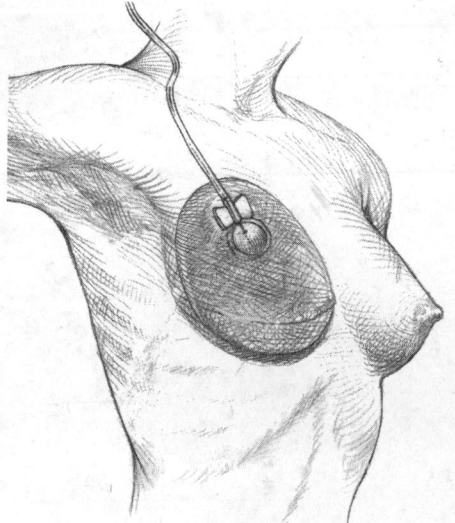

Textured anatomic-shaped expander
with integral valve inflated
with saline solution

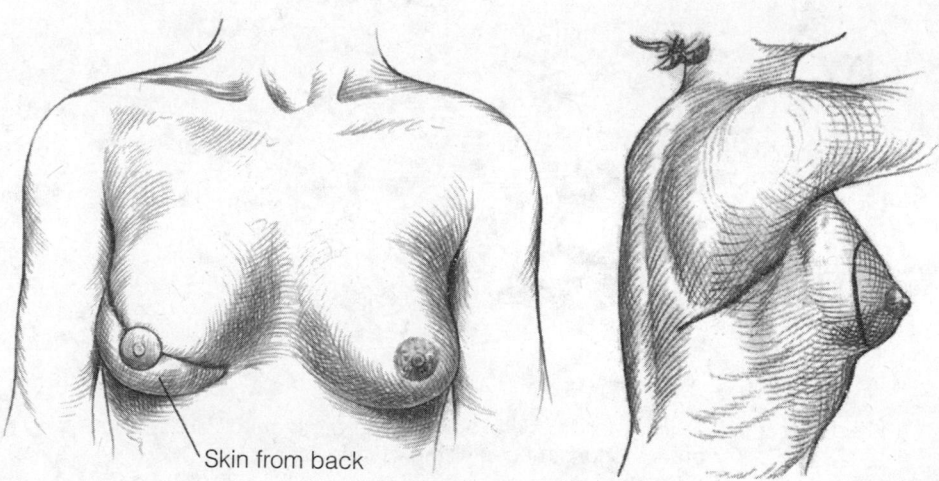

Skin from back

Nipple-areola reconstructed several months later

## Skin-Sparing Mastectomy and Immediate Breast Reconstruction With Endoscopic Latissimus Dorsi Flap and Tissue Expander or Implant

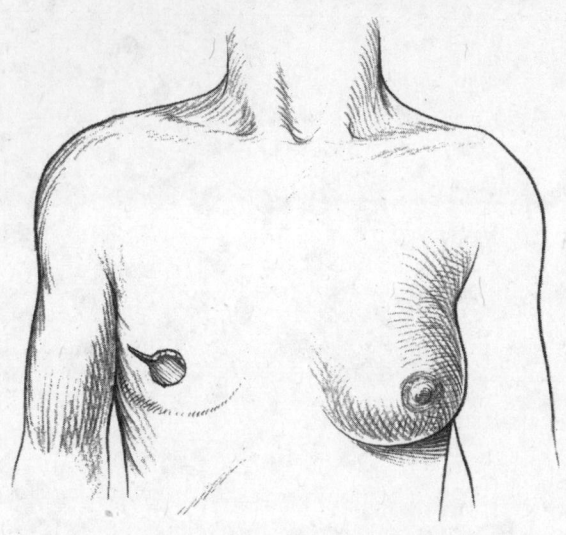

Skin-sparing mastectomy deformity after removal
of breast and nipple-areola

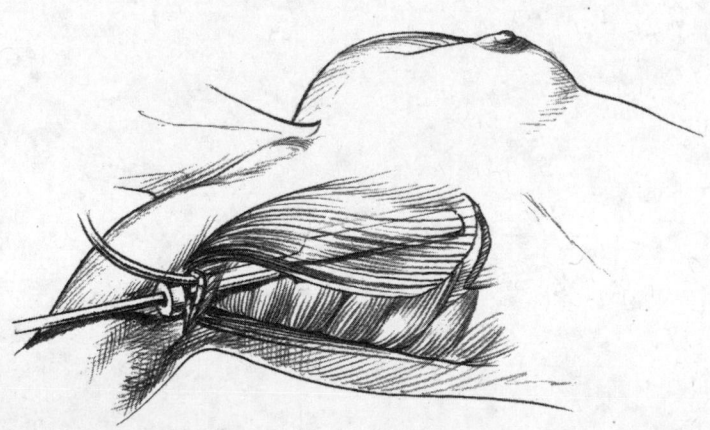

Endoscope used for pectoral muscle release through an axillary incision
for breast reconstruction with expander or implant

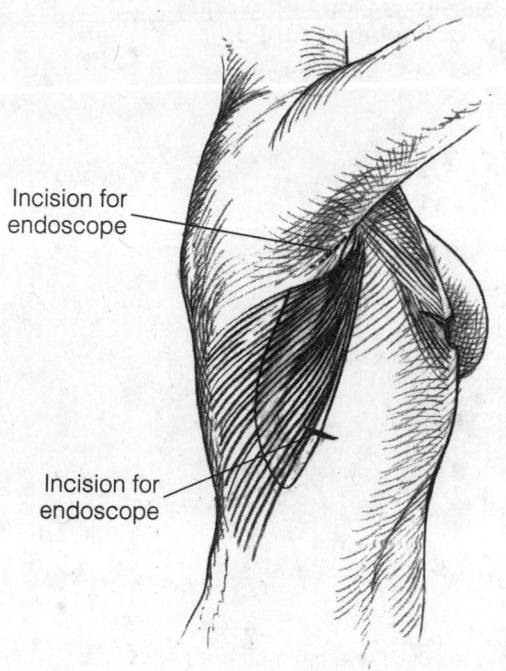

Incision for endoscope

Incision for endoscope

Latissimus dorsi flap designed on side with incisions shown for endoscopic harvest of latissimus dorsi muscle

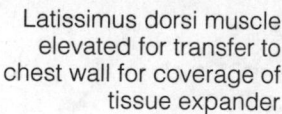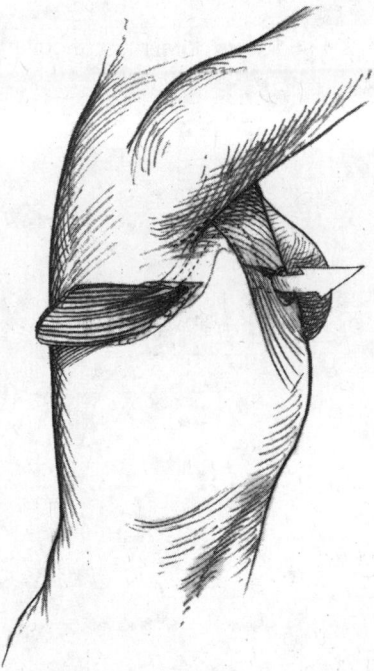

Latissimus dorsi muscle elevated for transfer to chest wall for coverage of tissue expander

## Skin-Sparing Mastectomy and Immediate Breast Reconstruction With Endoscopic Latissimus Dorsi Flap and Tissue Expander or Implant—cont'd

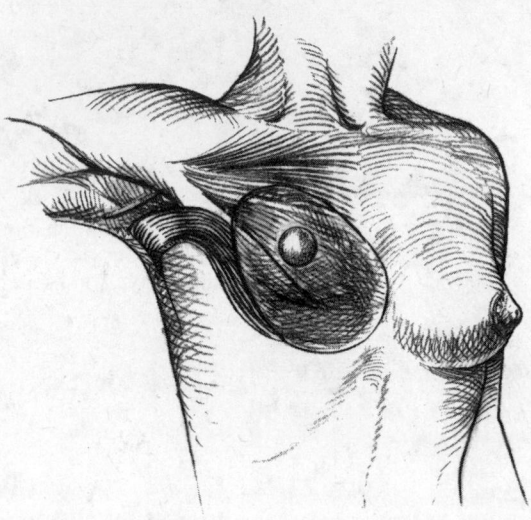

Latissimus dorsi muscle covering textured anatomic-shaped expander

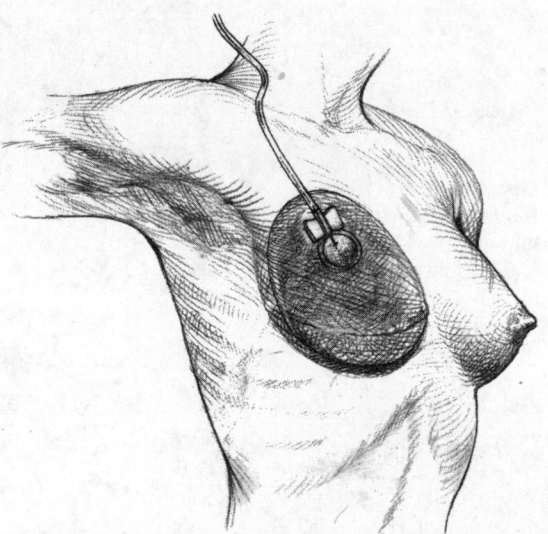

Textured anatomic-shaped expander being inflated with saline solution

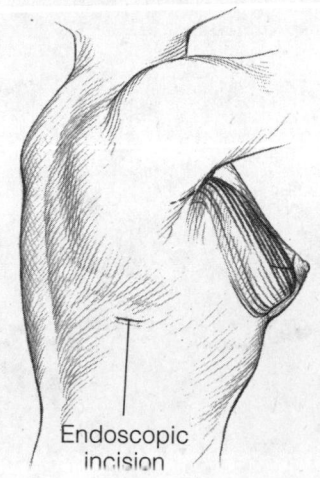

Endoscopically harvested latissimus dorsi flap over expander

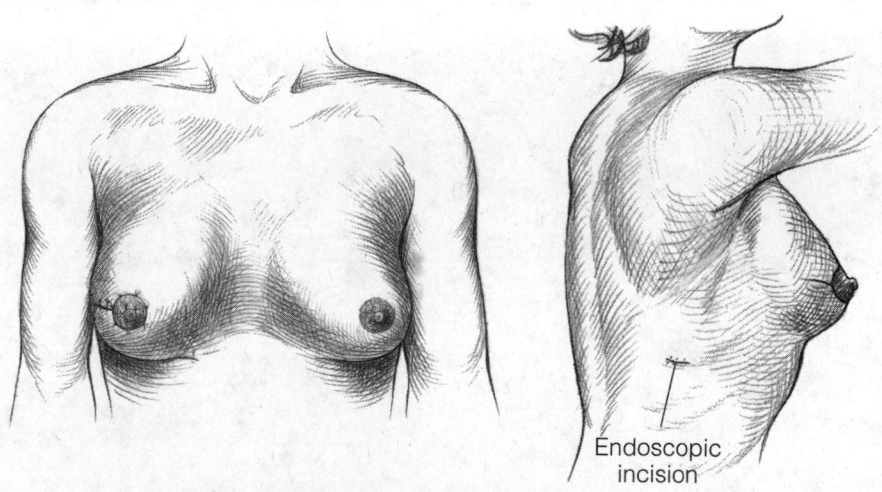

Nipple-areola reconstructed several months later

## Delayed Breast Reconstruction With Latissimus Dorsi Flap and Tissue Expander or Implant

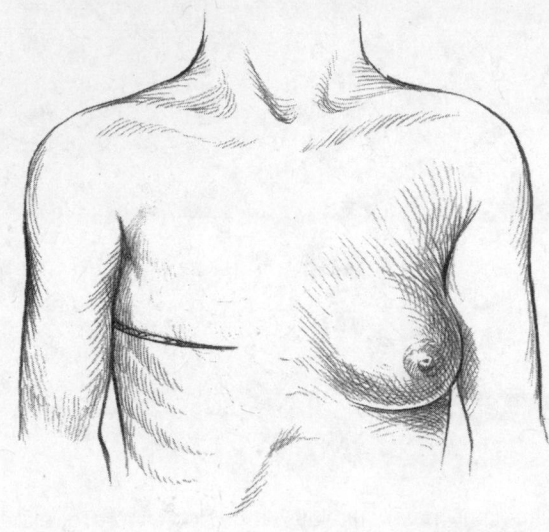

Modified radical mastectomy scar opened

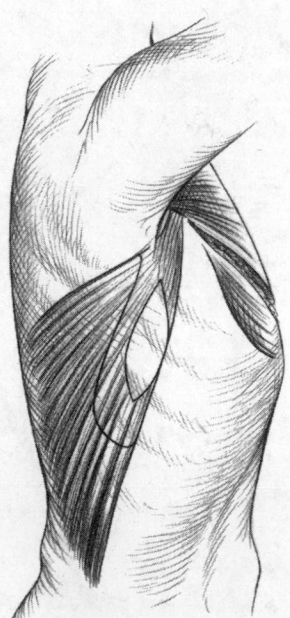

Latissimus dorsi flap
designed on side

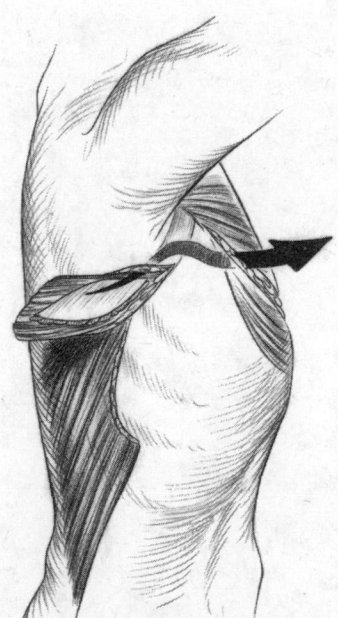

Skin and strip of latissimus dorsi
muscle elevated on side of chest

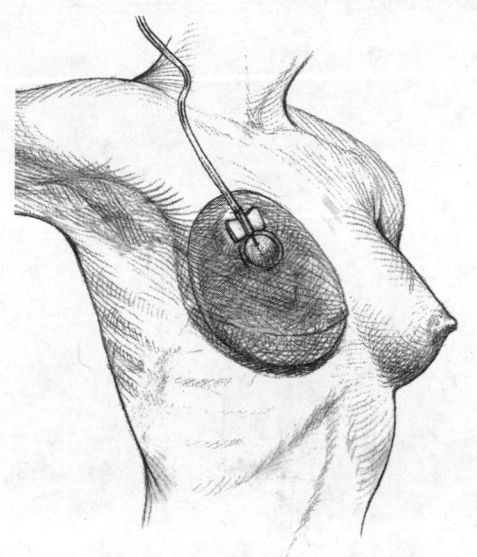

Textured anatomic-shaped expander
inflated with saline solution

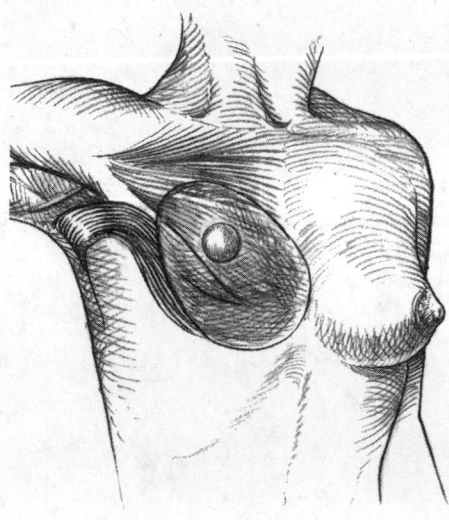

Skin and muscle to supplement deficient
tissue in lower breast and expander
implant to restore breast shape

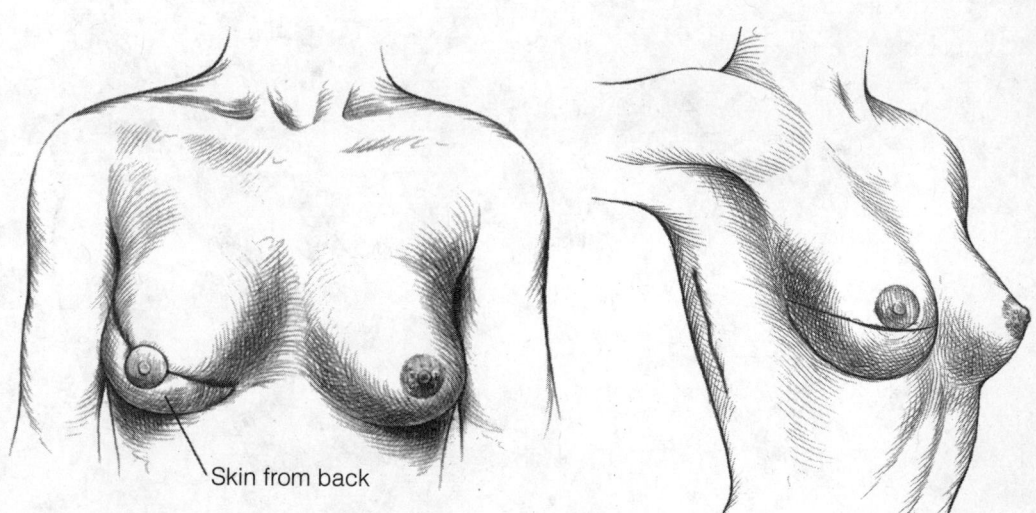

Skin from back

Nipple-areola reconstructed several months later

## Breast Reconstruction With Latissimus Dorsi Flap Without Implant (Autologous Flap)

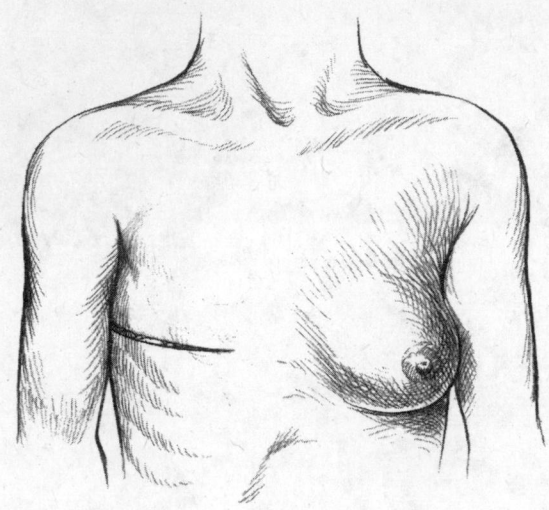

Modified radical mastectomy

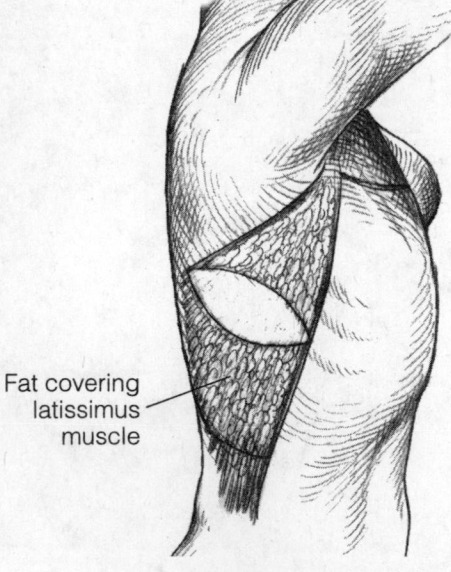

Fat covering latissimus muscle

Latissimus dorsi flap designed on back

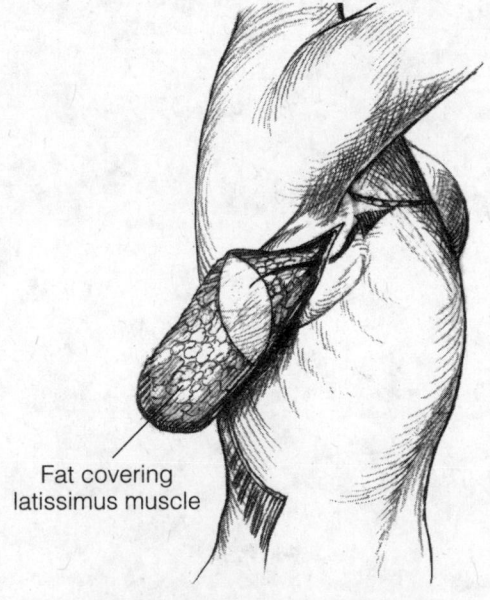

Fat covering latissimus muscle

Autologous latissimus dorsi skin and muscle flap elevated from back

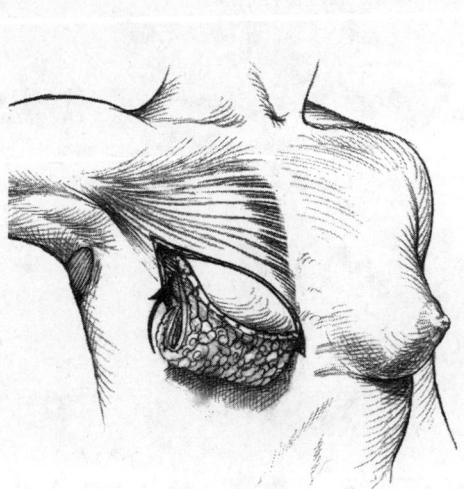

Fat and muscle folded under and
fashioned into a breast

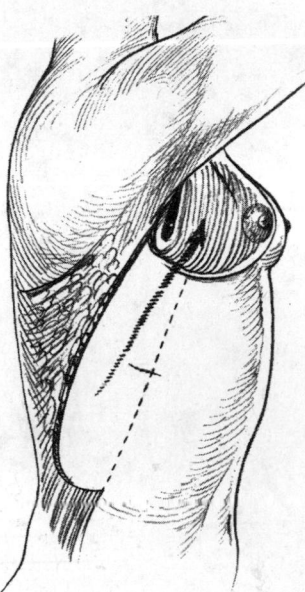

Autologous latissimus dorsi
flap inset

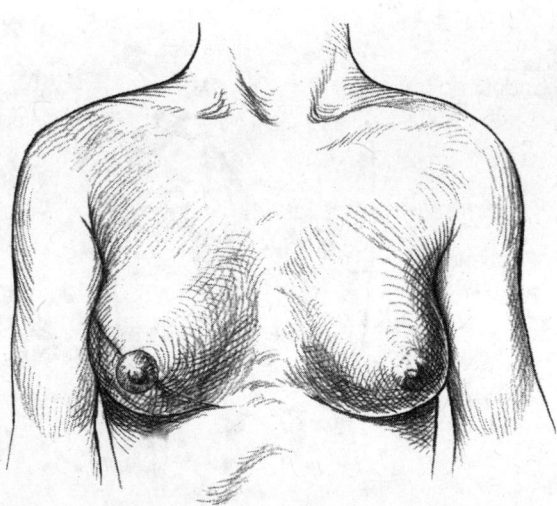

Nipple-areola reconstructed several months later

## Partial Breast Reconstruction With Endoscopic Latissimus Dorsi Flap

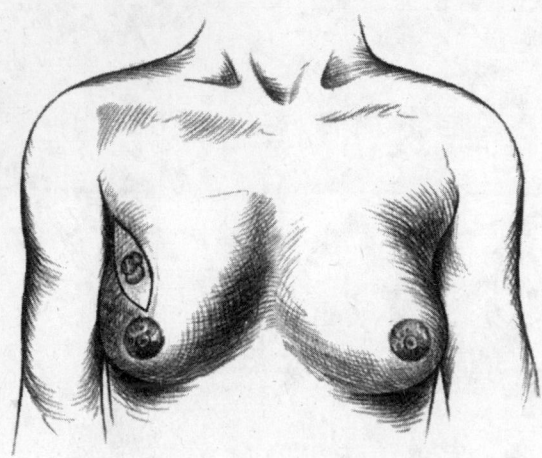

Quadrantectomy defect

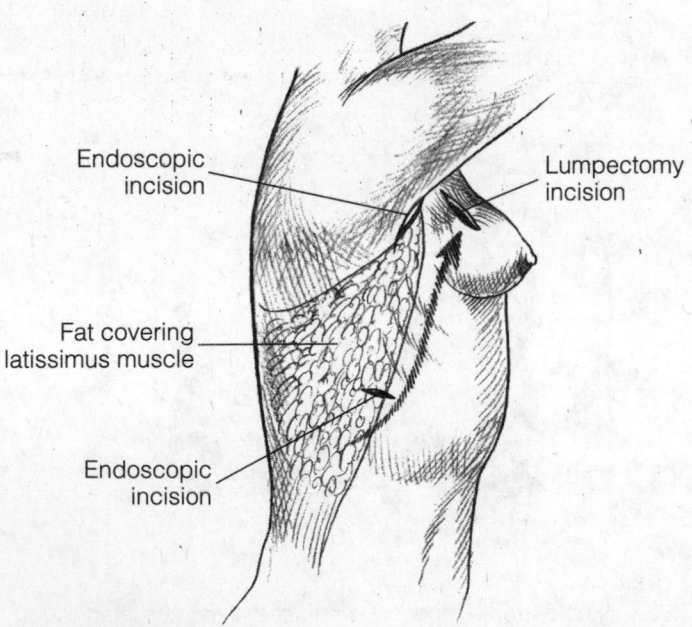

Endoscopic incision

Lumpectomy incision

Fat covering latissimus muscle

Endoscopic incision

Harvesting of latissimus dorsi muscle and fat through short endoscopic incisions to fill in large lumpectomy or quadrantectomy defect

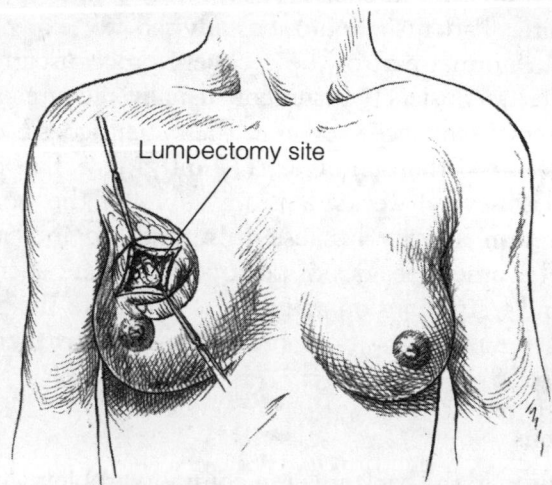

Endoscopically harvested latissimus dorsi flap in place in upper quadrant of breast after large partial mastectomy

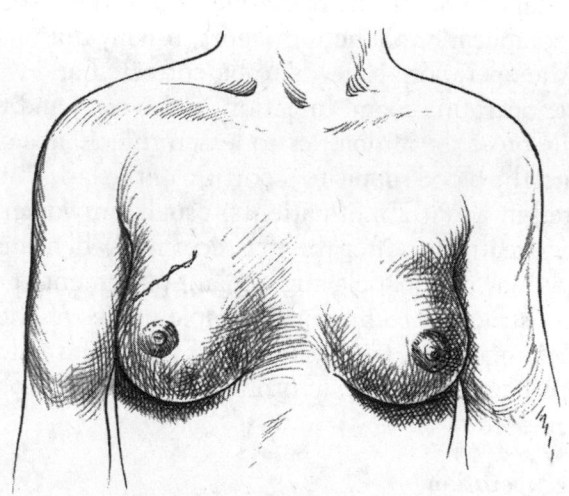

Incision closed

## Postoperative Care

After the operation the plastic surgeon inserts surgical drains into the reconstructed breast and back area to remove excess fluid from the operative site. Patients should be advised to expect significant drainage as a normal part of the recovery process, particularly with this flap. The reconstructive surgeon usually recommends that the back drain remain in place even after the patient goes home and until the drainage is less than an ounce (30 ml) a day. This drainage can sometimes last several weeks. It is advisable for the woman to limit shoulder or arm activity because this tends to increase the fluid drainage. The other specifics of postoperative care such as stitches, dressings, and restrictions on activity are similar to the postoperative instructions for patients whose breasts are reconstructed with implants (see p. 261).

## Complications

Fluid collection in the back area is a common problem after latissimus dorsi flap surgery. Sometimes fluid can accumulate after the drains are removed. It usually is reabsorbed by the body and disappears after several weeks. When this fluid buildup becomes uncomfortable, the surgeon may need to drain it with a syringe or reinsert a drain. Blood accumulation (hematoma) in the operative sites of the breast or back is an unusual complication. When it occurs, usually during the first 24 hours after the operation, it needs to be corrected and the blood removed in the operating room. Infection is also rare, and the surgeon will ordinarily prescribe antibiotics to lessen the chance of infection. Problems with the blood supply to a portion of the latissimus dorsi flap have occurred in about 2% of patients, usually in women who have had radiation treatments after the mastectomy. When this complication occurs, it may require delaying implant placement or selection of another reconstructive technique. Complete loss of the latissimus dorsi flap because of poor blood supply has been seen in less than 1% of patients. When this occurs, another method of breast reconstruction will be needed.

## Pain and Recuperation

This operation is more painful than reconstruction with available tissue. There is normally some pain in the back and underarm area where the flap was taken. The back and arm areas are sore for 2 to 3 weeks; the pain subsides as the arm regains motion. Endoscopic surgery with reduced skin incisions seems to reduce the postoperative pain. The drains are also usually uncomfortable and occasionally painful, particularly when they are removed. This discomfort is similar to that experienced after a mastectomy.

Hospitalization of 2 to 6 days is required. Recovery time is 3 to 6 weeks to return to work and 2 to 4 months to resume exercise or sports such as aerobics, tennis, and golf. If the woman's anterior axillary fold has been recreated, she needs to avoid strenuous arm activity for 6 to 8 weeks while this area heals.

The latissimus dorsi flap is generally not accompanied by loss of arm and shoulder function even though a muscle has been used. The muscle is still functional. It is simply transferred to the front of the body to provide tissue for rebuilding the breast. Some women report, however, that the muscle transfer makes it more difficult for them to keep their shoulder erect on the side of the muscle transfer. Exercise will help alleviate but may not totally eliminate this problem.

### Results With the Latissimus Dorsi Flap

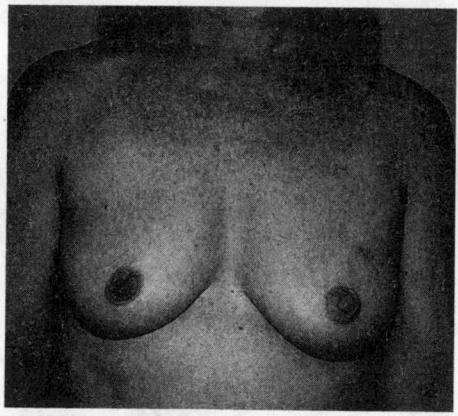

This 38-year-old woman with reasonably symmetric breasts requested lumpectomy to treat the cancer in the upper outer quadrant of her left breast. To get a local resection with clear margins the entire breast quadrant as well as some additional tissue was removed from beneath the nipple-areola. The significant deformity that remained was filled in with harvested latissimus dorsi muscle using endoscopic techniques that created no additional breast scars. She is shown 1 year after partial breast reconstruction and subsequent radiation therapy.

## Results With the Latissimus Dorsi Flap—cont'd

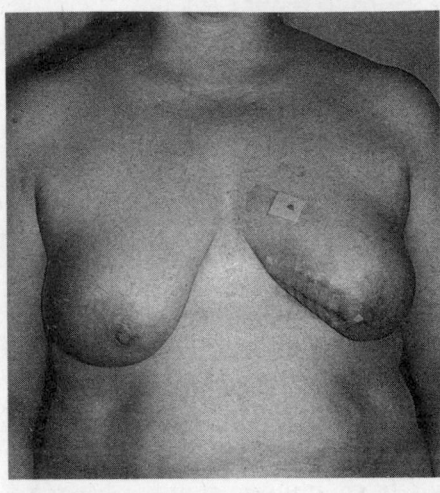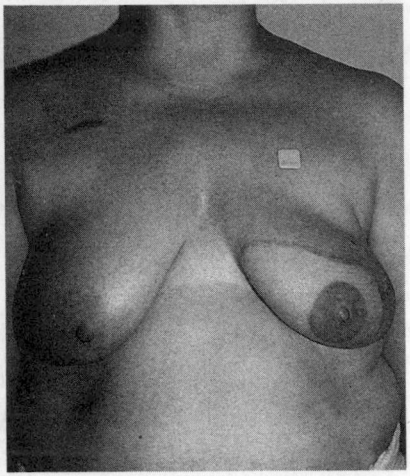

When cancer was detected in the upper inner quadrant of this 48-year-old woman's left breast, she requested treatment with lumpectomy. However, after two local resections were unsuccessful in obtaining clear margins, a mastectomy was performed. She had an immediate breast reconstruction with a latissimus dorsi musculocutaneous flap and the fat over the muscle. No implant was required. Her nipple-areola was later reconstructed with a local flap and a tattoo. She is shown 1 year after breast reconstruction.

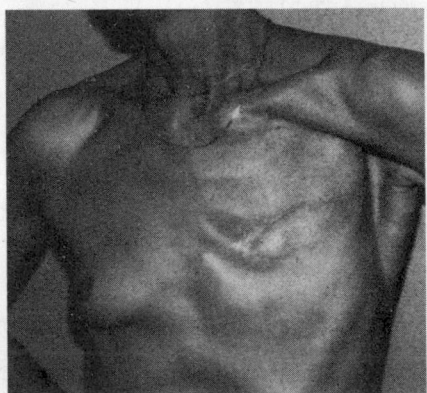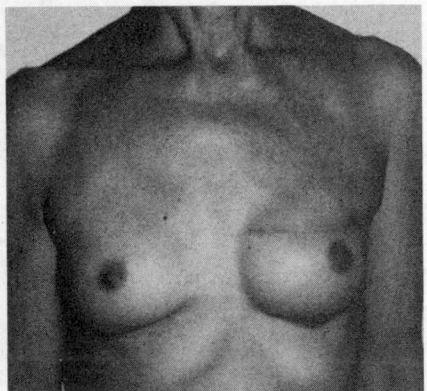

This 61-year-old woman had a radical mastectomy many years earlier and now requested breast reconstruction with augmentation of her other breast. She is shown 1 year after a latissimus dorsi muscle flap reconstruction with implant placement and another implant inserted behind her right breast for augmentation.

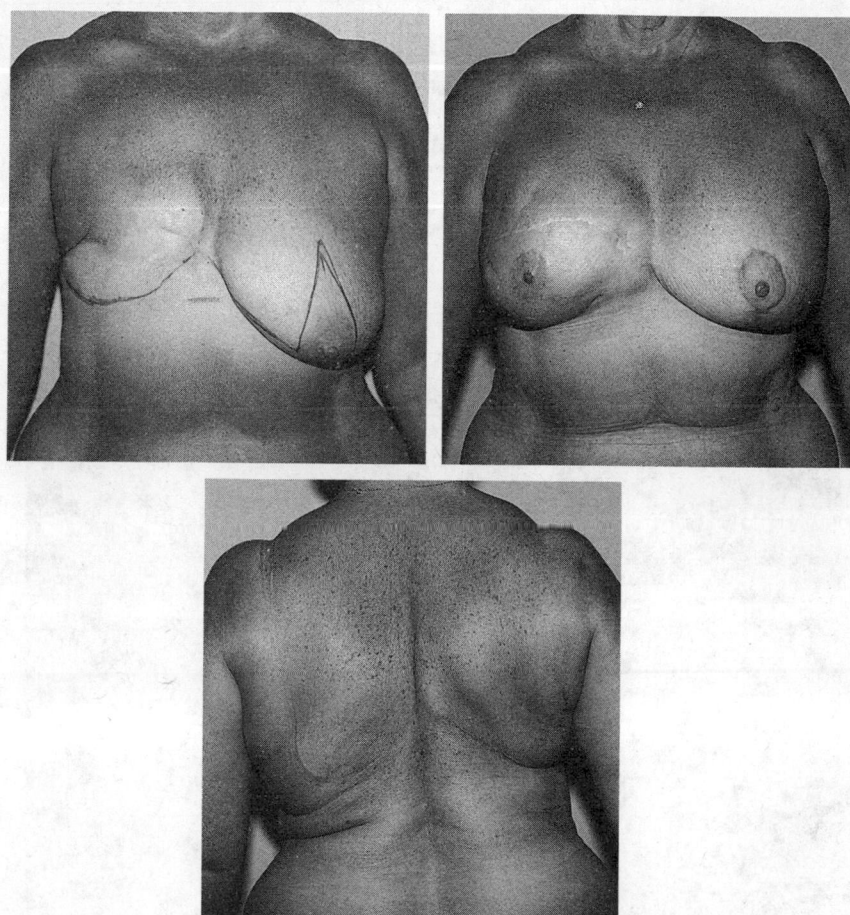

This 58-year-old woman had a modified radical mastectomy of her right breast and delayed breast reconstruction with a TRAM flap. Her opposite breast was ptotic and heavy and she requested a reduction mammaplasty for symmetry. She is shown 1 year after breast reconstruction and reduction mammaplasty of her opposite breast. Her nipple-areola was reconstructed with a local flap and a tattoo.

## Results With the Latissimus Dorsi Flap—cont'd

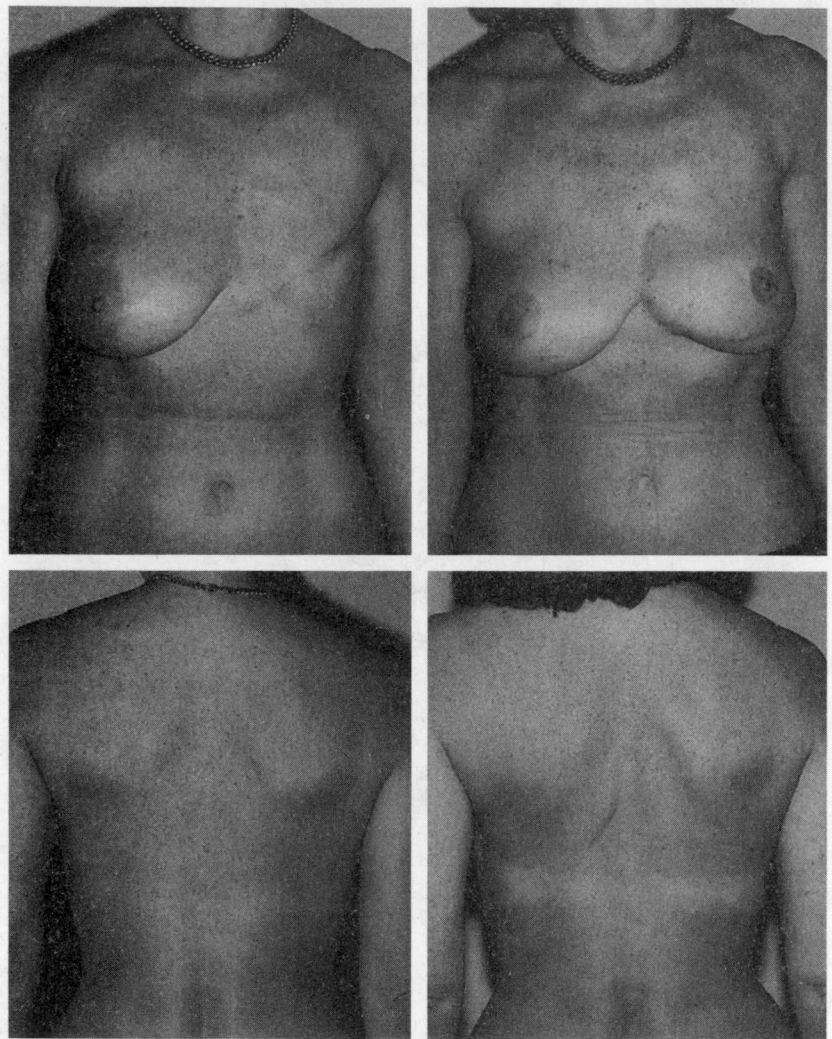

This 42-year-old woman had a left modified radical mastectomy. Since she did not want a lower abdominal scar, her breast was reconstructed with a latissimus dorsi flap and a tissue expander. Her other breast was reduced for symmetry. She is shown 2 years after breast reconstruction.

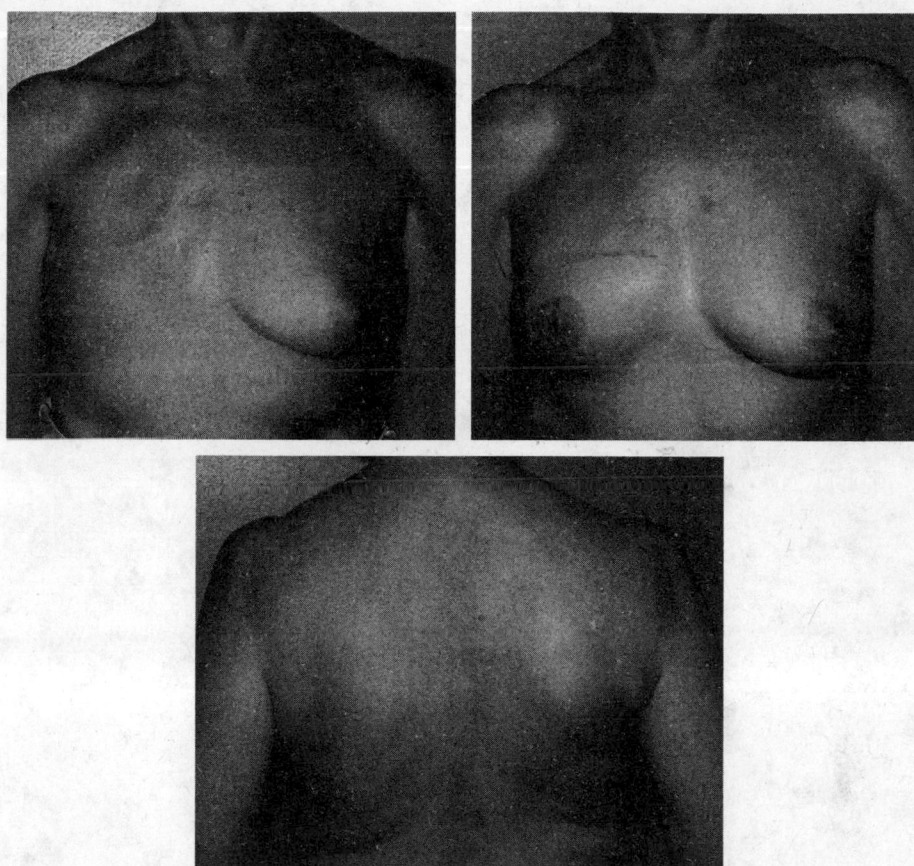

This 54-year-old woman had a right modified radical mastectomy. She did not want a skin island on her reconstructed breast or modification of her opposite breast. She is shown 1 year after her breast was reconstructed with a latissimus dorsi muscle flap and a tissue expander. Her opposite breast was not modified.

## Results With the Latissimus Dorsi Flap—cont'd

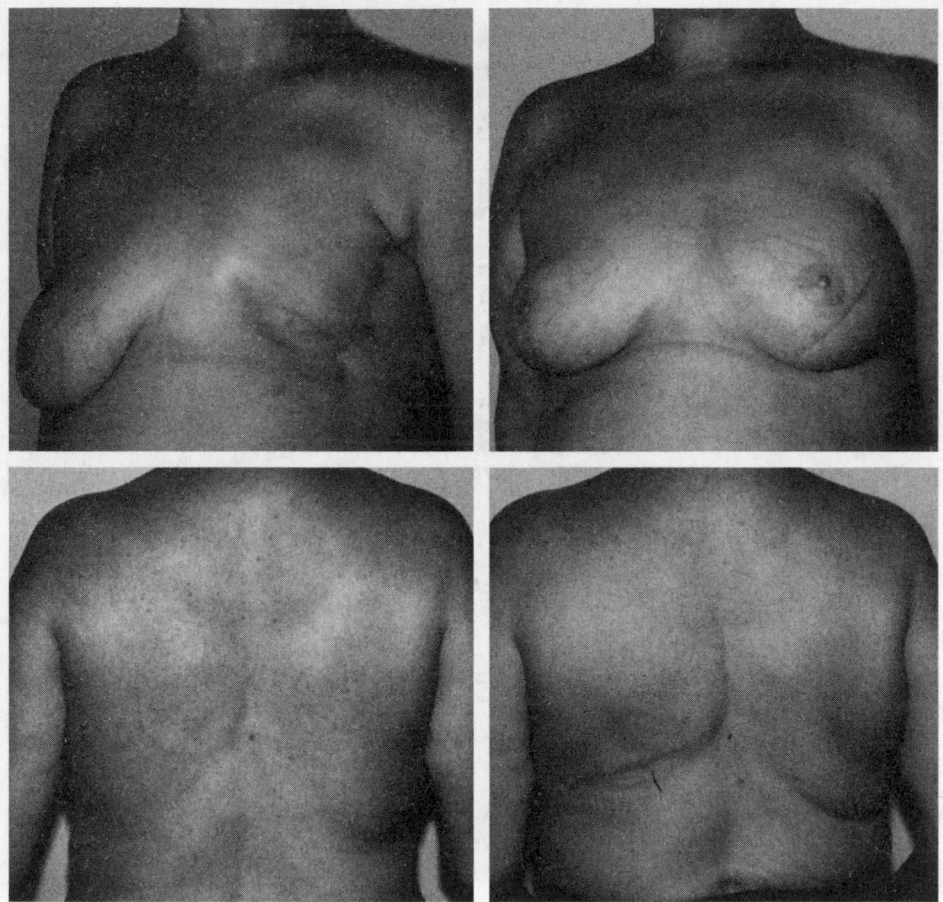

This 48-year-old woman had a left modified radical mastectomy. She is shown 2 years after latissimus dorsi flap breast reconstruction with tissue expansion and nipple-areola reconstruction and reduction mammaplasty of the right breast.

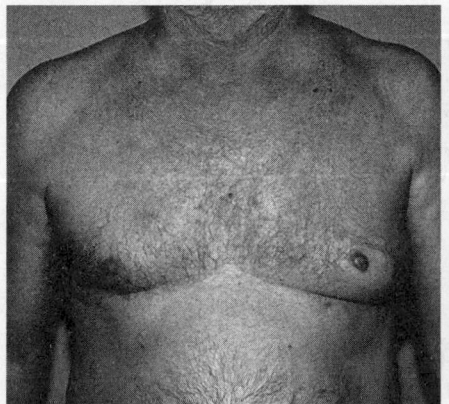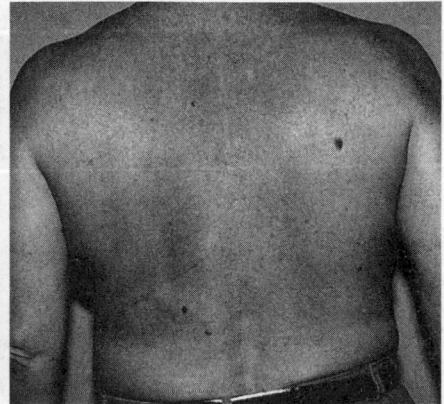

This 54-year-old man was diagnosed with cancer of his left breast. He had a modified radical mastectomy and immediate breast reconstruction with a latissimus dorsi flap. He is shown 1 year after breast reconstruction and a subsequent nipple-areola reconstruction with a local flap and a tattoo. The thin back donor site scar was acceptable to him.

## MICROSURGERY FOR BREAST RECONSTRUCTION

One of the more significant advances in reconstructive surgery during the past 25 years became a reality when surgeons began to suture and repair tiny blood vessels under the magnification of the operating microscope. This skill enables surgeons to move tissues from one part of the body where there is an excess of tissue to a deficient area that needs rebuilding. Because these flaps of autologous tissue (the patient's own body tissue) are separated and freed from the donor site and transferred to the new area where the blood vessels are reattached, they are often referred to as free flaps. This technique brings added choices to breast reconstruction. The reconstructive surgeon can rebuild a woman's breast by transferring her own fully mobilized tissues usually without the need for a breast implant. The most common and popular free flap donor tissues are the lower abdominal (TRAM) and the buttock skin and muscle (gluteus maximus musculocutaneous) flaps; they provide abundant tissue for a well-contoured reconstructed breast from a donor site that is often enhanced by tissue sculpting. The latissimus dorsi free flap is also a possibility but is used less frequently because abdominal and buttock free flaps provide more abundant tissue with more acceptable donor sites for the patient. The lateral hip region can be used if the TRAM flap tissue has already been used. The upper inner thigh or outer thigh can be used for free flaps, but most patients find the donor site contour and visible scars objectionable.

The freedom and flexibility this procedure offers is balanced in part by the level of surgical support and expertise required. This is the most complex and demanding of all of the reconstructive procedures. It is also prone to more serious complications, takes longer to perform with the attendant risks of greater blood loss, and usually requires a more extended hospitalization and recuperation period than implant or expander breast reconstruction. It is not for the inexperienced surgeon nor the patient who desires a simple, easy route to breast restoration. The patient should fully understand the extensive nature of this operation before she selects it. She needs to be physically and psychologically prepared for the extended convalescence it requires. Even under the best of circumstances these techniques are not 100% successful. Since the standard pedicled latissimus dorsi flap and TRAM flap have more than 99% reliability, if a free flap is chosen, the surgeon should have a high level of expertise and success with the technique because, if complications of blood flow develop, a reoperation will be needed and the transferred tissue can be lost. The patient should have an idea of the surgeon's success rate with this operation before choosing it.

Immediate TRAM free flap reconstruction has some advantages over delayed free flap reconstruction. Because the oncologic surgeon exposes the vessels for suture of the free flap during the axillary dissection, they are readily available to be sutured to the tissue moved from the lower abdomen.

For microsurgery to be successful, a woman should be healthy and have normal blood vessels. Excess scarring and radiation to these vessels may reduce the chance of a successful result. Patients with radiation damage to the chest wall and patients in whom previous flaps have failed are prime candidates for free flap breast reconstruction, as are women in whom the traditional pedicled TRAM or latissimus dorsi flap is unavailable or inadequate. This would include women with abdominal scarring that precludes the TRAM flap or patients in whom the nerve and blood supply to the latissimus dorsi muscle has been severed or the area damaged by radiation. It is also crucially important for a woman who desires this technique to have a skilled microsurgeon experienced in performing microsurgical breast reconstruction with an equally skillful and experienced breast management team.

## The TRAM Free Flap

The TRAM flap is usually the first choice when additional tissue is needed for breast reconstruction. Sometimes the TRAM flap cannot be transferred safely in the usual manner, that is, by moving the lower abdominal tissue to the breast region while maintaining its blood supply within the strips of the rectus abdominis muscle. When the abdominal wall is scarred or when the upper abdominal vessels are judged not to have sufficient blood supply to keep the lower abdominal tissues alive, as in the woman with a long-standing history of cigarette smoking or the woman who is overweight with evidence of diminished flow from the vessels from the upper abdominal muscle (rectus abdominis), then a TRAM free flap is indicated. Some surgeons experienced with this technique advocate it for most TRAM flaps.

### Surgical Procedure and Postoperative Appearance

Reconstruction with the TRAM free flap is a major operation and takes approximately 3 to 8 hours in the operating room, on some occasions even longer. This operation is done under general anesthesia and requires a hospital stay. As with the pedicled TRAM flap, this operation can only be done once, and the patient should be advised that if another breast reconstruction is needed at a later date, another technique and tissue source will have to be used. The TRAM free flap is designed on the lower abdomen, similar to the design used for the standard TRAM flap. After the flap from the lower abdomen is transferred to the breast region, the vessels in the lower portion of the abdominal flap are sutured into the blood vessels of the armpit region under the operating microscope. The chest wall is prepared by remov-

ing and reopening the mastectomy incision (if it is in an inconspicuous position) or creating a new incision that will permit a more aesthetic reconstruction. The incision is extended into the underarm or
a separate incision is made to permit access to the vessels in that area
for microsurgical hookup. The flap is then transferred to the chest
wall area. The highly technical hookup of the small vessels of the flap
to the breast region is performed under the magnification of the operating microscope.

After the vessels have been connected and checked, the transferred muscle is firmly sutured to the underlying chest wall tissue. The
overlying skin and fatty tissue is shaped and inset to form a breast
mound to match the other breast. The breasts are checked for symmetry and shape and the flap is stitched into place. The nipple-areola
reconstruction is performed in a second or a third procedure, depending on the amount of contouring that still needs to be done to the reconstructed breast.

Microsurgery can also be combined with the pedicled TRAM flap.
This has been called the supercharged or turbo TRAM flap. With this
procedure the lower blood vessels along with a strip of lower abdominal muscle are transferred for the reconstruction, and these blood vessels are hooked into the blood vessels of the underarm. Sometimes
just suturing a vein or artery in conjunction with a standard TRAM
flap is adequate for this supercharged approach. The results of this
procedure are similar to those of the traditional TRAM flap with its
pedicle intact.

The operation for an immediate breast reconstruction with a
TRAM free flap is basically the same as that described for the delayed
TRAM free flap reconstruction. Technically it is an easier operation
because the axillary vessels are already freed up and there is no scarring. Results of this procedure are quite acceptable, but as with the
immediate pedicled TRAM flap, the woman must be fully prepared
for the donor deformity and scar and the additional breast scars required for placing the TRAM flap. Again, some delay in the immediate surgery might be required to enable the woman to donate blood
for this procedure.

The description of the scars and postoperative appearance for a
free TRAM flap is similar to that described on p. 281 for the standard
pedicle TRAM flap.

## Skin-Sparing Mastectomy and Immediate Breast Reconstruction With TRAM Free Flap

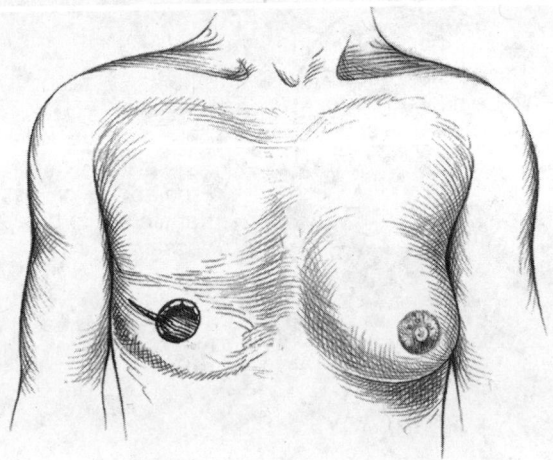

Skin-sparing mastectomy deformity after removal
of breast and nipple-areola

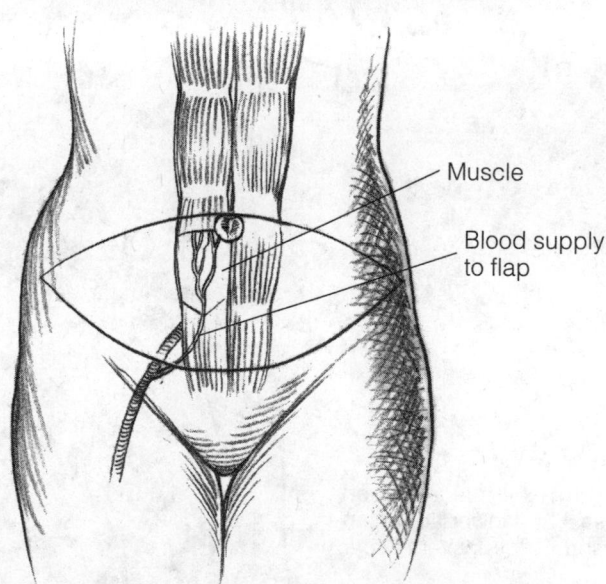

Muscle

Blood supply
to flap

TRAM free flap designed on lower abdomen

## Skin-Sparing Mastectomy and Immediate Breast Reconstruction With TRAM Free Flap—cont'd

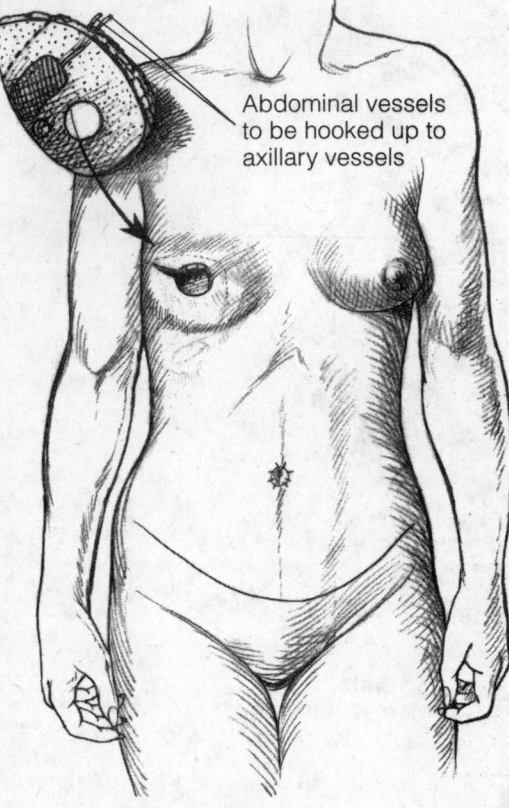

Abdominal vessels to be hooked up to axillary vessels

Free abdominal tissue transferred to breast and vessels

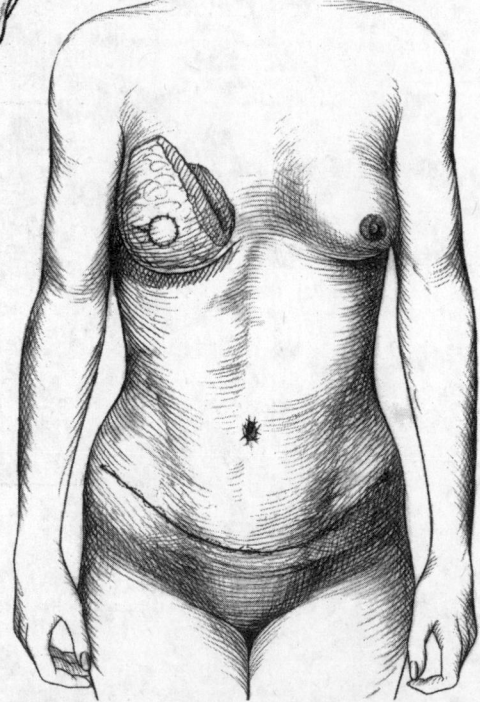

Abdominal tissue fashioned into breast and lower abdomen closed as a transverse scar

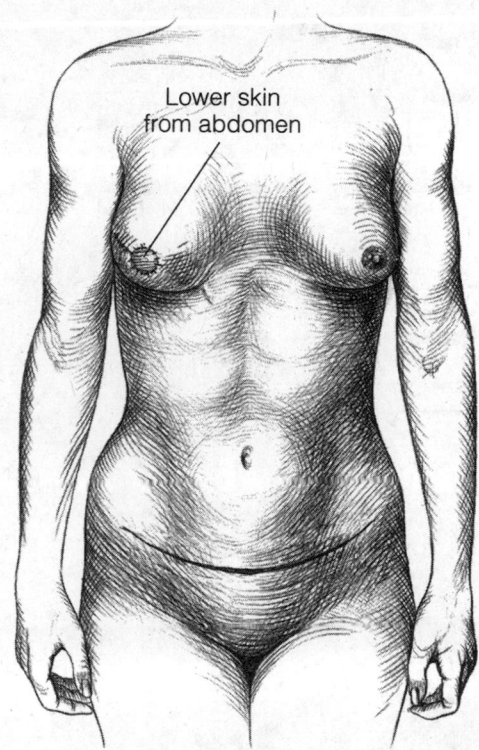

Lower skin
from abdomen

Breast reconstructed
and incision closed as
short incision encircling
areola with extension
to side

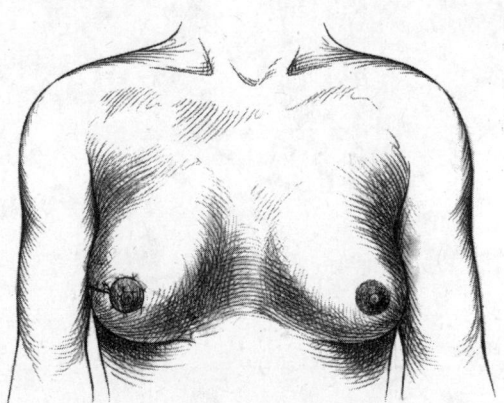

Nipple-areola reconstructed several months later

## Breast Reconstruction With TRAM Free Flap

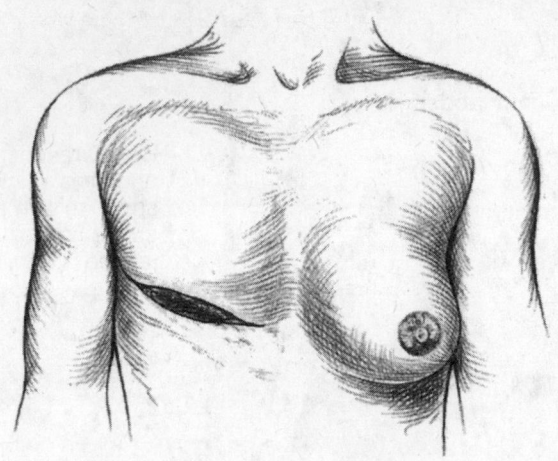

Modified radical mastectomy

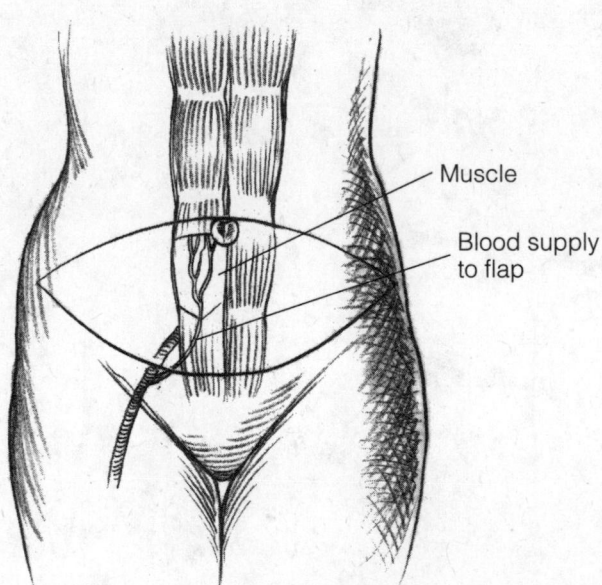

Muscle

Blood supply
to flap

TRAM free flap designed on lower abdomen

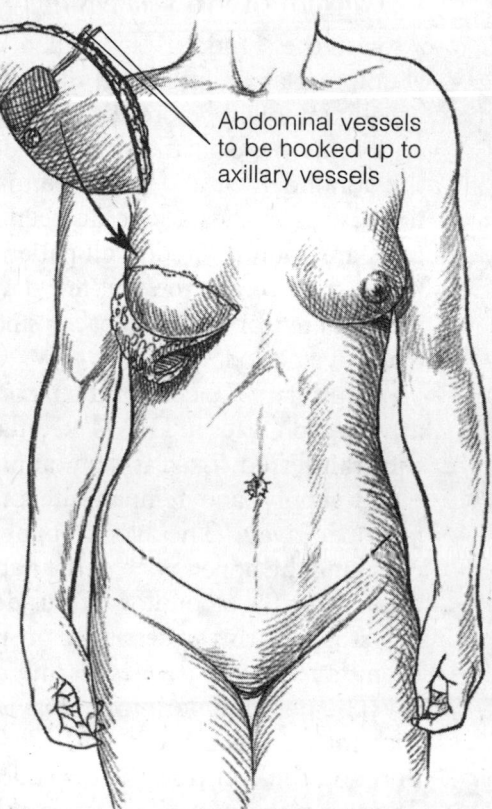

Abdominal vessels to be hooked up to axillary vessels

Free abdominal tissue transferred to breast, vessels reattached by microsurgery, and abdominal tissue fashioned into a breast

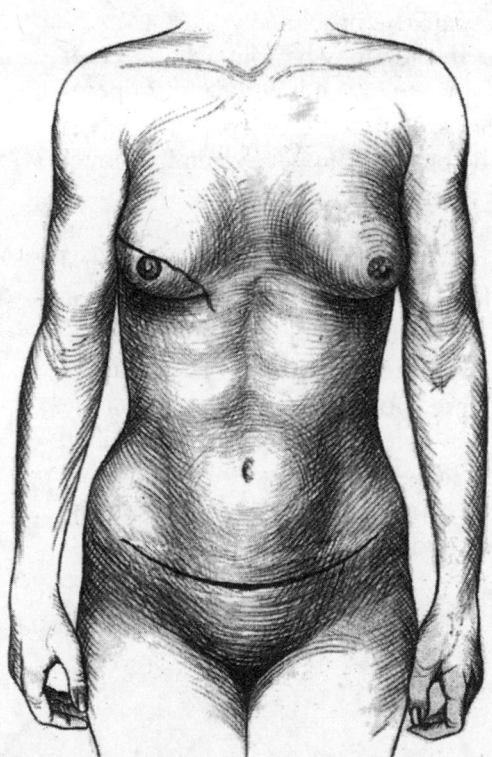

Nipple-areola reconstructed several months later

## Postoperative Care, Complications, and Pain and Recuperation

As with the standard TRAM flap, drains are placed in the breast and abdominal areas for 3 to 4 days after the operation. The drains are usually removed before the patient leaves the hospital and after the antibiotics have been discontinued. Sometimes serum accumulates in the donor defects and may need to be drained during a subsequent office visit after the patient has been released from the hospital. Antibiotics are administered to all patients undergoing microsurgical breast reconstruction for the first few days postoperatively. Cigarette smoking and environmental tobacco smoke are prohibited during the postoperative period.

A primary concern of the reconstructive surgeon in the postoperative period after a TRAM free flap is that the vessels are open and the transferred tissue is maintaining a good blood supply. The color, blood supply, and temperature of the flap are carefully monitored postoperatively. The blood supply to the flap can be assessed by checking the appearance of the flap and by pricking the flap with needles to test for blood flow. If it is determined that the flow to the flap has stopped, this necessitates an immediate return to the operating room to reexplore the vessels and repair the problem.

The potential for blood clots in the leg may be somewhat greater with microsurgical reconstruction because of the length of this operation and the fact that the dissection is nearer the veins in the pelvis. To protect the transferred vessels the patient's upper extremity movements are restricted for 5 to 6 days after the operation.

A hospital stay of 4 to 8 days is required. The patient usually can get out of bed 1 to 2 days after the operation, but it can take several weeks before she can stand upright. Most women gradually resume normal basic activities over the next 4 to 6 weeks. They can often return to work in 4 to 6 weeks and participate in sports in 3 to 6 months. All other aspects of postoperative care, potential complications, and recuperation for the TRAM free flap are similar to those described for the standard TRAM flap on pp. 286-287 and implant reconstruction on pp. 261-264. However, since the muscle is removed with the TRAM free flap, there is usually less abdominal pain.

## Results With the TRAM Free Flap

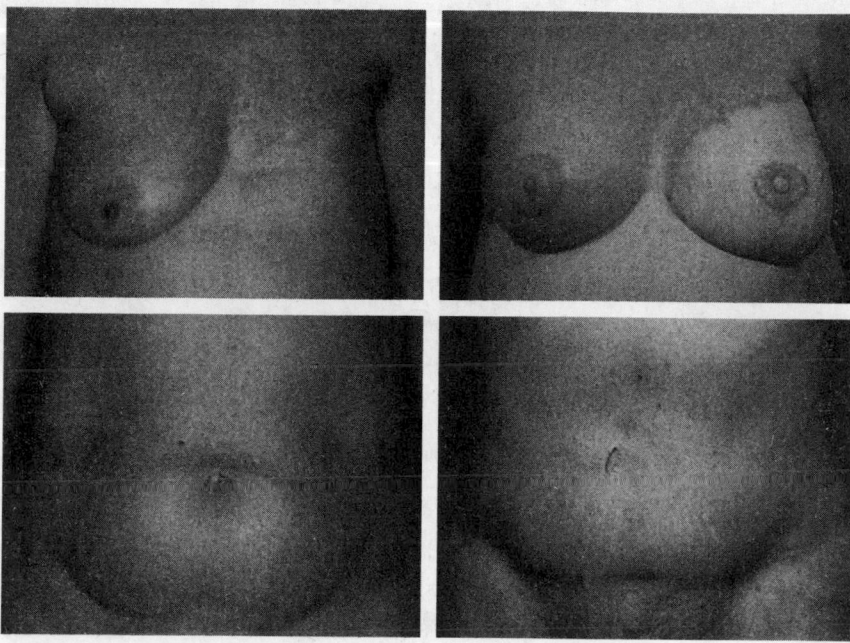

After a left modified radical mastectomy this 52-year-old woman requested breast reconstruction with a TRAM flap. Because most of her lower abdominal fat and skin would be required to match her opposite breast, a TRAM free flap was selected to provide additional volume. At a second operation her nipple-areola was reconstructed and a mastopexy was performed on the opposite breast to improve breast symmetry. She is shown 10 months after her nipple-areola reconstruction and mastopexy.

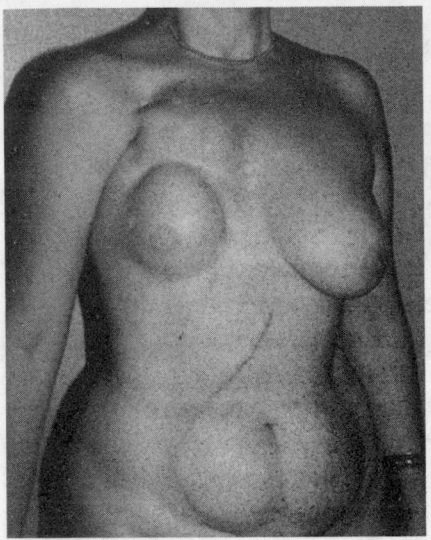 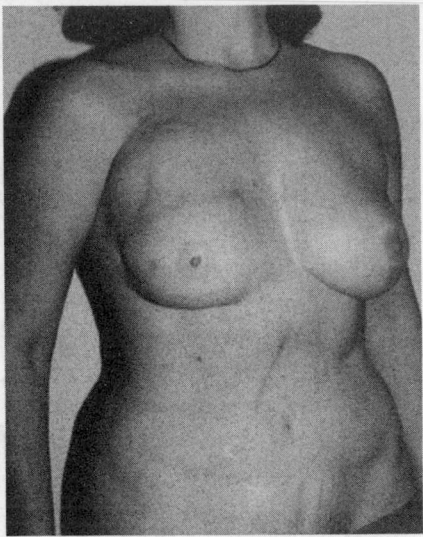

Five years earlier this 43-year-old woman had a right modified radical mastectomy deformity reconstructed using a breast implant. Breast firmness and asymmetry developed over time. Previous abdominal scars precluded a standard TRAM flap breast reconstruction. Her breast was therefore rebuilt with a TRAM free flap. She is shown 4 years after her second breast reconstruction.

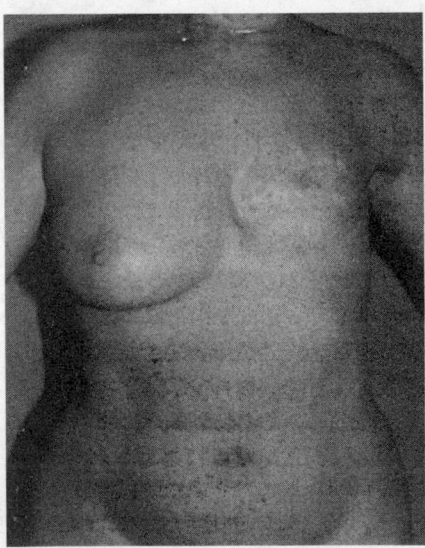 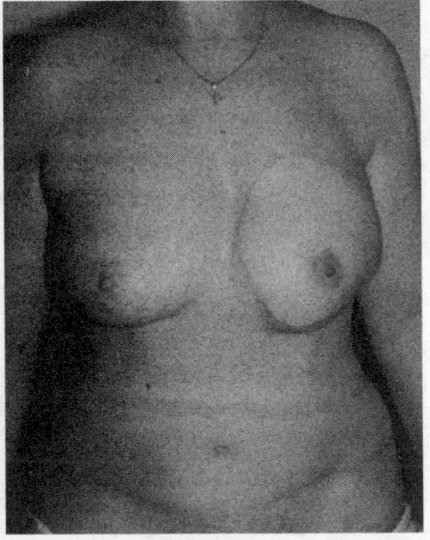

This 54-year-old woman had a modified radical mastectomy of her left breast. A standard TRAM flap breast reconstruction was ruled out because she was a heavy smoker. She is shown 1 year after TRAM free flap breast reconstruction.

## The Gluteus Maximus Free Flap

When the TRAM flap is unavailable or of insufficient size, the tissue for the breast reconstruction can be supplied by transferring a portion of the buttock skin and muscle to the breast region and resuturing the vessels of the buttock tissue to the vessels in the axilla or in the mid-chest region under the ribs. The buttock skin and muscle can be taken from either the midportion of the buttock (superior gluteus free flap) or more often from the lower buttock crease (inferior gluteus free flap). The advantage of using the lower crease is that this is the region of greatest excess tissue. Removal of the tissue from the lower buttocks can actually reduce and flatten a large buttock, and the scar can be placed in the crease where it is less obvious and can be covered by a woman's undergarments. In addition, the vessels of the lower gluteus flap are often better suited for microsurgical hookup.

### Surgical Procedure and Postoperative Appearance

Patients selected for this technique must be healthy and able to undergo a procedure that takes a minimum of 4 to 8 hours and possibly longer. This operation is done under general anesthesia and requires hospitalization. The success of the operation depends on the microsurgeon's skill and artistry in designing and shaping the buttocks into the new breast.

The surgeon designs an elliptical flap along the buttock crease, either along the fold, where the buttocks meets the thigh, or slightly higher, depending on where the greatest concentration of fatty tissue is located and on the quality of the vessels. The flap of skin, fat, and a small portion of the gluteus muscle is obtained along with the small blood vessels going into the muscle that nourish the tissue. The flap is then transferred to the chest wall, where the mastectomy incision has been opened and extended and the recipient vessels have been located. Next, the flap is connected to the vessels in the underarm or occasionally in the midchest region using microvascular techniques performed under the operating microscope. The vessels and flap are checked to ensure that there is good blood flow. Then the transferred muscle is sutured to the underlying chest wall and the flap of skin and fat is shaped and inset to match the opposite breast. During a second procedure it is sometimes necessary to further perfect the breast shape and contour both buttock and hip regions using additional surgical revisions and/or liposuction.

The procedure for the immediate gluteus flap is similar to that described for the delayed gluteus free flap. This procedure is not per-

## Breast Reconstruction With Gluteus Maximus Free Flap

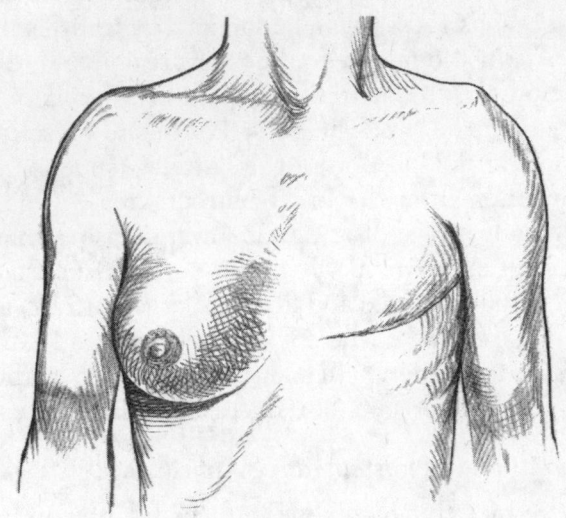

Modified radical mastectomy

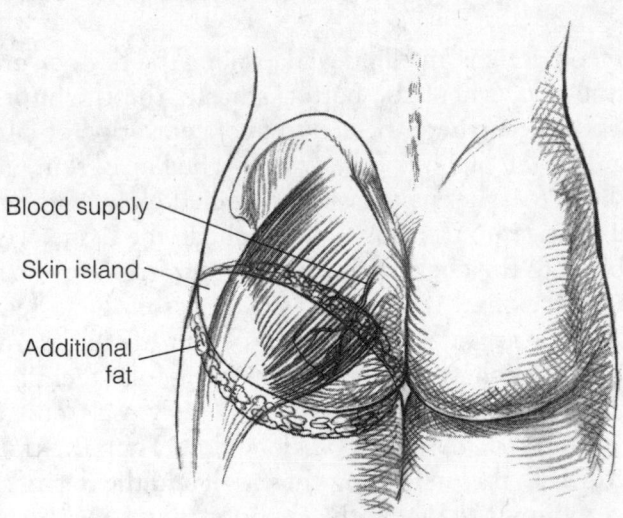

Blood supply
Skin island
Additional
  fat

Gluteus maximus free flap designed on buttock

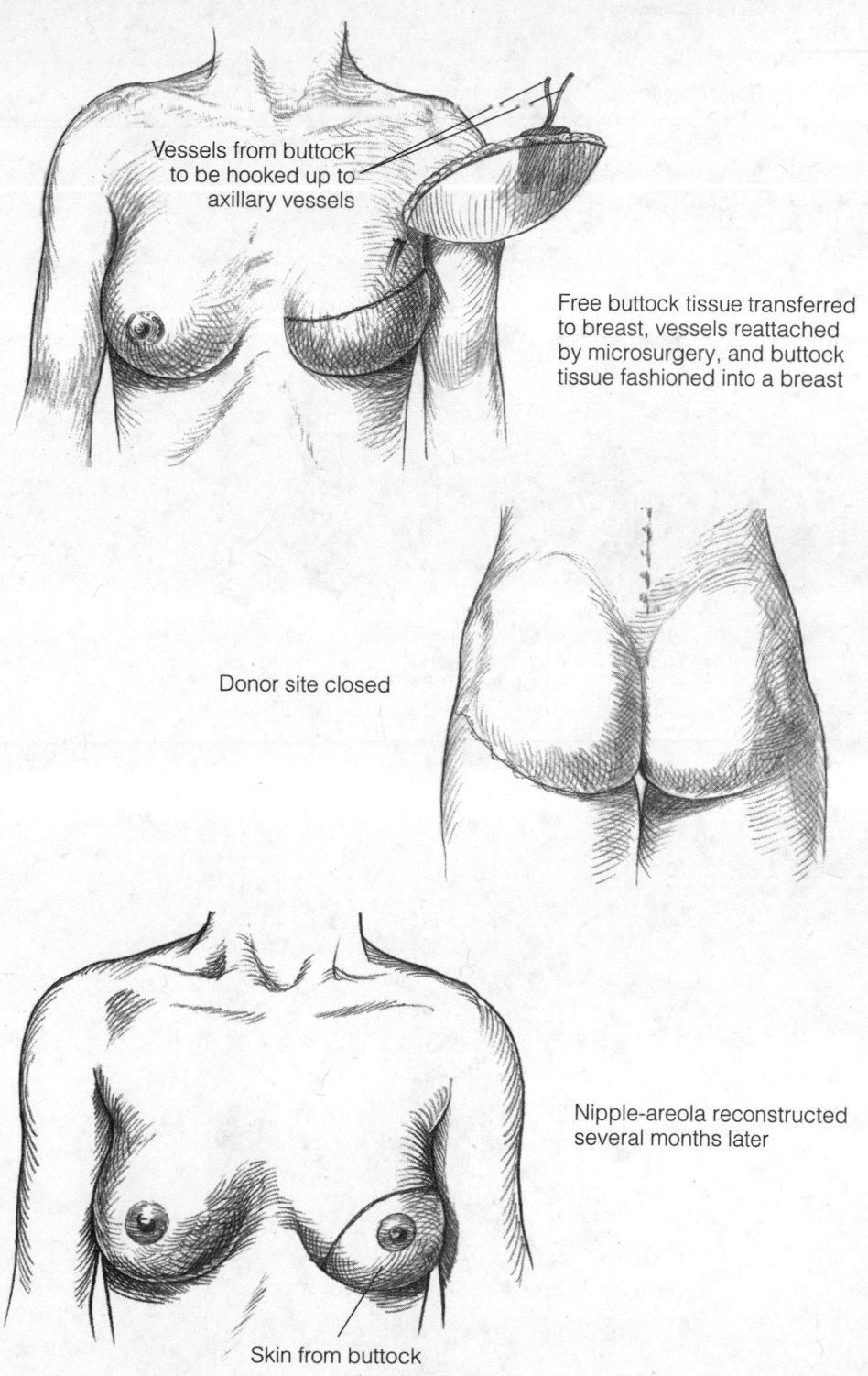

Vessels from buttock to be hooked up to axillary vessels

Free buttock tissue transferred to breast, vessels reattached by microsurgery, and buttock tissue fashioned into a breast

Donor site closed

Nipple-areola reconstructed several months later

Skin from buttock

## Skin-Sparing Mastectomy and Immediate Breast Reconstruction With Gluteus Maximus Free Flap

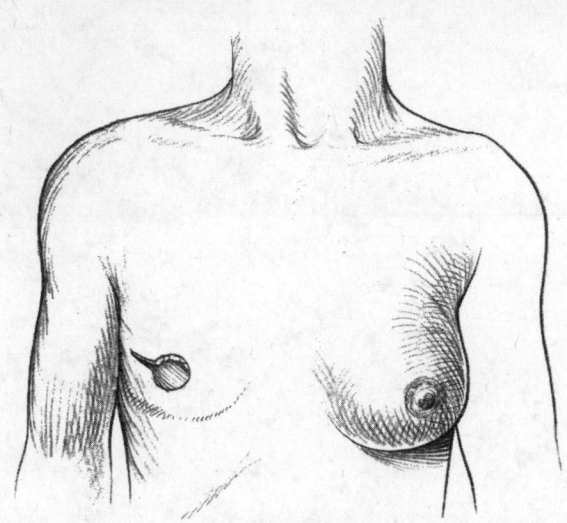

Skin-sparing mastectomy

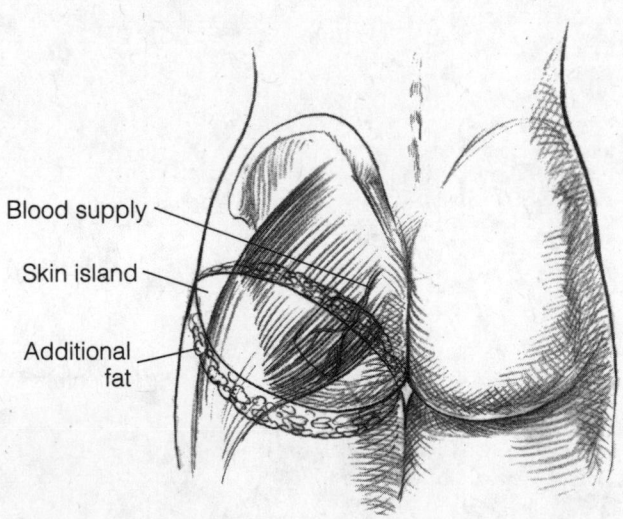

Blood supply

Skin island

Additional fat

Gluteus maximus free flap designed on buttock

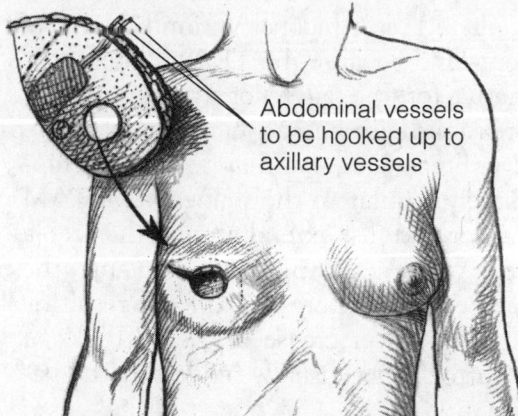

Abdominal vessels to be hooked up to axillary vessels

Free buttock tissue transferred to breast, vessels reattached by microsurgery, and buttock tissue fashioned into a breast

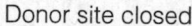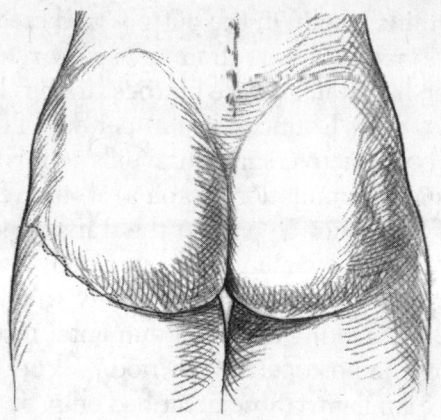

Donor site closed

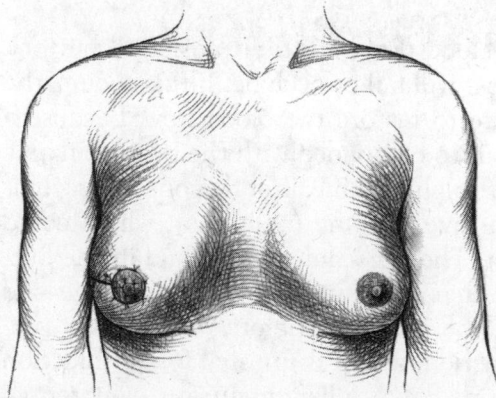

Nipple-areola reconstructed several months later

formed as frequently for immediate breast reconstruction because of the additional time requirements and because the TRAM flap is usually considered a better alternative for free flap reconstruction.

Postoperatively rebuilt breast usually has an elliptic pattern of stitches running along the lower breast crease and up toward the nipple area. When done immediately, similar to the immediate TRAM flap, the skin patch can be smaller and just extend around the areola and toward the underarm area. When used to replace implants, the entire gluteus free flap is buried beneath the breast skin. The resulting donor scar is positioned across the lower crease of the buttocks or across the midportion of the buttock. It is usually hidden by the patient's underpants.

## Postoperative Care

Drains remain in the buttock and breast for 3 to 4 days after the operation. The breast drain is usually removed before the patient leaves the hospital, and the buttock drain is left in place until the fluid loss is less than 1 ounce (30 ml) per day. This may take several weeks. The reconstructive surgeon avoids removing the drain too early because fluid accumulation (seroma) would require aspiration or replacement of the drain. To protect the transferred vessels the patient's upper extremity movements are restricted for 5 to 6 days after the operation. Antibiotics are administered for the first 4 days postoperatively. Cigarette smoking and environmental tobacco smoke are prohibited during the postoperative period. All other aspects of postoperative care are similar to those described on p. 326 for the TRAM free flap, p. 286 for the pedicle TRAM flap, and p. 261 for implant reconstruction.

## Complications

The greatest risk is that the blood flow into the transferred buttock tissue that forms the new breast will fail or occlude. If this occurs, the surgeon will need to reoperate to restore the blood flow. Because a nerve in the back of the leg has to be divided with the buttock flap, a portion of the back part of the thigh is numb after this operation. This nerve can also develop a sensitive swelling (neuroma), which could necessitate another operation. The accumulation of fluid in the buttocks can require drainage either intermittently with a syringe and needle or by replacement of the drain. Antibiotics are usually prescribed in the postoperative period, and it is unusual for an infection to develop after the operation. For a fuller discussion of potential complications, see pp. 286 and 326.

## Pain and Recuperation

Since the donor site is in the buttock region, the patient will have to lie supine or on her opposite side after the operation. The pain and discomfort from this operation are usually not as severe as that experienced with the TRAM flap but more than that experienced after breast reconstruction with implants and expanders. The PCA unit is used to relieve the postoperative pain. To alleviate pressure on the buttock area where the flap was taken, some surgeons use a low air loss type of bed. Pain when sitting can be relieved by using an inflatable donut pillow for the first few weeks after surgery. As with other free flap breast reconstructions, care is taken to monitor the flap after surgery to ascertain that there is good blood flow to the transferred tissue.

A hospital stay of 4 to 8 days is required. The patient gets out of bed the following day. Most women gradually resume normal basic activities over the next 4 to 6 weeks. They can return to work in 4 to 6 weeks and can participate in sports in 3 to 6 months.

## Results With the Gluteus Maximus Free Flap

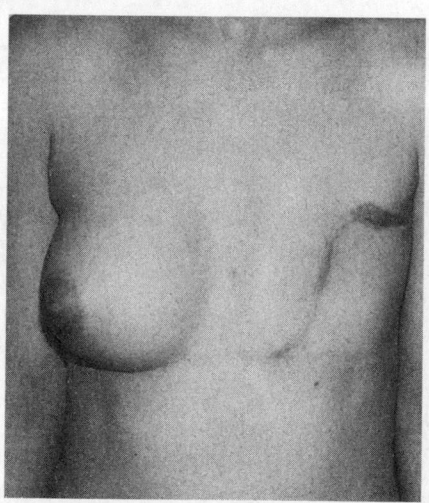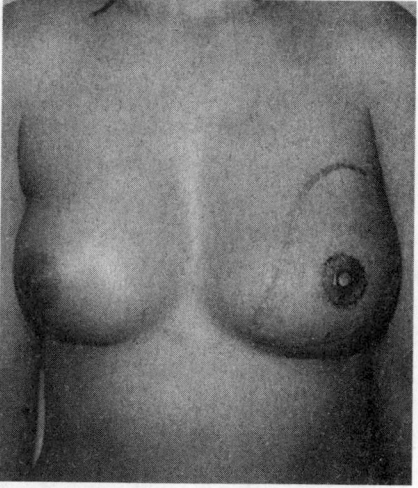

This 28-year-old woman had a left modified radical mastectomy. She decided to have a delayed breast reconstruction and requested a technique that would provide enough tissue to match her opposite breast. She did not want a TRAM flap and requested a gluteus maximus free flap breast reconstruction. She is shown 2 years after the reconstruction and later nipple-areola reconstruction with a local flap and a tattoo.

## *Results With the Gluteus Maximus Free Flap—cont'd*

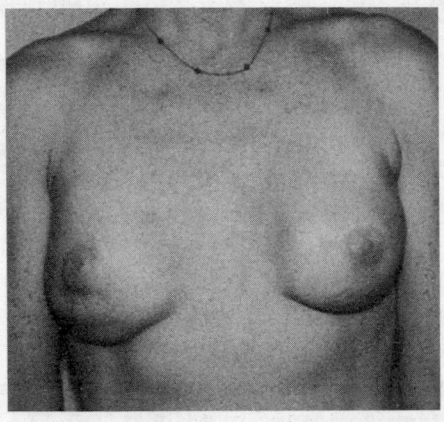 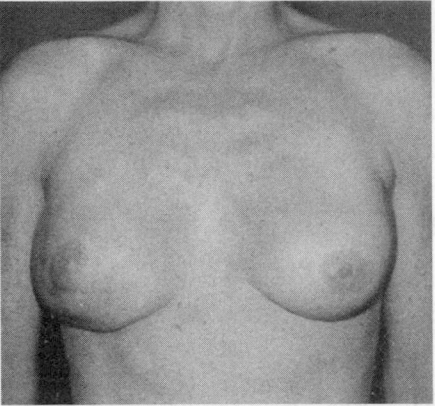

This 39-year-old woman requested bilateral flap breast reconstruction because she was dissatisfied with the results of her previous implant reconstruction. She is shown 6 months following reconstruction with lower gluteus maximus free flaps.

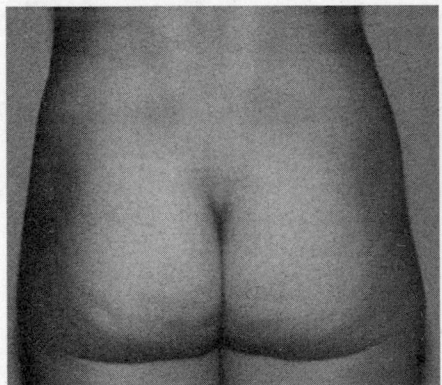 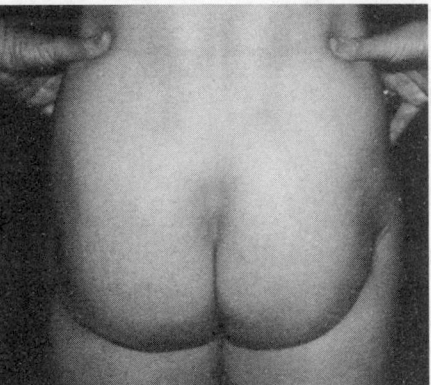

The buttock region is shown before and after the procedure.

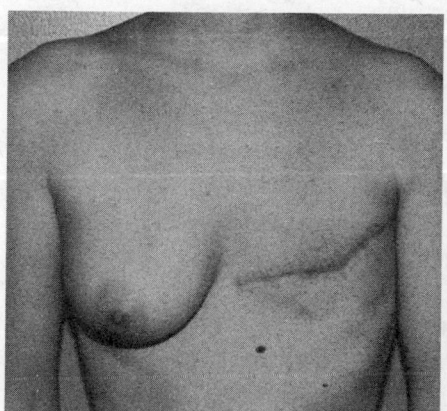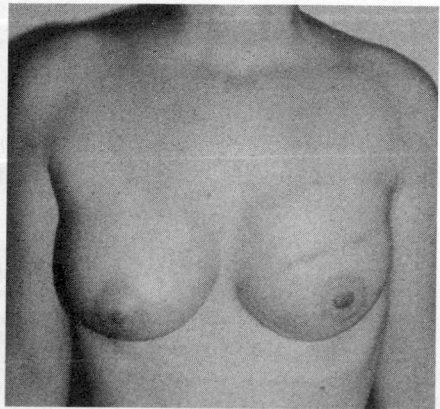

This 24-year-old patient had a left modified radical mastectomy. She wanted a breast reconstruction to match her unmodified opposite breast. Since her lower abdomen was thin, scarred, and irradiated, an abdominal flap could not be used. The patient did not want a back scar. She is shown 18 months after an inferior gluteus maximus free flap.

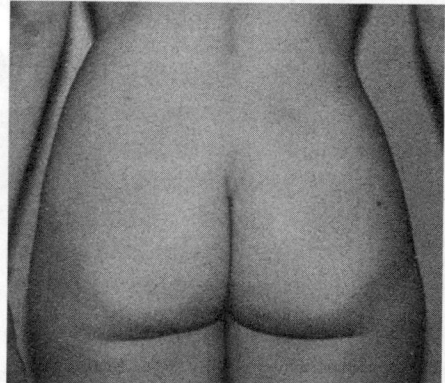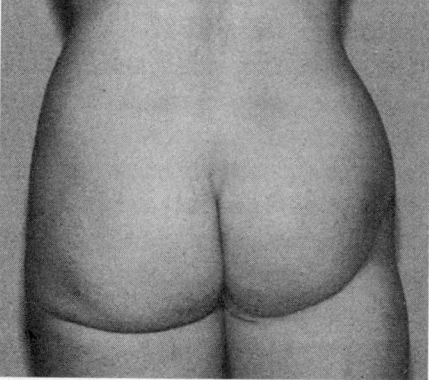

Her donor scar is located in the right buttock crease. Her opposite buttock was suctioned at the time of nipple reconstruction.

## Rubens Free Flap

The lateral hip or Rubens free flap is used when the TRAM or buttocks flap is not available. The technique, complications, and postoperative care and recovery are similar to that described for the TRAM free flap and the gluteus maximus free flap. This flap does not provide the abundance of tissue supplied by some of the other donor sites and many patients find the donor scars objectionable. It is technically demanding and takes tissue from only one hip area.

## FOLLOW-UP OPERATIONS

While it would be ideal for breast reconstruction to be completed in one operation, thereby creating a superbly shaped, symmetric breast, in practice this is expecting too much. The usual breast reconstruction can often be enhanced or improved with a second refining procedure. At this time the scars can sometimes be improved, excess tissue can be removed or deficient tissue supplemented, and if necessary, an implant can be inserted. Reconstruction of the nipple-areola is usually accomplished during this second operation. (A detailed explanation of nipple-areola restoration is given in Chapter 16.)

Proper timing for the second operation to place the nipple-areola should be determined once the breast appearance after the first operation is evaluated; the woman's breasts should look as similar as possible. If they are not symmetric, the surgeon may need to modify the size, shape, and position of the reconstructed breast, either before or at the time he creates the nipple-areola. Usually it is best to have the breasts optimally formed and shaped before placing the nipple. The need for a second operation does not indicate that the first procedure was a failure. The second operation presents the woman and her doctor with an opportunity to obtain the best possible result.

When a significant modification of the reconstructed breast is necessary at the time of the second operation, it is best that the nipple-areola reconstruction be delayed until a third procedure to ensure that it is accurately positioned on a stable breast reconstruction.

The timing of the second operation is also determined by the need for additional treatment such as chemotherapy. This is particularly true for the patient who has immediate breast reconstruction and then must have chemotherapy. Her second operation should usually be delayed until chemotherapy is completed. It is wise to wait at least 2 to 3 months after chemotherapy for the woman to feel her best and her general metabolism and blood count to return to normal. Because of unforeseen complications such as unpredictable healing or an especially extensive mastectomy defect, sometimes additional operations are necessary in addition to the two procedures.

A common secondary operation after implant or expander reconstruction requires the replacement of one implant with another to improve the breast contour, size, or position. The new implant is inserted through the incisions that are already present. Conditions of recovery are similar to those described for the initial implant placement (p. 264), but pain and recovery time are frequently less than for the initial procedure. If capsular contracture persists after several operations, the implant can be replaced with the fatty tissue from the lower abdominal area, a TRAM flap.

After a TRAM flap reconstruction it is often necessary to shape the breasts further, especially in the lower inner area where the abdominal (rectus abdominis) muscle is transferred. The patient's overall body contour can also be improved at the second operation with some finishing touches. These include liposuction or ultrasound-assisted liposuction of the reconstructed breast if it is larger in some areas than the opposite breast. The abdominal wall and hips may also be recontoured with liposuction or ultrasound-assisted liposuction to give a more aesthetic appearance. Similar corrections may be needed after the gluteus maximus free flap to contour the breast or the buttocks and hip area so that they are symmetric. When there is not enough tissue to create the ideal size breast reconstruction or the breast lacks projection after a TRAM flap, an implant or expander can be inserted at the time of the second procedure. Many women, however, who choose these procedures do so to avoid implants and prefer the flatness to the use of a foreign material in their breast. The back flap can be used to supplement a TRAM flap if more tissue is needed and the woman does not want an implant. Sometimes thickened areas of fat occur in the reconstructed breast after flap surgery; when this happens, these areas may need to be excised or biopsied both to confirm their diagnosis and to remove them. If the thickened tissue is determined to be thickened fat, then it can be excised or treated with standard or ultrasound-assisted liposuction.

## REOPERATIVE BREAST RECONSTRUCTION SURGERY

Reoperative breast reconstruction is secondary surgery performed to improve a previous breast reconstruction. It may be performed for a variety of reasons. Some women who have had breast reconstruction are disappointed with the results. Others may have experienced complications or find that the appearance of the breast reconstruction may have deteriorated over time. Some women who had implant reconstruction want their implants removed and their breasts reconstructed with their own tissues.

Reoperative breast reconstruction can include any of the operative approaches or combinations of procedures mentioned in this chapter. Possibilities range from exchanging a breast implant for another of a different size, shape, or texture to replacing a breast implant with the woman's own tissue from her lower abdomen or buttocks. Sometimes a back flap can also be useful for augmenting a breast reconstruction or filling in a defect with additional tissue.

Reoperative breast reconstruction surgery is challenging. Before pursuing this course, a woman should consult with her reconstructive surgeon about her options. Sometimes the plastic surgeon may tell the woman that under the circumstances she has the best possible result that he can achieve and no further operations are advisable. Alternatively, the reconstructive surgeon may suggest that she see another plastic surgeon with extensive experience in reoperative breast reconstruction procedures.

Today, the woman requesting breast reconstruction and the plastic surgeon performing this operation have a number of options to choose from. Local tissue reconstruction with implants and expanders and reconstruction with abdominal, back, lateral thigh, and buttock flaps are all means of restoring women's breasts. Endoscopic techniques provide new options for reducing scar length and for filling defects or correcting asymmetries after lumpectomy or quandrantectomy. A woman's personal needs and the specifics of her deformity dictate which procedures are most suitable. It is very important for the woman to communicate her desires for this surgery to her plastic surgeon so they can examine the different procedures together and decide on the simplest and most reliable operation that can meet these expectations.

# WHAT TO DO ABOUT THE OTHER BREAST: AESTHETIC BREAST CORRECTIONS

After losing one breast to mastectomy, a woman finds that her remaining breast assumes a special importance to her. It is a reminder of the breast she lost and a symbol of her once unscarred chest. She fears the development of a second tumor in her breast, but she also is protective of this lone survivor, not wanting to alter or touch it unless she has no choice.

When a woman contemplates breast reconstruction, her feelings about her remaining breast must be thoroughly discussed with her plastic surgeon since this will affect the type of reconstructive procedure she chooses and ultimately the success of her operation. Both she and her doctor are understandably concerned about the development of a new tumor in the remaining breast, and this possibility should be discussed with the general surgeon. Because the remaining breast will be used as a model for reconstructing the new breast, it must be carefully evaluated. If its appearance is difficult to match or if the woman wants it altered, the plastic surgeon may suggest an aesthetic surgical procedure to change it. Then the woman must decide whether she is comfortable with this suggestion.

Most women having a breast restored want to avoid an operation on their remaining breast. Some women absolutely refuse to submit to any surgery, which always entails some scarring. Usually these women were happy with their breast appearance before the tumor developed, and under ordinary circumstances, they would not have changed their breasts in any way. Therefore they want a reconstructive approach that will leave their surviving breast untouched but will still produce a balanced, aesthetic result. Fortunately, refinements and advances in mastectomy and reconstructive techniques have made this goal attainable for most women. With skin-sparing mastectomies and immediate reconstruction, breasts can be created that closely match the ones they replace. Reconstruction with autologous tissue or with textured, anatomic implants and expanders also faciliates symmetric breast reconstructions without opposite breast modification. If a woman's remaining breast is of average size (B- or C-cup brassiere) and the skin at the mastectomy site is not particularly tight, then reconstruction with an expander or implant will be sufficient to match her breast without further surgery. If a woman does not want her existing breast changed and it is relatively large or sags (ptotic) or the tissues at the mastectomy site are tight or irradiated, the missing breast will usually have to be rebuilt with a flap of extra tissue from her lower abdomen or from her back or buttocks, resulting in additional scars in one of these locations. This is also the case for the woman who wants her breast built with her own tissues and prefers not to have a breast implant for breast reconstruction.

Sometimes, however, the size or shape of the remaining breast cannot be easily duplicated, although with newer reconstructive surgery techniques, this does not happen as often as it once did. Or the woman may request that her breast be altered. In this scenario aesthetic alterations of the other breast are not as essential for obtaining symmetry and become more of a positive option for the woman who wishes to incorporate an aesthetic breast alteration into her breast reconstruction. In those instances when symmetry is difficult to achieve or when a change is requested, the woman may want to consider an operation on her opposite breast if it will ultimately produce breasts that more closely resemble each other and that she will be happier with. An operation on her remaining breast is preferable to feeling lopsided after her reconstruction and perhaps even having to wear a prosthesis. In this situation the plastic surgeon uses one of the procedures developed for aesthetic breast surgery to augment, reduce, or lift her other breast. The final decision for breast size is made by the woman herself, and she needs to clearly explain her expectations to her plastic surgeon before undergoing breast reconstruction.

## BREAST AUGMENTATION

If the woman's existing breast is small and flattened, she may want to consider having it enlarged to make it fuller and rounder. Then her reconstructed breast can be created to resemble this larger breast. This is particularly true if her breast reconstruction will be done with an implant or expander; implantable devices currently on the market come in a limited number of shapes and sizes and tend to produce breasts that are round and full. It is therefore difficult for implant reconstructions to match natural breasts that are small, flat, and droopy. Breast augmentation is a relatively simple procedure; however, it does require a breast implant, usually a silicone elastomer envelope filled with saline solution at the time of the operation. As with any operation, the patient should be fully informed about the benefits and risks of implant surgery before choosing this option. (See Chapters 11 and 13 for detailed information on implant surgery.)

To perform this operation the surgeon makes an incision, usually under the breast, in the axilla, or sometimes around the lower portion of the areola, and inserts a breast implant behind the breast tissue and pectoral muscle layer, thereby enlarging the breast shape. With endoscopic-assisted (minimally invasive) augmentation, shorter incisions can be used and the surgeon has better visualization of the submuscu-

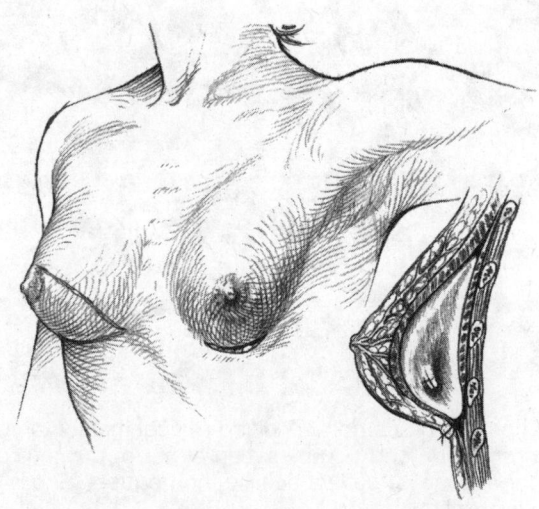

Breast augmentation with implant placed under muscle

lar region for optimal placement of the breast implant. It is then easier for the plastic surgeon to reproduce this larger and fuller breast
contour.

Breast augmentation may serve a psychological as well as an aesthetic need, giving a woman's self-confidence a boost at a time when
she needs an emotional lift. Fears that breast augmentation will hide
the development of a new tumor are unwarranted. Because the implant is placed behind a woman's breast and pectoral muscle layer, it
does not cover her breast tissue, which still can be accurately and effectively checked for any new lumps or tumors. A baseline mammogram is recommended before augmentation mammoplasty and 6 to 12
months after the operation for women over 30 years of age who have
developed breast cancer on the opposite side. Mammograms also may
be taken, and even a breast biopsy can be done without disturbing the
breast implant. Although some have expressed concern that a breast
implant can impair mammography, most breast imagers feel that
appropriate views of the breast permit satisfactory imaging. (See
Chapters 11 and 13 for detailed information on implants and expanders.)

## Results

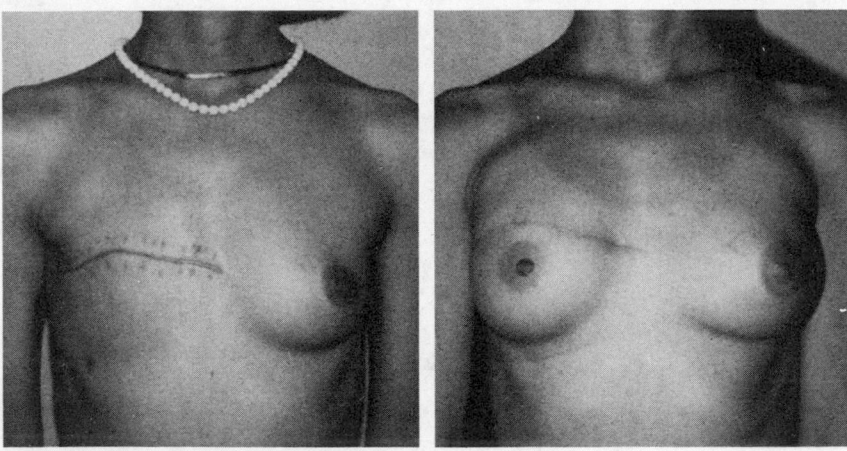

This 30-year-old patient had a right modified radical mastectomy. She requested implant reconstruction and augmentation of her opposite breast. Both procedures were done on an outpatient basis at her request. She is shown 2 years
after breast reconstruction.

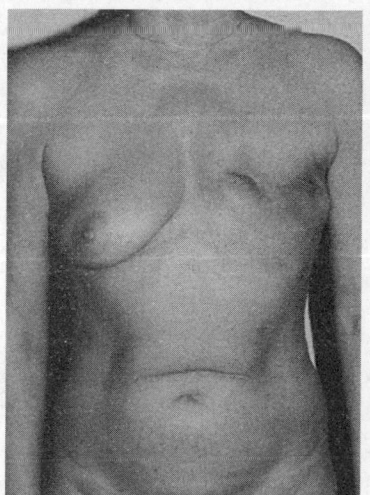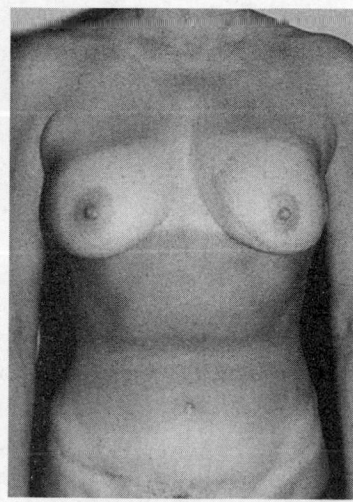

A TRAM flap was used to reconstruct this 52-year-old woman's left modified radical mastectomy deformity; her right breast was augmented for symmetry. She is shown 15 months after her breast reconstruction.

## BREAST REDUCTION

When the woman's remaining breast is large, she may require an autologous flap reconstruction to match it. (The TRAM flap often provides enough tissue to produce symmetry with most large breasts.) As an alternative, she may need to have her remaining breast reduced and/or lifted if the rebuilt breast is to match it. A reduction also may make the reconstruction easier to perform because less tissue will be needed for the new breast and it can be shaped to better match the reduced breast. Many women with large, heavy breasts that cause problems are only too willing to consider having their normal breast reduced to allow them to feel more comfortable and balanced and to mitigate functional problems caused by large breasts. In addition, tissue removed during a breast reduction is checked for tumors, and this information helps the surgeon assess this breast's status. Current breast reduction techniques are very reliable and have a high level of patient satisfaction and acceptance. A baseline mammogram is recommended before a reduction mammoplasty, for patients over 30, and 6 to 12 months after the operation.

The plastic surgeon does not want to reduce a woman's breast too much; he must know what size to make the breast because, above all, he does not want her to feel as if she is losing another breast. Therefore the expected size of her reduced breast must be carefully explained and the woman must understand how it will look before the reduction of the remaining breast is done. The decision for final breast size should be made by the woman herself and must be clearly communicated to her plastic surgeon. To avoid overreduction it may occassionally be necessary for the surgeon to perform an extra reconstructive operation later to expand or add an implant to the reconstructed breast. By reducing a woman's existing breast the plastic surgeon may be able to rebuild her missing breast without a flap procedure; however, a flap should be used if the woman is worried that her breasts will be too small. Most women with a full breast requiring a reduction will have better long-term symmetry if the breast reconstruction is done with a flap of abdominal tissue, but tissue from the back or buttocks can be used as well.

The incisions used for breast reduction result in permanent scars that usually resemble an upside-down **T**. When only a small or moderate reduction is needed, newer reduction techniques can produce shorter scars, either around the areola or around the areola with a vertical scar extending down to the inframammary fold. These scars

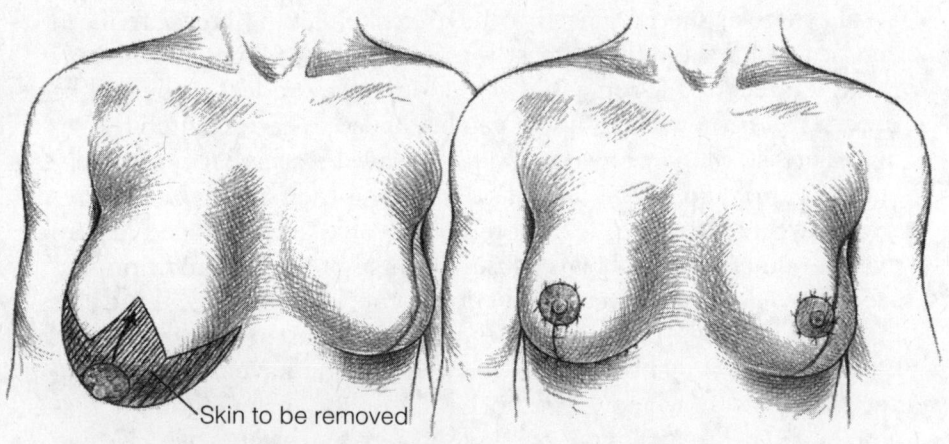

Reduction of the other breast to obtain symmetry with the
reconstructed breast using inverted T incisions

are easily covered when a brassiere is worn. As with all scars, they are often red for the first months after the operation but will usually fade and lighten after 1 to 2 years. Breast function is also a consideration during reduction mammaplasty. The nipple ducts are left intact to permit the possibility of future breast-feeding if this is a consideration. Even though there may be temporary numbness after this procedure, breast sensation and nipple-areolar sensation are usually not permanently affected.

During this procedure the surgeon removes the excess breast tissue, usually in the lower portion of the breast, to reshape the breast to a smaller size and narrower, more uplifted shape. Extra breast skin is excised, and the final skin closure leaves a scar around the nipple, down to the crease below the breast, and in a line in the crease.

During the postoperative period the reduced breast is often somewhat swollen and firm. The patient may also note decreased sensation in the breast and nipple-areola. The sensation usually returns during the first few months after the operation. As the sensation returns, the nerves may have heightened sensitivity, occasionally accompanied by shooting pains through the involved breast. When this occurs, the patient is instructed to massage her breast with different textures of cloth and during a bath or shower to use different water temperatures on her breast so that the sensory response can return to normal.

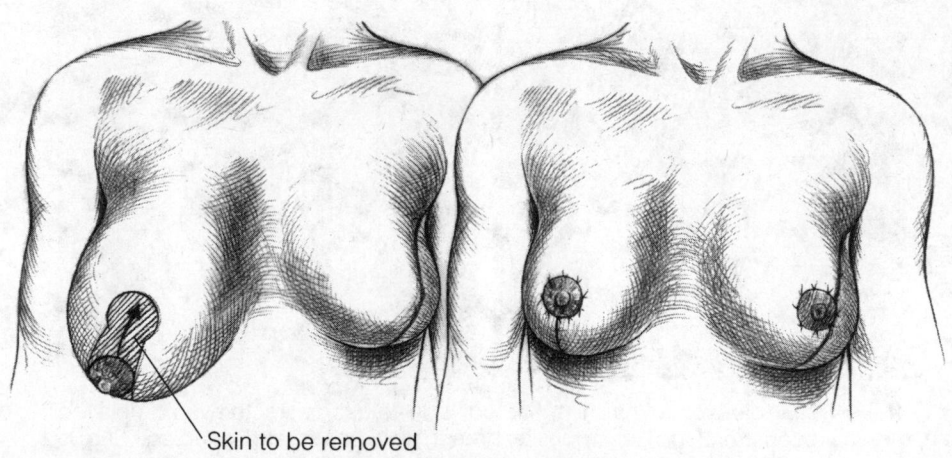

Skin to be removed

Alternate vertical short scar breast reduction technique
without leaving scar in inframammary fold

## Results

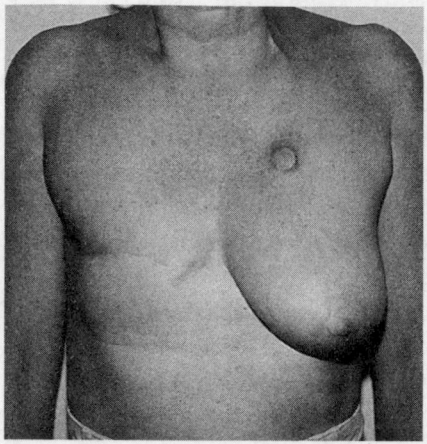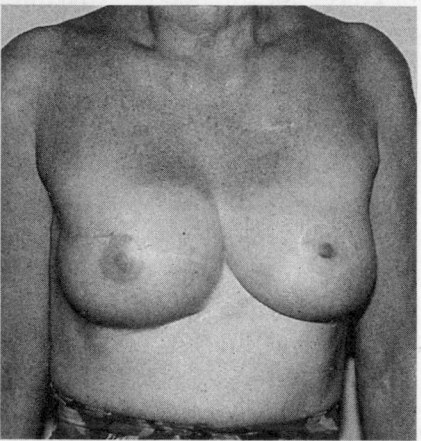

This 43-year-old woman had a right modified radical mastectomy and delayed breast reconstruction with tissue expansion. Her opposite breast was ptotic and heavy and she wanted reduction mammaplasty. She is shown 1 year after breast reconstruction with breast implant placement and a reduction mamma- plasty of her opposite breast. Her nipple-areola was reconstructed with a local flap and a tattoo.

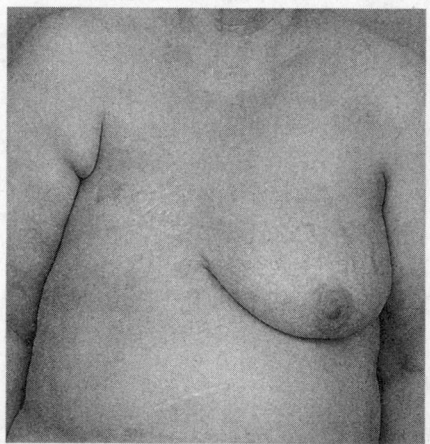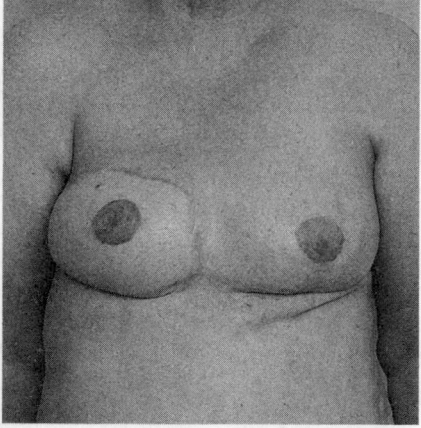

This 54-year-old woman had a right modified radical mastectomy and delayed breast reconstruction. Her opposite breast was heavy and sagging. She is shown 1 year after breast reconstruction with a TRAM flap and a small reduction mammaplasty of her opposite breast. Her nipple-areola was reconstructed with a local flap and a tattoo.

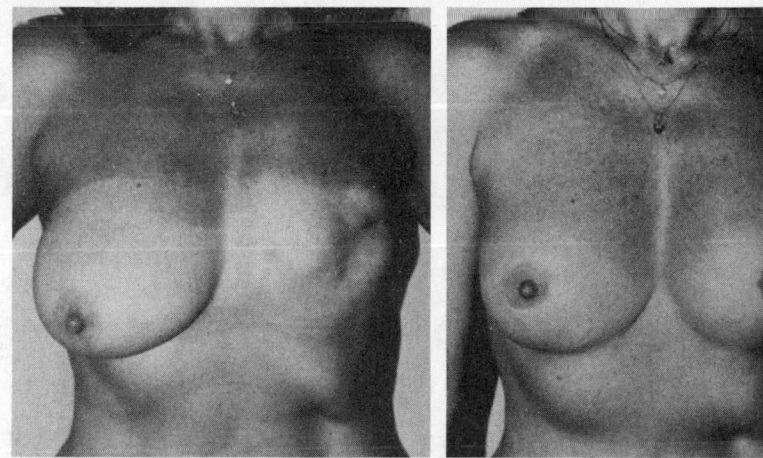

This 38-year-old woman had a modified radical mastectomy. She wanted her large opposite breast reduced and a smaller breast reconstructed to match. She is shown 2 years after implant breast reconstruction and reduction of the other breast.

## BREAST LIFT (MASTOPEXY)

If the opposite breast is of reasonable size but sags from the weight of excess skin and loss of support, the surgeon may find that the skin remaining after the mastectomy or available as a flap is insufficient to allow the stretch necessary to match this sagging breast. In this case the plastic surgeon may suggest a breast lift, or mastopexy, for the remaining breast. Many women are pleased with the prospect of altering their drooping breasts to give them a fuller, more uplifted, youthful appearance.

With a mastopexy, the surgeon moves the nipple-areola upward on the breast to a new position and removes some skin below the nipple. The breast lift incisions are similar to but often shorter than those used for breast reduction. When the breast does not sag very much, these breast lift (mastopexy) incisions can often be limited to the area around the areola with a vertical line extending to the lower breast crease. Many women who are considering a breast lift have considerable flatness in the upper breast region. Simply lifting the breast will not restore fullness to this area. It is best done with a breast implant. For the woman whose other breast is being reconstructed with an implant or expander implant, insertion of a matching implant behind the normal breast is often a good means of providing the most balanced, aesthetic result because bilateral implants behave more symmetrically over time.

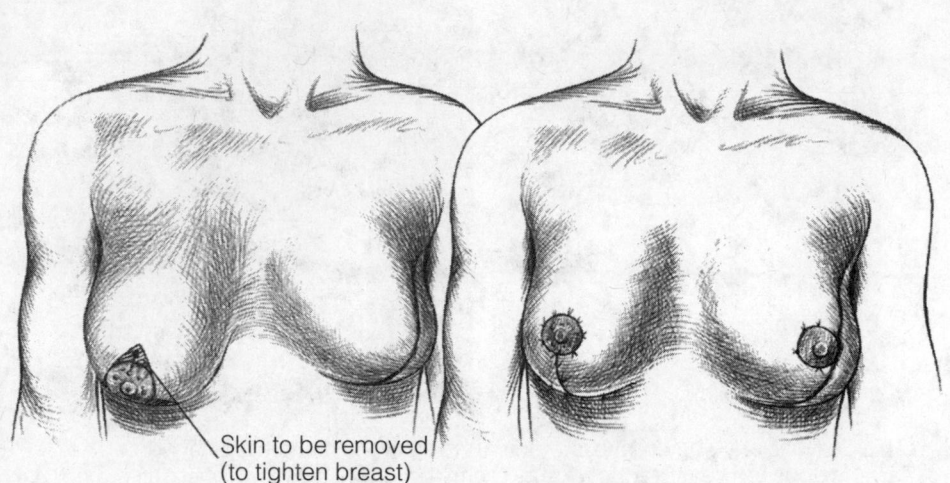

Skin to be removed
(to tighten breast)

Mastopexy (breast lift) of the other breast with inverted T scar
to obtain symmetry with the reconstructed breast

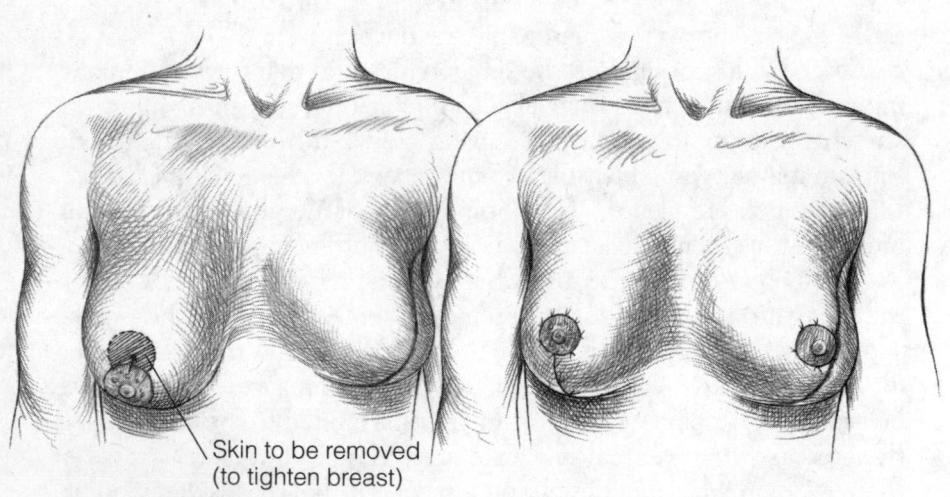

Skin to be removed
(to tighten breast)

Alternate vertical short scar mastopexy technique
with inframammary scar

# Results

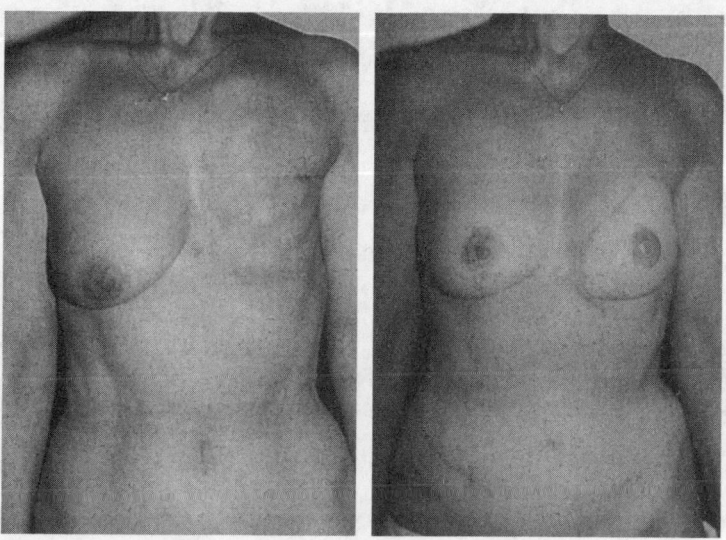

This 46-year-old woman had a modified radical mastectomy. She had breast reconstruction with a TRAM flap and her opposite breast was lifted for symmetry. She is shown 1 year after breast reconstruction and mastopexy.

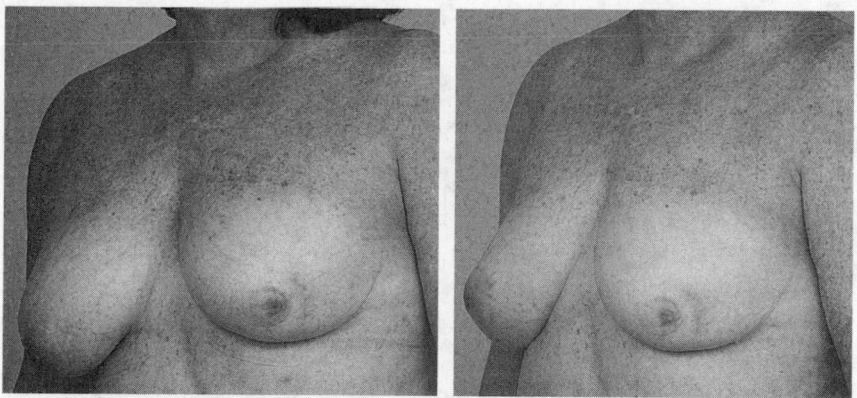

This 39-year-old woman had lumpectomy of her left breast followed by irradiation. After several years the left breast had become firm, contracted, and somewhat elevated. She was concerned with the asymmetry. She decided to have a vertical scar mastopexy to correct the ptosis of the right breast. She is shown a few months later and is pleased with the improved appearance.

## Results—cont'd

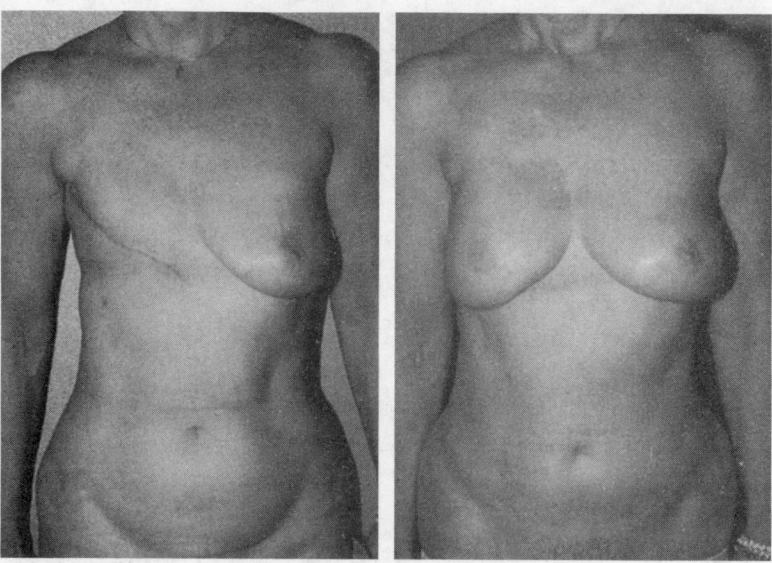

After a right modified radical mastectomy this 48-year-old woman's breast was reconstructed with a TRAM flap; a mastopexy was performed on her left breast to obtain a better match. She is shown 5 years after breast and nipple-areola reconstruction.

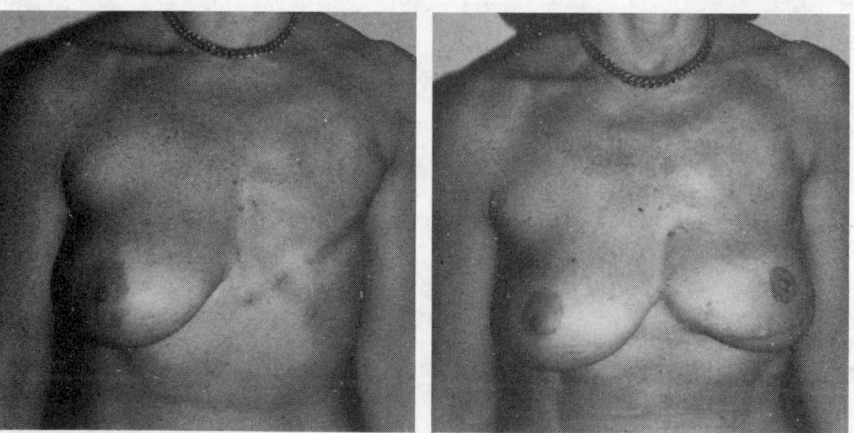

This 48-year-old woman had a left modified radical mastectomy. She is shown 2 years after breast reconstruction with a latissimus dorsi flap and tissue expansion and a mastopexy and small reduction on her right breast for symmetry.

The broad spectrum of techniques currently available to the surgeon permit breast reconstruction that closely approximates a woman's remaining breast without having to alter it. Skin-sparing mastectomy with immediate reconstruction, autologous flap reconstruction, and tissue expansion are all positive methods for creating fuller, more natural, symmetric breast shapes. When a modification is planned because the patient requests it or the shape and contour of the woman's breast makes it a consideration, the reconstructive surgeon can usually alter the remaining breast and reconstruct the missing breast shape during one operation. The new breast then can be built to match the existing altered breast. When there is some question about the necessity for changing the remaining breast or when the woman has doubts about this surgery, it should not be modified at the time of the breast reconstruction. In this case only the missing breast should be restored during the initial operation. Then, later, after the results of surgery are evaluated, a decision can be made about whether the natural breast should be changed or left alone.

# PROPHYLACTIC MASTECTOMY

Breast cancer is an overriding fear for some women, not merely a statistic. Some have witnessed the suffering and even death of mothers and sisters from this disease; others have themselves fallen victim to breast cancer. They have become sensitized to the life-threatening danger it poses. We read daily about the growing incidence of breast cancer among U.S. women as well as the recent discovery of breast cancer genes that indicate a strong inherited tendency for breast cancer. This only serves to intensify these fears. Realizing that they are in a high-risk category for developing a malignancy, some women seek a way of reducing the odds.

A prophylactic (also called risk-reducing) mastectomy with reconstruction is an operation that is performed with the intent of decreasing a woman's risk of developing breast cancer by removing most of her breast tissue and then rebuilding her breasts. By its very nature such preventive surgery is highly controversial and often raises more questions than it answers. The decision to have this operation with the goal of diminishing the woman's risk of getting breast cancer also involves removing a healthy breast that may, in fact, never develop a malignancy. The crucial question is whether this operation actually prevents cancer and whether other nonsurgical treatments could accomplish the same purpose.* Unfortunately, there are no clear-cut answers or definitive scientific data available at present. New infor-

---

*Initial results of the National Institutes of Health (NIH) study to determine if tamoxifen can be used to prevent breast cancer in high-risk women have shown some compelling evidence that this drug may prove to be an effective prophylactic treatment in the future. Other studies are investigating the role of raloxifene and of Taxol as cancer combatants. If the final results of this study prove tamoxifen to be an effective prophylactic treatment, this may obviate the need for preventive mastectomy. (See Chapter 6 for more updated information on this clinical trial.)

mation on the breast cancer genes and the availability of genetic testing to identify high-risk women who are carriers have further complicated this decision-making process. Some cancer surgeons are skeptical about the efficacy of this surgery. They believe that many prophylactic mastectomies are unnecessary. As one renowned surgeon stated, "The decision whether to perform a prophylactic mastectomy is difficult for the patient and surgeon because methods for predicting cancer development are still inadequate and there are no certain methods for preventing cancer."

Others question performing a mastectomy (total breast removal) before breast cancer develops to prevent a cancer that can be treated with conservative surgery and irradiation if it occurs. If one waits for cancer to develop, however, there is always the possibility that it may have already spread systemically before it is detected locally within the breast.

Only a woman in a high-risk category with more than one risk factor present should even consider prophylactic mastectomy. Furthermore, the motivation for this operation should be based on her level of concern about cancer. Is she terrorized by her fears of malignancy and subsequent death or can she be reassured that her breasts can be carefully and adequately monitored without surgery? The vast majority of women at high risk are managed by careful evaluation by their physician, breast self-examination, mammograms, and biopsies of any suspicious breast areas (see Chapters 3, 4, and 5). (The use of minimally invasive biopsy techniques is decreasing the need for open biopsy of these suspicious breast masses.) Women need to be fully informed about their risks and their options. Although an operation is usually not recommended, it is sometimes presented as a option if the patient's risk is very high and her anxiety level is so overriding that it cannot be allayed by continued monitoring.

If a prophylactic mastectomy is considered, the specifics of the operation should be carefully explained and fully understood. This is major surgery. Afterward, the reconstructed breasts have less sensation than normal breasts and can actually feel numb; their appearance often is not as attractive, and complications may develop that require additional operations and increase the potential for disappointment. Some women who have prophylactic mastectomies later regret their decision because the result does not meet their expectations. Physicians are understandably circumspect about an operation that can decrease the aesthetic and functional aspects of a woman's breasts while offering no guarantee that it will prevent breast cancer. A woman considering this approach is already anxiety ridden about her risk of developing cancer; it is therefore crucial that she understands the limitations of this surgery and does not expect it to exactly duplicate the breast that she is having removed. Most likely her breasts will not look or feel as they did before. A decision to have a prophylactic mastectomy should only be reached after a thorough discussion by the woman, her physicians, and her surgeons. Her doctors need to explain her risk status and the full ramifications of this operation, both positive and negative. A consultation with a genetic counselor may also be helpful in fully evaluating a woman's risk status and understanding its implications for her health. She also needs to discuss this operation with others with whom she is intimate. Finally, input from other physicians involved in her care and second opinions from other surgeons are recommended to ensure that this option is weighed carefully before making a final decision for or against it.

## HIGH-RISK FACTORS FOR DEVELOPING BREAST CANCER

Three main factors are believed to contribute to an increased risk of breast cancer. Many women fit into at least one of these categories, but that does not mean they will necessarily develop breast cancer and thus should have their breasts removed. What they do need is good information about their risk status, particularly those women who fall into any of the three high-risk categories.

### Family History in a Mother, Sister, or Daughter

Having a first-degree maternal relative such as a mother, sister, or daughter develop breast cancer increases a woman's risk by two or three times, with a lifetime risk of about 20%. If the cancer developed before menopause, her lifetime risk increases to about 30%. If the cancer was bilateral, the risk may approach 50%. Some women with these family histories also carry a heritable breast cancer tendency, such as women who have tested positive for the breast cancer genes BRCA1 and/or BRCA2. These two genes are thought to account for the majority of instances of breast cancer caused by inherited genetic errors. When these genes are changed or mutated, they lead to an increased susceptibility to breast cancer (in the range of 50% to 70% over a lifetime for women with mutations in BRCA1). Other families simply have random occurrences of multiple sporadic cancers. Increasingly, laboratory testing can define which of these two situations accounts for a particular woman's family history.

### Previous Personal History of Breast Cancer

If cancer develops in one breast, the chance of a new cancer occurring in a woman's other breast increases. If she is over 50, the risk is about 4% for the remaining years, and for those under 50, there is a lifetime risk of approximately 14%. If several cancerous areas are found in the first breast, the risk to the second breast is greater. These risks are further increased if the woman who had one breast cancer also has a family history, especially if her mother or a sister had this disease and particularly if it occurred before menopause. In addition, those women who have a small tumor that has not spread to the lymph nodes are more likely to live longer and therefore are at risk of developing a second tumor over a longer period of time. The pathologist's report on the first breast cancer can suggest an increased risk for the remaining breast. For instance, if the changes of LCIS (lobular carcinoma in situ) are noted, the patient's risk for another tumor increases by a factor of 2 to 3. The risk of this happening is about 1% for each year of life. If a woman develops breast cancer before the age of 40, the chance that she will develop another cancer in her opposite breast is somewhat increased.

### Advanced Age

Although recent statistics suggest that more younger women are now affected by breast cancer, the overall incidence rises with age. About 85% of breast cancers are clinically detected in patients over 45 years old. Advances in mammography have made it easier to detect early breast cancer in women over 50 and in postmenopausal women whose breasts are less dense.

## RELATIVE RISK FACTORS

Women in the following categories have a slightly increased risk of breast cancer:

- History of breast cancer in maternal or paternal grandmother, father's sister, or mother's sister
- Excessive exposure to radiation, particularly before age 20 (currently used diagnostic x-ray examinations [even cumulatively] do not reach these levels), and women who received radiation of the chest for previous malignancies such as Hodgkin's disease

- Early menarche (beginning of menstruation)
- Birth of first baby after age 30
- Never having borne children (nulliparity)
- Late menopause
- Obesity
- History of some types of fibrocystic change
- High fat diet
- Some ethnic groups such as Ashkenazi (Eastern European) Jewish woman who are at higher risk for developing breast cancer
- Use of estrogen supplements and estrogen replacement therapy

(For the convenience of our readers a similar, but more detailed discussion of risk factors is also included in Chapter 6.)

## PROPHYLACTIC MASTECTOMY AND RECONSTRUCTION: WHAT TO EXPECT

The objective of a prophylactic mastectomy (also known as "total, preventive, and risk-reducing mastectomy") is to remove as much glandular breast tissue as possible while preserving the skin covering so that the breast may be reconstructed to an attractive appearance. Today, these operations are usually done as skin-sparing mastectomies, which seem to provide the best aesthetic results. Because breast tissue is close to the skin, removal can sometimes impair the blood supply to the skin and nipple-areola. The surgeon usually will request that the patient refrain from smoking cigarettes for several weeks before the operation and after surgery to prevent any further compromise of the blood supply.

Heavy cigarette smoking causes the small vessels in the skin to constrict, thus increasing the possibility of complications. Problems ranging from changes in the skin, possible scarring, loss of flap tissue, loss of the nipple-areola, or implant exposure (requiring removal) are all possibilities. A review of patients with major complications after prophylactic mastectomy shows that the common link and contributing cause of these complications is cigarette smoking. Women who smoke are also at greater risk for developing lung cancer. It therefore seems illogical for these same women to undergo prophylactic breast removal because of their fear of breast cancer while they continue to smoke and risk lung cancer.

When the breast is of normal size, the nipple-areola skin can be left on the breast after the breast tissue beneath the nipple is removed. Some surgeons and patients, however, prefer to remove the nipple-areola during prophylactic mastectomy. The surgeon then reconstructs the breast with the woman's own tissue or by placing an implant or expander implant under the pectoralis major muscle layer (for information on reconstruction with available tissue, see p. 253). This muscle cover will help ensure that the implant remains soft and does not become exposed through the skin. Experience with the textured-surface implants and expanders indicates that they provide equally soft results regardless of whether they are positioned under the remaining skin or muscle. However, for patients with thin skin cover (that includes most of the women who have this prophylactic operation), the implant's contour and folds may be seen and felt through the thin skin and thus it is best placed under the muscle. If the patient is concerned about using breast implants and still requests prophylactic mastectomy, breast reconstruction with bilateral TRAM flaps can be considered. Autologous tissue is a good alternative for these women who decide to have their breasts removed out of fear of cancer and do not want to use a foreign material that might be a source of further anxiety. If the woman's breast is large and pendulous, it will require either a flap reconstruction (Chapter 13) to provide sufficient fill for the remaining breast skin or modification of the remaining breast skin so that the breast appears smaller and more uplifted. In the latter case the plastic surgeon temporarily removes the nipple-areola and excises the breast tissue and ducts from beneath it. Then he replaces the nipple-areola as a graft in the proper position on the newly reconstructed breast.

After the surgeon removes the breast tissue, he uses one of the methods described in Chapter 13 to reconstruct the breast. Prophylactic mastectomy and the subsequent reconstruction usually are performed in one operation (as described for immediate breast reconstruction), even though some surgeons advise delaying the reconstruction for a few days to months. Delaying breast reconstruction after prophylactic mastectomy is recommended routinely by some surgeons, and others delay it only for the patient with increased risk factors such as cigarette smoking or breast scars from previous breast biopsies, which could compromise the primary healing of the skin and lead to postoperative complications.

## WHERE ARE THE INCISIONS PLACED AND DO THEY SHOW?

A number of incisions can be used for prophylactic mastectomy, and the patient should discuss these variations with her surgeon. Today, many surgeons remove the tissue through a skin-sparing incision that encircles the nipple-areola and may have a slight horizontal extension to ensure complete tissue removal. Some surgeons perform this operation through an opening in the crease beneath the breast. These incisions produce the least obvious scars. Another option is to use a second axillary incision in addition to the one at the inframammary fold. Other surgeons have difficulty gaining access to the upper axillary breast tissue through this approach and use an incision lateral to the areola. Sometimes this incision is extended over the nipple to elevate it when the breast sags.

The presence of biopsy or other breast scars can influence the safety and position of the prophylactic mastectomy incisions. When the biopsy scars are relatively long, the mastectomy can often be done through these scars, thus avoiding additional breast incisions and causing less risk that some of the breast skin will not survive. When the breasts are large or there is excessive breast skin, the surgeon removes the extra skin from below the nipple-areola and just above the crease, leaving an inverted T scar, or through the middle of the breast, leaving a scar on the lower midportion of the breast. The woman considering prophylactic mastectomy who has larger breasts that also need to be lifted or made smaller should know that she has an increased chance of having problems and complications from the operation. The nipple-areola skin often has to be taken from its low position on the breast and either grafted to its new position or reconstructed at a later operation. Removal of a larger amount of breast tissue and the need for larger skin flaps also increase the risk that the skin will heal poorly. In some cases the breast implant used for reconstruction may have to be removed and replaced a few months later.

## WHAT IF A BREAST CANCER IS FOUND AT THE TIME OF A PROPHYLACTIC MASTECTOMY?

The breasts should be carefully evaluated for breast cancer before the decision is made to have a prophylactic mastectomy. Occasionally, either during the operation or later after the pathologist evaluates the tissues removed during the mastectomy, a breast cancer is found. Because of this possibility, a total mastectomy should be performed with breast tissue removed according to recognized cancer treatment standards and guidelines. However, to determine if the breast cancer has spread, an axillary dissection with removal of the axillary lymph nodes may still be needed to provide more information about the stage of the tumor and the advisability of chemotherapy or hormonal therapy. These possibilities should be considered prior to preventive mastectomy and an agreement reached as to how to proceed should breast cancer be found. When cancer is discovered during the prophylactic mastectomy, the axillary lymph nodes can be removed in the same procedure. If a breast cancer is found later by the pathologist during his evaluation of the mastectomy specimen, a secondary axillary lymph node removal may be advised. If the breast cancer is found near a preserved nipple-areola, it can be removed during a subsequent operation.

It is not possible to totally remove all of a woman's breast tissue during a prophylactic mastectomy; therefore some risk still remains. Estimates put this risk at no more than 0.5% or less. (Approximately the same risk that men have for developing breast cancer.) The woman who has had a prophylactic mastectomy should, therefore, continue to be vigilant about monitoring her reconstructed breast; if any changes are noted, they should be reported to her surgeon.

## HOW WILL MY BREAST LOOK AFTER A PROPHYLACTIC MASTECTOMY AND RECONSTRUCTION?

Breasts reconstructed with insertion of a breast implant under the muscle after prophylactic mastectomy are usually not as soft, sensitive, or mobile as natural breasts. Scars from the operation will be visible, and the recreated breasts often will not exhibit the flow and mobility of natural breasts. They are also usually flatter and do not have normal conical projection in the area under the areola since the tissue in this area has been removed. This flat appearance often improves during the first few weeks after the operation.

When prophylactic mastectomy is followed by breast reconstruction with the patient's own tissues, the appearance and feel of her breasts are more natural, but she must also endure a more involved flap procedure that usually takes tissue from the lower abdominal wall and leaves a long abdominoplasty scar in addition to the breast scars. Breasts reconstructed with autologous tissue often have greater sensation than those reconstructed with implants (which usually feel numb). Up to 70% of these autologous breast reconstructions demonstrate some sensation after a year's time. The unique sensitivity associated with the nipple-areola is not restored with any of the currently used methods of breast reconstruction, which is a major drawback of the procedure for many women.

Despite the obvious limitations of prophylactic mastectomy and reconstruction, women having this procedure usually are satisfied with their decision to have the operation because their main purpose has been accomplished: they have alleviated their overriding concern about their high-risk status by removing most of the breast tissue at risk.

The woman considering prophylactic mastectomy must be aware that even though only one operation is planned, additional procedures may be needed to correct asymmetry, treat a complication from the initial procedure, or to improve breast appearance if it does not meet the patient's expectations as to size or shape.

## Results

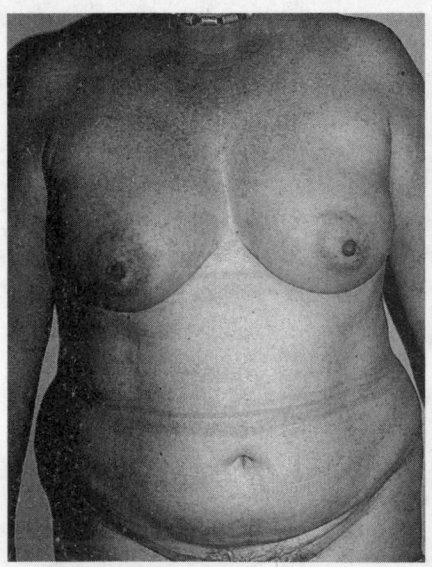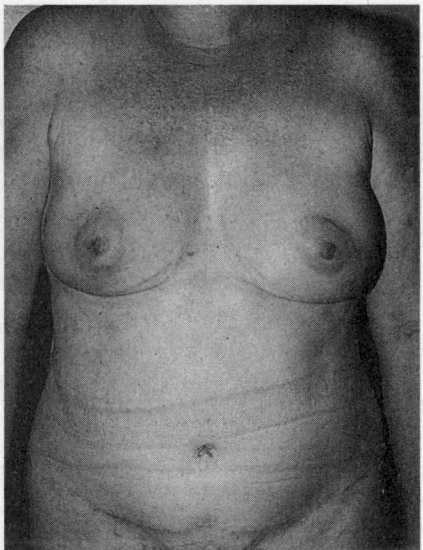

This 46-year-old woman had significant risk factors for breast cancer (her mother and two sisters had developed breast cancer before age 45). She decided to have prophylactic skin- and nipple-sparing bilateral mastectomies with immediate breast reconstruction using TRAM flaps. She is shown 3 years after breast reconstruction. Her anxiety concerning breast cancer is reduced and she is pleased with the improved abdominal wall contour.

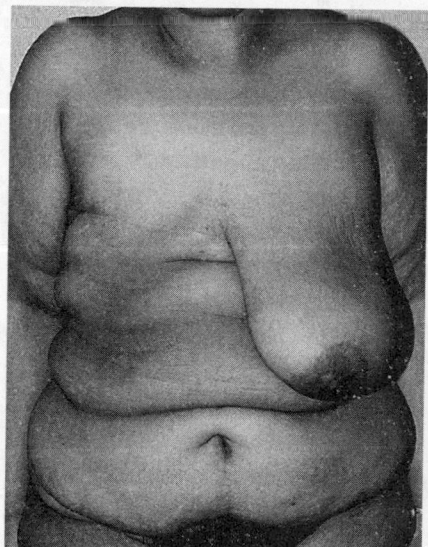 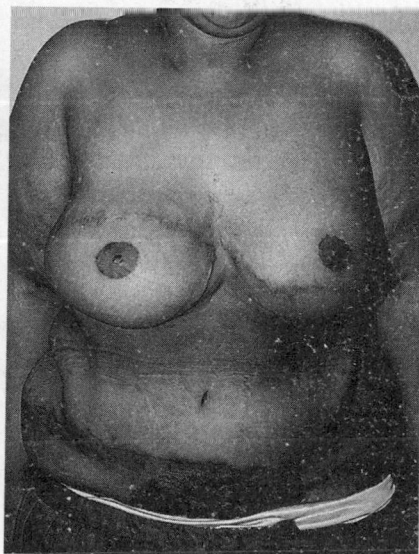

This 34-year-old woman had a right modified radical mastectomy and delayed breast reconstruction. Her opposite breast was heavy. Because of her increased risk factors she requested a prophylactic mastectomy. She had a left total mastectomy and immediate breast reconstruction with bilateral TRAM flaps. She is shown 2 years after breast reconstruction. Her anxiety about breast cancer has diminished and she is satisfied with the improved symmetry and abdominal wall contour.

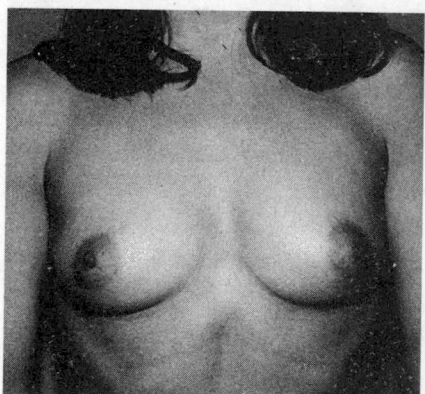 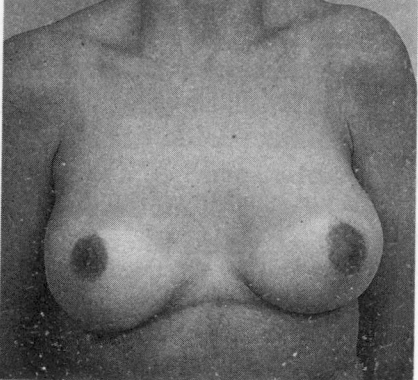

This 32-year-old woman had several significant risk factors for breast cancer. She decided to have bilateral total mastectomies with skin- and nipple-sparing mastectomies and immediate breast reconstruction. She did not want additional scars and elected to have breast implants. She is shown 8 years after breast reconstruction.

## Results—cont'd

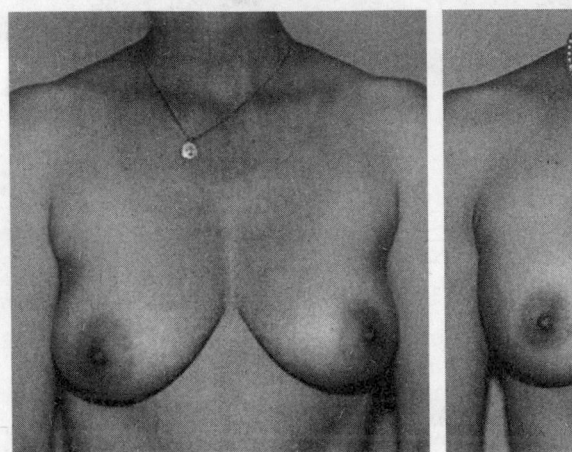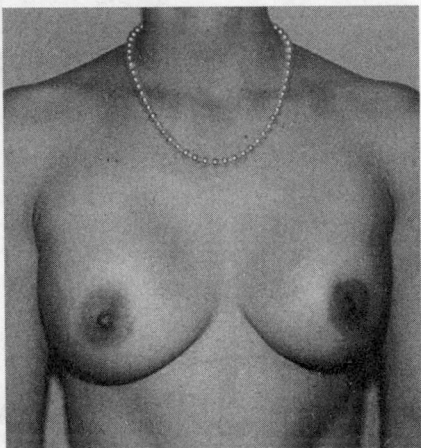

This 34-year-old woman lived in constant fear of breast cancer because her mother and 38-year-old sister both had premenopausal breast cancer. She is shown 3 years after bilateral prophylactic mastectomies and immediate reconstruction with implants.

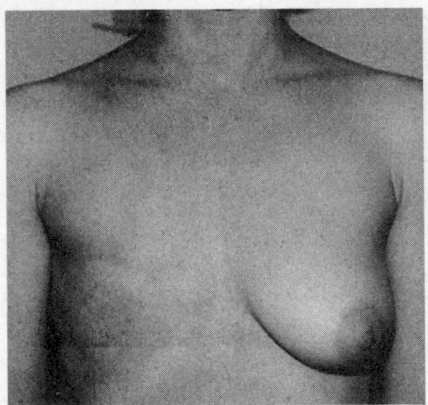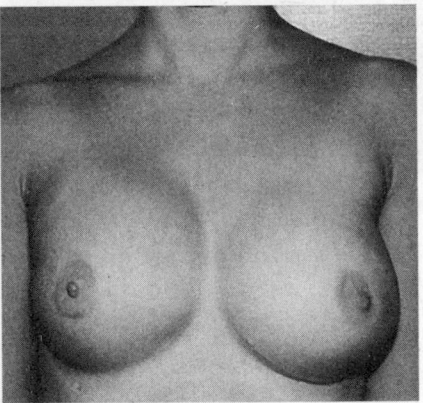

This 34-year-old woman with a family history of breast cancer had an earlier mastectomy. Terrified at the prospect of developing breast cancer in her other breast, she had a left prophylactic mastectomy with nipple-areola preservation and immediate reconstruction with tissue expansion. Her right breast was also reconstructed at the same time and her right nipple-areola was rebuilt several months later. The result is shown 1 year following breast reconstruction.

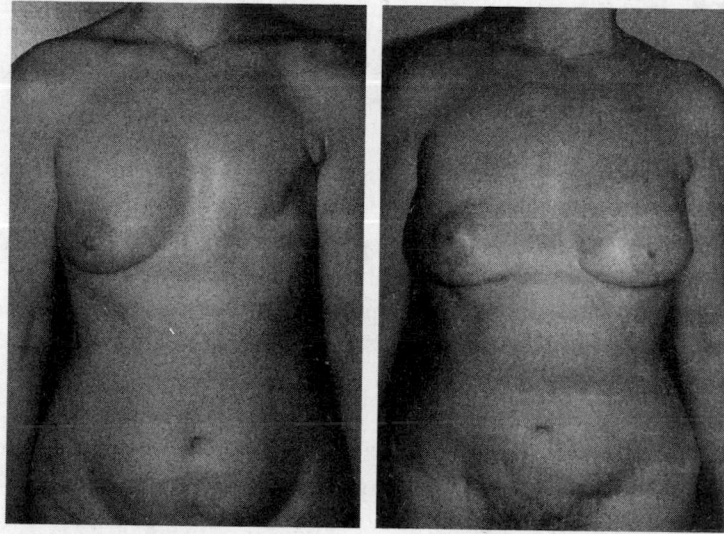

This 34-year-old woman with a strong family history of breast cancer had a modified radical mastectomy several years earlier. She later had a left prophylactic mastectomy and bilateral TRAM flap reconstruction. She is shown 3 years after breast reconstruction.

## PROS AND CONS OF PREVENTIVE MASTECTOMY AND RECONSTRUCTION

Although recent advances in technique have made a prophylactic mastectomy and reconstruction more aesthetically predictable, serious complications can still occur. To help a woman make a more informed objective decision she needs to question her surgeon about the positive and negative aspects of this procedure.

### Pros

- Decreases the fear of breast cancer by removing most of the breast tissue.
- Decreases the risk of breast cancer. The effectiveness of this preventive surgery remains a source of controversy. There is no definitive evidence to prove that a prophylactic mastectomy reduces a woman's risk of getting cancer, even though any tumors occurring in the thin layer of breast tissue remaining after this procedure are

usually easier to detect while they are quite small. Available reports do indicate, however, that the incidence of subsequent breast cancer is very low (less than 1%) after prophylactic mastectomy in women initially determined to be at high risk of developing breast cancer.

- Reduces painful symptoms caused by fibrocystic breast changes; however, breast pain alone should not be the primary indication for the operation. There are many other reasons for breast pain, and these are not improved by prophylactic mastectomy. In fact, some additional pain is always a possibility whenever a breast operation or any operation is performed.

## Cons

- Subject to operative risks associated with any major surgical procedure, including those from general anesthesia as well as complications of bleeding, infection, skin loss, nipple loss, capsular contracture, and implant loss. Additional abdominal complications can occur if a TRAM flap is used for breast reconstruction. Correction of these problems often requires additional operations.
- Frequently does not produce a reconstructed breast that is as attractive as the original breast. Permanent scars and a lack of normal breast flow and projection can be expected. Additional operations may be needed to improve the appearance of the breasts after prophylactic mastectomy and immediate breast reconstruction.
- Results in decreased sensation or loss of sensation in the reconstructed breast, especially the nipple-areola, because of the division of the sensory nerves when the breast is removed. Even though breast sensation does not return, the woman's breasts may feel uncomfortable, even painful.
- Often requires more than one procedure to achieve the best result or manage complications.
- Still leaves a small percentage of breast tissue as a potential site of breast cancer.

A woman's decision for a preventive mastectomy and reconstruction requires input from the general surgeon and other members of the breast management team. These specialists can advise her concerning her particular risks of developing breast cancer as well the normal, expected results of a prophylactic mastectomy for a woman with her type of breasts. She needs to be examined and counseled by at least two physicians who can evaluate her risk factors and their implications for her future health status. Prophylactic mastectomy is not an emergency procedure. If there is a suspicious breast mass or indication that breast cancer is present, this question should be resolved before a decision is made for prophylactic mastectomy. Most women at high risk are monitored most effectively by breast self-examination and regular physician examinations and mammograms. A woman should carefully consider all of her options and all aspects of her situation with the greatest of care before a final decision is made for preventive surgery.

# CREATING A NIPPLE-AREOLA

When a woman has her breast reconstructed, she also must decide whether she wants her nipple and areola (the circular pigmented area surrounding the nipple) reconstructed. Some women only desire to have their breast shape restored so that they feel balanced and symmetric. For them, the nipple-areola is of little consequence. To others, however, a nipple-areola is an important component of reconstructive surgery. This represents the finishing touch that makes their breasts look and feel more natural.

In interviews and surveys with women who had breast reconstruction we discovered an interesting correlation between the success of the initial procedure to build the breast and the woman's subsequent desire for a nipple. When the rebuilt breast does not meet her aesthetic desires, she usually does not want her nipple restored, no matter how simple the procedure, because it merely emphasizes a poor result. The attitude of these women is "enough is enough," and they are content to be able to fill out a bra. Women who have satisfactory aesthetic results frequently have the opposite reaction. They want a nipple-areola reconstruction as the final phase of their operation to create a more natural breast appearance and to provide a good match with their breasts. The fact that simpler techniques are now available makes the option of nipple-areola reconstruction even more appealing. The creation of the nipple-areola seems to complete a rehabilitation program for them. As one woman explained, "It becomes the icing on the cake; it is not absolutely necessary, but it is so beautiful when it's there."

Although reconstruction of the breast and nipple-areola is possible during one operation, the best results are obtained when the ideal breast shape is achieved first. Most plastic surgeons prefer to wait a few months after the first operation or after tissue expansion has been completed until the newly created breast is stable and symmetric with the remaining breast. Then the plastic surgeon and patient can more accurately determine the proper position, size, and projection of the nipple-areola. It is important for the woman to participate in this decision-making process. Once the nipple has been built, it is very difficult to change its position later without removing and regrafting it or starting over. She is going to have to live with it and it should look right to her. Unless additional corrections of the reconstructed breast are needed, the actual reconstruction often can be done on an outpatient basis under local anesthesia.

Significant advances have been made in nipple-areola reconstruction techniques during the past few years, and there are a number of techniques for women to choose from. It is now possible to rebuild a woman's nipple with the local tissue already present at the site of the new nipple-areola on her reconstructed breast. The color of the nipple-areola is then defined a few months later with a tattoo. Alternatively, when the skin on the reconstructed breast is thin and the opposite nipple is large, another option is to use a nipple-sharing technique in which a portion of the large opposite nipple is used for the nipple reconstruction. The areola can be created with excess skin at the lateral portion of the mastectomy scar, or if the patient had a TRAM flap breast reconstruction, it can be grafted from excess tissue at the end of the abdominal scar. The circular area of the areola can also be simulated with a tattoo of the approximate color and size to match the opposite areola without the need for taking a skin graft to form the areola.

Most women choose to have their nipples reconstructed from the local tissue on the breast and then have their nipple and areola tattooed later. These new techniques are often more appealing than previous approaches that created the nipple and areola from two different types of tissue transferred from other areas of a woman's body. These older methods are still used for some patients when appropriate, and they continue to give excellent results. The newer methods, however, are simpler, frequently less painful, and are often preferred because they seem to fit in more readily with most women's active lifestyles.

## NIPPLE RECONSTRUCTION

When a woman chooses to have her nipple reconstructed, she does so to complete her reconstruction, to enhance the appearance of her reconstructed breast, and to make it more symmetric with her remaining breast. Projection seems to be a key issue with many women who elect to have their nipples reconstructed; they want the freedom to wear T-shirts and swimsuits without being self-consciousness that one nipple is more prominent than the other. A woman should not decide to create a nipple for sensation or for milk production potential; these functions are impossible for the reconstructed breast.

Presently several primary methods of nipple reconstruction use local tissue at the site of the future nipple-areola to build the new nipple—the "C-V" flap (thus named because the design of the flap resembles two V's connected by a C), the skate flap, and variants of local flaps that are spiraled or turned to give a projecting nipple. With these techniques, a layer of skin and fat on the reconstructed breast is shifted to the center of the future nipple-areola area and formed into a nipple. The skin is used to create the nipple and the underlying fat contributes bulk, fullness, and permanent shape. The skate flap uses much of the skin at the site of the future areola for the nipple reconstruction;

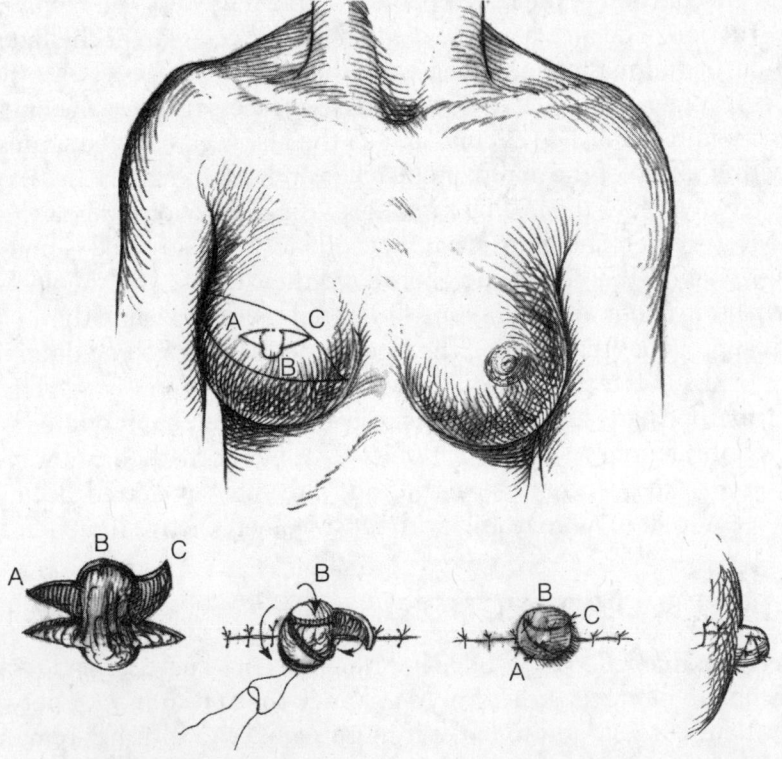

The C-V flap using tissue of reconstructed breast to create a nipple, which a few months later will be tattooed along with surrounding areola

the areola is then reconstructed from a graft of skin taken from another site such as the outer portion of the mastectomy scar. With the C-V flap, not as much local tissue is used and consequently it may not produce as large and projecting a nipple as the skate flap. However, the donor site for the C-V flap can be closed with two short scars; therefore an areola graft is not always necessary with the C-V flap operation. A tattoo can be done later for nipple color and areola reconstruction.

Although a nice-sized nipple can be created from breast skin, often its color is not dark enough to match the remaining nipple. In this case a tattoo provides a better color match. (See later discussion on tattooing.)

The opposite nipple can also be used for nipple reconstruction when there is not enough local tissue to build a symmetric nipple; however, this is not a popular choice today. It is often not acceptable to either the patient or her husband or significant other, and other sources of tissue for nipple reconstruction are selected. However, when the remaining nipple is very large and projecting or when the skin over the implant reconstruction is thin and tight and there is not enough extra tissue for a satisfactory nipple reconstruction, this method is still the best way to create a nipple that is symmetric in size, color, and texture. With this technique, a portion of the lower end of the remaining nipple is used for the nipple reconstruction. The donor area of the normal nipple is not significantly changed or scarred; it usually heals in 1 to 2 weeks without any numbness and little pain. After the nipple has healed, it does not lose its sensitivity or feeling.

## AREOLA RECONSTRUCTION

Methods for recreating the areola range from simple tattooing to the more complex graft techniques. The decision as to which technique is appropriate depends on a patient's lifestyle and preferences, although today most women seem to prefer tattooing the areola as the easiest and least time-consuming approach.

Some women do not care if the color is exact; they want the simplest, safest, and least painful method for creating a semblance of an areola. Tattooing, which may not always produce a realistic result, may be the solution that these woman desire. Although the texture and projection of the natural areola will be lacking, the color match of a tattooed areola can be quite good and an areola graft is not needed. Many women appreciate the convenience of this approach.

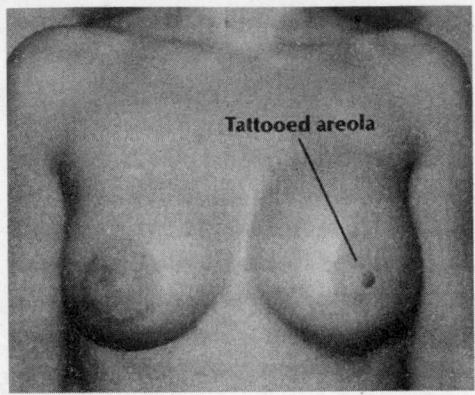

Tattooed areola

Tattoo without areola grafting was satisfactory for this woman who preferred a simple, nonsurgical procedure that produced the semblance of an areola.

When local breast skin is used for the nipple reconstruction, the tissue for the areola graft can be taken from the lateral portion of the mastectomy scar or the lateral portion of the abdominal scar if the woman had a TRAM flap. (With new skin-sparing mastectomies, the residual scars are now shorter and there is less available scar tissue for areola reconstruction.) When sufficient tissue is available, this technique is very acceptable to most women and it avoids additional scars; it is also effectively used in combination with the skate flap. The mastectomy scar and the excess skin at the lateral end of the scar can often be improved when the areolar graft is removed. Since this area is usually numb from the mastectomy, little pain is experienced when taking the graft or afterward. The main drawback is that the skin graft is not pigmented, and although it will appear pink during the initial weeks to months after grafting, it usually fades and a tattoo may be necessary to obtain a better color match.

A graft of tissue from the upper inner thigh crease is another means of reconstructing the areola, but this technique involves a painful donor site and has become unpopular with the advent of the newer, less painful techniques just described. Although this method is not preferred by most patients, it still produces excellent results and is still used for some patients. The tissue obtained from this area is pigmented and usually provides a good match with the opposite areola without the need for an areola tattoo. A round areola skin graft is removed from the upper thigh crease, and the remaining thigh skin is brought together as a thin scar line in this crease; this scar is practically invisible when healed and does not show, even in a bathing suit. The groin area is usually painful after this procedure and will feel tender for about 2 weeks.

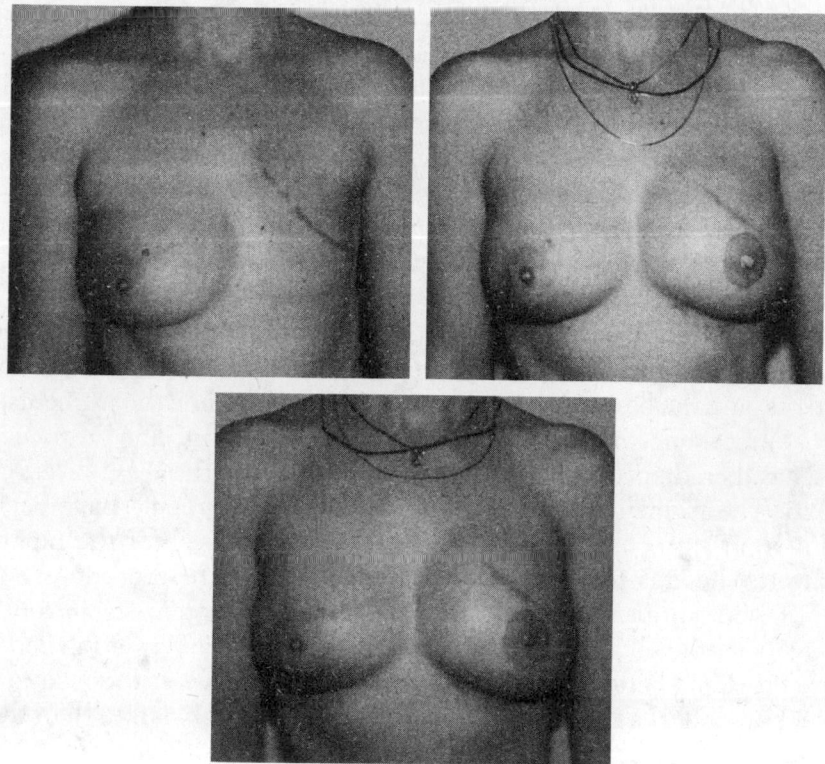

This 33-year-old patient had nipple-areola reconstruction with local skin used for nipple reconstruction and an areola graft taken from the lateral end of the mastectomy scar. Her nipple-areola was tattooed 2 months later. She is shown 1 year later.

Once the areolar graft has been obtained, the actual placement of the new areola onto the breast area can be accomplished. If the upper inner thigh graft has been used, a very thin circular layer of surface skin needs to be removed first to make room for this new areola. (In the skate or C-V flap operation this skin layer has already been removed to build the nipple.) The areola skin graft is then positioned on this area.

## NIPPLE-AREOLA TATTOO

Many times the color of a nipple and areola created from breast skin is not dark enough to match the remaining nipple-areola. In this case a tattoo provides a better color match. A tattoo is the most direct and permanent method for pigmenting the reconstructed nipple-areola. It is also effective, as discussed earlier, in creating the appearance of an areola for the woman who does not want to have another surgical procedure or for a woman whose opposite areola is so large that it is not practical to reconstruct a matching areola using a skin graft. Tattooing is used to create a pigmented circle to match the other areola without resorting to a large skin graft.

Many plastic surgeons who do breast reconstruction can perform the tattoo in their office as an outpatient procedure or can arrange to have the tattoo done by a qualified professional. The procedure is quite easy. The patient participates in determining the proper color for the new nipple-areola. The natural nipple-areola has a wide spectrum of colors, and the best color match is achieved by blending the pigments.

A local anesthetic is often used prior to tattooing. The tattoo device is then dipped in the pigment and placed into the outer layers of skin. The pigment is applied until the areola and nipple have been uniformly tattooed. Slightly darker pigments are used for the nipple tattoo. The area is a little raw for a few days after the procedure. An antibiotic ointment is used to keep it moist. If a woman's skin tones have a lot of yellow, the match may not be as close. Newer pigments are providing better matches for these individuals. Over the next few weeks to months the tattooed nipple-areola may look darker than the color selected; however, with time it fades, usually to an acceptable color. The woman should be warned that initially, because of the healing process, the tattooed nipple-areola will appear much darker than the natural one so that she will not be unnecessarily alarmed. Even so, some women are disturbed by the early disparity in color and are anxious for the color to fade so that it matches the remaining nipple-areola and does not stand out "like a beacon."

To protect the nipple and areola after surgery a protective dressing is taped over the nipple and stabilized with surgical tapes. The reconstructed nipple-areola tends to be dry after surgery; the application of a moisturizing cream can improve this condition.

• • •

Although the creation of a nipple-areola is not an essential component of a breast reconstruction, it adds a realistic finishing touch. By creating a nipple-areola on a woman's new breast a surgeon can transform her surgically created mound into a natural and aesthetic breast form.

# BREAST CANCER AND ITS
# EFFECT ON RELATIONSHIPS

## WHAT WOMEN WANT: MALE SUPPORT

"It is always hard on the man. He stands there, outside, and he sees all of the problems down the road. He is both frightened to death and threatened. But the patient, somewhere along the way, comes to terms with herself because she has no choice."

These words express the feelings of one breast cancer patient as she reflected on the predicaments that this disease creates for men and women. Her statement typifies the type of answers that we received when we surveyed women about this topic. Drawing on the responses of over 800 women who had breast cancer, we have summarized their feelings and thoughts about the problems they encountered in their relationships as a result of this disease. Issues addressed include the response to diagnosis, recovery from cancer surgery, the response to lumpectomy, the reaction to mastectomy, issues of intimacy and sexual relationships, common fears of the breast cancer patient, the single woman's special concerns, and male support for breast reconstruction. Although there are no prescribed rules for a man to follow under these circumstances, many of the women we surveyed had suggestions about what had been most helpful for them. This chapter incorporates these suggestions. In addition to information gleaned from our questionnaire, we have also included a short section written by a general surgeon on the topic of the patient-surgeon relationship and three interviews, two with men and one with a couple.

### Facing the Diagnosis

The discovery of breast cancer provokes many fears in a couple and these fears need to be shared. Both are worried about the prognosis of cancer and its effect on their relationship. They worry about possible treatment options and the effects of chemotherapy, radiation treatment, or surgery. Their concerns may not surface immediately, however, since there seems to be a tendency for couples to hide true feelings behind a cheerful, "make the best of it" facade. These true feelings can be damaging to a relationship if they are not brought into the open and examined. All of the women we contacted believed in and stressed the need for open and honest communication. As one woman said, "I asked my husband if he could allow me to feel what I was feeling, and I would try to allow him his feelings. I didn't want pity. I just wanted him to listen when I talked because it was a release to say how I was feeling." This need for unfettered communication was also echoed by single women involved in dating or in committed relationships. As one woman explained, "Naturally when you are dating you are always trying to present yourself in the best light, and sometimes that means not allowing the other person to see all of your hidden flaws. That's why you still wear makeup to bed. But cancer changes that dynamic forever. It gets down to bare essentials. If there is to be any hope for a long-term relationship, subterfuge must go out the window. It is a time for sharing and for honesty. Ultimately that is the test of a relationship. If a man runs at this point, he probably wasn't worth the investment of time and love in the first place."

Women also stressed the importance of physical closeness and contact accompanying this communication process. The value of hugging and holding was mentioned in virtually all of our surveys and interviews. One woman expressed this feeling most poignantly when she said, "Sometimes when the words wouldn't come, my boyfriend would just hold me, hug me, stroke me, and I would cry. That was real communication. Even though he told me he loved me, and I loved hearing it, his touch revealed all I needed to know. The physical closeness made me feel loved and accepted. Hugging makes a big difference."

Women emphasized the ameliorative effects of talking about their problems with someone else. It was crucial to have someone close to share the burden. Sometimes they just needed someone to listen to them and to hold them without "trying to make things right." As one woman explained, "During the tears, the anger, the insecurity, the fear, the ups and the downs, there is really no need to give advice or try to cheer a woman up. A man just needs to allow her to have all of these feelings and be understanding, even if none of these feelings make sense. More than anything else a man needs to listen to a woman's feelings, her fears, her hopes without judging or trying to 'fix' things." Another woman wrote, "There is no way that anybody can really understand what you are feeling when you have cancer, unless that person has experienced it himself. What can you say to someone, 'I'm sorry?' Sometimes you just need a one-way conversation with somebody. Men can help us by just letting us get upset and release some of the tension."

The time between the diagnosis of breast cancer and the selection of treatment is a tense one for both a man and a woman. For a man, the fear of his loved one's death from cancer usually far overshadows her possible breast loss. Understandably, his priority is the woman's health and survival. It is important, however, for him to acknowledge her concerns and be careful not to minimize her attachment to her breasts. Together they need to define their priorities and investigate her therapy options.

The first priority is for the woman to get the best care for her tumor. She often feels confused and depressed by all that is happening to her. By accompanying her to medical consultations a man can actively demonstrate his concern and help a woman focus on the issues being discussed. Together they can learn about and critically evaluate the various treatment options. Most of the couples we interviewed had taken the time to inform themselves about breast cancer and about breast reconstruction. They had read articles and books on these topics, attended lectures, and even seen movies and slide presentations. They agreed that this process helped them cope and also gave them a better understanding of what the future held. Repeatedly, in both our surveys and in our discussions with men and women, couples stressed the beneficial value of this educational process. As one man related, "By learning about my girlfriend's cancer we at least were able to understand our choices and make some decisions based on knowledge instead of fear. I actually think it brought us closer together."

## The Patient-Surgeon Relationship
ROGER S. FOSTER, Jr., M.D.

It is normal for a woman diagnosed with breast cancer to react to her disease and to the surgeon responsible for her treatment with mixed emotions. Feelings of desperation, rage, and hopelessness may coexist with feelings of courage, hope, and determination. She may be angry with fate, God, or even herself. Some of her resentment will naturally focus on her surgeon. Frequently he is the messenger delivering the bad news about her cancer and her prognosis. Furthermore, his treatments inflict pain, create scars, and may deform her body, all good reasons for her to react negatively. In addition to these negative feelings, however, most women also experience positive feelings for their surgeons. Because a woman is dependent on her surgeon, having entrusted her life and body to him, she feels vulnerable and exposed. She needs to reassure herself that he is a skilled professional and that he is a particularly sensitive and caring individual, personally interested in her welfare. Her intense feelings about her cancer and its treatment may lead her to attribute laudatory qualities to her surgeon that are really more reflective of her emotional needs than of the actual character of the surgeon himself.

These conflicting emotions of resentment and admiration are difficult to deal with, particularly for an already stressed woman trying to cope with a life-threatening disease. Her strong feelings are not wrong, but it helps if both the woman, her loved ones, and her surgeon are able to recognize these feelings for what they are. Her anger and hostility should not be personalized by the surgeon and taken as an affront. Similarly, a woman should not feel guilty about experiencing these negative reactions. Perhaps the surgeon has been lacking in tact and diplomacy. Maybe his people skills need some polishing. Even so, a woman and her loved ones need to understand that her anger is not necessarily attributable to the surgeon's personality. Much of her rage is situational, a reaction to circumstances beyond her control. The positive feelings of affection and even adulation that she may develop for her surgeon should also be recognized as situational in nature and should not be misinterpreted by the woman experiencing them or the man who cares about her. The patient's affection or even "love" for her cancer surgeon or plastic surgeon is not the same as the love she may feel for a husband or significant other, where reciprocity of affection is expected. Even though a man may experience moments of jealousy or resentment because of his loved one's seeming transference of affection to her doctor, he should realize that with time and recovery this affection as well as the anger she feels toward her doctor will diminish and she will view her relationship with him from a more balanced perspective.

## Recovery From Lumpectomy

After a lumpectomy a woman's recovery is usually relatively quick and easy. Many times this procedure can be performed on an outpatient basis. She goes home, breast intact and cancer eliminated, without significant pain or the need for a prolonged recuperation and time away from work. This relatively seamless transition between cancer diagnosis, treatment, and return to normal daily activities may cause others to overlook the seriousness of her situation. Many of the lumpectomy patients who responded to our surveys made mention of their frustration at the seemingly dismissive attitudes they encountered, particularly from the men in their lives. As one woman so aptly explained, "I sometimes feel just like Rodney Dangerfield. 'I get no respect!' For god's sake, I have cancer. I still worry about my life and about the very real possibility of a recurrence. Yes, I have my breast, but that doesn't mean that I don't still worry about it. I don't have to be mutilated or look like I am dying for people to take me seriously. My boyfriend keeps saying, 'Isn't it great that you are all okay now and it's over.' He treats me as if I am recovering from a cold. Well, it isn't okay and it isn't over. Yes, I kept my breast, but the trauma of my cancer diagnosis haunts me every day."

Most of the lumpectomy patients we interviewed stressed the need for a man to be sensitive to the complex emotions that a woman must deal with after lumpectomy. Although her physical appearance may seem virtually unchanged, it masks an inner turmoil. Whether a woman has had a mastectomy or a lumpectomy she still has faced the grim reality of breast cancer. The seriousness of her surgery or of her cancer must not be minimized. Her full recovery requires the same grieving process confronted by any patient dealing with a life-threatening disease. Breast cancer will live in her mind, if not in her breast, long after the tumor is removed and the scar has faded. As one woman so poignantly explained, "People think I shouldn't be upset about having cancer because I *only* had a lumpectomy." Another woman complained, "My boyfriend keeps telling me to 'Cheer up. You only had a lumpectomy; you are really lucky.' Well, I don't feel cheerful; I need some time to cope with this, to feel sad, to cry. Men sometimes look at lumpectomy as an excuse to avoid emotionally confronting the cancer issue." It is clear from our surveys and interviews that women who choose lumpectomy desire and need the same emotional support and understanding that is afforded to women who have mastectomies.

## Recovery From Mastectomy

After a mastectomy a woman commonly experiences a period of "peak" stress as she attempts to recover from the physical and psychological effects of this operation. Her physical recuperation usually takes 2 to 3 months but may be prolonged if chemotherapy or radiation therapy is necessary. At this time she may be weak, tired, irritable, and possibly ill from the treatments. Lifting a vacuum cleaner or carrying groceries might be too much strain for her, and she may need someone to assume some of her physical responsibilities until she feels better. (Women who have had lumpectomies and are undergoing radiation therapy may experience similar stress and fatigue. They also appreciate help with the daily household responsibilities.) A man's attitude when helping is crucial. Women stressed the importance of a man offering assistance willingly and not begrudgingly so that the woman does not "feel needy or as if she is nagging him to help her." Many women said that their arms felt sore and stiff for the first few weeks after surgery, and they appreciated having someone accompany them on trips to the doctor so that they did not have to worry about driving the car and possibly straining themselves. It also was helpful when a man could assist with some of the organizational and parenting responsibilities of the household, seeing to the children's appointments and schedules, attending recitals and athletic events, paying bills, arranging for repairmen, and filling in when necessary. As one woman explained, "My man was there when I needed him most, yet we were thousands of miles apart physically during portions of my treatment. He cared for our children, and his phone calls were sufficient to help me through." By doing the heavy cleaning, driving the carpools, or doing the grocery shopping a man can provide very positive support for a woman during her recovery.

There is a delicate balance between willingly assisting a woman until her strength returns and actually doing everything for her. Most women we surveyed appreciated the physical assistance men provided during their initial recuperation, but they were quick to resist any attempts to take over. Even though some of the men that we interviewed felt that they could best help their wives by relieving them of all worries and responsibilities, their wives did not agree. Most women were uncomfortable with this treatment. "Don't put us on pedestals. Help us, if we need help, but don't cure one thing and start something else. We do not want to be treated as invalids." Getting back into the mainstream of life seemed to be the focus for most of the women we surveyed. They actively feared being left out of life. They wanted to feel useful and to participate as they always had. They did not want people to "whisper and tiptoe around them."

## Reactions to a Woman's Changed Physical Appearance After Mastectomy

A man's response to her changed physical appearance worries the woman who has had a mastectomy. Above all, she fears his expressing shock at her missing breast. Many women worry that they will appear less feminine and lovable. Fearing rejection, they desire physical attention, love, and continued reassurance of their desirability. As one woman explained, "No woman is less feminine or intelligent or attractive because she has had a mastectomy, but sometimes it helps to be reminded."

The problem of how to react to a woman's altered appearance is not an easy one. In some cases the woman cannot adjust to her missing breast and does not want the man to see her. Some of the women we surveyed are "still dressing in the closet so no one sees them." Some have never shown their scars to their husbands or boyfriends for fear they will be disgusted at what they see. Some even avoid intimate relationships and possible exposure of their scarred chests. In other cases the woman is willing to show her missing breast to her loved one and allow him to help her change bandages, rub ointment on her scar, or reassure her that she still looks okay. Many of the women responding to us suggested that problems could be avoided if the scar were seen as soon as possible after surgery. One woman wrote that many of her worries had been eliminated because she and her boyfriend had viewed the scar together in the hospital in the presence of her doctor. They shared the shock together, recovered from it, and went on to concentrate on other matters.

## Impact on Relationships

Although many of the women we contacted felt that men were usually supportive of women cancer patients, not all of the stories we heard were positive. Some relationships ended. Boyfriends left and divorces occurred after mastectomy, after breast reconstruction, and even after lumpectomy. Some men could not adjust to their wife or significant other's status as a cancer victim or to her changed physical appearance. They "could not handle the tumor" or stand to "look at her lopsided chest with a breast on one side and a red scar on the other." Others could not cope with the added responsibility of worrying about a life-threatening illness. Some men found that the woman in their lives had changed and now had difficulty relating to her. They tired of "hearing about her cancer" and found her so inwardly directed after this experience that they did not feel that she could talk about anything else.

The missing breast itself, however, did not seem to be the actual cause of divorce or breakup after a mastectomy. Sometimes it inhibited a woman sexually or made a man more timid in his sexual approaches, but these inhibitions were often overcome with time. Interestingly, both men and women seemed to agree that divorces or breakups after a mastectomy or a lumpectomy were usually the culmination of a history of problems that had previously existed between a couple. These men were temporarily supportive through surgery and recovery, but when the fear of death had subsided and life returned to its status quo, the old unhappiness was evident again and often the relationship ended. In most cases, where there was good communication, common interests, and a deep abiding affection, the cancer diagnosis only served to strengthen the ties between the individuals. Relationships that were strong before the surgery became even stronger afterward.

## Intimacy and Sexual Relationships

Romance and intimacy is another sensitive area for women after mastectomy and even after breast reconstruction and lumpectomy. Worried about how their identity as breast cancer survivors or their changed appearance will affect their sexual relationship with a man, these women, no matter how close to their husbands or boyfriends, express fears of rejection. Men also have concerns; they worry about making the wrong moves, saying the wrong things, or pushing a woman before she is ready. Most of the women we surveyed desired a return to normal sexual relations as soon as possible. Keeping an element of romance in a relationship was very important to all of the women and men we interviewed. It helped them infuse a feeling of normality into their relationship. As one woman candidly explained, "Even though I was missing a breast, I still wanted to be treated as a sexy and romantic woman. I wanted to be flirted with. I wanted him to do romantic things to help me to feel loving and sensual. I wanted my man to touch my body, to tenderly caress me, and to look at me in such a way that I knew it didn't make any difference to him. As a woman I needed to know that I was still sexually attractive."

Many of the women we spoke to also agreed that women will differ in their readiness for intimacy and a man should "take the lead from the woman and try to encourage but not to rush sex." That cautionary note also applies to the woman who has had breast reconstruction. As one woman advised, "I think that men should not expect sex too quickly after a woman has had reconstruction. Women need some time to recuperate both mentally and physically. They still feel protective of their bodies. I know that I still protect my body and breasts during intercourse." Obviously this is a problematic situation; a man straddles a line between expressing his affection too forcefully or remaining aloof and standoffish. Each couple needs to work out their own individual method of relating and dealing with questions of intimacy; they need to talk about these problems and understand them.

The value of foreplay and afterplay was frequently reinforced by women as they divulged their personal desires in lovemaking. Many felt that a man should initially be more gentle and stroking, and this caring should continue. "He should not pull away physically after orgasm but should tenderly embrace her and tell her he loves her." A man should not be afraid to touch the woman as he did before. Stroking during lovemaking and after was judged vitally important for a woman's self-esteem both before and after cancer surgery and reconstruction. "My significant other was and is fantastic. He didn't care if I had reconstruction or not. In fact, my new breast is caressed as lovingly as the old one." One woman suggested the need for a man "to learn new sexual techniques to help a woman achieve arousal." As she explained, "With the loss of a breast and even after reconstruction, a major hot spot is irrevocably gone and all of the sexual sensitivity that accompanies it. Breasts are a 'turn on.' You lose that after a mastectomy and reconstruction does not fully restore it. You can't get that special sexual sensitivity back; there is a numbness now where you used to feel titillation. You need a good relationship with your sexual partner to compensate for this loss. And sometimes you need to be creative."

## A Woman's Fears

Understandably, the mastectomy patient has many questions and fears to cope with. Knowing about her doubts sometimes helps a man to be more sensitive to them. One woman poignantly summarized these worries when she sent us a series of questions that she felt needed to be answered:

- How can I face my husband or male friend?
- Will sex ever be the same?
- Will I be afraid for him to touch me?
- How will I feel about myself?

- Will I be the same person?
- Will I have the same outlook on life?
- Will my sex life be affected?
- Knowing that my man fell in love with my body as well as me, how will he feel about my body now?
- After I get a prosthesis, will people look at me and wonder which breast was cut off?
- Will people pity me, feel sorry for me?
- If I seek reconstruction, will people think I am vain and self-centered?

## Concerns of the Single Woman

For the single woman involved in dating, her breast cancer status represents a daunting obstacle to a relationship. Many of the single and divorced women we surveyed were frankly perplexed and somewhat distressed over what to tell a man in this circumstance. This confusion reigned regardless of the type of treatment that a woman had.

However, for the mastectomy patient, her missing breast presented special problems, particularly in deciding how to inform a suitor when a more intimate relationship was desired. As one woman revealed, "The worst part of having a mastectomy is that you just don't feel feminine. My male friend didn't make me feel that way; those feelings were self-inflicted. The first time we made love I didn't want to expose myself and I was terribly self-conscious. He just said, 'It doesn't matter to me,' but I said, 'It matters to me.' I always wore a nightgown. I just couldn't do it without it." Many of the single women we spoke to said that they were self-conscious about having a man see them totally undressed or in full light. One woman explained how she "always had a nightgown on and the room was always darkened." Some women, although not as many, even expressed feelings of embarrassment after reconstruction because of their scars, the telltale signs that they had surgery. As one young girl revealed, "For a long time I wore a shirt to bed or I took it off in the dark, but he was patient with me until I reached a point where I didn't feel self-conscious." Learning to relate intimately is not always easy for a couple under the best of circumstances; after a mastectomy, with or without reconstruction, it is particularly challenging.

Most women agreed that a straightforward approach was probably the best. Numerous scenarios were described in which the woman sat the man down and explained about her cancer diagnosis and treatment or her changed physical appearance and what it meant. Generally, men accept this news far better than women anticipate, sometimes even better than the women themselves. This is as true of mastectomy as it is of lumpectomy.

This is a very emotional time for a woman, and in many ways she feels that her femininity and her self-esteem are on the line. Patience and understanding are required of a man, and she in turn must be willing to communicate her feelings and fears to her partner in order to reach a level of comfort and fulfillment.

Fear of rejection was cited by all of the women we surveyed as a reason for not telling. As one woman explained, "The dating scene today is difficult enough without adding breast cancer into the equation. Men are just frightened of commitment. If a man learns that a woman had breast cancer, he may not want to take on the added burden of a possible recurrence or future illness. Not everyone is brave or caring. So I worry about telling someone early on because I don't want him to be scared away before he has a chance to really get to know me and to develop an attachment. On the other hand, if I wait too long, he will think that I am dishonest and may leave anyway. So I just haven't told anyone, and I have been very tentative in forming new relationships until I really decide what to do." The uncertainty described by this woman was typical of a number of the woman we spoke to. There was no one solution for handling this problem. Women were as puzzled over when to tell a man as over how to tell him. Ultimately, much depended on their intuitive sense of the man and their desire to have this relationship grow into something more meaningful. Many of the single women we spoke to chose to avoid disclosure intially, unless they had some special interest in the man. At that point, however, they felt that an honest, heart-to-heart explanation was called for. For the mastectomy or breast reconstruction patient, that disclosure might also involve baring her breasts, although most women felt that verbal communication should always procede any "show and tell." Then, as one woman explained, "I just sit back and see what kind of man I am dealing with." Not all of the responses were what these women had been hoping for, but as she explained, "I want to know upfront rather than invest a lot of myself in a relationship that is going nowhere. I don't want a jerk in my life. I value myself too much for that."

## Support for Breast Reconstruction

When a woman decides that she wants to have her breast reconstructed, she often looks to a man for encouragement. Frequently, in our surveys, women explained that despite their strong personal motivation for reconstruction, they still needed a man's emotional support. They wanted to be reassured that reconstruction was okay and that they were not being vain or selfish because they desired more surgery to restore their missing breasts. If a woman seeks breast reconstruction, a man's support helps to enhance this experience and contributes to her rehabilitation.

Some men will resist the idea of breast reconstruction, hoping to shield their loved ones from additional pain, operative risk, and hospitalization. Judging from our questionnaires, we found this initial negative male reaction to be very common. Most of these men felt that the woman had suffered enough and they wanted to get on with life. Most of the women we surveyed understood these male concerns but felt that if a woman's commitment for reconstruction were strong, a man should respect her desires and encourage her.* Unlike the mastectomy, breast reconstruction was regarded as positive surgery meant to restore what the mastectomy removed. As one woman explained, "It is important for a man to support a woman's decision about breast reconstruction because it is her body, her feelings, her life. He should avoid making decisions for her. She needs to feel that she is in control."

A woman may not be as pleased with her new breast immediately after breast reconstruction as she had anticipated. It will not fully resemble the original breast and will bear a scar and feel numb to the touch. At this stage of her recovery she is extremely sensitive and vulnerable to criticism. She does not want to hear that her new breast is not as nice as her normal breast; she cannot tolerate negative comments or criticism of her appearance.

• • •

The man's role in dealing with a woman's breast cancer experience is a difficult one. It requires sensitivity and understanding of the special needs that a woman has as she confronts a life-threatening disease and the physical and mental adjustments that accompany treatment and rehabilitation. There is no way that he can ever really understand the full impact that breast cancer has on a woman's life. Yet his support and empathy are essential to help her cope and heal from this experience. Playing the role of supporting player is the best position he

---

*Most plastic surgeons are pleased to see a man accompany a woman for a consultation about breast reconstruction. His presence usually indicates that she is not alone in her decision and has someone to support her.

can take. He needs to listen to a woman's concerns, communicate with her, and try to understand her desires. His attitude and assistance can have a beneficial effect and can contribute to a woman's return to good feelings about herself, about him, and about the future.

## THE MAN'S ROLE: TWO PERSPECTIVES

The following two interviews further investigate the man's role in the breast cancer experience. Dean Sterling and George Johnson tell their stories and offer suggestions for other men confronting similar situations.

### Dean Sterling

Beth Ann* and I have a special relationship and a long involvement with each other. When she was diagnosed with breast cancer in 1992, we had been together as friends since 1966, as lovers and companions since 1972, and as a married couple since 1980. We were friends long before we were lovers. We have always tuned in to one another. Consequently, breast cancer proved an intense bonding experience for us. It was almost as if I had been diagnosed along with my wife; that's how close we are.

My wife's cancer was discovered during a routine physical. It came as a total shock. She takes good care of herself. I am proud of that. She has never smoked and is an extremely light drinker. She has been that way her whole life, sort of wimpy when it came to the college drinking scene but a great designated driver. She has never done drugs and has always exercised and eaten well. She looks as great now as she did 25 to 30 years ago. We were not expecting any difficulty with breast cancer because there was no family history. During her routine physical, her doctor noticed that the consistency of her left breast was different from that of her right breast so he sent her for a mammogram. The mammogram revealed a tumor and calcifications. He wanted to do a lumpectomy before Christmas to get a definitive diagnosis.

I was working at home the day she got the news. Whenever she comes home she sings out "hello" right away; it is a joy to hear her voice. I heard the door open, but she didn't say anything. All I could hear were the cats meowing. I went, "Hmm that's odd." When she came back to where I was, she stood looking at me from the hallway. I

*Beth Ann's interview is included in Chapter 18.

said, " How are you doing?" And she goes, "I am not so sure. I went to the doctor and he found something in my breast. They took a mammogram and it was highly suspicious for carcinoma." Then she started crying. That's when I knew that this had really shaken her. She is always upbeat, never dwelling on the negatives. I don't think the full impact really hit her until that moment. We both read the report and understood its seriousness. She cried for several hours. Then she looked at me and said, "Well, there is nothing we can do about it, so let's deal with it." She actually baked cookies that night to keep busy. She doesn't let herself get too down.

I was a wreck, but in her presence I kept a close rein on my emotions to show her that she could depend on me. I also felt that we couldn't afford to lose control now; our energies had to be totally focused on what we would do. We needed to consider all the possible scenarios. That night we started to work up game plans on a big paper tablet. We did decision trees—positive, negative, surgery, no surgery—to eliminate as many unknowns as possible. I also tried to be more attentive to her and more romantic. We went out for supper afterward and then went shopping; she bought a dress. Over the next few weeks I spent a lot more time with her. Behind the scenes when I was alone, I would get misty-eyed or cry because I knew what was coming up. But when we were together, I was strong and sympathetic so that she felt she could let me absorb some of her pain. I tried to support her by maintaining a confident, upbeat, let's-go-get-em attitude and that worked well for her.

They did the diagnostic lumpectomy right before Christmas. The pathology report indicated ductal carcinoma in situ. This diagnosis inspired an in-depth research effort on our part to find out as much as we could about this cancer and the treatment options available. We were able to tap into a wealth of breast cancer resources and the extensive cancer community that is out there. We were never aware of this network before because breast cancer had not touched us personally. All of a sudden there were magazine and newspaper articles popping up everywhere. The mere mention of the topic in casual conversation would elicit a knowing response as well as a story about a mother, sister, or friend who had it. My medical background as a med tech and a physician's assistant came in handy. I was familiar with medicine and brought some of that knowledge along with my computer expertise to bear on our investigation.

We quickly discovered that a vast array of quality information is available through many different sources. The local library provided articles from popular periodicals such as *Woman's Home Journal, Reader's Digest,* and *Cosmopolitan,* whereas research libraries at local universities or medical schools contained medical books and journal articles on the disease, its prognosis, and more technical information on new drugs, therapies, and operations. The computer terminals in the libraries were really helpful and should not be overlooked. They provided us with access to newspaper articles and other reference materials that were in the library itself or on the Internet. Local bookstores also yielded a wealth of consumer health books, self-help books, and alternative medicine titles.

On the Internet we found a wide range of articles and resources from popular consumer to highly technical scientific articles. It lists cancer societies, cancer organizations, medical schools, books, and articles. It also has testimonials, chat rooms, and Websites with feedback from women who have experienced breast cancer, research findings, information on clinical studies, support groups, you name it. So if someone has the skill and the access (or knows someone who can help), the best place to start is the Internet.

The Internet has search engines to help you locate the information that you are seeking. You just type in a subject you want to investigate. For example, you type in *breast cancer* or *cancer* or *breast.* Sometimes you have to be creative and use different types of search criteria. However, if you just want to look up breast cancer you will probably get over 30 pages worth of materials, maybe even more. Then you start refining your categories. You can type in *breast cancer surgery, breast cancer chemotherapy, breast cancer mortalities,* or *breast reconstruction* if you want to narrow your focus. The Internet is an amazing resource.

We found that there wasn't just one source that gave us everything we wanted to know. Medical books provided great scientific information, but not the human interest perspective on what women experience. We found that "touchy-feely" input in bookstores and the public library or on the Internet. I found little information directed at the significant other on how to address this problem. I wanted to know what men do. I was forced to develop my own game plan. I spent many hours documenting what I was going to do. So by the time it came time to do it I would grab my notebook and flip pages to the right stage of therapy. "Let's see. This is surgery day so I want to make sure I have a medal of St. Michael on her wrist." This helped me keep track of all these little things that needed to be done.

We both felt that the time invested in researching our options was well spent. When we went to see the surgeon, we had a solid knowledge base to help us understand what he was saying. He recommended a full modified mastectomy with no breast reconstruction. We agreed with his diagnosis, but Beth Ann told him that before she made a decision she wanted a second opinion to explore alternative treatment options.

One of Beth Ann's friends recommended a surgeon at the university hospital and we went to see him. He examined her, took another set of mammograms, and showed them to us. After looking at the breast x-ray films, we were convinced that a modified radical mastectomy was the safest way to remove all the cancerous tissue. The surgeon suggested that Beth Ann might want to consider having a skin-sparing mastectomy with immediate breast reconstruction. That way she could have less skin removed and the reconstruction would provide a very nice result. He felt that she would be a good candidate for this combined procedure. He called a plastic surgeon that he works with and had him come over to examine Beth Ann. The plastic surgeon agreed with the surgeon's treatment recommendation and explained the various options for breast reconstruction. Beth Ann was particularly interested in a flap procedure that would not require implants; she was delighted to learn that she had enough fat on her tummy to make her breast look nice and full.

For Beth Ann, the breast reconstruction was very important, more so for her than for me. My first thought was, "Oh gosh, get rid of it, get rid of the cancer. Your breast has never held a good conversation with me, so I don't care. Let's just save you." She is more to me than a breast. But for her it would have been a constant reminder of the cancer that was in her body. Now when she blow dries her hair in the morning and looks in the mirror, she can see her breasts and she feels whole. She is very pleased with the results. As a man looking at her reconstruction, you know sexually, it is pleasing also. It looks normal and she is still as much a turn-on after surgery as before.

We debated whether she should have an immediate reconstruction or wait and have a delayed procedure. We shared the same philosophy of attack, attack, attack. That is the way we deal with things. Some people want to sit back and take time to emotionally adjust and work through their feelings of anger and grief; we try to bypass some of the early stuff quickly so that we can get to a resolution. We wanted to attack the cancer just as rapidly as we could. So the debate was do we wait till after the chemotherapy and then go back into surgery and have reconstruction and more hospitalization or do we do the mastectomy and reconstruction all at the same time and then have the chemotherapy right after? If the breast did not heal properly, they would have to delay the chemotherapy and that might be risky. However, if it did work properly, we would not have to worry about going back to surgery again and would not have that dread hanging over us.

We are very much into positive thinking, so we opted to have the reconstruction at the same time and are very glad that we did. Therefore we were really excited, really pumped after talking to the plastic surgeon and the cancer surgeon. Three weeks later Beth Ann had the skin-sparing mastectomy and immediate breast reconstruction with a TRAM (abdominal) flap. Next she had chemotherapy, and after a healing process, she had nipple reconstruction and later her nipple and areola were tattooed. Unfortunately, the tattooing did not take well and the breasts are two different colors, but it is close enough so that individually each breast looks normal.

Back to the day of surgery. We arrived early in the morning on a Wednesday and she stayed in the hospital through Monday, about 6 days. She went into surgery about 7:30 A.M. First, the general surgeon did the mastectomy, which took about 3 hours, and then the plastic surgeon took over. She was back in the room by about 1:30 P.M. There were no major complications. She was somewhat coherent by 2:30 in the afternoon.

She did not have a lot of pain. We were very lucky in that. She did have a morphine pump that she could tap whenever she needed a dose of painkiller. Prior to surgery we listened to a number of audiotapes by Dr. Bernie Siegal for cancer patients getting ready for surgery. They were very helpful. In addition, we had some subliminal tapes on reducing pain and staying motivated. We put a Walkman on her during the entire surgical process. It played the same tape over and over the entire time she was in surgery. I brought a boom box into the hospital, chained it to a washstand, and put earphones on her; we continued to flip the tape over whenever she felt bad. I learned meditation years ago in Southeast Asia. Whenever she had any type of pain, we would focus on where the pain was and then tell it to go away. I think it was the combination of the morphine drip, the tapes, and all the support and positive vibes that helped her. Her attitude was that this discomfort was temporary. We had already spent many hours at home prior to surgery outlining all of the possibilities of what could happen, ranging from absolutely no pain to death. We left no stone unturned, and we did it in a positive manner. "Well you could die you know or you could come out with no pain at all." We wanted no unknowns. I think the combination of being open about what was happening along with our confidence in our doctors and the medical staff at the hospital led to a very easy surgery.

When she came out of surgery, I looked at her breast right away even though I didn't know if that was okay. I was sort of peeling the bandage off the front of the breast so I could look at it when I got caught by the nurse. She was just great. She laughed and said, "Let's go ahead and take it off." I was fascinated with what I saw, from a mechanical, technical point of view as well as an aesthetic one. Beth Ann had a round white disk of skin where the nipple was before. When you pressed on it, blood flowed back and forth. It didn't look bad; I mean it just looked like the breast was winking at you because there was a white circle where the nipple had been. All I could do was heap praises on her and tell her how wonderful it looked. So, I think that Beth Ann felt good that her new breast looked okay. In fact, it looked so good that I got in the habit of wanting to show it to everyone. Beth Ann had to slap my hand and tell me to stop. But it looked great.

While we were in the hospital I did a lot of her maintenance. I gave her baths. We went into the shower together, and I hosed her off. She even considered trying to make love in the shower, but it wasn't a good idea because she could barely stand up straight. I said maybe we better curtail this activity. Even so she still wanted to cuddle in bed, so we stayed pretty close.

The surgery did not pose an intimacy problem for us. However, I understood that she might have concerns about what was happening to her body. I also felt that she knew me well enough to know that this would not be a problem for us. It isn't like some relationships that are already in trouble and this is the last straw for the guy who just can't deal with it. She had enough confidence in me to know that it was not going to affect me one way or the other. However, at the same time my concern was her psychological state; I know that as individuals we tend to be more critical of ourselves than others are of us. So prior to surgery I talked to her about it. When we found out about the breast cancer, I made sure I spent more time talking with her and not doing the newspaper thing over the dinner table. I bought her dresses that were a little more risqué, a bit more sexy. We had romantic evenings at nice restaurants. We had more private time together, and I tried to reinforce those loving feelings. The night before her surgery I bought her a new boom box and that Whitney Houston CD "I'll Love You

Forever.". That was our dedication song for the surgery. We actually danced in the living room the night before and it was great. She was really misty-eyed and we were both filled with good feelings. We also did an excitement jump. We got pumped up, raised our fists, and literally shouted, "Go, go! We're gonna go get it; let's charge, let's get it!" This was to clear out any negative vibrations.

She had surgery on Wednesday morning. She stayed in bed all day on Thursday, and I helped her sit up in bed periodically. I got my hand slapped by the nurse for letting Beth Ann sit up too many times. On Friday she was allowed to get up and sit in the chair for a while. After breakfast I gave her a sponge bath, and then we sneaked her into the bathroom, propped her in a chair, and I washed her hair in the sink, blow dried it, and washed her face. She was delighted to get her hair done; it made her feel totally clean and refreshed and it looked great She wouldn't let me put her makeup on (said I would make her look like a Kabuki dancer), so she did it herself and put on a bathrobe. Except for the IV and the fact that she was a little bit stooped over, you could not tell that she had anything done 2 days before. She looked totally uplifted and she felt terrific. This is something that I would highly recommend to any man whose loved one is in the hospital. As soon as she is able to get up, help her get cleaned up, wash her hair, and put on makeup. It will do wonders for her spirits. The nursing staff is just too busy to take care of the aesthetics; they do what's required and what's needed. The little niceties like washing your hair or putting on makeup do not fall into the crisis mode, yet these things are really uplifting.

After her bath they told her that she could go for a walk. So we started walking the hallways. She was happy to stretch her legs. We also went down to the cafeteria two or three times before they gave us the go-ahead. The fact that Beth Ann was pushing ahead of schedule on a lot of things was encouraging and inspired confidence in her ability to recover. She knew when she was tiring out and tried not to overdo it.

We developed motivational strategies to help her cope with this experience. I hung posters in her room. One showed a big waterfall in a lush forest and was reminiscent of pleasant experiences we had shared backpacking. Every time she felt any pain she would focus on the waterfall and it would help her remember the good days. She would put herself there and it would ease the pain. I also taped up posters of colorful birds because she is a bird watcher and a poster for people to sign when they came to visit. We had a lot of trinkets in the room to make her feel positive. We made it our environment, not the hospital environment.

Looking back on the hospital experience, I can honestly say that we made the best of it. We converted a difficult situation into a good experience. We actually had some fun with it. We didn't think too much about the negatives; we just concentrated on the positives. We had a special time because we spent 5 or 6 days together in the hospital just talking and laughing and sharing. We really valued that time. The only thing that was bothersome to her was that the morning of surgery she started her menstrual period, which is common after surgery and likely due to stress. I told her not to worry, we'll deal with it and she goes, "Well, now what else?" So the whole time she was in the hospital I changed her pads and washed her whenever the blood leaked. It was actually pretty funny. She said, "I can't believe you are changing my pads."

After we came home from the hospital it took a few days before she was moving around and going for walks. She was sort of hunkered over and we didn't push that too hard. I hung a plant hook on the side of the wall and attached a rope to it so that she could tie it to her hand and hoist her affected arm up in the air. She was supposed to elevate her arm to exercise it, but she couldn't so we used this pulley system to mechanically help her raise her arm up and down.

At home I told her, "It's up to you now. You can either lay in bed and feel sorry for yourself or you can get off your ass and go get it." We even used the term "carpe diem," seize the day. I said that every day is a day of recovery to be seized. She was great. I was so proud of her. I would come home from work and find that she had walked almost a half mile around our entire apartment complex. She continued to do that every day. She would go until she couldn't go any further, and then she would rest and continue to push. The only time she ever got in trouble was when she went a little bit too far and ran out of energy. She actually had to call a taxi cab to bring her home. She did not allow herself to be restricted very long. Within a week she was out running around doing things. She took 7 weeks off work. She had a lot of sick leave and her boss encouraged it. That time off gave her a chance to focus on her recovery.

I tried to be helpful whenever I could. There were certain tasks such as grocery shopping that were more difficult for her. She couldn't lift the bags, do the dishes, or handle the housework. These are things that women do naturally and most guys don't even notice after a while. But I think the guy needs to take a proactive approach to the housework and laundry and not let things get dirty. One of the best and most appreciated things a man can do for a woman in this condition is to assume responsibility for the household chores. Laundry and cooking are easy enough to do and are things that will prey on her mind unless they are attended to. It is up to the guy to do them before she gets a chance. Otherwise she might overextend herself by trying to do these things.

It is hard for a man to know how to act in these circumstances. One of the problems we encountered early on occurred because for the first time in my life I couldn't make things better for Beth Ann. I couldn't fix things for her. I have thought about this quite a bit. Previously, if her car broke down or if there was something she couldn't do, even though she tries everything, I could always handle it. But not this time. I could not take her place in surgery, even though I wanted to, badly. I empathized so strongly that sometimes I would actually eclipse her. I asked the first surgeon more questions than she did. It was as if I were the one that was undergoing the mastectomy, to the point that sometimes I would say, "Do I need to have this done?" I was almost absorbing her psyche, and I had to learn how to back off and let her be the driving force. That was the big challenge, trying to lay back and listen. At the same time she made me aware pretty quickly that she had things to say and thought processes that needed to be respected. She was a little bit steamed at me over that. So for me and for all men dealing with women who are coping with breast cancer, listening is a major thing. You have to understand that you cannot do this for her. That was the only psychological hurdle to overcome. The rest was trial and error. Some things work and some don't. Like having sex. It has to be approached carefully. You must remember that she had an operation and you don't want to hurt her; yet, you also don't want to back off too dramatically because you want her to still feel sexually desired.

We had no problems relating sexually after the surgery. She is probably going to kill me for saying this, but we have always had a hot relationship from the first day I saw her in 1965. She was walking down the street with her sister and she turned me on at that moment. We have always had a super relationship both as friends and as sexual partners and it has never changed. There was some concern on her part, but it wasn't whether I would be interested. Her concern was more focused on her ability to have sex, whether she would feel the same, and what body changes she should expect?

Our plastic surgeon told us it was okay to resume sexual intimacy 2 weeks after surgery; that was our official go-ahead. However, we had sex before that time but we were cautious. I did not want to be a pig and she wanted to be careful because of her surgery. She was concerned that uterine contractions during orgasms might cause pain because of her abdominal surgery. So we were very tentative at first. We had to learn new positions to accommodate our special situation. I couldn't be on top of her because she had just had major chest surgery. We had to be creative.

We are cuddlers at night; we have always been. She is just an absolute delight to sleep with. It's like having a teddy bear in bed. It's wonderful to sleep against each other. If she is not cuddling into me I am cuddling into her, and we are touching all night long. After surgery, however, when you throw that leg over the top or you reach over and just sort of grab, you can do damage or cause pain. We had to figure out a way to prevent me from doing that. I didn't want to sleep in another bed because we didn't want even the illusion of separation. So we took big bath towels, rolled them up, and put them between us so I would hit them before I bumped her. We could still hold hands, I could still carress her, but I couldn't throw my leg up over her.

After she could almost stand up straight so she didn't feel awkward or uncomfortable going out in public, she got dressed up in an evening gown, and we went out to a good restaurant featuring fine dining, nice wine, and good music. Then we came home and had an intimate evening in front of the fireplace. Those romantic touches were very important for her psyche and for mine. I was thrilled to have her back. In a situation like this it is very important for a man to woo his woman again with the romantic gestures that won her in the first place. Small things like leaving love notes and cards in books for her to find or drawing hearts or smiley faces on her mirror help her to know that things haven't changed; it is even more romantic now than it was before.

It is easy to be overwhelmed by all the concerns associated with the various treatments. To cope, we segregated them into tasks; it was a form of project management. We took one task at a time and just dealt with it. Therefore, as soon as the surgery was over, we put that behind us and turned our attention to the next stage of treatment—

chemotherapy and its potential side effects. Again we took an attack approach. Let's investigate the problem and let's confront it. We put on the Bernie Siegal tapes for chemotherapy and talked about chemotherapy as our friend, not our enemy. So we got geared up for that too. We took posters into the room where they give chemotherapy, the same ones from the hospital. When we went in for the first treatment, we felt really pumped up. We did another jump up and down and shouted, " Let's get excited, let's do it." We arrived a half hour early for the blood work and were anxious to get going. Beth Ann took her first treatment without too much difficulty. She was surprised that she did not feel sick right away, only a little tired. So we went out for lunch and shopping. We knew the clock was ticking and the nausea would set in. We got home about 2:00 P.M. and watched TV. At 3:00 she was feeling a bit light-headed and nauseous, so she went into the bedroom. By 4:00 she was really nauseous and she put the earphones on with music tapes; I gave her a heating pad; then I left her alone. She doesn't like me to be in the room when she is vomiting; it's an ego thing. This was the routine we followed for each of the treatments. We viewed it as a day that we spent together rather than a day for chemotherapy.

She was fine after that incident, and she lay there and just zoned out. She slept listening to the tapes. By Saturday morning she was still feeling tired, but she was able to get out. We took it easy the rest of the day. She stayed at home all that week, and there were no major repercussions from the first chemotherapy treatment.

Two weeks later she started losing her hair. We had talked about the possibility. I was hoping she would lose it because I wanted to see her bald. In the early *Star Trek* movie there was a bald lady who looked great. Beth Ann did not share my enthusiasm for hair loss. However, she also knew that I would not be repulsed if she did go bald and we talked about that. She decided that she wanted to save the hair that fell out so that she could match her old hair color in case something changed. She would use it as a reference point. She got ready with a plastic bag for the day she would start shedding her hair.

Before her hair loss we went wig shopping; she wanted a wig to replicate her own hair. For some reason, the wig that we found made her look like Loretta Lynn. I mean it was like a big hair Momma! Even when she got it cut and trimmed it looked too big. It was like," Holy smokes this wig looks like hell. A woman at the wig shop recommended a frosted blond wig in a short hairstyle. Beth Ann has never been a blond, so she said, "Let's try it." It looked absolutely great on her. We bought it before her hair fell out so she would be prepared.

Her hair started coming out one weekend when friends were visiting from out of town. She would grab clumps of it and just lift it right off her head and put it in a plastic bag. By Monday she still had a lot of hair, but it was thinning down the middle and on the sides and not looking good. It continued to fall out until Wednesday. Then we decided to shave the rest of her head. She looked great bald. I never could talk her into going public that way, but it looked terrific.

We celebrated after the last treatment. We went out and had a big dinner. Although chemotherapy was not easy for her, we tried to reduce its impact by diverting attention to more pleasant thoughts.

When something like this happens in a relationship, a man has to look himself in the mirror, put his macho tendencies aside, and recognize that he is a partner in this experience. Most men still engage in old-time role playing. They think that diseases and health problems are for women to worry about, not men. They should grow up, take a more mature attitude, and get involved. Too many of them bale out when a crisis like this occurs; they don't know how to deal with it so they run. They need to deal with it and participate. That's the big one—participation. Men need to get in touch with their emotions.

One of the regrets I have is that I was too aggressive initially. I was more aggressive than she was during our first visit to her surgeon. (Maybe it was my military training kicking in.) Suddenly I was acting like it was my breast when it was hers. I went, "Wait a minute, this is her decision about her treatment; it is not mine." I was ready to do whatever the first surgeon recommended because my concern was to get rid of the cancer and that was all I was focusing on. Then I realized that I had overstepped my bounds because this is her life, her decision, her breast. Although I am a part of it, it is not my place to make it. That's when I had to back away; that was the hardest thing for me to do. It was really tough trying not to control things because I really wanted to help her. I wanted to shield her from as much as I could. But it was still her decision, and afterward when I thought about it, I was proud that she cut me off and said, "Nope I want to get a second opinion. I want to see what else is out there." I thought this was great she was taking charge and not letting me bulldoze her through the situation. If she weren't such a strong person, I might have overshadowed her. For most men, this is one of the hardest parts of dealing with breast cancer. All the guys I have talked to say the same thing, "We feel so helpless; we don't know what to do. You know we have always fixed things before. We want to fix this thing, but we can't do it and we can't even be involved." But that is not true; a man can be involved, but his role has to change. He has to understand that he is a supporting player now, not the main actor. It is the woman who must take center stage.

## George Johnson

Jenny's lump was discovered 1½ years ago during her regular checkup. Her mammogram revealed a possible mass within her breast that had not shown up on her physical examination. She had three other biopsies before, but they had always been benign. When she entered the hospital, the doctor told us that this lump might be cancerous and a decision needed to be made about therapy: whether to go ahead and have a frozen-section biopsy and do a lumpectomy or mastectomy right away or come back later for treatment. Her physician also informed her of other treatment options, including breast reconstruction.

When cancer was diagnosed, it was her decision to have a mastectomy and to do it immediately. I had mixed feelings about having it done right then, but she seemed determined to get it over with. Her decision may have been prompted by her sister's recent death from breast cancer. Her passing created enormous concern on both our parts. Since then, whenever Jenny has any kind of problem, no matter how minor, cancer is the first thought that comes to mind because it apparently is in the family and has been present all along. Therefore, considering her family history, she was anxious to get rid of the breast and the cancer and to protect herself from her sister's fate.

I tried to be supportive after the mastectomy. I must admit that I was distressed by seeing her body with only one breast on one side and a scar on the other side. She takes such pride in her appearance that I hated for her to have this done to her. It was painful for me to know that she was unhappy. The mastectomy had little effect on our relationship. Initially, maybe, there was some constraint there, particularly in lovemaking, but it was quickly overcome. There really was no problem.

When a couple confronts this type of trying situation, it's important for them to have a deep love for each other, and obviously, after 35 years of marriage, Jenny and I have this feeling. Coping with breast cancer and a mastectomy might be more difficult for a couple who is just dating or in a new relationship. They wouldn't be sure of each other and would be uncertain about what the future would hold for them. I would also think that cancer and mastectomy would be more traumatic for a younger individual because of the sexual implications. If people love each other, however, no matter what their ages or the length of their relationship, they will talk about their problems and try to help each other. If a man leaves a woman over a mastectomy, there wasn't much love there in the first place.

My wife was not happy with her appearance after her mastectomy. She felt that she did not look right in clothes, even though with a prosthesis an observer cannot tell the difference. But I could tell she felt uncomfortable. When she put on a bathing suit, she would stretch and pull it to make it cover more of her body. Just by looking at her expression I could see how displeased she was because she felt her deformity was noticeable. I tried to reassure her that she looked just as good as she always did, which she did. I felt she looked fine in her clothes, but I don't think she really believed me. Her prosthesis was also uncomfortable and she complained about it. The inconvenience of the prosthesis probably speeded up her decision to have reconstruction. Emotionally, I could tell that she just didn't feel right. She was not satisfied with the way she looked.

I believe that my wife had already made up her mind to have breast reconstruction even before she had her mastectomy. Almost immediately after she came home from the hospital she started talking about reconstruction and reading about it. But we really hadn't discussed this topic before. To get more information Jenny and I talked with a physician friend of ours who lived in Virginia. At that time he did not recommend more surgery. He was not really sold on breast reconstruction. But I could tell before the end of our conversation with him that Jenny really wanted this surgery.

I had mixed feelings about breast reconstruction, but I did not make any suggestions one way or the other. My feelings were somewhat negative because I worried that she wanted this done for my benefit. I also didn't want her to undergo any more surgery with its pain and discomfort. I felt that she had suffered enough. I gradually changed my mind as she helped me to realize that she actually was enthusiastic about this operation and she wanted it for herself and not for me. After I understood her determination to have breast reconstruction, I got on her side 100%.

If a man feels that reconstruction will make his woman feel happier or as if she were more of a woman, then he should encourage her, be supportive, and go along with her wishes. That's really all he can do because she will have to make the decision herself, if this is what she wants done. He needs to talk to her about her needs and really listen to what she has to say. If anything, reconstruction might enhance their relationship. If a husband or boyfriend is totally against reconstruction and discourages his loved one from having it done, their relationship might suffer. Once he sees that she is determined to proceed with this operation and that it will make her happy, he should encourage and help her.

In order to learn more about reconstruction, Jenny secured a number of pamphlets, and we read them together to understand the nature of the surgery and the various types of reconstructive procedures. Some of this material was really graphic and showed exactly what the plastic surgeon would be doing and how the new breast would look. It's important for a man and woman to get literature before reconstruction and decide what will be done. They also need to consult with a surgeon together and determine what procedures will be used and what the expected recovery period and restriction on activity will be.

After much research, Jenny got our friend in Virginia to check with a well-known surgeon who could suggest a plastic surgeon for breast reconstruction. We also got a local recommendation for a plastic surgeon. Both doctors recommended the same plastic surgeon, so we felt very comfortable because his name had come up twice. This vote of confidence was particularly reassuring for Jenny. She made the decision to have reconstruction and set up an appointment for us to go interview this plastic surgeon.

Needless to say, we were very impressed with him. He seemed concerned for her and interested in doing what she wanted. His first question to us when we came in for the visit was, "Well, what do you want to talk about?" This is really how the conversation started. We discussed our interview at great length, later, and I don't think we could have been more pleased with him. He is a gentle person and did not try to push us in any way. After meeting with him, Jenny went ahead and made the necessary arrangements to have the plastic surgery done.

Her breast was reconstructed with a flap of tissue from her back. It was called a latissimus dorsi flap reconstruction. She also had surgery on her other breast as a preventive measure. My wife is at high risk for developing another breast cancer. Over the years she has had breast biopsies for lumps in both of her breasts, and these biopsies have been very anxiety provoking for us. Our plastic surgeon knew of Jenny's cancer status and of the constant fear that we lived with. So he suggested that when her left breast was reconstructed she might also want to consider having the mass of tissue inside her right breast removed and replaced with an implant. He felt that this operation might reduce her risk of developing another cancer. Jenny decided to have this preventive surgery to help alleviate some of her preoccupation with cancer.

Jenny also had a nipple-areola created as a second procedure. She wanted her breast to be complete. Knowing my wife, I don't think that she would have been satisfied without going the full way and having a nipple put on. She has been delighted with it and so have I.

After reconstruction her recovery was rapid, with no complications. Initially, she could not drive for 2 weeks, but the inconvenience to me was minimal. There were times when I had to chauffeur her somewhere, and I assumed responsibility for certain chores around the house that she could not do physically, but none of this was a problem. A man should plan on offering some extra help during this time.

Jenny's physical condition contributed to her speedy recovery as much as anything. She is conscientious about taking care of herself and has always been in very good shape. She was this way before any problems developed and is even more so now that she has had reconstructive surgery. I think she looks great. Until she healed completely, she was limited initially in what she could do with her arms. Now she is fully recovered and participates in aerobic exercises twice a week. She was never confined much. I think she was determined to recover quickly because she knew that I did not originally want her to have this surgery, and she was trying to prove something to me.

Breast reconstruction has totally changed Jenny's attitude about herself and her appearance. It makes me feel good to see how pleased she is with herself. For all practical purposes, she is just like she always was before she started having trouble. She is active now with the American Cancer Society as a Reach to Recovery volunteer. She visits and counsels other women about her experiences. She is grateful because her surgery was so successful, and she wants to reassure women who have had mastectomies or who are considering reconstruction that everything will turn out okay.

Her friends around her age and even younger are all interested in her reconstruction. During our vacation with some other couples the girls got together and they had show and tell. They wanted to see her breast, even though none of them have had breast cancer. One of our friends who lives in Nebraska and might need to have a mastectomy is very interested in Jenny's experiences. Our friends can hardly believe that she went through what she did, because she looks so good. They are impressed with the results, with her great attitude, and, I daresay, that anyone who does not know that she had the surgery would not know. There is no way.

I give my wife credit. She changed my attitude about reconstruction. I really think it's something special now.

There is one final point I didn't touch on that might be interesting for people to know, and it has to do with a person's age and what makes you "too old." When Jenny wanted to have this surgery, nobody discouraged her necessarily, but I think there was some feeling, "Why go through with this at your age?" She was 54 years old, and they felt that if she were younger, say in her twenties or thirties, that this would be fine, but at her age, why bother? But that is not so. She is still just as much of a woman as she was when she was 20, and I hope women considering reconstruction will keep this in mind. If you are over 50, so what! Forget about your age; it really doesn't matter. Do it for yourself if it makes you feel good. My wife did and it has done wonders for her and for us.

## HOW COUPLES RELATE

The final interview in this chapter is with a young, unmarried couple: Scott Meyers and Sheila Andrews. Together, they relive their experiences from the diagnosis of Sheila's cancer, through her mastectomy and chemotherapy, to her present decision to have her breast reconstructed. Discussing the problems that a couple faces when the woman develops breast cancer, they offer insight into the various methods they have used to help them cope with this disease and the trauma associated with it.

### Sheila Andrews and Scott Meyers

*Sheila:* It all started when I went to my gynecologist for what I thought was a cyst, nothing big. When he checked me and said, "I want you to see someone else," the alarm went off. He assured me that it was nothing to worry about, but when I wanted to wait a month to make the appointment, he wouldn't let me; he insisted I go the next week. I went to see the surgeon that he recommended;

he did a needle biopsy and said he would call me in a few days with the results. When I didn't hear from him, I called his office because I was getting anxious. It was the day of our Thanksgiving dinner at work. I asked the nurse for the results, and she gave the phone to the doctor who asked me to come in to talk to him. I said, "No, that is worse than you telling me right now, over the telephone. Tell me now, and then I will come in later today and we can talk." He told me that the lump was malignant. My head was spinning from the news; I felt as if I were in another world. I was just 30, recently divorced with a teenage daughter, and I had no idea that it would be cancer. There was no breast cancer in my family. I was trying to get myself together, so I went into a private office to cry. I was hysterical . . . and then I thought about Scott.

Scott and I had only been going together for 3 months, and we were very new into our relationship. All of a sudden, I was finding out that I had cancer and not only did I have to cope with that, I had to deal with trying to tell someone who I had only known for a short while. I called him on the phone and told him.

**Scott:** After I got off the phone from talking with Sheila, I fell apart. When I managed to pull myself together, I picked Sheila up from work and we went for a drive. Cancer was something that I had never dealt with or been exposed to before. I'd never known anyone that had it; it was all new to me. I was scared for her, not knowing what she was going to have to experience. Ours was a new relationship at the time and I didn't know how this was going to affect it and really how I felt about it. I don't know that Sheila knew either. Neither one of us was aware of what was going to happen in the next few months, or even the next year. It was a matter of waiting, talking to doctors, and slowly finding out.

**Sheila:** When I went to see the doctor, he told me that he was going to put me in the hospital and schedule surgery. Before doing the mastectomy, he would do another biopsy while I was under anesthesia. He had all the consent forms ready for me to sign, because he felt that it was better for me to sign the papers ahead of time so he would not have to wake me to confirm that I had cancer. I signed the papers and went in blindly. I just said, "Yes, yes, yes." I did not know anything.

After I knew that I had to have a mastectomy, Scott and I were just wasted. Saturday night, before I was to go into the hospital, we went through several bottles of champagne, drowning our sorrows.

We decided to have a going-away party for my breast. We put on music, got loud and crazy, and poured a bottle of champagne over my breast. Scott kissed it goodbye. It was a wild thing to do, but it made us feel better. Now that I am thinking about reconstruction, I guess we will probably have to christen the new one, too, when I get it. It will be like having a new boat, only I'll be getting a new breast. That night we just lay in each other's arms and cried half the night. We hardly said anything. We just got everything out, all the tears that might have been held back. We cried and cried and cried.

**Scott:** It is essential to be open with each other. You just can't keep your feelings hidden. From a man's perspective, you need to express yourself. You can't be afraid to cry. If you can't cry about this, what can you cry about?

**Sheila:** I was terrified before surgery. I broke out in hives and went white. I had never had an operation in my life. The only time I was in the hospital was when I had a baby, 13 years earlier. I never had a sick day. This was the first time I had been sick, and that really threw me. It had been such a little problem.

I went to the hospital a week later and when I woke up I did not have a breast. It was that fast. They did a modified radical mastectomy, and I didn't even know what a modified radical was. At that time I didn't know anything. The only thing I knew was what I was told; I put my entire life in the hands of a doctor who I had never met before, and I said, "Just do what you have to do."

**Scott:** I don't think I thought so much about the mastectomy or her losing a part of her body. I just wanted to see her recover her health. My main concern was her survival.

**Sheila:** After surgery the doctor told me that my cancer had spread; I had three positive lymph nodes. I was in stage II of my breast cancer, which I didn't understand. Then he started talking about chemotherapy, and that was another whole trip. Everything you hear about chemotherapy is devastating, and all of a sudden, the focus wasn't on losing my breast, but it was on chemotherapy. I thought, "God, how am I going to survive this?" Then the oncology nurse talked to me and gave me brochures on chemotherapy. All of this time when I was in the hospital, Scott took care of my daughter and ran my house. He did all of the cleaning.

**Scott:** I did all of the housework. There were some habits formed there that are very hard to break.

**Sheila:** I have a high tolerance for pain, probably abnormally high. The evening of my surgery I took no pain killers, and by the time I was released from the hospital, I was reaching over my head. I was determined to block out what had happened to me. "You know," I said, "there is not a damn thing wrong with me. Life will resume as normal." In fact, I ran the vacuum cleaner when I got home, just to prove that nothing was going to stop me. I caught the wrath of God when Scott got home and found that I had vacuumed the bedroom. After that scene, I just gave up vacuuming forevermore.

**Scott:** That was a good example of her proving to the world that she wasn't sick. I said, "Don't prove it to me, and don't prove it to the world either. You don't need to be vacuuming this house. You don't need to have that attitude." We talked about that for a long time.

I was asking myself many questions during this period, and I was questioning many values. I had to go back and think about the way I regarded Sheila before she developed cancer. I had to determine how I felt and then ask myself why I should feel any different now. I mean, I love this woman, and at the time I decided that I would see her through this experience, just because of my feelings for her; I didn't think they should change because she had this disease. If anything, this experience probably strengthened my feelings for her in helping me give her the support that she needed.

**Sheila:** He helped me cope with my problems all the way through. The day after surgery, he said, "Okay, let's see what we are dealing with." He just opened my gown and looked down and said, "Uh, huh." I was the one who looked at my scarred chest and passed out. All he did was go, "Uh, huh, okay." He changed my bandages when I got home and rubbed lotion on my scar, even when I couldn't do it. He helped me with my bra, he helped me get dressed, he did everything for me. I was never embarrassed or ashamed in front of him.

**Scott:** It didn't bother me at all. It was just something she had to go through. I knew she didn't want it; who would? I certainly didn't enjoy it, but we had to live with it. I'm also not a squeamish person. Scars don't really bother me. I wanted to see her scar, not merely from curiosity, but from a real interest in her.

I also knew that she was worried about how I would feel about her body, but it really didn't affect our sex life. We had sex the day after she came home from the hospital. I was worried about hurting her, sure, but it worked out just fine.

**Sheila:** Even though Scott never made me feel ashamed, I was self-conscious about my body, and I probably still feel some self-consciousness. It's hard, even now, to have a romantic candlelight dinner, put on a beautiful gown, and have one side totally flat. Whether you like it or not, breasts are very, very important in sex and in the way you present yourself. I'm sure they also affect the way he looks at me. He says it doesn't bother him, and it probably bothers me a lot more than it does him. It is tiresome, looking down there and seeing no cleavage.

You have to realize that I had only been with Scott for 3 months when this occurred. There were still many things I didn't know about him. We became very close, immediately, but I still wasn't completely comfortable. Even now, there are times when I am shy about the way I look, and I have a hard time dealing with it. I'll tell him, "Kill the lights; I'm coming to bed." I know that is absurd. You would think that your feelings are somehow attached to your eyesight. But, when you are missing a breast, there is definite comfort in darkness.

When I went back to see my surgeon after I had been released from the hospital, I had many questions for him. I wanted to know about the chemotherapy: Who would administer it and would it be done in his office or in the hospital? He referred me to the university hospital and to a whole new set of specialists. That scared me. I didn't know these people, and I didn't know what to expect from them. He gave me names of the doctors at the hospital and handed me my pathology report in a sealed envelope.

I went home and immediately ripped open the report and read through it. I came to the part that said, "Prognosis: poor" and I went bing! I had no business reading that report. I didn't know what I was reading and I did not know how to interpret it. It scared the hell out of me.

**Scott:** We both read through the pathology report, but I didn't understand most of it, only words here and there. At the bottom, it read: "Prognosis: condition poor." That, everyone can read; it was black and white and simple language. It was also very difficult to take. We had both just been through her surgery and were trying to remain positive. Then to have something like that come along is demoralizing. It is like having someone tell you that all of your effort is not worth shit; it doesn't matter what you do, because this is the way it is.

***Sheila:*** Six weeks after my surgery I went to the hospital to see the doctors about chemotherapy. They told me that the type of cancer I had was poorly differentiated and had a high recurrence rate. That was another blow. I went into a rage. I cursed them and screamed, "Bullshit. You are not telling me that I am dying. I am only 30 years old. I have a daughter and my own house. For the first time in my life, after a terrible marriage, I have a man that I really love; I have everything to live for: a new job, a new relationship, a child, everything." I really fought it, and I've continued to fight it. I have bad moods, but I am not going to let it get me.

***Scott:*** I think the chemotherapy was even more of an adjustment for Sheila than the surgery itself. Chemotherapy required a great deal of patience and understanding from me and from everyone around Sheila, especially her daughter. The drugs affected her poorly. She was moody and short-fused. She had a temper and she cried all of the time. She stayed in bed a lot. I could deal with that and her daughter handled it well. Her daughter showed real understanding and patience for her mother and what she was enduring; I think she knew that Sheila was not always going to act that way and there would be an end to it. We were all relieved when the chemotherapy was over. It really pushed everyone to the maximum. I had to keep telling myself that the drugs were making her react the way she was. She said many dumb things during that time. I think her logic and reasoning were not as clear as they normally were, and she was very emotional.

***Sheila:*** You go through so many emotions with cancer, and chemotherapy does trigger those emotions. You are high at one moment and then lower than a snake the next. My moods were up and down. I don't think I was really rational for many of the things that I did or said. I wasn't altogether there and I wasn't in control all of the time. Despite my actions and the way life was treating me, Scott moved in with me during my chemotherapy. I really knew he loved me if he could move in at that time.

Chemotherapy was terrible for me. I had very long, luscious blonde hair, and after the first chemotherapy treatment, it started coming out in handfuls. During the second week I had big clumps of hair falling out of my head. I made an appointment to see wigs, and they matched me with several long, blonde wigs. Soon, I was practically bald. I looked like Bozo the Clown; I had a strip of hair running along the edges of my scalp. I not only lost the hair on my head, but I also lost the rest of my body hair, every bit, from head to toe. I still had a few eyelashes, but my eyebrows were almost nonexistent. I had to wear a lot of makeup to look normal. I also gained 18 pounds on chemotherapy, which I am having a hard time losing. So, besides being bald, not getting into my clothes, and losing a breast, I kept saying, "What is next?" It is a tremendous amount to deal with.

**Scott:** Hair loss was traumatic for Sheila. She seemed to have an enormous amount to cope with, and it was sometimes hard for me to help her.

**Sheila:** With a breast, you can camouflage your loss, but with hair loss, what can you do? I mean, I couldn't wear wigs to bed. Talk about romance. He had to look at this woman who had one breast and was bald as a billiard ball. "Oh my God, I looked like I just stepped out of a circus." We can laugh now, but at the time there were many tears. Finally, all this hair was falling out and he made the ultimate decision. He said, "Sheila, you are clogging all of the drains. I have to cut off every bit of your hair because it is falling out, and it is getting all over your clothes. Let's just get it over with once and for all." I said, "Okay," and he got the scissors and just snipped off the rest; that was probably the best thing he ever did. He just got rid of it, and I stopped worrying about it falling out.

**Scott:** There were times when I needed someone to confide in. I have one or two close friends that I can talk to, but they didn't really understand what was happening.

**Sheila:** We often talked about our relationship. In fact, there were times when we weren't sure that it would last. It had nothing to do with my cancer; it was just his own feelings. He has other commitments; he goes to school, he works, and he loves to travel. It's hard to commit yourself to a woman who has cancer, who is going through chemotherapy, and who has a 13-year-old daughter and a house. That's a lot to ask of anyone. He had to be absolutely sure how he felt about me before he made any kind of commitment to me.

**Scott:** I needed to work through my own feelings and think about my life. I thought about how I felt about Sheila before surgery and before she had cancer. I had to decide what I was feeling now. I had to confront myself: "Am I staying with this woman because I pity her or because I love her?" There were times when I really couldn't answer that question. Finally, I decided that if I left I would never know, and if I stayed, I would have to be very careful about why I stayed. I decided that I wanted to stay. I love her and I wanted to give her 100% of my support and love and see her through this experience. If there were anything that I could do to help her, I would do it. That meant taking care of her, her surroundings, and her daughter. It meant providing moral support and letting her know that she was going to get through this okay. I was determined to keep as optimistic an attitude as I could and to show some strength for her.

*Sheila:* He was always planning for the future. That was important for me because when all of this first happened, I didn't take any interest in the house or even in balancing the checkbook. I owned my own house, and we talked about painting it. But I would say things like, "Why should I paint this damn place if I am going to die? Why should I buy anything?" I didn't want to buy anything: clothes, furniture, paint, anything. Why should I, if I weren't going to be able to enjoy it in 6 months? Toward the end of my chemotherapy, many of these feelings disappeared; we repainted the house, and I started buying clothes again.

*Scott:* She started living a normal life again. She joined a support group through the American Cancer Society and she started taking dancing lessons. By remembering that there were other things that she needed to do with her life, she began to get out again and not let this hold her back.

*Sheila:* You can allow yourself to get depressed and let everyone feel sorry for you. It's easy to have a sad face and then people will say, "Oh, I'm so sorry." I didn't want that crap. I just wanted to be happy and to laugh. Scott and I had funny experiences and we tried to keep our sense of humor. Our laughter has helped me survive this experience. When I go to my support group, I tell people about the funny things that happen. Like the time I forgot to put the toilet seat down and my wig fell in. I had to shake it out, wash it, and hang it out in the sun to dry. Then I realized that I couldn't go anywhere because I was bald, my other wig was being fixed, and I only had this one. You must laugh at things like that.

*Scott:* I wanted to take her to a loud dance studio in town, with her dressed like the lady in *Star Trek*. She wouldn't have it.

*Sheila:* He wanted to dress me in silver tights and makeup. He wanted me to be a Trekkie. He told me it would be the chance of a lifetime.

Actually, we did have fun with it. We went to a Kenny Loggins concert in June and I was still pretty bald at the time. I had ⅛ inch of hair all over my head, so I decided to dress in style. I bought myself a bright lavender headband and put on a black jumpsuit with high heels and makeup. I wore lavender and black jewelry, earrings that were as big as my head, and beads. I didn't wear my wig. We went to the concert and people did double and triple takes. I'm sure they were talking about that bald woman. "A good-looking man like that with a bald woman, yuck!" It was really interesting. The women made derogatory comments about my head, but the men seemed to be complimentary. It was very, very strange. If they had only known why I looked the way I did.

Getting involved with support groups has also helped me to adjust. Women need to know that there are self-help groups available and that we are not alone. The American Cancer Society has a number of these groups going. Reach to Recovery is one and I am now a volunteer. I'm also in another support group that meets once a month and we swap stories about our experiences. It's one of those meetings where you can cry, especially with the women who have just come out of it. We cry, we hold each other, we laugh. You can face a lot of things together.

One of the women in our group just had a recurrence. She had her surgery the same time I did, and she was just getting ready for her yearly checkup when they found an inoperable mass in her chest. She only has 6 months to live. You have to learn that when you are working closely with people, not everyone is going to make it and that's hard to take. I had to come to grips with that reality this month with her.

We share everything in these meetings. We talk about sex and looks and feelings. Many of these women are single and are dating. They ask, "How do you tell a man that you've had this surgery? Maybe you've only gone out with him two or three times, and it gets to a point where you might end up in bed. What do you do then?" That's a problem that you need to broach and you need to know what to do. Even with Scott it was difficult for me because I was still self-conscious.

I learned about breast reconstruction in my support group. One of the women had it done and she told me about her plastic surgeon. I had no idea that there were any alternatives. My surgeon never said anything about reconstruction. After I heard about it though, halfway through my chemotherapy, I started asking doctors at the hospital about breast reconstruction, and they said, "Go for it." They were very supportive. But they also told me that I would have to wait until the chemotherapy was over. Then they said, "Do it. You're young and you want your breast back. It would be a great thing for your mental attitude."

**Scott:** I really didn't like the idea of her doing it. I'm not comfortable with it. I don't want her going into an operating room again. We have talked about it quite a bit, and I am concerned because I feel that she is doing this entirely for me, and there is no need.

**Sheila:** Probably he is right to a certain extent. I am doing this partly for him, but it is also for me. I think that if I have breast reconstruction, I'll feel better about myself and the way that I look. After a mastectomy, every time that you look at yourself in the mirror, it's a reminder of cancer. Personally, I don't feel I have cancer anymore; I really don't. It's something I had to deal with at the time, but now it is time to go ahead and get my breast reconstructed and stop worrying about it. I don't want to look down any more and see that there is a breast missing. I miss wearing regular bathing suits and nice lingerie. Actually, the more I think about it, the more I realize that I am doing it for myself. It is to help me forget this disease.

I like to sleep on my stomach, but with a missing breast this position becomes awkward and off balance. I am also uncomfortable with my prosthesis. I'm an accountant, and just moving my arm to the calculator makes the prosthesis rub; it bothers me. The first thing I do when I get home from work is kick off my shoes and throw out my prosthesis.

In my mind, I made a commitment to investigate breast reconstruction the minute I heard that it was a possibility. I decided that I wanted it if I could have it.

I was really scared when I went to see the plastic surgeon. The first time he saw me, he told me to take off my clothes so he could take some photos. He got out his camera and took about 20 pictures of every angle of my breast. He was also taking pictures of my stomach and my hips. Meanwhile, I'm thinking, "Oh my God, Blackmail!" I felt like I was posing for *Playboy*. But he needed those pictures to decide what to do, and he said that with the weight I had gained during chemotherapy and after having had a child, he felt an abdominal flap was the best operation for me. You see, I don't have an 18-year-old stomach anymore, and yet my remaining breast has a nice size and shape. If I had this flap surgery, he wouldn't have to touch my opposite breast. He felt he could get the best match for my breast with an abdominal flap reconstruction; and I would be more pleased with it, knowing that I could get rid of my stomach and also get a breast to match my remaining breast.

I had to think a long time about having this operation. Not only am I going in for more surgery, but I am having a major operation; this is the most complicated form of reconstruction. It is a big deal to decide. When you have cancer, you don't have a choice. You go into the hospital, and you get surgery. I'm going into a major operation that is by choice and that is hard. I am saying, "Okay, Doc, I'm going to let you rearrange my entire body and I'm putting it in your hands." If I didn't trust my plastic surgeon, I wouldn't be able to say that. It shows you how much faith I have in him. I am saying, "Do your best. I totally trust you with my life."

**Scott:** She isn't making this decision based on ignorance, however. Since her mastectomy, we've taken time to learn about reconstruction.

**Sheila:** Several weeks ago we invited a girl over to our house. She had this same operation by another surgeon, and we wanted to see somebody else's work. She came over 8 weeks after her surgery and she showed Scott and me her breast. She just stripped down and said, "Okay, this is what I look like." It was nice seeing another breast. When you go into this, you have to understand that your body is never going to look exactly the same as it did before. There are going to be some concessions. There are going to be some scars; I will have a scar across my stomach. My main concern is my appearance in clothes; now I will be able to wear a bra and will not have to wear a prosthesis. I will be able to fill something out again.

**Scott:** I'm still having problems with her having more surgery. It's another operation and it worries me. But if it's going to help her psychologically and improve her self-image, then I want her to have it. It has to be important to her.

**Sheila:** I am looking forward to breast reconstruction. I am not interested in having a nipple-areola put on right now; it's not a priority for me. I can always go in later and have it put on. I'm not in a hurry. No one would really see the nipple, except Scott. If I feel deprived, I can probably just cut out brown construction paper and stick it on.

I want to be able to wear a normal bathing suit this summer. In fact, the night before my surgery I'm meeting my plastic surgeon at the hospital with my bathing suit. It has a French cut to the legs, and instead of a straight line cut across my abdomen, he is going to give me a "happy face" scar so that I can still wear this suit. I'm going to try on my suit for him so he can plan my scars to fall in the right area. Women don't understand that the scar doesn't have to extend straight from hip to hip; it can be curved up. It's nice to know that even these details can be individualized.

Women need to know about breast reconstruction and about the different options for cancer treatment. They need this information before it happens to them. Every woman should be informed about breast cancer. She should know about mastectomies and reconstruction before she has to worry about them. I went into this experience so ignorant. I just said, "Do what you want." I didn't know anything. I didn't know that there were alternatives; I didn't know that there was breast reconstruction. I think if women knew about reconstruction and knew the results, they might not be so hesitant to go in if they felt a lump. I really think that detection is the key, and knowledge about alternatives and treatment will encourage women to report problems as soon as they discover them.

**Scott:** I agree with Sheila 100%. I think women should be educated. They should know their options, and they should get involved in them. Once you've experienced what we have experienced, you learn to be happy and to make the most of life. You learn that one of the most effective ways of coping with a situation like this is by remaining positive.

# FOURTEEN WOMEN TELL THEIR STORIES

Women are the inspiration behind this book; their voices permeate our writing. Many of these women have been transformed by the specter of breast cancer and have shared their thoughts and feelings to help make this book a reality. Their input has been invaluable and their sensitivity and generosity are reflected in the stories they have to tell. Following are 14 stories of women who had mastectomies and in two cases lumpectomies for breast cancer and sought breast reconstruction. Six of these interviews are new, replacing five of the ones published in the previous edition. As difficult as it was to leave those five stories behind, it was a necessity. Procedures for breast reconstruction have changed and improved over the past 4 years, and we wanted our readers to benefit from others' experiences with the latest technical advances. Therefore this time we have added information on reconstruction to fill contour defects after lumpectomy, endoscopic techniques, microsurgical buttock (gluteus maximus) flaps, skin-sparing mastectomy and immediate reconstruction, and autologous back (latissimus dorsi) flap reconstruction. Although some of the narrators of these stories have changed, we have tried to retain the spirit behind the interviews and capture the courage and honesty that typified all of these women. Interestingly, as we compare the original interviews with the more recent ones, many of the same phrases, comments, fears, and emotions are echoed. The operative details may differ, but the concerns remain surprisingly constant. Most striking is the similarity of responses given to questions probing women's reactions to breast cancer, motivations for seeking breast reconstruction, and satisfaction with this operation. We have also been impressed that over the years women have become better informed about breast cancer and its treatment, and increasingly they have become their own health advocates. As in the previous editions, we have altered names and personal details to protect the privacy of these women.

From the many taped interviews, we have purposely selected those women who underwent different reconstructive procedures, some immediately after mastectomy or lumpectomy and others delayed until various times after surgery, to give you some idea of the reconstructive possibilities available and the potential benefits and problems. These women range in age from 29 to 60 years and represent diverse social, cultural, professional, and family backgrounds. We have included single women, widowed and divorced women, and married women with and without children. The questions asked each woman were varied in the interest of providing a wider coverage of topics. Thus one interview focuses on the issue of self-image for the woman seeking breast restoration; another examines the loss of control that is associated with a cancer diagnosis, still another discusses the predicaments that a single woman with a mastectomy faces when dating. Patient self-advocacy, the power of positive thinking and spirituality, and the importance of being an informed consumer are also explored. Certain subjects, however, are dealt with in each dialogue, including reasons for deciding on breast reconstruction, timing of reconstructive surgery, pain and recuperation after reconstruction, physical and psychological results of reconstructive surgery, and benefits and limitations of reconstructive surgery. An attempt has been made to present an honest, balanced discussion of this option so that women contemplating breast reconstruction will have a realistic understanding of what this surgery offers. Because the female half of this writing team did the firsthand interviewing to facilitate a free and candid discussion, these stories and the questions and observations are presented in the first person.

We begin with Debbie whose medical background gave her an unusual insight into the life-threatening disease that abruptly altered her life and reshaped her perspective.

## DEBBIE: CONTROL IS JUST AN ILLUSION

"A lot of positive things have come out of this year, particularly how I view life and treat other people. I think I am more sensitive, but I live with much less illusion that I have control over my life. Loss of control was very difficult for me. I always thought I could manage everything. Breast cancer has a way of bringing you up short and making you face reality."

Control is a big issue for Debbie. Although she expressed a desire to slow down and enjoy life, she is still "going like gangbusters to catch up with many of the things I didn't finish last year." Despite her heavy travel schedule, she has managed to finish her Ph.D. and pass her medical boards all in the same month. Clearly life is still frenetic, but breast cancer has made her feel vulnerable. It has interrupted her routine and forced her to examine her life. Before she thought she could handle everything. "I was the total self-contained woman. But breast cancer has changed all that."

Debbie is a pretty, petite, 41-year-old. Her short red hair frames her slender face, making her look younger than her years. Her black metal glasses, however, lend an air of seriousness. Debbie was only 39 years old when her breast cancer was discovered. An M.D. with a busy career and hectic schedule, Debbie "just didn't have time for breast cancer." As she relates, "I didn't have time for much routine health care. I have always been extremely busy in my work and I travel a lot both in the United States and overseas.

Despite her medical background, she knew little about the disease and was shocked when her cancer was diagnosed. As a young single woman, breast loss was a major threat to her. However, her tumor was over 2 cm and a mastectomy and breast reconstruction seemed the best treatment option, that is, until she heard of neoadjuvant chemotherapy. After further investigation she opted for this new treatment in which chemotherapy is first given to shrink the tumor and prevent spread. Then she had a lumpectomy followed by another course of chemotherapy and radiation therapy. Even so, a *partial breast reconstruction with an endoscopic latissimus dorsi flap* was necessary to correct the defect left after tumor removal. Debbie is delighted with the somewhat unconventional choice that she made. She came out of surgery feeling "normal" again.

Our interview traces her story from the time she first heard the shocking diagnosis.

### How was your breast cancer discovered? What specialists did you talk to?

I noticed an area in my breast that felt a little different. My doctor said it was fibrocystic disease. So I put it out of my mind. I was doing breast self-exams once a month, but I didn't suspect I had a problem until 9 months later when I thought I felt a cyst in that area. It was movable and seemed to be filled with fluid. I was too busy to go in to have it checked. Sitting at my desk 3 months later, however, I felt a strong sense of urgency to have the lump checked immediately. This occurred 3 days before I was preparing to present a talk at a major meeting. I saw my physician on Friday and she sent me for a mammogram. After the mammogram the radiologist met with me. He said, "I think that you have a malignancy. I don't see this kind of pattern with anything but cancer." I was stunned.

I decided to see a breast surgeon at the university hospital. I convinced myself that there was nothing to worry about. I would get a biopsy and everything would be fine. After all, I didn't have a family history of breast cancer and I was only 39 years old, too young for breast cancer. Lurking in the back of my mind, however, were nagging worries about other risk factors. I was single, had never been pregnant, and was raised on a typical southern diet.

I was referred to a woman surgeon who had a curt, business-like manner. She was just what I needed. She was a no-nonsense physician who was not prone to mincing words. She said, "Let's do a needle biopsy right now and if it is negative we will do an open biopsy."

The needle aspiration was one of the most painful procedures I have experienced. I don't know why. Other women don't find it painful. They didn't get any cells with the first aspiration and had to repeat it. I left for lunch while awaiting the results. When I returned, the nurse, who had been friendly earlier, avoided looking me in the eye. Being a physician I knew what that meant: the tests must have been positive for breast cancer. So I wasn't totally surprised when the surgeon confirmed the diagnosis.

My breast surgeon called a plastic surgeon in to confer. They determined that they would have to remove most of the breast to get clean margins. At least the whole top part of the breast would have to go, leaving a significant defect. That was devastating to me. I had at least hoped that I could have breast-conserving surgery, now I would have to face mastectomy. I asked the plastic surgeon about immediate breast reconstruction. I did not want to come out of surgery without a breast. He reviewed my options. I was too slim to have a whole breast constructed out of my latissimus dorsi back muscle. A TRAM flap taken from my abdomen would be a better alternative. He asked me to come by his office later for further discussion and to meet some of his breast reconstruction patients.

*How did you react to the news that you had breast cancer? What did you do after you heard the diagnosis and treatment options?*

I kept busy. I spent the entire day talking to different specialists. I suddenly remembered that I had a hair appointment at 6 o'clock and I felt compelled to keep it. "I'll be damned. I'm going to get my hair cut despite all this." While I was at the beauty shop I called my mother to tell her I had breast cancer. The whole scene was surreal. Why would you get your hair done on the day you find out you have breast cancer? But it seemed a normal thing to do and I needed that. It was a way of maintaining some semblance of control.

*Did you seek a second opinion?*

I called a colleague who is a research director for an oncology group in Indiana. She asked me what treatment I had chosen. I told her I was scheduled for a mastectomy and immediate breast reconstruction the next Wednesday. The large size of my tumor and small size of my breast ruled out lumpectomy. She cautioned against making a hasty decision. She said "Get on a plane. I will schedule appointments for you to talk to the doctors here."

Instead of going to the meeting I flew to Indiana where I met with a number of specialists. The diagnosis was the same, but they told me about another option called neoadjuvant therapy (also induction chemotherapy). With this approach, chemotherapy is given before surgery for women with late-stage or an aggressive form of cancer that is likely to spread (such as inflammatory breast cancer). The chemo-surgery is administered early to shrink the tumor and halt possible spread.

I was already scheduled for surgery in 2 days. I thought why change things now? However, why not get chemotherapy now instead of waiting 4 to 6 weeks after surgery? Nobody can predict when cancer will spread. It could be in 2 days or 2 weeks or even 2 years. So I had some difficult decisions to make.

*How did you make your decision?*

I went with my instincts. I called my surgeon back home and asked her opinion of this new therapy. She said nobody was doing it there and there were no statistics on its effectiveness in treating the stage II breast cancer that I had. All the statistics were compiled on women who had more advanced stage III and IV cancer.

The physicians in Indiana referred me to a local oncologist experienced with neoadjuvant chemotherapy. I went to see him and decided to try this new approach. I called off surgery, and on the next Tuesday I started chemotherapy.

### Did being a physician make this decision-making process any easier?

It made it harder. Being a physician, I was an integral part of the decision-making process in a way that most patients aren't. Instead of doctors talking to doctors, it was doctors talking to me. I was the person in between. My doctors assume I know more than I do. I'm a really good immunologist, but I don't know a thing about breast cancer. I suppose I can understand what I read better than most patients, but still. . . . My doctors gave me enough information, but I am not sure it would have been sufficient for most patients.

I have tried to pick good doctors whose advice I trust and let them do their job. When I first talked to my oncologist, he starts off with, "I know you've read all about this." I stopped him right there and said, "No, all I have read is some basic material. I haven't read all the medical oncology literature. Yes, I have an M.D. degree, but I don't have any training in that area and can't make critical decisions on whether this or that was a good study. I need you to be my doctor and I will be the patient. I will ask questions when I don't understand things." Sometimes, however, I do find myself feeling a little intimidated and hesitant to ask questions when I perceive that my doctor is busy. That is a bad attitude; patients need to ask questions because doctors need to know when a patient is confused.

### Was the neoadjuvant (induction) chemotherapy successful? How did this therapy affect your plans for cancer surgery and plastic surgery?

During the first week of chemotherapy I didn't even touch the lump. I thought you can't be examining yourself every day to see if the chemotherapy is working. When I finally did touch it, I could barely feel it anymore, and this was a palpable 2.5 to 3 cm lump. That actually frightened me. I don't know why; it was just so amazing to me that it could work so rapidly. I called the oncologist and said you need to tell me what is happening here. I thought I was losing touch with reality. I didn't believe that it could happen that quickly. I was sure that I was in denial. But I wasn't. The tumor was shrinking after only the first round of chemotherapy. I had three to four more sessions to go before the surgery.

At this point I decided to see a radiation oncologist at the medical center to inquire if I would be a candidate for breast conservation now that the tumor was shrinking.

### How did the radiation oncologist react to your request for breast-conserving surgery instead of the mastectomy?

The radiation oncologist basically told me I was crazy. He said there weren't any studies that showed that neoadjuvant chemotherapy was going to work; there were just some unknown protocols. I could tell he was worried about me. He thought I should stop the chemotherapy now and have the mastectomy as planned.

I am usually a pretty confident person, but this time I became almost hysterical. I had been told by the medical oncologist that what I was doing was no worse than standard therapy and may be better. But here my radiation oncologist tells me I am nuts. It was very upsetting.

The sad fact is that most women have the surgery first and then tumor markers and tumor characteristics are used to determine whether they will need chemotherapy. But nothing guarantees whether a particular chemotherapy is going to work for a particular tumor. These therapies are based more on a global perspective that in a particular study it worked for 90% of women.

Earlier I had asked my medical oncologist why women have surgery, go through chemotherapy, receive a clean bill of health, and then 5 years later they find cancer everywhere. He said that the chemotherapy regimen probably was not effective for the tumor. I knew my chemotherapy regimen was working. I could *feel* my lump going away. That was the most valuable input I could get.

I called my medical oncologist in Indiana and told him the radiation oncologist here wanted me to stop chemotherapy now after only one dose and have surgery immediately. The medical oncologists had recommended three or four rounds of chemotherapy before surgery. He said, "Don't do it; you are setting yourself up for chemotherapy failure. You need to complete the course and then have your surgery." I decided to stay with my decision.

### Did you talk to your breast surgeon about changing your therapy from mastectomy to breast-conserving surgery? What was her response?

I told her that I was thinking about having breast-conserving surgery instead of a mastectomy because my tumor had shrunk so much I couldn't feel it anymore. She examined me and couldn't feel it either. We bargained back and forth. She was hesitant to acknowledge that my tumor was smaller. She still wanted to take out a relatively large area of tissue even though it would be smaller than originally planned. Now she would only remove the area of the tumor, not a wide margin of tissue surrounding it. However, it would still leave me with a big defect and I would need some type of breast reconstruction. She suggested I talk to the plastic surgeon before I made a final decision.

### What did the plastic surgeon recommend?

I went to see the plastic surgeon. Previously he said that I didn't have enough tissue on my back to build a whole breast after mastectomy. Now, however, my tumor was much smaller, and I was considering having a lumpectomy. So I told him how my situation had changed and asked if he thought I had enough back muscle and tissue to fill in the lumpectomy defect? Would I be a candidate for the endoscopic back (latissimus dorsi) flap technique? I learned of this procedure when I visited his office the first time. I had spoken to a woman who had an endoscopic back flap to fill in a lumpectomy defect. She let me see what her reconstruction looked like and it was amazing. There were only three small scars and it looked very natural. I thought this might be something that would work for me if I have breast-conserving surgery. He listened carefully, examined my breast, and finally said, "Okay, if you decide to have the lumpectomy, we'll do it."

### Did you decide on a mastectomy with immediate TRAM (abdominal) flap reconstruction or lumpectomy with immediate endoscopic latissimus dorsi (back) flap reconstruction followed by radiation therapy?

Two weeks before I had the surgery I was still vacillating between lumpectomy and radiation therapy and mastectomy. Although the survival rate is equivalent for both approaches, local recurrence is about 10% higher for lumpectomy and radiation therapy. I had to decide whether I was willing to risk a higher recurrence rate.

My breast surgeon said it depends on what kind of person you are. If you develop a local recurrence after this procedure and can say, "Well I tried. It seemed like a good option for me at the time." Then go for the breast-conserving surgery and the latissimus flap. If you are a person who is going to berate yourself for making a wrong decision, then go with a mastectomy and a TRAM flap. Even then, your recurrence risk doesn't go down to zero.

So I weighed the options. With breast-conserving surgery, my risk for recurrence is 10% higher, but I will have my breast intact and it will match the other side a lot better. I also will avoid the major surgery and recovery associated with mastectomy and TRAM flap reconstruction. I tend to be an optimist. I thought this breast-conserving surgery seems to be a better approach for me. So I went for it. I had a lumpectomy with immediate endoscopic latissimus dorsi flap reconstruction. Then I had a follow-up course of chemotherapy and later 6 weeks of radiation therapy.

### Was axillary node dissection necessary since you already had chemotherapy?

I agreed to the lymph node dissection even though I had to be convinced it was necessary. I worried about developing lymphedema. Even though I wasn't at high risk for lymphedema because I wasn't elderly or overweight, I still worried. I thought this is my right arm and I just don't have time to deal with lymphedema. A woman in my support group developed lymphedema and had to spend about 4 hours a day in a pressure cuff. So I asked my breast surgeon why I needed to have the nodes resected when they would probably be negative because of the chemotherapy. Couldn't I just forget the node dissection? She told me I needed the dissection in case I still had a number of positive nodes and a bone marrow transplant would be necessary.

### Tell me about the operation. What was it like? How long did it take? Were you prepared?

The surgery involved three basic steps. First I had needle localization to zero in on the exact location of the tumor. Then I had a lumpectomy to remove the tumor and axillary node dissection to obtain a sampling of lymph nodes in my armpit area to check for tumor spread. Finally, I had breast reconstruction using endoscopic techniques to harvest a portion of my latissimus dorsi back muscle and tunnel it through the axillary incision to restore my breast contour.

The surgery was probably more difficult for me because of the four courses of chemotherapy. I had taken only 2 to 3 days off work during chemotherapy and I had traveled when my white blood cell count permitted. I went into surgery quite tired. The night before I stayed up until 3 A.M. in the morning to get a paper off to a colleague. I thought, "Great, I'm going to have general anesthesia and can catch up on the sleep I lost. What a misconception that was. I wasn't prepared for the needle localization procedure before the lumpectomy.

### What does needle localization involve?

The mammogram taken before I had chemotherapy was used to accurately pinpoint the location of the lesion and to guide needle placement. The needles are inserted into the breast and then they take other mammographic views with the needles inserted. It is quite painful.

### Do they give you local anesthesia?

No. Sensation is necessary to ensure the breast can be maneuvered correctly for the mammograms and the needles positioned accurately. Each time they insert a needle they have to do a mammogram. I needed three needles inserted. My breasts are fibrous and there was a lot of scarring from the chemotherapy, so it was difficult to get the needles in far enough. It was so painful that I passed out.

Once the needles were inserted, dye was injected into them, a wire was inserted, and the needles were pulled out over the wire. At this point I was beginning to get the idea that this was not going to be a piece of cake. I was thankful that I was going to be asleep for the rest of it.

### What happened after the needle localization?

Before the general anesthesia was administered, the plastic surgeon made preoperative markings. I have scoliosis; the right side of my rib cage bows out a little. He said, "You're probably going to be the only woman I have done this procedure on that I am going to even out." That made me feel a bit better, although he was partially kidding me. My breast surgeon did the lumpectomy and axillary node dissection and my plastic surgeon performed the breast reconstruction. Afterwards my breast still looked and felt like me.

### How long did the operation take? Did you experience much pain?

My operation took 3 hours. I was hospitalized for 2 days. They wanted to send me home after the first day, but I wasn't feeling well. I was dizzy and couldn't stand up. So I stayed an extra day. My mother stayed with me the whole time, which helped. I had pain every time I moved my arm and probably should have requested more pain medications.

### What was it like being in a teaching hospital? Describe your hospital stay? Did you have any problems?

This was my first experience having surgery at a teaching hospital; before I was in private hospitals. Even though I have traveled that route myself during training, I forgot what it is like for medical students to come in at 5 o'clock in the morning to look at your wound. At 6 o'clock a resident comes in, at 6:30 the chief resident checks on you, and then the attending comes in. So you have four or five people coming to see you.

I didn't like being on display. I knew that the medical student who came in didn't have a clue as to what she was looking at. Anyway, I was feeling very paranoid. I know that one of the factors that contributes to lymphedema is infection; and I didn't want a lot of people opening up my dressings. There are just so many people all of the time.

I also understand why the plastic surgeon had to take so many pictures of me. But it is difficult. You're standing naked and having pictures taken with this little paper panty on. My distaste for all of this was tempered by knowing why it was necessary. I also knew that some of this routine is not really necessary. There is really no reason for a medical student to wake you up at 5 o'clock in the morning. Why aren't rounds made with at least the resident to cut down on the disruptions. I know that the students need to come in to write the notes in the morning before the resident comes in, but by the end of the first morning I was ready to slap a few hands and say, "You do not know if this looks good or bad. The only person who can come here and tell me this is okay is my plastic surgeon."

### How long did they leave the drains in? Was it painful when they were removed?

I left the hospital with two drains. The first drain came out within a week. If I had to rank painful, that is number one, number two is needle localization, and number three is fine-needle aspiration biopsy.

They clip the sutures and say take a deep breath and hold it because this is going to hurt. Then they just rip the drain out. You have no idea that something that long was inside your back and your scapula. You can't cry because you have no breath left. It is absolutely excruciating, but it is over quickly, thank goodness. The second drain in your side comes out in 2 weeks; it is not as long as the first one and for some reason is not as painful. Maybe it's because you have more numbness in that area.

### Did you have any problems or complications?

After the drains were removed, fluid accumulated all the way up to the scapula. It was like a bag of water. I had to come in every week and have them aspirate it. That wasn't as painful as I would have thought because I didn't have much sensation there.

*Why did you need more chemotherapy after surgery when you had chemotherapy before surgery?*

They split the whole course of treatment because they wanted me to have some kind of mop-up chemotherapy after surgery. Then I had the radiation therapy.

*How long did you have radiation therapy? What was involved?*

Every day, Monday through Friday, for 6 weeks. They place a big target thing around you, like X marks the spot, to focus the therapy. The radiation produces an intense sunburn on your breast that is initially sore and painful to touch. It is red, inflamed, and swollen and then it tans. They draw marks over your breast area and cover them with plastic to keep them from rubbing off. So you walk around for 6 weeks with lines all over your breast. The redness on my breast has faded now, but the nipple is still somewhat red. For a while the nipple was very sore and inflamed. You couldn't touch it at all.

I actually went to an aesthetician and had her apply superficial peels to this sunburned area on my breast to bleach it. We did six sessions and I also did home bleaching as well, which improved the skin damage from the radiation therapy. The radiation shrank the breast slightly, and I understand that it will continue to shrink a little more over time.

*How long was it before you could get back to your normal activities?*

I went back to work 2½ weeks after surgery. In another 2 weeks I started physical therapy twice a week. I lifted weights and did exercises to improve my shoulder mobility. The therapists worked with me to try to loosen the adhesions under my arm and improve mobility. My plastic surgeon recommended this. I waited until the radiation therapy and postsurgical chemotherapy were over and my hair grew back before I started playing tennis. It gets hot playing in a wig. Now I am back to tennis and back to aerobics. The only reason my schedule is less demanding is because I have chosen to start taking weekends off and not working so late at night. It's a life choice.

My plastic surgeon also recommended massage therapy. Unfortunately, insurance doesn't pay for massage therapy, but I did it anyway.

*How often have you had massage therapy? Has it helped?*

I have therapy once a week, and I've continued it during my trips to Maine, California, Indiana, and even China. Everywhere I go now I locate a therapist. Before the therapy my scapula was really bound from adhesions. I was stiff and tight—tight to the point where my muscles and ribs hurt. So I have been aggressive with my physical therapy and message therapy, and it has helped enormously in restoring mobility and flexibility.

Every time I come in the residents comment on how good my donor site looks. Well, it ought to look good; I've paid thousands of dollars for massage therapy. I recommend it to everybody. It has been one of the best things I have done to keep myself mobile.

### Are you pleased with the aesthetic appearance of your breast?

It looks really good. Overall, my breasts are smaller, but they are symmetric. They have the same droop and they look very much alike. The scars have faded and you really have to look to see them. Anybody who didn't know that I had the surgery wouldn't be able to tell.

### What do your scars look like?

There is a semicircular incision around the areola. Another incision extends across the axilla or armpit area. It was used for the node dissection and had a drain in it. It was also used at the time of endoscopic surgery to pull the latissimus dorsi flap through to the chest area. You can barely see that scar anymore because it is in the tissue folds. I also had a 1-inch scar on my side with a drain across my ribs. There is a 1-inch vertical incision on my scapula that I suppose was used to insert the endoscopic instruments. It was sewn up at the time of surgery and did not require drains. The drains were really pretty painful, particularly the one in the armpit. Everytime I moved my arm I felt like I had a hot poker in my armpit.

### How does your reconstructed breast feel? Is it sensitive?

Most of the sensitivity in my breast has returned. My nipple is not as sensitive as it was. My breast surgeon made an incision around it and dissected under it to do biopsies at the margins of the tumor. During that procedure some of the nerves were cut, especially around the top of the nipple. The nipple still has sensation, but it doesn't always react like the other nipple does, for example, when it's cold. It is still sexually responsive. For a while it was very sore. I didn't want to touch it. Part of that soreness was from the radiation therapy.

I didn't realize that the muscle transferred to my chest has its own blood supply, which means that it is still innervated. When I do something that moves the latissimus muscle in my back, my breast moves. When I contract the muscle in back, the muscle in my breast also contracts. The first time I reached up on a shelf to pick something up, this muscle contracted. I thought, "What is this?" Then I remembered that a woman in my support group told me that the muscle continues to function as if it were still on my back. That has been difficult to adjust to; it is a constant reminder that I have had the surgery. I can't do aerobics or cleaning or reach up for something in a cupboard without it contracting. My plastic surgeon tells me this is something that is not going to go away. If I raise my arm in a certain way, it pushes the breast up.

My reconstructed breast is warmer and somewhat firmer than the other one. I guess that is because the muscle is transferred with its blood supply and that healing is going on. The massage therapy helps to soften it a bit.

### Do you notice any other physical changes related to your surgery?

My armpit area is flatter and firmer now. It is numb, and yet it feels like something is under my arm. It is a strange sensation because you can't really feel when you are shaving. I worry about cutting myself. I actually bought a special shaver.

### Why did you decide to have immediate breast reconstruction? Did being single influence your decision?

It never crossed my mind not to. Being a single woman, I thought that I would be able to cope better with all the changes if my body image stayed intact. I didn't want to wake up from the surgery without a breast. I also felt immediate reconstruction would produce a better cosmetic result because the scars would be shorter.

### If you had it to do over again, would you have breast reconstruction? Would you choose the same procedure?

Yes, I would do it again and I would choose the same procedure. The scarring is minimal and I like the look of my breast. I think that I look the closest to the way I looked before surgery. I don't have scars that anybody is going to notice. I've been to the beach since then, and you can't tell. Most of the scars are behind the strap or on my side. Most of the time I don't think that much about having had breast cancer. It only hits me every once in a while. But everyday I am reminded that I have had reconstruction. But even that memory is fading. I have been told that it takes a year or so for those tissues to loosen up and become more normal.

### How do you tell a man in your life about your breast cancer or breast reconstruction?

I was involved in a relationship when this happened. I told him when I was going in for the biopsy. He knew about it when the lump started nagging at me, even though I was saying it was nothing. I actually had him feel it. I said, "Do you feel that? Doesn't it feel different to you?" He didn't know, but it felt different to me, so he told me to do something about it.

I called him when I was waiting for the results of my biopsy and I called him afterward. He was very supportive the whole time. He said it didn't matter and I really believed him. I know what your body looks like does matter. And it matters to your partner, but I really got the impression that that wasn't why he cared about me. I really wished at that point that I was either married or that this friend was my partner, but we had both talked about it and we knew we weren't going to be lifelong partners before this even happened.

I don't know how I am going to handle this in the future. I don't know if I am going to tell somebody up front. That is why I wanted to look as much like I did before surgery so it isn't an issue. It is amazing to me how women have complete mastectomies and choose not to have breast reconstruction. They must be truly strong and have an amazing sense of their own self-worth to go through all that and then experience all those body image changes. I didn't want that. I still worry about it. I know I don't look quite as good as I did. I don't think anybody else would really notice, but I know. Even though I am to the point of thinking I look pretty good now, what would somebody else think about it?

### How did your breast cancer therapy affect your desire for intimacy and your sexuality?

During therapy I really did not want any sort of relationship, any sort of intimacy. It just wasn't something that was of interest to me during that time. When I started having radiation therapy, it was very painful. Also, when you are having radiation therapy you have marks drawn all over you. If a woman is sensitive or hesitant about pulling her gown off in front of strangers, this would send her through the roof. You go in there every morning and you sometimes see the same technician, sometimes not. I just wish I had a buck for everybody I pulled my clothes off for in the last 18 months. But you become very unemotional about it. It turns the sexual part of it off too. Plus its very painful during that time. The skin hurts during radiation therapy. You feel like you have a bad sunburn, you're swollen, you have marks all over you, and they put plastic on you so that the marks don't come off.

During that time this man and I were still friends, but the relationship just went by the wayside. This is the time you find out if a person is supportive. After this type of experience you know whether you want to spend the rest of your life with a person. My friend and I had already agreed that we did not. So I can't say he left me because I had breast cancer.

### What advice would you give to a woman considering breast reconstruction?

For me, the process of dealing with having cancer, facing major surgery, and undergoing chemotherapy and radiation was much easier knowing that I could come out of it perhaps cured and with pretty much the same body. You go into it very frightened. Part of the terror is not knowing exactly what you are going to look like. It was comforting to know that I had this option. To know that reconstruction at the time of the initial surgery would give me a better result was a bonus. I went home with a sense that not much had really changed. I still had my breast; it was just filled in with something different. I would recommend that a woman consider immediate reconstruction. I have never wished that I had waited. I have yet to hear a woman say that she is sorry she had immediate reconstruction, but I have heard some women say they regretted waiting.

It's also important for a woman to know, however, that as good as your doctor is and as many of these procedures as he has done, he has not experienced the surgery himself. There is a tendency for surgeons to minimize the length of recovery and the discomfort that you will feel. Somehow saying, oh, you're going to have this discomfort or you're going to have this tightness doesn't cut it. I am always hearing women in the support group say, "I just didn't realize how much pain there would be or how long it would take until I felt better or until I could return to my normal level of activity!" So I would advise women to consider the recovery a year-long process that you really have to work at to get back to feeling like you did before surgery.

*What advice would you like to give to other women?*

As a child, when I had something unpleasant to do, I would always say, "I wish it were next week and this was over with." I remember my mother saying, "Deborah, you are wishing your life away." I thought of that when I started therapy, and then I realized that I do not know how much longer I have to live. Nobody does, but once cancer is brought into the equation it makes life more real. I was so determined during therapy. I thought I had no idea what percentage of the remainder of my life this year represents. It could be half the rest of my life; it could be all of the rest of my life. I am going to try to live it and enjoy it. I am going to try to get something out of every day and give back to people what they have given to me. I have been wishing my life away. I had been putting things off until I was less busy. I think I've learned to treasure the experiences that I have, good or bad, because I learn and grow from them. I have learned to treasure the people that are in my life and to tell them today because I might not be here tomorrow to say it.

I have also learned to give myself a break. I was hard on myself and afraid of not having control of everything. I wanted perfection, but this experience has taught me that all those things are really an illusion. You never really have control. Things are never really perfect. You might as well go with it and enjoy what you can and try to make it better. Use the resources that you have around you, including the people in your life, and let them help you through this. I was the epitomy of the self-contained woman who didn't really need anybody or anything. I could do everything for myself. I didn't need support. I found out through this that I do need support and I tell people that I need it now. It has become a very freeing experience. I am not sure I would say, "Gee, I'm glad I had breast cancer." And I have heard women say that. It is a terrible experience. And fear will stay with you for the rest of your life. But on the whole many more positive than negative things have come out of it for me. It has helped me to open myself up to life.

## SANDRA: YOU JUST NEVER THINK IT IS GOING TO BE YOU

"I was standing in the room undressed from the waist up. The technologist came in with my film, and I held it up to the light. I took one look at it, and I saw the breast cancer. I just stood there, and I thought to myself, I have breast cancer. I cannot believe this; I never thought it would happen to me. I have breast cancer." I was almost paralyzed, and I said to her, 'I have breast cancer!' She said, 'You can't know that.' But I knew.

"I got dressed quickly, ran to my office to get my old films, and banged on Jill's door. She is the other radiologist I work with. I banged on her door and I said, 'Jill, get over to the breast center. I have breast cancer!' I ran back over to the center and then I just collapsed and cried while she looked at the films. I kept thinking to myself, and saying over and over again, 'You just never think it is going to be you.'"

Interviewing Sandra is an electrifying experience; she is animated and intense, and I sense that she has already anticipated my questions and formulated answers long before I pose them. At 40 Sandra is a slender, energetic brunette whose straight shiny hair bounces as she talks. She has a busy career, a happy marriage, and three young children. As a radiologist at one of the country's leading medical centers, Sandra spends her working days interpreting breast x-ray films for other women. She is more knowledgeable about breast cancer than most women and has ready access to some of the leading specialists in this field.

As she speaks of that day 2 years ago when she diagnosed her own breast cancer, she is still overwhelmed by a sense of disbelief. A biopsy several days later confirmed her diagnosis. Drawing on her knowledge of breast cancer, she carefully planned her own therapy, choosing to have bilateral mastectomies: a modified radical mastectomy to treat the cancer in her left breast and a prophylactic mastectomy on her right breast. Although cancer had not yet been detected in her right breast, she knew that her odds of developing a new cancer in her opposite breast were good, and she preferred to have both breasts removed rather than live with the fear of a more serious cancer. She also knew about breast reconstruction and felt that her chances for breast symmetry would be improved if both breasts were reconstructed simultaneously. Because her cancer was localized, she did not have chemotherapy.

Six months after her cancer surgery Sandra had bilateral breast reconstruction. Her decisions about breast reconstruction were made with the same care and intelligence that she had applied to her cancer therapy. She interviewed four different plastic surgeons and explored the surgical options for breast restoration. She chose the plastic surgeon and the reconstructive approach that would achieve her personal goals. Although she originally considered a TRAM flap, a major reconstructive procedure, she eventually selected a much simpler technique, *intraoperative expansion with implant placement*. This approach required less recovery time, promised good results, and allowed her to get back to living a normal life in the shortest period of time. Her story is a compelling one.

### Did the fact that you were a physician make it easier for you to deal with your breast cancer and your decisions about treatment?

Most women have to go through a learning phase first. They start out knowing nothing about breast cancer and suddenly they are diagnosed with it. They struggle with weighing one expert's opinion and recommendation against another; they don't know what to expect next. I knew all that. I was one step ahead of where other women would be. I was trying to guess the pathology, to see whether I had an invasive cancer. I knew exactly what I wanted to know: the good prognostic signs and the bad prognostic signs. I wanted to move as quickly as possible to find out my prognosis. I wanted to know exactly how far along my cancer was, how big it was, and whether there was invasion so that I could feel comfortable with what I had to face. This waiting period was not easy for me, perhaps because I knew so much. It was one of the most intense experiences that I have ever been through. I was anxious every waking moment; I barely slept until I knew my pathology. At one point I was so tense that I just wanted to cry as loud as I could. But I knew that the kids would hear me and want to know what was wrong. So Bob took them to McDonald's and then I just cried and cried. I felt much better after that. It is amazing how crying can make you feel better. The unknown, the waiting was very tough for me. Once I knew the pathology I was fine and it was not difficult for me to make a decision about therapy.

### How did your family react?

I called my husband right away. I said, "Bob, I just had a mammogram and I have breast cancer, but I don't think I am going to die from it." He was totally speechless, then almost hysterical. We didn't tell the children until after the diagnosis was made.

### How did you tell your children?

The biopsy report was back on Monday and I was in the hospital having my cancer surgery by Thursday. I didn't waste any time because I knew what I wanted. We told the children on Wednesday night. We sat down in the family room, Bob and myself and these three little boys. They knew this was a big deal because we were having a family conference. Before we said anything, Jonathan, the little one, said, "Okay, who's dying?" Bob and I looked at each other. We thought we had kept a good secret. We tried not to let them know, but they knew anyway; they could sense the tension. We said nobody is dying. Then Bob said that I had a mammogram and Jonathan said, "And you have breast cancer, right?" He knows that mammograms are to find breast cancer. And so we said yes. We told them that there were good kinds of cancer and bad kinds of cancer. Lung cancer, for example, is a bad kind of cancer; breast cancer can be bad or good, but I had a good kind and we expected that I would be cured of it if we took care of it right. I was going to go into the hospital to have surgery to get rid of the cancer. That would be the end of it. They wanted to know if I was going to get new breasts. I said yes, but at a later time.

They wanted reassurance. They wanted to know if I was going to die? How long was I going to be in the hospital? We told them that I would go into the hospital and the doctor would take my breasts off and that would take care of the problem. I also told them that they would have to help out after I came home from the hospital since I wouldn't be feeling well for a while. I would be home for a month and that was good, because I wouldn't be working and they would get to see me a lot. They would have to be very patient and easy on me and soon I would be strong and feeling well again and that would be the end of it.

### Why did you choose a mastectomy over a lumpectomy with irradiation?

I was diagnosed with intraductal carcinoma of the comedo type. Because this type of cancer tends to have a higher recurrence rate, it doesn't do as well with lumpectomy and radiation therapy as it does with mastectomy, especially if the margins of the resected tumor are positive. Even before I knew that the margins were positive, I elected to have mastectomy because I didn't want to take a chance or worry about the possibility of local recurrence. My decision was also influenced by the fact that this tumor has an excellent prognosis if the whole thing is removed.

*Why did you choose a prophylactic mastectomy to remove the tissue from the normal breast before any diagnosis of cancer?*

I know, realistically, that people who have had one breast cancer are at higher risk for developing another breast cancer in the other breast. I wanted to minimize the chance of developing a worse lesion on the other side. This lesion that I had was theoretically curable or highly curable. Why take the risk 5 years from now of developing an invasive cancer in the other breast that might become systemic and threaten my life? That was a compelling reason for me. As it turns out, the prophylactic mastectomy was a smart move. When they removed the opposite breast and biopsied it, it showed atypical hyperplasia, a high-risk lesion. That meant I had quite a significant risk of developing breast cancer on the other side.

The fact that I am a breast imager also factored into my decision. I see women with breast cancer and I see women with second breast cancers all the time. I just couldn't have it on my mind. I wanted to do it and get it over with. I didn't want to wait year after year to see if I was going to get a second breast cancer. I also see many women with breast reconstruction. I know how difficult it is for a plastic surgeon to make the reconstructed breast and the original breast look symmetric. To me it wasn't a big deal to have the other breast removed. I wanted my breasts to match, and I wanted to minimize my chance of having a second breast cancer. So I decided to have both breasts removed and then to let a plastic surgeon reconstruct both at the same time to make them symmetric.

*How long did it take you to recover from your mastectomies?*

In 4 weeks I was back at work and able to function. I couldn't move my arms very well, but I could drive a car; I certainly could read films. I was glad to be back because I could interact with people. I worked part-time for a few weeks. After 2 months I was back in full swing, although not feeling completely well yet. That took about 3 months.

*Did you join any kind of support group?*

I didn't really need a support group. I desperately needed people; there's no question about it. I needed the support of people in my daily life. I needed them to visit me, to call me, to be solicitous, to stroke me, and to tell me they were hoping that I recovered. I had lots of support from the people that I work with. They relieved me of any clinical responsibility; I wasn't forced into stressful situations. That's the most people can do for you. It helps enormously to have people tell you that they are thinking about you and wishing for the best.

### How did your husband help you cope with this experience? Was he supportive?

He helped me by listening, taking me everywhere I needed to go, and not making any demands on me. He totally relieved me of responsibility for the kids. He interfaced with them because he knew that it would be difficult for me and they would sense my anxiety. As it turns out, they sensed it anyway. He did whatever he could for me. After all, there wasn't anything much he could do.

### Why did you decide to have your breasts reconstructed?

I had my breasts reconstructed for convenience, for my own self-esteem, and to look good again in clothes, whether or not I looked perfect in the nude. I wasn't after the perfect cosmetic result. I was annoyed with wearing prostheses. It is difficult to get comfortable prostheses, especially after a bilateral mastectomy. I got the smallest size that I could find, so they were as light as possible. Despite my efforts, they were hot and heavy and they didn't feel natural. If I wanted to go on a trip, I had to worry about how I was going to pack all this stuff; it was not convenient at all. I bought bilateral prostheses that cost over $600 ($300 apiece, plus the price of the bras, a swimsuit, etc.), and I wore them five times in 6 months. A friend of mine said, "Sandra, if you're so uncomfortable in those prostheses, don't wear them. Everybody that knows you, knows that you don't have any breasts, and we don't care. The people that don't know you, don't know if you were flat-chested before or what. Just don't wear them." So I didn't.

I walked around flat-chested for 6 months because I was symmetric and could get away with it. I did not wear my prostheses, and I felt perfectly fine and comfortable, except that I looked absolutely dreadful in clothes. There is no way that you can get clothes to drape on you; women's clothes are not made for a total flat-chested look. And we are talking about more than the normal flat-chested appearance of a woman with small breasts. With bilateral mastectomies, there is actually less subcutaneous tissue in front. I decided that I wanted to look more natural and normal and feel good about myself and the way I looked—not necessarily at home, in the nude, but in clothes to walk around every day of my life. I did not want to wear prostheses to accomplish that purpose.

### Was it difficult to face more surgery after you had just had your mastectomies?

Yes it was. I hurt and I was uncomfortable for so long. You can't sleep very well when you have bilateral mastectomies. I was flat on my back; I could not roll over in bed for 6 weeks. I was just trying to get better. I wanted desperately to be able to hug my children again and to cuddle them; they needed me to be able to do that. And I really didn't want to hurt again. I was also very tired for at least 3 months. I am a fast-moving person who likes to accomplish a lot of things in a day, so it was very annoying to me to spend 3 months dragging around. The prospect of giving up another few months of my life was not appealing. Actually, it was the experience of recuperating from the initial surgery that helped me decide what type of reconstructive method I was going to select. I wanted breast reconstruction, but I also wanted to minimize the time I had to spend recuperating.

### Did your husband support your decision to have breast reconstruction?

My husband did not want me to have reconstruction. He said, "You've been uncomfortable enough. Why would you want to have any more surgery?" He made it perfectly clear that if it was for him, not to do it. It didn't matter to him. He didn't care. But I told him that it was really for me. I didn't want to wear prostheses. I wanted to feel comfortable in clothes without having to wear a harness (that's what it feels like). It was entirely for me and not for him. Then he accepted my decision and was supportive.

### If you were interested in minimizing your recovery period, why didn't you have immediate breast reconstruction at the time of your cancer surgery?

I investigated that possibility before I had my mastectomies. I consulted with a plastic surgeon about immediate reconstruction. I decided against it primarily because the surgeon could not guarantee that I would not need blood. My surgeon assured me that he had done bilateral mastectomies for years and never had required a transfusion just for mastectomies alone, but he couldn't guarantee that I wouldn't require blood if I had bilateral reconstruction on top of that. Getting blood these days is risky. If I needed a transfusion for my reconstruction, I wanted to bank my own blood. I did not want anyone else's blood. So that was the primary factor that influenced my decision-making process.

### How did you select the method of breast reconstruction and the plastic surgeon to perform it?

I saw a total of four plastic surgeons because there was a question as to whether I was a good candidate for all the procedures. I wanted to know about all my options so I could make an informed decision. There are a variety of different methods of reconstruction.

I investigated having the TRAM flap, but found that it would be very difficult because I did not have enough abdominal fat. I went to see several plastic surgeons about this. One told me that with as little abdominal fat as I had he would probably have to put implants under the bilateral TRAM flaps to make my breasts large enough. I decided that if I was going to go through major surgery for the TRAM flap, probably more major than the original mastectomy with a much longer recuperation period, then why put implants under my reconstructed breasts. That would defeat the purpose of natural reconstruction with my own abdominal tissue. In addition to that, I wasn't willing to sacrifice a year of my life: 3 months off work, 3 months feeling lousy, and 6 months of not feeling myself. That was too much. Time is very precious. I feel a sense of urgency to get on with my life and enjoy what I have. My priorities were totally reestablished after facing a cancer operation.

Tissue expansion was another option that I explored. Two plastic surgeons that I consulted suggested that I have tissue expanders placed bilaterally and then later, in a second procedure, after my tissues had been stretched, have the expanders replaced with implants.

Then I went to see another plastic surgeon out of town who reviewed all of the options for me, listened to my expectations, and suggested a different approach. He said that he could use intraoperative expansion and put the implants in to reconstruct my breasts in a single operation, rather than the two-stage reconstruction required for tissue expansion. If I wanted to have nipple-areola reconstruction, I could have that at a later time as a minor outpatient procedure. I elected to have the one-stage intraoperative expansion with implant placement. I felt more confident with that particular surgeon, but also it was an easier, one-step procedure with a shorter recuperation time.

### Was your reconstructive surgery painful and how long did it take you to recuperate?

After reconstruction I had lots of nausea from the narcotics they were giving me. I never pushed the PCA (patient-controlled analgesia) button to get more pain medication; it was already giving me more than I could handle. As soon as I weaned myself from that, I felt much better. Tylenol worked just fine, without the nausea. My level of pain and discomfort, while still significant, was not nearly as bad as with my mastectomies, and I was able to go back to work in 10 days.

### How did your breasts look and feel during the first few weeks after surgery?

I have seen so much breast reconstruction that I thought that I would know exactly how I would look and feel when I had it done. But I was wrong. I didn't expect my breasts to be as swollen, tight, and shiny as they became.

The swelling and blueness didn't show up during the 3 days I spent in the hospital. Then my husband and I went to a hotel so that I could be watched to make sure everything was okay before I flew back home. In the hospital I was elevated in this nice hospital bed, sitting almost erect, and there wasn't much swelling. At the hotel I just propped myself up on a couple of pillows; I could barely get out of bed because I was sore and bruised. When I woke up the following morning, my reconstructed breasts were so swollen and tight that I was afraid that they were going to just burst open. (This from someone who is informed . . . who knows what happened to her.) I had dreams that if I sneezed or coughed the seams would open up and the implants would go into orbit. I had this vision of them popping out, so I was afraid to sneeze or cough. Of course, that was totally unfounded. But that's how tight my breasts felt.

They also became totally blue, like two giant ripe blueberries. That wasn't immediate; blue took about a week. They were so swollen and blue. My husband was horrified looking at them. I was blue from my chest above the incisions down to my hips. I spent the weekend looking at those tight, blue, swollen breasts and worrying about them.

### Was your plastic surgeon responsive to your concerns?

Yes. He was very responsive and reassuring. In fact, the reason we stayed in the hotel was to see the plastic surgeon before we went home. When I told him how I had imagined the implants popping out, he laughed and said, "You know too much to think that's going to happen. This is fine, a normal postoperative course; your breasts will do just great." Then, of course, I was relieved. And he was right. That all resolved, everything softened, and my breasts have turned out fine.

### Did you have any late problems or complications?

I had some sutures coming through the skin when I was on vacation. That was a little bit difficult to handle, but it turned out to be relatively minor. I called my plastic surgeon on the phone, and he told me to clip the end of the exposed stitch and that problem was handled very well. Other than that I have had no problems. I have healed as expected, and over time my breasts have softened and become more natural looking.

### Was your reconstructive surgery covered by insurance?

Yes, it was, and we have several policies, but insurance companies are not happy to pay for breast reconstruction. It makes me very angry. When I first called my insurance company (my husband has coverage with a different company), they gave me the run-around. The first person I spoke to said that they would not cover breast reconstruction because it was cosmetic. I said, "I know better—I am a physician. You are not correct. How dare you say this to anybody on the telephone. Of course it's covered. Let me speak to somebody else." Then they referred me to somebody else. And I said, "I am contemplating having reconstructive breast surgery and I want to know what you pay. I want to know what my out-of-pocket expenses will be." And they said, "We can't tell you what we pay. We pay 80% of the usual and customary fee." I said okay, "What is the usual and customary fee?" They said, "We can't tell you that." I said, "What do you mean you can't tell me. I am contemplating very expensive surgery. When I buy a car I want to know what it is going to cost before I buy the car. I don't expect to get a bill after I buy the car to find out then how much it is going to cost me. I want to know ahead of time." They refused to tell me. So I called the CEO's office, and I told him who I was and I described the run-around that I had gotten. I asked him how they dared to treat people this way. Didn't they realize that there are many people who might forego breast reconstruction because they fear being saddled with enormous bills. It was terrible to do this to people. The CEO said that he would call me back, and he did 48 hours later to tell me the usual and customary fee they paid for breast reconstruction. It was pitifully poor. Then I called my husband's insurance company to find out what they would pay. They also told me they couldn't tell me, but they did, sooner than my insurance company. And they provided better reimbursement for the surgeon. So my breast reconstruction was covered by two policies that we had, major medical in addition to my husband's policy. But I was incensed at the way it was handled.

### Have you had your nipple and areola reconstructed?

Initially I thought, yes. I'm going to do the whole wad. I'm going to do everything. I'm going to do anything that I feel like doing. But I changed my mind. I feel comfortable with my breasts as they are now. It accomplishes what I wanted. I look good in clothes. I don't have to wear prostheses. I don't have to go through any more surgery, and I don't want to. I don't need it; my breasts look very symmetric. They're soft. They look great in a bathing suit, in a nightgown, and in clothes. That is what I wanted.

### Has reconstruction affected the way you feel about yourself?

In terms of self-esteem and self-image I can't say that reconstruction has made that big a difference. I value myself enough, with or without my breasts. I did it more for convenience and physical appearance, to feel good about the way I look. I don't feel that my breasts, before or after the surgery, are what makes or breaks me.

### Are your reconstructed breasts sensitive? Are they warm?

They're not sensitive. There is pressure sensation, but it's not the same sort of discrimination that you have when you touch the rest of your skin that has normal nerve endings. They are also a little bit cooler than the rest of the body.

### Are you satisfied with your breast reconstruction? If you had to do it all over, would you choose to have breast reconstruction again?

Without a doubt, yes. It was worth it for me. It was relatively easy compared to the original surgery, and I am pleased with the results. My breasts are symmetric, soft, and squeezable. My kids like to snuggle up. I know that when they get cuddly against my chest, they are thinking those are Mom's new breasts and they feel nice and soft. Nobody can tell. If somebody came up and touched my chest, there is no way to know. My breasts feel very natural and normal.

### What advice would you like to give to other women considering breast reconstruction?

Become informed. Investigate all of the options so that you can make a choice that meets your personal needs. Identify your goals. Why are you considering breast reconstruction? What do you expect to get out of it? Do you want to look as natural naked as you possibly can or just to look good in clothing? How much time do you want to invest? If you are thinking about a more lengthy procedure, you need to assess what it will cost in time and money. How are you going to pay for it? It is crucial to know what your expectations are. Once these questions are answered, you need to know about all of the different reconstructive procedures before choosing a particular method. You can't just go to somebody and have him tell you this is the surgery for you. There is no such answer. You must have input. First, you must be able to state what your goals are. How do you want to look? How much are you willing to go through to achieve that look? Then, when you feel informed, when you know all of your options, and only then, can you make the best decision for you.

## MAGGIE: A WOMAN'S SEXUALITY

"Flamboyant" was the word she proudly used to describe herself, and I had to smile at the accuracy of her self-assessment. An imposing woman of 5 feet 8 inches, Maggie has an air of self-assurance that dominates her conversation. She is also somewhat of a flashy dresser, which only serves to complement her personality. The day of our interview she was dressed in a bright red blouse draped in comfortable folds over her ample bosom. Her waist was cinched by a gold belt, several gold chains encircled her neck, and her long fingers tapered into finely manicured nails, lacquered in bright red to match her lipstick. She wore black slacks and black high heels and her black hair was carefully coiffured in a short, bouffant style. Her gold bracelets clinked as she talked to me about the importance of breasts and sex appeal to women of all ages and why she, as a widow in her early sixties, felt it was particularly important to have breast reconstruction.

Maggie's striking appearance is consistent with her open and appealingly honest personality. She likes herself and the image she portrays; she was determined not to let breast cancer diminish her body image or make her uncomfortable interacting with others. Her cancer was discovered when she was widowed after 34 years of a happy marriage; one married daughter lived in a nearby town. Even though she was involved in a busy career in retail lingerie, she did not want to spend the rest of her life without a partner. She liked socializing and also frankly admitted that she liked her breasts just as they were. She had always worn clothing that was "sexy" and she "didn't want to change her image now." Of particular importance was her desire to be able to feel free to engage in an intimate relationship without inhibition. Therefore, when she was diagnosed as having breast cancer, she was determined not to delay breast restoration any longer than necessary.

Living in a small town, she did not have an experienced reconstructive surgeon available to consult, so she undertook her own research to find out all she could about the different types of reconstructive operations and the best surgeons to perform them. She decided to have a *delayed TRAM flap breast reconstruction*. Although this was one of the more complicated procedures, she selected it because she did not want an artificial substance in her body. As Maggie explained, "I'm an original and I want everything about me to be real." Even though immediate breast reconstruction was not an option for her, she was determined that the delay would be as brief as possible to curtail the period of breast loss. Her deadline was to have her breast reconstruction completed and be totally recovered 1 year after her mastectomy. She set about this goal with style, humor, and determination. Now, 3 years later, this gutsy lady has remarried and is enjoying life more than ever. Sometimes Maggie even forgets that her reconstructed breast is not her original one.

### How did you discover your breast cancer?

I found a lump while I was examining my breasts in the shower. I had fibrocystic breasts, so I had lumps before, but this one felt different. It seemed to be attached to the skin; with the others the overlying skin was more movable. I decided to follow up with my gynecologist. He referred me to a surgeon who sent me for a mammogram and suggested a biopsy. When I came out of the anesthesia after the biopsy, my daughter was there and she told me they had found a malignancy.

### What was your reaction to your cancer diagnosis?

I wanted to know how bad my cancer was and what was going to happen to me. When my doctor told me that I was going to need a mastectomy, I told him that I couldn't have one. I was alone. I was unmarried. My breast was a very important part of my body. I felt that I needed my breast if I was to get on with my life. I just couldn't have a mastectomy, but he said that I must. That's when I started my research. I needed to find out quickly what my options were.

### What type of research did you conduct to investigate your options?

I got on the phone and started calling people. I had heard of a lady in my town, a friend of a friend, who had a mastectomy and breast reconstruction; I called her. I contacted everybody I could think of. I even called people in other states. Somebody would know of somebody and I would call. This was all new to me. I am the kind of person who wants to know what lies ahead of her and what is the best direction to go. In 3 days I did quite a bit of research, and I learned about cancer treatment and breast reconstruction.

### *Why was reconstruction so important to you?*

My mother's oldest sister had breast cancer. She had her mastectomy many years ago and she never had reconstruction. To me it was a horrible sight. I felt that I would have to change my image if I lost my breast. I am a flamboyant dresser. I have always liked low, revealing clothes. I am that kind of person, that's just me; I have been that way from the age of 16. I didn't want to lose my breast. I liked me. Even though I was not involved intimately with a man at that time, I did not feel that I could ever be comfortable with the opposite sex if I had only one breast.

### *How did you learn about reconstruction? What type of reconstructive technique did you select?*

I heard about reconstruction through my phone calls to women with cancer. I would call these people and ask them questions. "Did you have reconstruction?" "Where did you have it?" "What was it like?" "Who did your surgery?" "Were you satisfied?" I never spoke to anybody who had anything but implants, but I knew flaps were being done because I had read about these techniques in some books. I decided early on that I didn't want implants. I am not that kind of person. I've never wanted false teeth. I've never wanted anything artificial if it was possible to have the other. I would settle for implants before I would do without, but I wanted the best, and I felt that my own tissue was best. I also wanted immediate reconstruction so I wouldn't have to go without my breast.

### *Were you able to have immediate reconstruction?*

No. As it turned out my cancer surgeon did not feel comfortable with my having a TRAM flap or with the idea of immediate reconstruction. At that time there was no local plastic surgeon who could have performed the tummy flap. My cancer surgeon's focus was on saving my life and getting all of the cancer removed. He felt that I shouldn't delay treatment but should go ahead and get my cancer taken care of immediately. Even though I desperately wanted my breast, I decided that I was putting the cart before the horse. I wanted my doctor at home to do my mastectomy because he had a very good name. I also felt that he would take a more personal interest in getting all the cancer. Since there really wasn't anyone in town who could have done the reconstructive surgery, immediate reconstruction was out of the question. So I had my mastectomy and then I was ready for reconstruction. And despite my cancer surgeon's warning that no plastic surgeon would touch me for 6 months, I was determined to get my breast back sooner.

### How long did it take you to recover from your mastectomy? What was your emotional reaction to the surgery? Did you experience much pain?

The pain wasn't too bad. I had my surgery on Tuesday and checked out of the hospital on Friday morning. The mental anguish was much worse than the pain. I didn't let anyone except my mother see me without a breast. I had the surgery at 9 o'clock in the morning and that afternoon I sent my mother out to get an artificial breast to put in my gown. I still insisted on wearing my low nightgown, and I lay there very straight so that nobody could tell that the prosthesis was pinned in my very sexy nightgown. I wondered if I could go on with my life. After all, I had lost something very important to me, something that made me a whole person. I couldn't concentrate on the pain; breast reconstruction occupied my thoughts. I'm impatient that way. If I have anything facing me, good or bad, I am anxious to get on with it.

### How did you find the plastic surgeon to perform your TRAM flap breast reconstruction?

I had heard about him from several of the women I talked to. He had a good name, and he was at a major medical center. I decided to consult with him. If I didn't like him, I could always go to someone else in the city. I live in a small town, and I just felt that a major medical center was the best place to go. I went to see the plastic surgeon just 3 weeks after my mastectomy. As it turned out, he suited me just fine, so I didn't need to consult with anyone else.

### What was your consultation like? Why did you decide to select this plastic surgeon to perform your breast reconstruction?

I came all dressed up and in my high heels. I was afraid that because of what I had heard about a 6-month delay, he wouldn't operate on me right away. My goal was to have everything complete, behind me, and out of my mind as much as possible within a year. When I was filling out my medical history, I would not write down the month that I had my mastectomy. I just wrote the year. I made up my mind before I went into the plastic surgeon's office that I had to stay in control. I wanted to tell him what I wanted and what I could stand; I wanted it my way. If he had not listened to me, I would have gone elsewhere.

At the beginning of our consultation he asked me why I had come to him for reconstruction. I said, "Because I heard you are the best and I won't have anything but the best. I don't want implants. I want a TRAM flap." I just told him exactly what I wanted. Later, when he saw me undressed, he said, "When did you have this done?" I said, "It doesn't matter when I had it done; I want this reconstruction done during your first opening. I want it now." He grinned. He is a quiet, laid-back person, so it was easy for me to stay in control, which I liked. I loved him from day one. A woman in this state of mind doesn't need sympathy, but she needs someone who is calm and gentle. I felt his caring from the time that he started talking to me. He smiled and said, "We'll have to see when I have the next opening." I said, "You're going to do me?" and he said, "Yes, but this type of surgery is not for everybody." He did not paint a very pretty picture.

### What did he tell you about the TRAM flap? Did he describe the risks and benefits? Did you understand that this was a major operative procedure?

He said that the TRAM flap was painful. You have to be in good health and it can be time consuming, possibly 6 hours of surgery with a long time for full recovery. He also said that several steps or different operations are usually needed to get the breast and abdomen to look just right. He explained that it would probably take close to 9 months to a year to complete it, the nipple and everything. I would need to have blood transfusions. I said I would give my own blood because I didn't want anybody else's blood. He thought that was a good idea. He told me that it was a hard surgery. He said I would have to be off work for quite a while. He told me about all the possible complications. He explained them in great detail so that I would understand what I was getting myself into. Of course, I didn't listen, not really, because I know me and he didn't. If he would do his job, then I could do mine. My plastic surgeon gave me a book to read when I left his office. Even with all of this information, I did not realize what I was facing; only experience can teach you that. As far as I was concerned, I felt I could tolerate anything for a few days in order to have peace of mind and to feel whole again.

### Did your plastic surgeon take pictures of you during your consultation?

My plastic surgeon took pictures of me from my first visit through my final operation; he took some before and then some each time I had another surgery. It is uncomfortable for any woman to be totally undressed in front of a stranger, no matter if it's your doctor, and have him taking pictures of you. I'd joke about it because I was uncomfortable. I'd say, "Why are you making all these pictures? Am I going to be in *Playboy*?"

### Was your plastic surgeon reluctant to perform your reconstruction just 3 weeks after your mastectomy? Did you have to make any special preparations to meet that deadline?

He said, "You know it's been just 3 weeks since you had this other surgery." I said, "I know but I am very healthy despite the breast cancer. I am also very headstrong and determined to do this." So he agreed to operate on me in 3 weeks; that made 6 weeks to the day since my mastectomy. But he let me know that I was pushing it. I would have to follow his directions to get ready or else my breast reconstruction would have to be delayed. I was happy with that. I said, "You tell me what to do and I will do it. I will be ready." Normally he asks a person to do sit-ups to improve blood circulation to the abdominal tissue. I would still have to do these exercises, but I would have less time. He also said, "You have to give 3 pints of blood in the next 3 weeks—that's going to be tough." He gave me iron tablets. He told me to eat all the raisins I could, the rarest meat, livers—the blood-building foods. I did exactly what he said and more. I did my sit-ups; I ate raisins at work all day. Every week when I went to give blood they would say I was on the borderline and probably wouldn't make it the next week. But I did. I was able to give my 3 pints, and in 6 weeks to the day I checked into the hospital to have reconstruction.

### How long did it take you to recuperate from your reconstructive surgery? Did you experience much pain?

The reconstructive surgery lasted $4\frac{1}{2}$ hours. Afterward, when they rolled me to my room, they bumped my bed. I knew then I was in bad shape. I hurt all over from my breast to my lower abdomen. The pain was concentrated more in my abdomen than it was in my breast, but it was all connected. When they transfer the muscle to the breast, they open a tunnel from the abdominal area to the breast area, so there is a large area that needs to heal.

I had four or five drain tubes coming out of my abdomen and breast, a catheter, a morphine pump for pain, and oxygen. The next morning when two nurses came to get me up, the pain was almost unbearable. One of the nurses, unfortunately, wasn't well trained in how to get a person back into the bed. She let me fall back, which was the worst thing. I had stitches and it hurt terribly. I know the morphine helped, but by the third day it was making me deathly ill and I told the nurse to take the pain pump out. I felt I could tolerate the pain better than I could tolerate the nausea. I told them I would ask for a shot if the pain got too bad.

Knowing that they had taken part of a muscle and transferred it, I had this horror of not being able to straighten up, like an old woman. So my next step was to get on my feet to see how far I could straighten up. I was looking forward to that although I knew it was going to be like death itself. I surprised myself when I did get up to go to the bathroom on the third day. I was still quite bent over, but I knew if I kept on I would be able to straighten up pretty soon because I wasn't as bad off as I expected. I am very tall, 5 foot 8 inches. A little person wouldn't have as far to stretch as I did. It was very important to me to be erect again, so I really worked on it. By the fifth day I was in the hall walking, taking tiny steps. I had to hold on to the rail, but I was straight.

I was in the hospital 8 or 9 days. When I left the hospital, I stayed with my mother for a week and a half. During that time I was not always able to dress because I was so sore that I could hardly stand for anything to touch me. Even so, I exercised. I found a flat place in my mom's yard, and five or six times a day, with just my night clothes and my tennis shoes on, I would walk one way and then another and then I would go lie down. Then I would walk again. Three weeks after my surgery my daughter asked me to go to a shopping center with her. I called a hospital equipment store, rented a wheelchair, and went shopping in a wheelchair. I was totally exhausted when I got home. I could hardly stand any bumps, but I did it. I still had on the stretch halter top they had given me in the hospital to wear over the bandage. I wore my clothes and jacket over that.

It took 2 to 3 months before I felt like myself again. As far as the pain was concerned, the first step of the reconstruction was the most painful. The rest was a breeze.

### What was done during this first step of your breast reconstruction?

I was cut from one side of my abdomen to the other, all the way in front. The abdominal skin was then grafted from the navel to the hairline to move up to my breast with the accompanying abdominal muscle (the rectus abdominis muscle) and fat to give me enough skin and tissue to build a breast. It is my understanding that this flap of abdominal muscle and tissue was threaded up through a tunnel into the left side; that's where my mastectomy was. Then my plastic surgeon shaped a breast from it. He also had to make a new navel. I have a very pretty navel, almost as good as Mother gave me.

### Was your breast what you expected after the first stage of reconstruction?

I had been told what to expect, but it's always a surprise when you see yourself after surgery. It was difficult to face the scars. I didn't expect my stomach to feel so hard; it was also numb and that lack of sensation was quite disturbing to me. It resembled the numbness you experience after you have Novocaine at the dentist; you know you are touching something, but it has no feeling. My breast was also numb, but I was expecting that. Even so, it still felt strange and it looked funny without a nipple.

I had more swelling than I had anticipated. Immediately after my operation the area under my breast where my flap was tunneled was swollen as big as another breast. I worried if it would ever go down. That was my first question to my plastic surgeon. He assured me that the swelling would go down, and if it didn't, he would take care of it during the next step of surgery. That eased my mind because I had all the confidence in the world in this doctor. I knew that after a few more operations he could make me look the way I wanted to. I was anxious to get on with it. I kept asking when he planned to do the next step.

### What other procedures or steps were required to complete your breast reconstruction?

I had some hardening under the arm; that's where my lymph nodes had been stripped. You could feel stitches. It felt like scar tissue. It was a hard knot and it pooched out. In the second step he took care of that; he reopened the incision, removed that tissue, and it was fine. It bothered me that he had to make another little scar on my breast to remedy that situation. When I looked at it I thought, "Oh Lord, another scar."

He also suctioned the swollen area under my breast that I was so concerned about. By this time it had shrunk to the size of a lemon, so there wasn't much contouring to do. In the lower abdomen on each side where he started and finished the incision, I had little areas of skin that seemed to hang over. He called them "dog ears." He told me not to worry about these dog ears because he planned to use them to get tissue grafts for my nipple-areola reconstruction. Fortunately, one side leveled out and we didn't disturb it; he got his graft from the other side.

### Why did you decide that you wanted nipple-areola reconstruction?

To make the reconstructed breast look like the other breast. It would not have been complete otherwise. I knew I had gone through the worst and I would never settle for an unfinished job.

### Did he tattoo your reconstructed nipple-areola, and if so, was it a good match with your opposite nipple-areola?

Yes, I had a tattoo and, no, the match is not good. I hurried too much for the first tattoo. I was so determined to get it all done. They told me that they felt they were doing the tattoo too soon. It might not take because the tissue had not healed enough. It didn't. I had to have it done over, but the match still isn't good. My plastic surgeon is not happy with the coloring on the tattoo and neither am I. It's too dark. I have a lot of yellow tones in my skin and that is one of the hardest colors to match. My plastic surgeon has said that he can take care of it.

### Did you have any complications, any problems?

No. It just took some time to recuperate, but I really didn't have any trouble.

### What were your primary goals in having reconstruction?

To be like I was. I never thought that I had the prettiest breasts in the world, but once I had lost one, I wanted a replacement just like the old one. Until you lose something, you never appreciate it; you take it for granted. I didn't really want any miracles. I didn't expect to mess with nature. Nature does a great deal for most people. But once I had lost my breast, then I felt I owed it to myself to find a way to restore what cancer took away.

### Are you satisfied with the appearance of your breast? Is it soft, natural? Does it have feeling?

Yes. I cannot tell now that it has not been there forever. I also cannot tell any difference in feeling. I was told by my plastic surgeon that I would not have any feeling in this breast, no sensation. But I am one of the fortunate ones; I do have feeling now, but no sexual feeling. The nipple has no feeling, but all around the breast and at different places on the breast I know when I'm touched. When they did the tattooing, they had to numb me. They were quite surprised because I had feeling.

### Where are your scars located and how do they look?

The scarring is disturbing. I have a scar completely around the breast on the left side and an inch long V-shaped scar extending onto my breast from my underarm. I also have a scar that extends across my entire lower abdomen. But now my scars are fading into hairline scars that are more acceptable.

### If you had the choice to make over again, would you choose to have breast reconstruction? Would you select the same technique? Was it worth the pain, the time away from work, the expense?

Yes. I think the direction I went was best for me. I don't know anything that I could have done to make it turn out any better. I have been totally pleased. I feel complete. I feel attractive again. I feel comfortable undressing in front of a man. I look good in my clothes again. I can go on with my life.

### How does breast cancer and breast reconstruction affect a woman's relationship with a man? Is it difficult when you are single and dating? What are the worries?

Divorced, widowed, or single women have mastectomies and reconstruction just the same as married women who have companions and support. At the time of my mastectomy I was not involved in a sexual relationship, and it would have been impossible for me to consider one with only one breast. Even though I had reconstruction, I wondered how I could explain what had happened to me. I wondered if a man would feel that I was complete, sensuous. Then I decided that any man that doesn't accept me as I am isn't worth my time. This sounded good, but I still had to give myself a pep talk every time I went out on a date. When I met a guy, I would think about how I would tell him. When you are dating, this is a worry. Most men like to love a woman and a woman likes to be loved; a breast is an important part of that. Even if you don't have a sexual relationship with a man, the first thing most men do after they get pretty well acquainted with you is fondle your breasts. I didn't tell anybody about my breast, however, unless our relationship developed and I saw that I was going to undress. Then before I reached that point, I would prepare him for what I had to say. I would begin by telling him that I had breast cancer and had a mastectomy and breast reconstruction. Sometimes I wouldn't go any further. It was surprising how the men related; I don't think it made a difference to anyone I became involved with. And men don't hide their feelings well. Usually they were shocked to hear about it at first, and then they would say, "Well, if it weren't for the scars, you couldn't tell you've had anything done." I said, "That's right, and in time it will be less visible."

### When you met your present husband, what was his reaction to your breast reconstruction?

I met him through a friend, and we had several phone conversations prior to our face-to-face meeting. Of course, I didn't tell him anything about my surgery at that time. I really didn't even like the guy the first meeting. He continued to call me though. Several weeks later I was coming to the city where he lived, so I called him and told him that I was going to be there. He insisted on taking me to dinner. At dinner we talked and found out we had mutual interests and that we both liked to travel. When he asked if I wanted to go to Nashville with him that weekend, I surprised myself by saying yes.

I like to dance and sing and I was looking forward to a good time in Nashville. It didn't worry me that I had this reconstructed breast and would have to tell him about it. That wasn't on my mind until the time came. That's the way that I handled it with everybody I met. So I didn't think the breast would make or break my relationship.

That night we checked into a motel and made dinner arrangements at a nice steak place. I thought, "Well, I like this guy and I'm probably going to wind up in the bed with him." Before we went out to dinner, I pointed over to the other bed and told him to sit down because I had a story to tell him. He sat down and I said, "I had cancer a year ago and I had to have a breast removed." I was always a little "hyper" about telling someone even though I never thought I was. As I was telling my story, I looked over and big tears started rolling down his face. He reached over embraced me and kissed me. I asked him, "What are you crying for?" Here's this big old 300-pound man crying and I'm the one who's had the surgery. He said, "You're just the most remarkable person that I have ever seen in my life." You know, I had several male friends that I dated after having my breast reconstruction who said the same thing to me. They said, "You're marvelous. I admire you, and there is nothing to be ashamed of." I always told them that I wasn't ashamed of it; I just felt that I should tell them in case they questioned the scars. I think that men accept this better than women accept it themselves.

## What advice would you like to give to other women considering breast reconstruction?

A woman at any age owes it to herself to consider breast reconstruction. It does wonders for you mentally. It helps you to bypass self-pity and move on to life.

## JEAN: THE FABRIC OF A LIFE

Jean arrived at our interview fresh from the health club still dressed in a black Lycra jumpsuit, an oversized purple T-shirt and running shoes. She wore no makeup and her short, light-brown hair curled softly with the perspiration from her recent workout. Her headphones were draped around her neck and she turned off her radio as she lowered herself into the chair. At 48, Jean is the picture of health—young, slender, and athletic.

From her demeanor and ready smile, few people would suspect the hardships she has faced. Jean is no stranger to breast cancer and grief. Her mother was diagnosed with the disease when she was still premenopausal, in her forties. She died 10 years later after two bouts with breast cancer, two radical mastectomies, and two courses of chemotherapy and radiation therapy. Jean vividly remembers her Mother's strength during her 10-year illness and marvels at how truly remarkable she was. Her example has fortified Jean during her own struggles.

Because of her family history of breast cancer, Jean was meticulous about breast monitoring. It was during one of her annual mammograms that her cancer was discovered. She underwent 3 years of treatment—a lumpectomy, bilateral mastectomies, two courses of chemotherapy and radiation therapy, and *bilateral breast reconstruction with gluteus maximus free flaps.* Throughout this long process she grew to rely on her own judgment, to research her treatment options, and to express her needs. Her assertiveness was not always welcomed. Her first surgeon made it clear that "he was the doctor and he would make the decisions." They came to a permanent parting of ways when he refused to perform the bilateral mastectomies she requested to treat her second breast cancer. He suggested that she was crazy to take such action and clearly did not know what she was doing. This was a particularly traumatic time for her. She and her husband had just suffered the unbearable loss of their 16-year-old daughter from cystic fibrosis. But she used her daughter's lifestyle example to move beyond her sorrow.

She refused to lose confidence in her ability to make decisions. She got a second opinion and found another doctor who was more responsive to her needs. He agreed with her decision for bilateral mastectomies and agreed to perform them. She had the bilateral mastectomies and later, after thoroughly investigating her options, decided to have *bilateral gluteus maximus (buttock) free flap breast reconstruction.* Jean took control of her health care decisions and gained a new sense of empowerment. As Jean explained, "For me, the ultimate satisfaction came from being knowledgeable. I participated and made decisions rather than allowing someone to tell me what to do and how to feel. There is a certain amount of power in knowing you are a partner in the decision-making process."

Jean is delighted with the decisions that she has made. When I asked about her satisfaction with her results, she slipped off her T-shirt, pulled down her jumpsuit, and proudly let me see for myself. Her story is a compelling one of courage and determination.

## How old were you when your cancer was diagnosed? How did you react?

I was 42 when I first learned I had breast cancer. It did not come as a total shock to me because my mother developed premenopausal breast cancer in her mid-forties. She had a radical mastectomy with radiation and chemotherapy. In the seventh year she developed a second cancer in the opposite breast and had the same treatment. She lived 3 years longer. I was 20 when I lost my mother. Breast cancer became part of my life at an early age. She was a wonderful example for me. She joyously marched through life despite the cancer. She was a golfer, and I don't think she ever missed a round of golf because of her illness. With that history, I wouldn't say that I was surprised by my diagnosis.

### Considering your family history, what was your routine for monitoring your breasts?

My first mammogram was at age 35 and I got them annually after that. I had small, thin breasts with lots of dense tissue, lumps, and bumps that were hard to read radiographically. When I reached 40, my OB/GYN told me that once a mammogram report becomes a paragraph, you know you're in trouble. He wanted someone besides himself checking me, so he sent me to a breast surgeon. From then on, in addition to my yearly mammograms I had two physical examinations.

### How was your breast cancer diagnosed? What was the proposed treatment? What part did you play in the decision-making process?

The cancer first appeared as a small area of microcalcifications on my yearly mammogram. You begin to learn about those little white spots, and I could see them clearly. Although my surgeon told me that it was highly unlikely that this was breast cancer, I insisted on a biopsy as a precaution. It revealed intraductal infiltrating carcinoma. With my family history, I asked for a mastectomy. Once again, he insisted it was the wrong thing to do. All the latest research showed that lumpectomy with radiation was as good as mastectomy. I did a literature search and found that to be true. But I still wasn't convinced, so my surgeon sent me to consult with other specialists who supported that treatment approach. They convinced me that I was too young to lose a breast, and the cancer was too small to justify a mastectomy. I had a lumpectomy with follow-up radiation and then started investigating chemotherapy. My oncologist and I reviewed the current research; chemotherapy was not advised for such a small cancer that was node negative. But I had a gem of an oncologist who knew my family history and my feelings. He agreed to support my decision for chemotherapy even though he wasn't in complete agreement. I felt very good that the decision was being left to me. Since my cancer was microscopic, I decided why not take every precaution, even if I only decreased my risk of recurrence by a small percentage. So I had the whole ball of wax. I had surgery, radiation, and chemotherapy. I was confident I had made the right decision. Later this decision was confirmed by reports from the breast cancer clinical trial indicating that young women with small, node-negative cancers did well with chemotherapy. I thought, yes. I did the right thing.

### How was your second cancer discovered?

A year later a follow-up mammogram revealed the exact same pattern of microcalcifications almost in the identical location, just next to the surgical margin. It was interpreted as normal with a recommendation for a repeat mammogram in a year. I had heard that story before. Those little spots looked exactly the same as the previous ones. I couldn't believe it! My brother is a radiologist and I asked him for a second opinion. He reviewed my films and saw the same pattern as before. He recommended follow-up with a biopsy. To confirm that he wasn't being an overprotective brother, he had four other radiologists view the films without telling them whose films they were. They all recommended biopsy. With the force of such unified opinion, my breast care team agreed to do a biopsy. Once again the biopsy revealed in situ cancer. This time I was adamant in my insistence that I wanted mastectomy, not a single mastectomy but bilateral mastectomies—a mastectomy to treat the cancer and a prophylactic mastectomy to remove the other breast as a precaution.

### What was your surgeon's response to your request for bilateral mastectomies? Was he supportive?

I had already had several head-to-head confrontations with my surgeon. He said I was still too young and he would not perform bilateral mastectomies when the cancer was confined to one breast.

### Why was your surgeon so resistant?

He didn't think I knew enough to be part of the decision-making process. I would not cooperate. We argued through every decision, starting with the original biopsy and the original surgery. When I read the literature and asked, "Should this test or that test be done? Was I a candidate for this or that?" he literally would get red in the face. One time he stood up and actually screamed at me over the desk that "he understood where I was coming from. He knew that women felt like they had to know all there was to know. When I went through medical school, read every journal, and knew how to do surgery, then he would have these types of discussions with me. Until that time I couldn't possibly know enough to make these decisions. *He* was the doctor and *he* would make the decisions."

### How did you handle these confrontations?

I told him that he misunderstood; I only needed to be a specialist in one teeny-tiny subject—my breast cancer. This was linked to one diagnosis, in one area, and I could get all the information I needed because I knew how to use a library. I didn't need to be a surgeon or an oncologist or to know everything there was to know. I only needed to know about my one problem, the clinical trials that were ongoing, and the options for treatment. With this information, I could participate in making decisions about my care. If he didn't want to participate with me, then this relationship was not going to work.

This confrontation was really hard for me. I was dealing with far more than cancer and an arrogant doctor. My cancer was diagnosed just 2 months after I lost my only daughter to cystic fibrosis. She died in my arms at the age of 16. I was in the midst of the most profound grief that anyone can experience. It was difficult to even focus on the problem, much less know what to do. My first thought was that it would be really easy not to deal with it at all and just let the doctors make all the decisions for me. My life was in turmoil then and it would be easier to take the path of least resistance. I seriously considered that route.

### How did your daughter's memory influence your decisions about your own health care? What was the turning point?

I thought about my daughter and how she would have dealt with those decisions. She lived a very full life for 16 years, despite the suffering from lung disease. No one who met her ever knew about her problems, nor did they ever stop her. She was fourth in her class and died as an honor roll student who had not missed a day of school that year. She was a person who did not give up; she was not a quitter. The legacy of her lifestyle wouldn't allow me to be a coward. That was a turning point for me. I decided to trust myself to determine what treatment was right for me. It was an affirmation of life. It ushered me through the grieving process and gave me the confidence I needed.

### Why did you get a second opinion?

When I chose my surgeon, I had hoped that he would treat me as a partner in my health care decisions. But here he was telling me that I was incapable of making decisions about my own health care. We had established a tenuous relationship to get through the first surgery. Now, with the second cancer, he is telling me that he'll only do a mastectomy on the side with the double cancer. I couldn't accept that. It kept coming back to me that I had asked him for the mastectomy the first time. Would it have been different if he had done what I requested? I decided I needed to work through this decision with someone who would listen to me and respect my opinions. I felt strongly about the need for bilateral mastectomy after watching my mother die. So I decided to get a second opinion.

### What did your second opinion reveal? Why did you decide to switch surgeons?

The surgeon I chose for a second opinion was highly recommended by three or four people whose judgment I respected. I was looking for someone who was thorough, yet conservative. When I went to see this surgeon, I didn't tell him what the other surgeon had said. I told him I wanted a second opinion to see if my request for bilateral mastectomies was wrong or misguided. I gave him my history, mammograms, and biopsy reports. I also told him about my mother and daughter. I wanted him to understand all of the factors that influenced my decision for bilateral mastectomies.

After evaluating this information he recommended bilateral mastectomies. His support for my decision confirmed that I really wasn't as far off the mark as the other surgeon would have me believe. I wasted no time in switching surgeons. My new surgeon agreed to do the bilateral mastectomies, and he welcomed my input in the decision-making process. I now had a surgeon who would listen to me.

### Did you consider having immediate breast reconstruction at the time of your mastectomies?

I chose to have the bilateral mastectomies first and take time to investigate whether I wanted breast reconstruction. If I decided to pursue this option, I wanted to locate a surgeon and decide on the best procedure. I have heard of women who cannot bear to come out of surgery without their breasts. I understand that feeling firsthand. I will never forget the shock I experienced when they removed my dressings and I looked at my concave chest. Even so, I do not regret my decision to take things one step at a time.

### Why did you decide to have breast reconstruction? What were your reasons?

It took some time to adjust to the fact that part of me was gone, but I got used to myself. I joked about my adolescent chest. I felt accepted by my friends and my husband. Having supportive friends helped me feel good about myself. It also freed me to take time to examine my motivation and decide whether I wanted to undergo more surgery.

Ultimately my reasons for deciding to have breast reconstruction had more to do with my lifestyle than it did with self-image. It was a positive statement about my hope for the future. Exercise and fitness play an important role in my life. Although I had adjusted to my body and had resumed going to the "Y" to exercise, I came to realize that the world was not ready for a mastectomized woman. It is different when you take off your clothes and there are no breasts there. I felt much like handicapped people must feel. People don't mean to stare, but they do. They don't mean to make this brief, audible sound, but they do. No matter what their motivations, people still stare and ask questions. I like the freedom to exercise without feeling that I am on display. I like being able to exercise in jumpsuits like this one. I enjoy going into the Jacuzzi afterward. I could do that comfortably without breasts. But I increasingly came to realize that people weren't quite ready for that. I couldn't just take off my clothes and walk in the Jacuzzi like everybody else.

Breast reconstruction also represented my proclamation to the world that I had a future and I was getting on with my life. I felt good when I finally decided to have breast reconstruction. I had invested the time to examine my motivation, to find a plastic surgeon, and to select the best technique for me.

### How did you select a plastic surgeon and decide on the best breast reconstruction procedure for you?

A number of excellent plastic surgeons with expertise in breast reconstruction practice in my area. I went to see several of them. I had read about the TRAM flap and asked if I would be a candidate. Even though they said I was a candidate for the TRAM flap, I noticed that they sort of wrinkled their noses when they said it. I did not feel particularly reassured. Finally, one plastic surgeon (he had gone through the nose-wrinkling phase also) said that he could do the TRAM operation. However, because my stomach was very flat, there wouldn't be much tissue available for a bilateral reconstruction, and he would only be able to create very small breasts. If that was acceptable to me, then he would do the operation. I needed to be fully aware of the limitations, however. I responded that I wasn't looking for size. It was really to be more natural.

After I left the plastic surgeon's office, I thought about what I had just said. What was I thinking? Why would I go through this major operative procedure to end up with something that's terribly small?

Surely there must be some other solution. At that point I hadn't investigated other options, so I started reading books and atlases and learned everything I could about the different reconstructive procedures. I discovered there is excess tissue in many areas of the body that can be used for reconstruction, not just the stomach. When I read about microsurgical breast reconstruction, it seemed the perfect procedure for me. I certainly had other areas to donate from if my stomach was inadequate.

I went back to the plastic surgeon who had been forthright about the TRAM flap and asked if I were a candidate for a microsurgical procedure. He suggested a gluteus maximus free flap (that's a microsurgical procedure using buttock tissue for the breast reconstruction) and called his partner in to examine me and give me his opinion. What followed was very embarrassing.

### Why was the examination embarrassing?

I told this plastic surgeon that I probably had plenty of tissue on my buttocks that he could use. He goes, "Okay, let' see. Just pull down your underwear and turn around." I did, but it was a horrible feeling. What was worse, however, was his reaction. I had barely turned around when he exclaims, "Oh yes, no problem." With all I had experienced, his reaction ranks up there as the ultimate embarrassing moment. So I had found the right procedure for me and the plastic surgeon to perform it. We agreed that I would have gluteus maximus free flaps. Because of the complexity of this procedure each breast would be reconstructed in a separate operation.

### What did your breast reconstruction involve? How long did it take? Was there much pain or discomfort?

I had been prepared for a long operation, knowing this was considered the most complex of reconstructive techniques. They were right; the first operation took over 10 hours. I do fairly well with pain, and I didn't think the procedure itself or the healing of the wounds was that painful. There was discomfort, however, because you lose the use of one hip and one side at the same time, so it is difficult to get comfortable.

After the operation, you are pretty bundled up; you've lost part of your buttock on one side. The anastomosis where they reattach the vessels restricts what you can do with your arm, how you hold it, how you move it; you are also restricted as to how you can lie down. It is hard to bear weight and sit on your hip. There is a good deal of discomfort, but it is not actually pain. I coped with these aftereffects just fine, but I was sick from the anesthesia and IV antibiotics.

### What was the problem with the anesthesia?

The anesthesia was the only part of my hospital experience that was unacceptable. You come in before the surgery, meet the anesthesiologist, and think you've made a connection. I explained that I did not tolerate drugs or medications well. He listened carefully and took profuse notes. I thought, great, he will make sure that everything goes off smoothly. When I got to surgery, I even checked to ensure that they had a record of my concerns about anesthesia. They said sure, but the anesthesiologist that I spoke with the day before was not there, and my special requirements went unheeded. I was put to sleep according to the standard routine. For me it was a disaster. After 10 hours of surgery, it was difficult to wake up from the anesthesia. I was nauseous and felt like I was in a fog. I was violently ill for 5 days; I couldn't eat and I was throwing up.

### What was the timing between the first and second breast reconstruction? Did your reaction to the anesthetic cause a delay?

They usually schedule the second operation after a long delay, but because of my work schedule, I wanted the reconstructions done one after the other. I asked if they could first operate on one breast and I would stay in the hospital for the usual 3 to 7 days. At the end of this time, if I was up to it, I wanted to have the second operation. My plastic surgeon agreed to that schedule because I was in good physical condition and could handle it.

If the first breast reconstruction had gone like the second one, it would have been a breeze. But the first one went so badly because of the anesthesia that I even considered canceling the other reconstruction. Before I was ready to come back for a second operation, I had to ensure the method of anesthesia would not have the same aftereffects.

I read about anesthesia and interviewed different anesthesiologists to figure what could be done differently. I consulted with another anesthesiologist. He called the hospital to suggest a different approach to avoid the severe reaction that I had suffered during the first operation. They agreed to start me off with a shorter acting anesthetic that would put me into a light level of anesthesia for as long as it was safe. They would put me into a deeper level of anesthesia for the middle of the procedure and then they would turn off the anesthetic before I came to. With this approach, I woke up right away, I was out of bed that night, and I asked to go home the next day. It was an amazing difference because someone had listened and acted accordingly.

### Did you take anything for pain after the second operation?

They gave me something when I woke up and after I got back to the room. That was all I needed. It was not a painful process because most areas were numb.

### Describe the recovery. What limitations did you have? How long did it take you to get back to your normal level of activity?

I was in the hospital for 7 days with the first operation and for 3 days with the second. Initially, it's almost impossible to get into a car or to sit comfortably anywhere. Your leg hurts a lot and you compensate by leaning back on couches and chairs because you can't sit up. It's also hard to go up steps. There is a lot of discomfort and tightness and your movement is restricted. It takes a considerable amount of effort to keep moving and to climb steps. It took a good 3 to 4 weeks at home.

### Did you experience any complications?

Fluid accumulated in the hip area after one of the operations. I had to wear a drain for 6 weeks, which I concealed with slacks when I went back to work. That was difficult. It's hard to bandage your buttocks and hips. There really aren't bandages you can put on your hips or strap around them in a comfortable fashion. I had to be really creative with how to wear great big fluffy bandages around my rear end. It was horrible sitting on the drain, moving with it, working with it for so long. I was told to stay home for 4 weeks or longer, but I went back to work both times in 3 weeks. I worked full time at a busy hospital clinic; there was a lot of activity and a lot of moving around, but I managed.

### How long was it before you felt you were really back to yourself, back to your normal activity level?

That took a very long time. It was great to be able to go back to work in 3 weeks, but it probably took at least 6 months, maybe even 8 months, before I felt like myself physically.

### When were you able to resume exercising? Have you returned to your former level of fitness?

I am a runner, and at the time I was also active in lifting weights. The reconstructive surgery greatly restricted those activities. I have never gotten back to the level I was at before. Now I sort of meander a mile or two. I've become a very slow runner; I literally plod. I do more walking outside and on the treadmill. I still lift weights but not as many or as heavy as I did before. I have backed off a little and try to do more cross training.

It has been important psychologically and physically for me to remain active, but sometimes I got tired of starting over. It took 3 years for me to finish all of the surgery and therapy. By then I had started over exercising about 15 times. I also was restricted in my weight lifting for quite a while. That was frustrating and I have never gotten back to my original level of fitness and energy.

### Did you choose to have nipple-areola reconstruction?

I almost didn't do that. I actually liked how nice and smooth my breasts felt and I didn't want to mess that up. Again, it had to do with clothes. I decided that I have gone this far so why not finish it off. I wanted my breasts to look normal under bras and slips and flimsier clothes. I'm glad I did it. The nipple was made from a local flap of excess tissue in the breast area. The areola was created by tattooing and the nipple was also tattooed.

### Are you pleased with the color of the tattoo?

The color needs to be darker, but it's my fault because they matched my normal areola, which was extremely pale, almost pink. They even commented that it was going to be very light, but I said, you told me to match my original color and this is it. My husband agreed it was the right color, and we decided not to make it darker at the time. It has never turned darker; in fact, it has faded a little over time. At some point I might do it again, but it doesn't matter that much to me.

### Are you happy you chose the reconstructive approach that you did? Would you do it again?

Yes, I would do it again. Even though the gluteal free flap was described as a long, difficult procedure with potential complications, I was willing to accept those conditions if I felt it would give me the result I wanted. I wanted my rebuilt breasts to be natural and my own tissue. That's what I got. The outcome was pretty perfect.

### Are you happy with the aesthetic appearance of your breasts?

Absolutely. They are natural, they are well contoured, and they are balanced. I got my wish. Now, when I go to the Jacuzzi at the YWCA nobody stares and I am no longer self-conscious.

*Are you pleased with the size of your breasts?*

It seems silly now, particularly since I investigated everything else so carefully, but it never occurred to me to think about my breast size. The subject didn't come up until my preoperative visit when the nurse said, "What cup size do you think she's going to be?" My first reaction was what a weird, invasive thing to say. I don't care. My plastic surgeon said, I think it will probably make a B cup. I thought, well, I was a B before so that's pretty good. Later, when I thought about it, I couldn't believe that I never asked. Then I realized how unimportant it was to me. As long as my breasts were somewhat even I was going to be satisfied. Well, I came out of surgery a size D! My husband to this day keeps saying, "They're just so big!" It's kind of funny that it turned out this way. I tell my husband that I have given him a treat.

*Do you have sensation in your breasts? Are they sexually responsive?*

If there's anything that I do mourn, it is the loss of my breasts as sexual organs. My husband and I had to talk about that and deal with it. It is a loss to me not to have sensitive breasts. Some feeling on the skin returned right away and I can feel fine touch in some small areas, but in most areas it is numb. My breasts will never be sexual organs again and that's a terrible loss.

If your breasts were a sensitive area and were a turn-on to increase your pleasure and stimulate pleasure in other areas, then that feeling cannot be replaced. It is just not there anymore. My husband knows that I have some feeling in some areas, but it's not the same, and he can't stimulate them because there's no feeling. But even knowing that I don't have feeling in my breasts, he thoroughly enjoys them and lovingly handles them, which gives me immense pleasure.

*What do your scars look like? Where are they placed?*

I ought to show them to you. They are hard to describe. You would have to be pretty close to see that there are scars around both breasts, and they are getting paler as time goes by. I am not bothered by them.

*How do your buttocks feel? Are they numb?*

My rear end is numb and uncomfortable. It's a different form of numbness; it's a parasthesia and it hurts. Since they cut a nerve down the back of the thigh, there's feeling on my skin but numbness underneath. It hurts when skin in the area gets caught or pinched, for example, when I am sitting on a vinyl car seat and my skin tugs or pinches together as I get up. That is enough to make me literally jump out of the car.

I still have residual muscle tightness in my buttocks and thighs as well as my upper body and breast area. This does not get any better unless I really stretch, lift weights, and move around to increase flexibility. This is not an operation for someone who isn't fully aware of what they will have to do to get back in shape. If I had only had one side reconstructed, it probably wouldn't seem as much of a challenge because then you could favor the operated side. We laugh about it, but we now judge restaurants by their chairs. I can't sit on wooden benches or picnic on the ground anymore. I can't sit on something flat. I'm uncomfortable because I've lost the cushioning that reduces the pressure on your buttocks when you are seated.

### Have you considered getting genetic testing for the breast cancer genes?

I really should be genetically tested and I want to be. I've listened to papers presented on genetic testing and I've attended lectures. The issue is insurability. I'm not as interested in having this information for me. It has already happened to me, and I've lost the young person in my life who needed this critical information. However, my brother has three children all in their twenties, and the one who's 25 already had a lump. It would be nice for them to know, and they can't get tested unless I get tested. I called the places that were the first to do genetic testing and they would be glad to do it for you, but you risk losing your insurance if you get tested. It's unfair not to be able to know something that could help you and your relatives because you fear having your insurance cut off. I have traumatized over this. They have discovered that if you carry the high-risk breast cancer gene you also have a greater risk of developing ovarian cancer, so I need to know, but who can afford to take the chance? You would never get insurance again.

### What advice would you give to women about dealing with breast cancer and breast reconstruction?

Dealing with cancer is no different from dealing with any other life calamity that everyone faces at some point. We all have losses—the loss of a family member, a relationship, a job. I don't believe anyone gets through it alone. I have spent a lot of time soul searching and questioning why these things happen. What is the use of being a good person who works hard, lives hard, tries hard, and cares about others?

What does it stand for? Something must come of it? Yet, after all that I had experienced, I sometimes feel like it makes no difference. It seems senseless and incomprehensible and the anxiety is unbearable at times. God cannot make this go away but can give me something back. He can give me the opportunity to experience life—a friend, a thoughtful gesture, an act of kindness, a sunset—all of the pieces that form the fabric of life. I am now strong enough to totally heal. I have always spent my life developing and investing in meaningful relationships. I didn't think of all those ties as a lifeline, but they were. When I see people who can't deal with trouble, it seems to always come back to the absence of a support system. They don't have a family, they don't have friends, the pieces are missing. You need to have a mutual, caring network to help you deal with life's surprises. That means giving of yourself to other people and knowing and accepting that no one can make it alone.

## LYNN: WHY WAIT?

"I didn't want to see myself without my breasts, and I didn't see any reason to wait. Why wait and heal only to be reopened and have to heal a second time? With immediate breast reconstruction, I never felt the terrible devastation of breast loss after bilateral mastectomies. The hard part was over once I had that surgery and from then on it was an adventure in rebuilding."

It was summer when I interviewed Lynn for the first time. Tanned and fit, she was dressed in a white shirt and shorts with her dark hair pulled back from her face. Married with two daughters, she has an active career as a communications expert at a local high school. Who would ever imagine that breast cancer could strike this beautiful, articulate woman of 47? And yet, true to the statistics, Lynn was diagnosed with breast cancer 5 years ago.

Her diagnosis, while shocking, was not totally unexpected. She had a family history of breast cancer and had herself been plagued with fibrocystic breasts, a long-standing problem. Lynn had been under close surveillance by her surgical oncologist for many years and had had numerous biopsies for suspicious lumps. Just 2 years before her breast cancer diagnosis, after she had three suspicious lumps biopsied at one time, her oncologist suggested that she consider prophylactic mastectomies and reconstruction to reduce the risk of developing breast cancer in the future. She had even seen a plastic surgeon

about this option, and he also recommended preventive mastectomies. But Lynn was still doubtful; she didn't have cancer and the
thought of having her breast tissue removed was not appealing. Re-
flecting on this early decision now, Lynn admits that "I should have
been smarter. My mom has breast cancer and I have a family history."
She went to another oncologist for a second opinion. He told her it
would be foolish to let them take her breasts off. She should wait until
she had cancer, if, indeed, she ever did. That was just the news that
she wanted to hear, so she decided to wait and see.

Two years later, shortly after her aunt had been diagnosed with a
breast malignancy, Lynn's breast cancer was discovered during yet another biopsy. This time she took immediate action. She had a modified radical mastectomy on the right side and a prophylactic mastectomy on her left breast, a procedure in which the breast tissue is removed and the nipple cored out. *Both breasts were reconstructed immediately with tissue expanders.*

Lynn's decision to have immediate breast reconstruction was partially explained by her mother's experience with breast loss. "I had
seen my mom with her concave figure and staples all across her chest.
I watched her battle with a prosthesis. I remember the day that she
threw it against the wall. She was so tired of hauling that thing
around. She had very big breasts, and after her one breast was removed, she needed a large prosthesis for balance; it weighed 7 or 8
pounds. That's a heavy load to carry. I knew that route was not for
me. With immediate reconstruction, I never had to experience breast
loss. I never mourned my breasts. My attitude was, 'Now that this is
out of the way, let's go.'"

Lynn's initial reaction when she woke after her operation was one
of relief. "When I woke up, I lifted the sheet immediately and all I had
was two little Steri-Strips on my body. I had expected massive bandages. I had these little mounds and it was like I didn't lose that much.
Even knowing that it really wasn't me under there, it was reassuring to
have something there."

### How long did it take you to recuperate?

I had my mastectomies and reconstruction on a Thursday, and I went
home on a Saturday, but it took a good 4 weeks before I felt like doing
much. My mom came and stayed for a week and helped out. I went
out in public right away; I attended my daughter's graduation a week
later. I went to the grocery store. Raising my arms was a little difficult,

however, and I didn't want my scars to stretch. So I was careful about lifting and moving. I didn't vacuum. In fact, I still don't vacuum if I can get out of it.

I was off for the summer and I didn't go back to work until late August. I was still having my breasts expanded then. The expansion was not hard once I got over the initial part. In October, when I had my expanders replaced with implants, I stayed off work 2 weeks. I really didn't need that full 2 weeks; 1 week would have been fine. But at that point my priorities were different. I decided that I was going to take all the time I needed to heal. I put myself first probably for the first time in my life.

When I had my nipple reconstructed, it was done the day before Christmas vacation, and I had another 2 weeks to recuperate.

### What type of anesthesia did you have for each of your surgical procedures?

The anesthesia was one of the hardest parts of the surgery. I was under general anesthesia for the original surgery when my expanders were inserted. But I also had general anesthesia when my implants were put in and when my nipples were done. It was all done under general anesthesia. It's hard for me to come back from anesthesia; it takes about 4 to 6 weeks to get it out of my system. I'm tired and drag around. That's why I took 2 weeks to recuperate each time.

### How did you choose your reconstructive technique? What considerations were most important to you in making this decision?

I chose tissue expansion with implant placement because that's what my plastic surgeon recommended. He told me about the other operations and about the tummy flap, but because I was so slender, he didn't think I had enough stomach fat to reconstruct both of my breasts. Today, there are even more options for the breast reconstruction patient. They can move tissue from other parts of the body with microsurgery. Even so, I really didn't want to go through the pain of a procedure that involved. And I didn't want all of the scars. So tissue expansion seemed to be the best option for me.

### Describe the expansion process. What happened when you had your breasts expanded? Who did it? How long did it take?

Two weeks after my surgery I met with my plastic surgeon and his nurse, and we started the expansion process. My plastic surgeon told her how much fluid to inject into my expanders and over what period of time. From then on his nurse usually took care of me, injecting about 100 ml of fluid into each breast during each session. Expansion proceeded pretty rapidly. It took about 15 minutes each time, and I went every week for the first 7 or 8 weeks and then less frequently. We never cut back on the amount of fluid injected, and we never stopped. But she always gave me the option. She was very responsive to my needs.

### Tell me how this nurse helped you? What did she do to make this process easier for you?

She was one of the greatest supports that I had. She allowed me to have control, to make some decisions about my body, and to decide how fast I wanted to have my breasts expanded. Each time she asked if I felt I could handle it. If I told her something didn't feel right, she never brushed me off or dismissed my concerns. Instead she would say, "Tell me how you feel. Exactly where is the problem?" Not all nurses do that. I've had experiences with other nurses during that process and I've never had that kind of compassion. If I was extremely tight, she allowed me to say whether I wanted to be expanded or not. And a lot of them don't. They say, "You have to get used to the tightness because the only way to stretch the skin is to expand it immediately." But that's not necessarily true; sometimes your skin doesn't stretch as fast as they think it should. Sometimes you need the time to allow your skin to relax and work itself loose so that it is more comfortable.

Tissue expansion involves some sense of being violated. This is true especially with the original surgery, but even with the expansion you are not in control of making decisions about what's being done to your body. My nurse gave me control.

### Was your plastic surgeon responsive during the expansion process?

My doctor's schedule was extremely tight, and I couldn't always reach him. But I could always see him when I had a problem. I understand from other people that their doctors don't see them during the expansion process. I saw him every single time. It was important to me that he was still going to check to make sure everything was okay. I needed to be in touch with my doctor during that time.

### How did it feel to have your expanders inflated? Was it painful?

I had more feeling on my right side where I had the preventive mastectomy. I always felt the pinprick of the needle being inserted into my expander port. Once it was in, I didn't feel a thing. The other side had no feeling. I could feel some pressure. I was not always comfortable, but I was never in pain.

After the first 4 weeks it felt like I had bricks put in my body. My breasts felt heavier, like I was carrying more weight. That's probably because my expanders were positioned behind my chest muscle and were exerting pressure on it. I just felt my breasts blowing up; I could actually see them as they grew. That was encouraging to me because I didn't want to be flat-chested. As a teenager I was fairly big-breasted. And I think I would have had a hard time being totally flat-chested. But I could see my breasts as they grew, and each time I would go home and think, "They're getting better."

### How long did the expansion process take?

Everything went like clockwork. I wore my expanders for about 5 months. It took me 4 months to have my breasts totally expanded and then a month to let my breast skin rest so my breasts would become comfortable.

### Was it inconvenient?

No, because it was summertime. Had I been in school it might have been. But my mindset was such that nothing would have seemed an inconvenience. I had tunnel vision with breast reconstruction. Other things went on in my life, but this was a goal; it consumed a large part of my life and my thinking.

### Why did you choose to have your nipple-areola reconstructed?

Because I wanted to be complete. I wanted my breasts to look normal and to match. The nipple on my normal breast was preserved after the prophylactactic mastectomy, so I wanted one on the mastectomy side also.

### How was your nipple-areola reconstructed and when was it done?

My initial surgery was done in May, my expanders were replaced with permanent textured-surface implants in October, and my nipple was reconstructed in December. The nipple reconstruction was done at a third procedure to allow my breasts to settle. My nipple was reconstructed from the scar tissue extending under my arm. They sit you up to graft the nipple, and they have to open a fairly decent-size scar to get the skin for the nipple graft. I also had my nipple tattooed as an outpatient procedure.

### *How do your breasts look? Are you satisfied with the appearance?*

My breasts are symmetric and I look terrific in my clothes. I asked to be big and I got bigger than I had planned to be, but I'm very satisfied. Sometimes I have to be careful about buying clothes because the top doesn't fit the bottom, but that is a minor inconvenience compared to my level of satisfaction.

After the modified radical mastectomy my armpit was hollowed out and it looked funny to me in clothes. Other people probably wouldn't notice if I kept my arm down, but I was self-conscious. To correct this problem my plastic surgeon removed a piece of muscle from my back (the latissismus dorsi muscle) and swung it under my arm, so I now have a fairly normal looking armpit.

My nipples still don't match, but that is because I had my nipple skin preserved on my normal side. At the time I didn't want to lose the nipple on my normal side if I didn't have to. That seemed very important then; it isn't now. Sometimes I wish I had gone ahead and had it taken off so there was a little better match. But that side is more comfortable because I have more skin.

Also, the color of the tattoo on my reconstructed nipple does not match the color of my preserved nipple. I have yellow-toned skin and yellow tones are difficult to replicate. I've heard that they now have tints with more yellow pigment available. After my tattoo fades, I am going to have my nipple-areola tattooed again to try to get a better match. It is hard to do it again. After all of that surgery, Band-Aids are a real turn-off.

### *How do your reconstructed breasts feel? Are your breasts sensitive? Are they soft? Are they warm?*

I have no feeling in about a 3½-inch diameter. I do have feeling around the outside of my breasts, but only in the skin. All of the good, warm sexual sensations are gone. I miss those most of all.

My breasts are cooler than the rest of my body. When it's cold, my breasts get cold. I'm a walker, and I try to counteract that by layering with lightweight clothes. Then my breasts don't get so frigid. On winter nights I use an electric blanket and flannel sheet to keep me warm. The rest of my body isn't cold; I just feel cold when I touch my breasts with my arms because I have no feeling there.

### *Is there anything you would change about your reconstruction?*

I would like to have the sexual feeling back, and I think someday they probably will know how to do that. If they do it in my lifetime, I'm going to be jealous. But that is the hardest part for me.

### Has the mastectomy and reconstruction experience affected your feelings of sexuality and femininity?

Yes. Breasts are important; they are a turn-on. Now that my breasts are no longer sensitive, I don't have that response. As you get older, turn-ons are harder to come by. You are without that and you have to have a pretty good relationship with the person you have sex with, whether it's a husband or another partner. The woman who goes through this has to know that this is a loss.

Your femininity goes with the mastectomy; the reconstruction rebuilds that femininity. I never get in the shower that I don't look at myself and smile. I never feel devastated.

### What are your scars like?

I don't scar badly. You would never even notice I had a scar on my right side. The one on my left side from the mastectomy is also faded and barely noticeable. It is a very thin line and the nipple is grafted right over the major part of the scar. I do have a red scar from when he redid my armpit. It will take several years, but I know it will eventually turn white like the rest of my scars have done.

### Did you have any problems or complications after your breast reconstruction?

No, none at all.

### What coping mechanisms did you rely on to help you get through this experience?

I went through this experience fairly humorously. When I went in, knowing hospitals the way I do, I wrote "prophylactic" on my right breast and "modified radical" on my left, so that they didn't do the wrong side. When I went in to have my implants put in, I communicated further by writing "big" on my breasts. And when I had my nipple tattooed, I also had a little heart tattoo put on my side. I figured it took a lot of heart to get through it all.

### Did you join a support group?

Yes, a breast reconstruction support group, and it was important to me. It has been a vital part of the healing process. You talk about this experience with your family, but they can't really relate. They've never had muscle spasms as the muscle adjusted to having a foreign body behind it. They don't know what it's like to lie on your stomach and feel like you are lying on rubber balls. They don't know when you move from side to side that you feel like you've got to push your breasts back into place, which you really don't. But it's a strange feeling because of the lack of sensation in your breast. I can go to my support group and I can talk all I want about my breasts and about reconstruction and nobody says, "Here she goes again." It's a group that wraps around you when you have problems. We share more than just our breasts: the good and the bad. With reconstruction, I knew everything that could go wrong. Women in the group share what has gone wrong with them. Doctors will tell you what might possibly happen, but in my support group I could see firsthand what did happen. Some people belong to the group for a short while and then leave because they don't need it anymore. I still need it, not just as a means to express myself, but because it is payback time. The women in the group were wonderful for me; if I can be there for somebody else, then I want to do it. I am one of the lucky people. My reconstruction was aesthetically successful. It looks fantastic. I've not had any major problems. Not everyone is so lucky. One of my good friends who I brought to the group died 2 weeks ago. That was tough to deal with. But that helps me stay in touch with reality. It scares me, but it helps me.

### In retrospect, do you feel that you made the right decision when you had a prophylactic mastectomy on your normal side?

Definitely. If I was allowed more hindsight, I would have done it 2 years earlier when my breasts were merely high risk. I would recommend that anyone who is diagnosed with precancerous breasts get them off. What you gain from early prevention far outweighs the loss of a breast. It is just not worth carrying the time bombs around. And that is literally what I did. As my husband said, "Somebody has to hit you with a 2 by 4 to get your attention." Second opinions are great. But if they are different, go for a third or a fourth and then weigh all of your information. I'm sorry I stopped at two.

### Was reconstruction worth the time, pain, and money? Would you do it again and would you choose the same reconstructive approach?

I would do it again in a heartbeat. And if something were to go wrong with my implants tomorrow, I would probably have tissue expanders and implants again. I know that 20 or 30 years down the road I may have different options, but I really don't want any other major surgery unless it's absolutely necessary. Tissue expansion and implant placement are not major surgery. I also know that the flap procedure is available to me if my implants should fail or if something should happen and I cannot have implants anymore.

Aesthetically, tissue transfer is not as pretty a result as you get with expanders and implants. With the TRAM flap there are more scars. Not only do you have the scar across your stomach, but you end up with two scars across your breast, rather than the one. The scarring bothers me.

### Has your mom had breast reconstruction?

My mom decided to have reconstruction after she saw me go through it; she had my plastic surgeon do her reconstruction. She was 72. She also had her second breast removed and had prophylactic mastectomy and reconstruction. She's had more problems with her reconstruction than I had. She had an infection and had to have her implant removed. She ended up having a latissimus dorsi back flap transferred to give her better skin cover for her implant. She is having some problems with her other breast right now and is scheduled to see her plastic surgeon.

### Is she happy she did it?

Yes, because she doesn't worry anymore about developing cancer on the other side. But she isn't as comfortable as I am. I feel somewhat guilty knowing that she did it because I did, even though I didn't pressure her. In fact, I tried to discourage her because I worried about surgery at her age. I wanted her to do the reconstruction for her self-image, but I didn't want her to go through any pain or discomfort. She came through it better than I did to begin with. But her aesthetic result has not been as successful as mine because of capsular contracture. She has one breast that is hard and she will probably have to have that implant replaced.

### How did your family react to your mastectomies and reconstruction?

They were with me all the way; they were as involved in it as I was. We engaged in a lot of humor to keep us all going. My youngest daughter is the funny bone in the family and she kept it light. She called the state department to get me a handicapped parking sticker as a double amputee. They didn't give me one. But that was her type of humor. Even now, she jokes, "Those are the biggest things I have ever seen, Mother; what do you do with them?" My husband chose to stay with me in the hospital and take care of everything, even though my aunt was director of nursing there and offered to stay. But I was more comfortable with him. It was a bonding time for us.

### Are your daughters concerned about the threat of breast cancer? How has this experience affected them?

It has brought us much closer together. It has also made us aware of what's in their future. They have to be careful. My oldest daughter is very open and talks freely about her body. She is very large-breasted, and she is a tiny person. She is aware that her breasts could be time bombs and that cancer could come earlier for her than it did for me. It seems to be hitting younger people all the time. My gynecologist has recommended that she come in every 3 months to have her breasts checked. My younger daughter is 19 and is very hard to work with. She is self-conscious about her body; no one sees her body. We found her a wonderful female gynecologist. Even so, my daughter said it was the most horrifying experience she's ever been through. She has even said things to me in jest, yet not really joking, "Thanks, Mom, look what you have given me to look forward to." I know that it hangs in her mind.

### Do your daughters do breast self-examination?

Yes. My oldest one does BSE. She told me she could not find any lumps. When I ask my other daughter, she'll say, "Mother, I'll take care of that." She really won't open up about it. I worry about her more. She probably is the one that checks the most because she is more frightened by it. I don't know if she knows what to look for. We have a friend who is 25 and was diagnosed with breast cancer in December. That brought it home, but my younger daughter still doesn't talk to me about it. I know that this experience has heightened both of my daughters' awareness of the threat of breast cancer. They talk about it with their friends. Their friends are all aware that I've had it, and when they come over to visit, they never meet my eyes when they are talking to me. Their eyes are right on breast level. They ask me a hundred questions about how it feels. What does it feel like inside? How does it feel to touch? I'll say, "Why don't you touch my breasts and see?" I don't ever push. They always want to.

### How have your friends reacted to your breast cancer and breast reconstruction?

It took my friends a long time to ask me if my breasts look right. I said, "They are beautiful; you ought to see them." My support group made it easy to do show and tell. I touched other women's reconstructed breasts before mine were ever finished. I knew what they felt like, I knew what they looked like. That was really important to me to know beforehand what it was going to feel like.

When my mom had her breast reconstruction, her friends thought she was ridiculous and vain. After all, she was 72. Since then three of her friends have had mastectomies, and now they want to touch and feel and see her breasts because they are considering reconstruction. These women are all in their late sixties or early seventies, but they see how great it's been for her.

### Did your plastic surgeon meet your needs? Could he have been more responsive?

When you are dealing with somebody on a very busy time schedule, you have to come prepared with questions written down or so well implanted in your head that you don't walk out and say, "Oh, I wanted to ask him this." My plastic surgeon hung the moon as far as I am concerned. He is probably the most caring man I've ever been around. He was responsive, but I wish he would slow down a little. He is in and out. He moves like a butterfly. Although all my needs were met, I would like him to sit down in a chair when he comes into my room. I would like him to talk to me after he has examined my breasts. I did learn to express these feelings to him. I would say, "I didn't get my money's worth yet; sit down, I want to talk." I didn't want small talk; I know his time is valuable, but I want to be able to express my concerns, to let him know when my breasts are uncomfortable. Some people are intimidated by doctors. And you can't be. You are paying their bills. You have a right to decide what's going to be done with your body. You have a right to tell your doctors how you are feeling about things and expect them to respond to that.

### What advice would you like to give to other women about breast reconstruction?

Most people think reconstruction is just going to be more surgery. But it is different. It is uplifting, upbeat; it's the healing process. You're back looking like you did. Don't let the threat of cancer stop you from doing it. I think people are so afraid once they have cancer that they worry that reconstruction is just an extension of their illness and it's not; it heals you. Cancer is terrifying, it is horrifying and I will live with that every day. Wondering what's going to happen next. But reconstruction is nonthreatening. It is a rebuilding process. Although I was a whole person without my breasts, reconstruction restored me physically to the person I was.

## SHARON: HOW DO YOU TELL A MAN THAT YOU HAVE HAD BREAST CANCER?

"Everyone sees me as so independent and I am. But sometimes you need to be able to lean on someone else. You need to confide in someone and not worry about rejection. Cancer puts you in a precarious position. You are both strong and vulnerable and it is hard to achieve the right balance." These mixed feelings were confided to me by Sharon as she told me about her breast cancer and breast reconstruction experience and the important role that friends and lovers can play in helping you to adjust to life after breast cancer. Sharon was treated for breast cancer 20 years ago when she was only 30 with two small children. There were few treatment options at that time. She went in for a biopsy and woke hours later to discover that she had a modified radical mastectomy. Fortunately, the cancer had not spread and no additional therapy was required. Since that time she has divorced, raised two boys by herself, gotten an undergraduate and graduate degree, had *two different breast reconstruction operations (first implant surgery and then a TRAM flap)*, and had a hysterectomy. She has also changed jobs and struggled with developing new intimate relationships.

Sharon is a small, slender brunette who exudes an air of self-confidence. Attired in a tailored black pantsuit, she looks professional and composed. Despite her outward composure, Sharon expresses her vulnerability in confronting some of the challenges that breast cancer has introduced into her life. She laughingly admits that she is puzzled by the dating game and still seeking the best way to tell a man about her breast cancer and reconstruction. It has been an awkward and uncomfortable experience and she remains frustrated and somewhat discouraged by the strange reactions and rejections that have greeted her when she has confided her secret to others. Sharon recently celebrated her fiftieth birthday. She sees it as another landmark and a surprisingly liberating experience, which she hopes will lead her to view life with more equanimity and to resolve some of the problems she has experienced. Her story begins when she was only 30.

*How did you discover you had breast cancer?*

I went in for a biopsy. When I woke over 5 hours later, I knew that I must have had a mastectomy. This was 20 years ago when I was only 30. No one suspected that the lump in my breast was cancer. I was too young. When my doctor asked if I had a family history, I said no. Later, when I asked my mother, she told me that my grandmother had died from breast cancer. From that moment on breast cancer was a daily reality for me.

*How did you cope with your cancer diagnosis? Was your age a factor?*

Breast cancer was a solitary experience for me. Back then people didn't talk about it. They didn't want to know. There was no one my age to relate to.

It was also an emotional time. I'll never forget the first time I looked at myself. I still get tearful when I think of it. That's what is so great about reconstructive surgery. After my first implant surgery I looked down to find I had cleavage again after being flat-chested for over a year. It seems silly, but it's not. You lose part of your body and you mourn for it.

*How did your husband react? Was he supportive?*

When I first had the mastectomy, my husband was very supportive. I was embarrassed when he saw me; he took it better than I did. But it didn't last. It was a long time before we had sex again, and then a year after the mastectomy he stopped touching me above the waist. That did something to me. It was a constant reminder that I had breast cancer. I don't know if he was turned off by it or what happened. I didn't realize at the time that our marriage was bad. He had been having affairs since our second year of marriage, but I didn't find out until much later. After we divorced, the knowledge of his long-standing infidelity helped me to understand that our lack of intimacy had little to do with my cancer.

*Why did you decide to have breast reconstruction?*

Initially I decided against reconstructive surgery to avoid having more surgery. I went the prosthesis route. I did this for 18 months until my prosthesis fell out in the car while I was driving carpool for my preschoolers. I leaned over to open the car door and my prosthesis just plopped out on the floor in front of these 4-year-old kids. That was it. I decided to have the reconstructive surgery. I was still young, and I didn't want to live the rest of my life that way.

### How did you choose your plastic surgeon?

The plastic surgeon was on staff at the hospital where my mastectomy was performed. My cancer surgeon recommended him because he was well known for reconstructive breast surgery.

### What type of breast reconstruction did you choose?

You didn't have many choices back then. I had an implant reconstruction and my nipple-areola was rebuilt during the same operation.

### Were you happy with the appearance and feel of your breast after the implant reconstruction?

Not really. Although it was better than being flat, it was not natural. The breast shape was distorted and the nipple was in the wrong place. It never did look right. I teased my plastic surgeon about taking before pictures but no after pictures. I said, "You are not happy with this either." He offered to fix it for free, but I said no. I did not want more surgery. So I lived with one nipple up and one down for years. I had to be careful about what I wore to make sure that it was lined to camouflage my asymmetric nipples.

### Did you experience any complications or problems from your implant reconstruction?

A capsule formed and my breast became hard and misshapen. I also had intermittent pain and discomfort. I told my plastic surgeon early on that the implant was causing problems, but he just kept telling me to massage it. That wasn't a solution for me. I was trying to forget that I had cancer, so I didn't massage it and I am not sure that it would have helped.

### Why did you choose to have a second breast reconstruction to redo your implant reconstruction after 20 years?

A few years ago I suspected that my implant had ruptured because my breast had suddenly gotten flat. I not only had a nipple in the wrong place, but one breast was noticeably smaller than the other. An MRI confirmed the rupture. The silicone was contained in the capsule that had formed. The rupture made the decision for me. I then had a TRAM flap.

*Why did you decide to have a TRAM flap for your second breast reconstruction?*

I had read about the TRAM flap. I even cut out an article about it. I knew if I ever had breast reconstruction again that was the operation for me. The breast is so natural. I did, however, worry about the recovery and the pain associated with flap surgery.

*Why did you decide to have the nipple-areola reconstruction?*

Why not? I have this mound of tissue on my chest; the nipple-areola reconstruction makes it look more like a breast.

*How long did the TRAM flap surgery take? How long were you hospitalized? Did you experience much pain?*

It took 5 hours. They had to remove the implant before they could do the TRAM flap. I was in the hospital for 7 days. Initially the pain is somewhat of a blur and you are grateful for that. You wake up bandaged and you feel more pressure than pain. For me, the pain came later, mostly in my abdomen. There was minimal pain in my breast area even after the mastectomy. It was pretty numb.

*Did you have any complications or serious problems?*

I had severe, incapacitating abdominal pain. My plastic surgeon says this type of reaction occurs in only a small percentage of patients. It felt like somebody was pinching me or jabbing me with a knife. If I moved, stood up, or tried to walk, it was excruciating. I was bent over, had to shuffle when I walked, and move very, very slowly. It took a full 3 months to recover, and even then I was weak. I couldn't walk upright. I became protective of my body. It changed my personality.

That's all gone now; I feel so good that it is difficult to imagine that I felt so withdrawn. I saw my breast surgeon after I was feeling better and he asked if they had prescribed an antidepressant. I said no. He said antidepressants may be helpful for pain problems similar to mine after some operations. In retrospect, I recognize that I was really depressed during this period, and an antidepressant might have been effective.

*What was the most difficult part of the recovery process?*

It's the inconvenience that gets to you. You are incapacitated. When you have been accustomed to doing so much, it's hard to slow down. You have to plan every act from eating to sleeping because you are restricted. It's difficult to get comfortable when you sleep. I put pillows under my legs and beside me. I used a recliner in the daytime. You do whatever makes you feel better. You learn to roll out of bed rather than sitting up to avoid the pull in the abdominal area. It was a thrill the first time I actually laid on my back or got out of bed without pain. You know you are recovered when you can move freely.

### What kind of restrictions did you have initially?

After the TRAM flap you are instructed not to lift things. They don't tell you that you are physically unable to lift things or do ordinary tasks. After my surgery my son stayed home for 2 weeks to care for me. When he returned to work, I had a more difficult time managing than I had anticipated. He left a casserole in the refrigerator, but I couldn't reach the shelf to get a glass or a plate. I couldn't even lift the casserole out of the refrigerator. It never occurred to me to just get a spoon and scoop out the food. Instead I decided to make a sandwich, but the bread was moldy. When my son came home, I was sitting in the recliner in tears. I hadn't eaten anything and I felt so helpless. I never realized that I would be so incapacitated.

It is important to plan for your recovery in advance. It will be a while before you can lift objects as simple as a gallon of milk. You need to store food in smaller containers and make other accommodations. I couldn't even lift my fluffy bath towels. I had to use a hand towel for my hair and a lighter weight bath towel.

### How long did it take after your TRAM reconstruction until you felt that you were fully recovered and able to resume your normal level of activity?

I went back to work part-time after 3 months, but I was still weak, which was frustrating. It took 6 months to a year to do most things easily. Five months after my TRAM flap I went on a 7-day sailing trip to Barbados. I couldn't help with the sailing, but I helped with the kitchen duties.

### When were you able to resume an exercise program?

I started walking short distances after 3 months. I went to the end of the street and I gradually increased the distance. I returned to the health club in September and began using the treadmill. I still cannot do step aerobics. I have never done sit-ups. I tried them before the TRAM operation to strengthen my abdominal muscles so I would be in shape for the operation. After the operation the nurse told me that now I would be able to play golf. I laughed and told her "that's great because I didn't know how before."

### Are you happy with the results of your TRAM reconstruction? How does it compare with your earlier implant reconstruction?

This time my plastic surgeon has done a better job. Techniques have improved. Unfortunately, I couldn't benefit fully from the new reconstructive techniques because I have the old kind of mastectomy scar. My breast shape isn't quite right either. My plastic surgeon has revised it twice with minor procedures that required only a local anesthetic. However, it looks fine in clothes and in a bathing suit and that is all I care about. The second revision made my breast look square and I wish I hadn't had it done. It still is not the way I want it to look, but the plastic surgeon has done the best he can with what he has to work with. I'm glad that I had the TRAM flap rather than an implant. Even with the scarring, the TRAM reconstruction looks so much better and more natural than the implant reconstruction. Best of all, it's permanent. I know that my breast is never going to go flat the way it did before. I look fine in a bra, but I still don't look at myself undressed. When I get out of the shower, the first thing I do is put on my bathrobe. I don't know that I am ever going to like looking at myself again.

### Do you have any sensation in your reconstructed breast?

I have very little, even though it is better than it was with the implant reconstruction. Because the mastectomy was performed 20 years ago, it was unlikely that I would regain sensation. When I had the implant reconstruction, my plastic surgeon grafted part of the nipple on my right unoperated breast to make the new nipple on my reconstructed breast. As a result, I also have no sensation in my right nipple.

### How does your abdomen feel? Does it have sensation?

I have some sensation to touch. That was a real concern for me. I was numb on one side of my body and worried that I would stay numb across the abdomen. I have also discovered that my muscles are sensitive to cold. The first time I went swimming I had horrible muscle spasms and had to get out. That is one of the things they don't tell you. Cold weather affects you. I still get muscle spasms across my abdomen when cold air hits it; it feels strange, but it goes away and you learn to live with it.

My abdomen feels stretched all the time, like a tightly pulled rubber band. If I gain 2 pounds I know it and it is an odd feeling. I don't know if it will ever go away. Someone suggested that I dwell on it too much. However, you can't understand how it feels to be stretched constantly. I asked the breast surgeon about it. He explained that my abdominal skin is not very elastic because I never was much overweight and my skin just doesn't stretch. So I really have to watch my weight, which is not such a bad thing.

### How was your nipple reconstructed this time? Are you satisfied with its appearance?

He took a little local flap of skin and used it to build the nipple. The nipple isn't finished yet; he is going to do the tattooing today to make the nipple darker and to create an areola. The nipple still looks too big, but I was told it would shrink. So I am going to have the tattoo and see how the size changes over time. I know that the results from nipple-areola tattooing can be very good. Yet women in my support group say it can take four or five times to get the color right. If that is the case, I am not sure that I want to bother.

### What are the scars like from your mastectomy and from your two breast reconstructions?

I have a diagonal scar across my breast from the mastectomy. There were no new scars with the implant reconstruction, but the TRAM flap left an elliptic-shaped scar on my breast. I also have a scar extending across my abdomen from my hysterectomy. The TRAM reconstruction was done through this incision without creating any new scars. I always disliked scars. It's ironic that now I have these huge scars on my body and it doesn't bother me.

### If you had it to do over again would you have breast reconstruction? Was it worth the time, pain, and money?

Yes, I definitely would. After the implant rupture my female gynecologist suggested that I just go flat again and not bother with another reconstructive operation. I said absolutely not. Who needs that daily reminder that you have had cancer. Anyway, when you are flat, you have such a problem with clothes. People who have never had a mastectomy don't understand. If you wear a prosthesis, you are always wondering how it will look with a particular outfit. It is a constant hassle. So yes I would definitely have a TRAM reconstruction again despite the pain and the time involved. It was worth it. I can put on just about anything now. That may sound shallow but it is not. It's the way life should be. Now I feel normal again.

### If you had it to do over, would you opt for immediate breast reconstruction?

If the option had been available to me, I would definitely have chosen an immediate TRAM flap. Some people say that you need to give yourself time to experience breast loss before you have reconstruction. I strongly disagree. Why should you have to deal with being flat on one side? You don't need a reminder that you have cancer; you already know it. It is enough to deal with a life-threatening illness. Why should you also have to cope with breast loss? It is a real boon to a woman's emotional health to have everything done at once.

### What role did your friends play in supporting you during your breast cancer and reconstruction experiences? Were they understanding? Did they help you cope?

Friends can really make a difference. I was fortunate in that most of my friends were sensitive to my situation. They were not only a source of psychological reinforcement, but they also provided practical assistance to facilitate my recovery. They brought me food and helped with errands. It was a relief to be able to lean on other people while I was recovering. It doesn't matter if you are strong and independent. I got through a divorce, went back to school, and raised two kids on my own. I'm independent. But I also have learned that there are times that you need the love and support of other people. Most people honestly want to help you.

I was touched and grateful for the help that I got, often from unexpected sources. A woman in my church group who I didn't know well called and wanted to bring breakfast by the first morning I was home from the hospital. It was such a neat thing to do. She showed up that morning, knocked on the door, brought breakfast for my son and me, and left. She didn't offer to stay so that I wouldn't feel obligated to entertain her when I was feeling so lousy. She doesn't live anywhere near me. Another woman brought some books over; she knows I love to read. Two men in my church group cooked dinner for me after the first 4 weeks. Even though I didn't feel great and the dinner was less than delicious, I was touched that these two single men made the effort to fix a special meal for me and bring it to my house. It helped to just know that people were thinking of me. A woman who went to school with me called me every few days, despite her hectic schedule. One of my oldest and dearest friends came to the house and took care of all the flowers and visited with me regularly.

### Were there any disappointments?

Not everyone is understanding or sensitive. Some people can't deal with surgery, with disease, with cancer. It hurts that they aren't there for you. One woman told me that if I hadn't thought about breast cancer I wouldn't have gotten it. Another friend told me that her husband was appalled that I had reconstructive surgery. It was people like me who ran up the insurance rates. One of the secretaries in our office who I had been close with never came to see me during the 3 months that I was home.

Some people were well intentioned but misguided. One neighbor came over 3 days after the TRAM flap surgery to announce that she was having a luncheon for me to "cheer me up." A woman who has just had a TRAM reconstruction is in no shape for socializing. I could hardly move and I hurt all over. It's major surgery after all. But she wouldn't take no for an answer. She plans a luncheon at my house and brings three women over while I sit there in my pajamas. They went to all of this trouble to prepare a lovely luncheon complete with wine, but I was in no condition to enjoy it. They chattered away while I sat there in pain wishing they would leave. My neighbor thought she had done a wonderful thing for me. She didn't understand that I needed to be left alone to recover.

### Why did you join a breast reconstruction support group? Was it helpful to you?

I started going to a support group because I wanted to talk to other women to learn more about the TRAM flap and what to expect during the recovery period. The reassurance and practical advice that I got from the women in this group were tremendously helpful. I met several women I could call and ask questions to make sure that everything was okay. I'd call and say, "It's 3 weeks now, but I still can't do such and such." They'd say, "Don't worry; everyone feels this way after 3 weeks. You are doing great." About 6 weeks after my surgery, when I could hardly walk, one of the woman took me aside and explained that women who are thin sometimes have a harder time recovering from this type of operation. After her TRAM flap she had been in the same condition at this stage. I would be just fine. I just had to give it some time. It was so reassuring.

### What type of practical advice did the women in your support group provide?

Women in my support group gave me the practical information that helped make my recovery easier. For example, one woman suggested that I rent or borrow a recliner to help relieve the abdominal pressure. She had one, even slept in it, and it had really helped. I was able to borrow one from a friend. Another women told me to put a chair by the bathtub and another chair by the bed to help me get in and out. She also suggested that I buy oversized underpants to take with me to the hospital. That was great advice. After a TRAM reconstruction you don't want anything touching you. Some women in my group even wear boxer shorts. I just got underwear that was several sizes too big. Sometimes, I still wear it, just because it doesn't cling.

### How does breast cancer and breast reconstruction affect a woman's relationship with a man? Is it difficult when you are single and dating? What are the worries? How do you tell a man that you have had breast cancer?

Dating is hard enough without breast cancer. Communicating with a man about this problem is difficult. You fear rejection. I have had a series of less then satisfying encounters. The world is made up of all types. There are wonderful men out there who are understanding and accepting and there are others who leave much to be desired. If you are a divorced woman who has had breast cancer and two breast reconstruction operations, relating to the opposite sex is a big concern. You worry about how you are going to tell a man about your cancer, about your body. I still haven't found the answer. It's an awkward situation.

The therapist I saw after my divorce thought I should tell men early and just get it out on the table. If the man couldn't take it, then he would just move on. My approach was more gradual—let him find out what a wonderful person I am first and then tell him. I've tried both ways with various reactions. It was not a problem for the first man I went out with. He was absolutely wonderful and that was good for my self-esteem. But then, after 6 months, he left and I was devastated. It wasn't related to the cancer. Our personalities didn't mesh, but it was still difficult to accept.

I used the therapist's approach with the next man. I told him after three dates. This man has a handicapped son, and I was sure that he would empathize and understand that because part of you is different that doesn't diminish your value as a person. His reaction was very strange. His behavior was so disturbing that I called him the next day and asked about it. I was floored by his response. He told me that "he can honestly say that ignorance is bliss." This is the same man who only days earlier had proclaimed his devotion to me. I was going to have a hard time getting rid of him," he had said. Well, all I had to do was admit that I had breast cancer and he was out the door. I probably should have just written him off at that point, but I needed closure so I wrote him a note explaining why I had confided in him. I wasn't expecting to sleep with him, I just wanted him to know where I was coming from. He returned my letter unopened with a computer-printed letter that read: "I do not wish to read your letter. It has nothing to do with what you told me. The timing is just not right." It was signed G. So I sent a postcard back to him so he would have to read it. It said "G, Bull shit." I signed it S.

I told the next man after we had been dating for 4 or 5 months. I related the other incidents to explain why I was hesitant about telling him. He responded by trying to convince me that he was okay. We had two more dates and everything seemed fine. We were scheduled to go out the following weekend when he called my secretary and canceled. I never heard from him again. So I'm thinking, this is a curse that I will have to bear forever. I guess I will just have to get used to it.

Then, with the next few men that I dated, it went more smoothly. I recently told the man that I am currently dating, and once again the response was puzzling. He cut me off and said something like, "We all have flaws." I said, "I don't consider this a flaw. It's something that nature did to me." Maybe I am approaching this wrong or maybe I just haven't found the right person.

I have only been intimate with three men other than my husband in the 10 years since my divorce. They have accepted me as I am. Unfortunately, I have had more bad experiences than good. Each time I tell a man about my cancer and reconstruction, I have this overwhelming fear that he will reject me. I am finally reaching the point where I can tell people and accept their reactions with less apprehension. Maybe it's because I'm 50 now, and I realize that there are a lot more people out there who have been touched by breast cancer. Men of my age are coming to realize that their bodies aren't perfect anymore, although they still want this perfect woman.

I accept the fact that if I never marry again it may or may not be related to breast cancer. Men are just men. Some are shallow. Others have more substance. I keep hoping that there is this really wonderful person out there.

It takes years to acknowledge the fact that some people cannot accept you as you are. I can't get into mens' minds to understand whether they don't like the scar or whether they fear losing you. It's irrational. You can get killed by a car just walking across the street. I had cancer 20 years ago; the chances of it recurring are slim. My new therapist suggested that I should just let the man see my breasts. Can't you just imagine that? After three or four dates you raise your blouse and bare your breasts. I don't think so. What would have happened if I showed this man that I am dating now? Maybe that would make the difference. I don't know. He won't even talk about it, and I am not even sure he is entitled to see. If he can't talk to me about it, why should I do a show and tell?

No one has seen the new me with the TRAM flap yet. I think the implant reconstruction looked so bad that I dreaded telling men because I felt misshapen. With my TRAM reconstruction, I look a lot better. It makes me more willing to show somebody, but I'm waiting for the right person.

## JOAN: FROM CATERPILLAR TO BUTTERFLY

"Cancer has taught me to live life to the fullest. I used to be a caterpillar watching life go by, crawling instead of flying. Cancer made me realize that life is to be *lived*. Now I am a butterfly ready to take flight."

Joan shared these words of wisdom and of triumph as she proudly displayed the brightly sequined butterfly, which was attached to her equally vivid green sweater. "It's a stick-on," she confided in me, "that goes with anything I wear. It's a sign of hope and it just makes me feel good. Butterflies are so beautiful. When I see them, I can't be sad." Joan was diagnosed with breast cancer over 5 years ago after a sudden bout of fatigue literally stopped her in her tracks during her morning walk. A trip to the doctor and a subsequent mammogram resulted in a cancer diagnosis. Joan was stunned but philosophical about the news. Although her doctor originally thought a lumpectomy would suffice, the pathology report showed that the tumor margins were not clear of cancer cells and she had one positive lymph node. She would require a mastectomy and subsequent chemotherapy. When she learned that she could also have breast reconstruction, Joan decided to have a mastectomy with *immediate breast reconstruction with a latis-*

*simus dorsi (back) flap of her own natural (autologous) tissue.* She chose this form of reconstruction because she did not want an implant and had sufficient back tissue to do the job.

Joan is a soft-spoken, no-nonsense individual. She works in a government office as an administrative assistant and is not a wealthy woman by any means. Now in her fifties, Joan is heavyset with streaks of gray highlighting her medium-brown hair. Although she is not an animated talker, there is an earnestness about her that makes you lean forward to try to embrace the many layers of her personality. Breast cancer represented a special challenge for Joan. As a single woman, she lacked the support system provided by husband, children, or significant other to help her cope with recovery or with the grieving process that usually accompanies this type of life-threatening illness. Other life events precipitated by her cancer led to changes that caused substantial stress. She was forced to give up her second job because of doctor's orders to slow down; she found herself strapped economically, unable to meet financial obligations without this supplementary income; and most recently, a job reassignment caused further concern.

Joan's story poignantly illustrates the complex emotions and life changes that breast cancer elicits and the special problems that single women may encounter. Joan prides herself on her optimistic and pragmatic approach to life. However, she also admits that once she let down her guard, fully one year after her cancer diagnosis and treatment, she was overcome by a deep overriding sense of grief and depression unlike any she had ever experienced. Her faith finally pulled her through this particularly dark period. As Joan recalls, "I just gave it to God. I said now you take it and do what you will." Since that time bouts of depression still overtake her, and she has had counseling to help her cope. She has also gone back to school to recapture her zest for life and her optimism about the future. Her hope is that by helping others she can also help herself.

### How did you discover that you had breast cancer?

We have a wellness program at work and are allowed time to exercise. I walked every morning and was up to 2 miles a day. One day, halfway into my walk, I started getting very tired. It just kept getting worse. I finally had to sit down on somebody's wall outside their house. I thought, "Oh, my God, something's wrong with me. I don't know if I am going to be able to get back to work." I sat there for over 20 minutes and then started back real slow. I went to my doctor's office the very next day. I told him, "Something is desperately wrong with me." The fatigue was unbelievable. I had never experienced anything like that. He did some tests, and when he got to the breast exam, I could tell by his face that he had found something. He sent me for a mammogram.

They found a large fast-growing cancer. I hadn't felt anything myself. Of course, I wasn't very regular about doing breast self-exam then, but I do it regularly now. As soon as they looked at my breast, they could actually see that it was dimpling, sort of pulling in. I thought that I knew all of the signs of cancer because my mother died of pancreatic cancer. But that was a new one for me. I also never realized that fatigue could be part of it. After examining my breast and looking at my mammogram, the doctors were 99% sure that this was cancer.

### How did you cope with your cancer diagnosis? What helped you to deal with this news?

Frankly, it was harder for my doctor to tell me than it was for me to hear it. I was sorry to put him through it, but that's life. I shed a few tears and then drove home. I thought, "Okay Joan, you have two choices. You can go home and cry all night, but then tomorrow you will go to work with red puffy eyes and a migraine. Or you can do something else." So I did something else. It was December 2nd and I put up Christmas decorations—the tree, the lights, the candles, the whole deal. I sat there and enjoyed the glow. I said to myself, "You are about to start a long journey. The only way to survive it is to have a positive attitude. Positive energy will heal you; whereas negativity and depression will only make things worse." To me there was no choice, there was only one way to go.

### What happened after the diagnosis? How did you find a surgeon?

My internist recommended a surgeon, but I didn't like him. He seemed cold and impersonal. He told me that he was 99% sure I had cancer. Whenever he saw dimpling like mine, it was always cancer. I thought to myself, "I deserve better. Cancer is enough to experience; I don't want to be treated like a number." I told this doctor I needed a second opinion.

A friend at work referred me to another surgeon. I went to see him and I took a pad of paper and tape recorder to help me remember what he said. I liked him right away. He was willing to talk to me as long as I needed, until all the questions were answered. He was the total opposite of the first surgeon. I said, "This is the one for me."

### Did he answer all of your questions and explain your options?

Yes. He told me that I would probably be a candidate for a lumpectomy or that I could have a mastectomy with breast reconstruction. He was pretty confident that the lumpectomy would take care of it. They would do that in place of a biopsy, in case that was all that I needed.

### What did the lumpectomy reveal? Why did you then have a mastectomy?

He did the lumpectomy as an outpatient procedure. When the pathology report came back, one tumor margin was not clear of cancer. My surgeon offered to go back in and clean it up, but I told him to "just take the whole breast. I don't need it. My life is more important." At this point I had entrusted my fate to God. I said "God, I don't know what to do. You guide me. I know you will show me what's best." And God did. Two weeks later I had a mastectomy with immediate breast reconstruction.

### How did you learn about breast reconstruction?

The surgeon asked if I were interested in breast reconstruction. I hadn't thought about it. To me, plastic surgery was something that was either done by women who were vain and wanted bigger boobs or smaller butts or it was for accident victims. You know—either vanity or trauma. After some thought, however, I decided I would like to consult with a plastic surgeon. My surgeon made an appointment for me to see one of the top plastic surgeons in our area.

### Why did you decide to have breast reconstruction? What reconstructive procedure did you choose? What did this involve?

I decided that if I could have my breast rebuilt naturally, I would go ahead and do it. It would be something that I would do for myself. When the plastic surgeon explained all of the different types of reconstruction, I was just blown away. I'm going, "Whoa, I didn't know you could do all that, even tattooing and nipples." I thought, "This is neat."

I was determined not to have implants. I had gotten rid of cancer. I didn't want anything else put in, particularly something that might cause further concern. Since I didn't want implants, a flap of my own tissue was the best option. I was not a good candidate for the TRAM (abdominal) flap because I was too heavy, and it would be a more dangerous operation for me. Fortunately, for once in my life, being overweight was a blessing. I had plenty of fatty tissue on my back. So I chose to have my breast reconstructed with an autologous latissimus dorsi (back) flap. It was a good choice. With this procedure, the plastic surgeon took a back flap of muscle and fatty tissue and tunneled it through my underarm incision to my chest wall to shape my new breast.

### Why did you decide to have immediate breast reconstruction?

I was excited that everything could be taken care of in one major operation and I would have a breast when it was over. That meant one less hospital stay. This was my very first experience in a hospital, and I was relieved that I could just get it over with at one time and at less overall expense.

### What was your primary goal in seeking breast reconstruction?

I wanted a rebuilt breast that looked like my natural one. I didn't want implants because they might need to be redone periodically. That didn't make any sense to me. Why not use natural tissue and save yourself a lot of trouble down the road? I joked about it with everyone at the hospital. I said, "Well I went into the hospital with me and came out with me slightly rearranged."

### How long were you hospitalized? Did you experience much pain? Was hospitalization as frightening as you imagined?

I was in the hospital for 6 days. The pain wasn't bad. With the latissimus dorsi flap, they have to make a mid-back incision that also cuts the nerves in that area. Therefore I had no pain to deal with, just the strange sensation of dead weight. My new breast didn't hurt; it was just heavy. The nurses had me on the PCA (patient-controlled anesthesia) pump so I could give myself doses of pain medicine. I only hit the button twice during the first day. I didn't need it after that.

I was out of bed the next day. From then on I spent little time in bed. People were surprised to see me roaming around. I don't know what they expected. When someone knows you are a cancer patient, I suppose they expect to see you lying in bed, pale, looking like you are ready to die. I wasn't. I was walking the halls, talking to the nurses, and waving to everyone.

I was pleasantly surprised by the hospital experience. I thought it would be horrible. I had always joked that if I ever had to go to the hospital, someone would have to knock me out and take me there before I had time to think about it. But it wasn't that bad. Anyway, I had so much to do that I really didn't have time to worry about the hospital stay.

### Did you go home with drains? How long did these stay in?

I had three drains inserted in the hospital. These bother a lot of people, but they weren't a problem for me. They took out two of them in the hospital. I went home with only one drain still in; it was removed after 3 weeks.

### Did you have any restrictions on activity after your surgery? Did being alone present any special problems during recovery?

Because my back flap was used to reconstruct my breast, I was not allowed to lift my arm above my shoulder for a while. I was also not allowed to drive for about 7 weeks. What struck me as funny is that I despise driving. I do it out of pure necessity. I really hate it. What I need is a chauffeur and that's not going to happen any time soon. However, when they said I couldn't drive during recovery, I felt a burning desire to get out there and drive. Boy, did I want to drive a car! I wanted out of that apartment and into my car. I bugged my plastic surgeon every time I came in. Of course, once there was no restriction, I didn't want to do it anymore.

My activity was generally limited for about 3 months. I had to forego exercises until I healed. I got carried away in the hospital with my exercises. I had surgery in the morning and that night they let me walk across the room. The next day I started walking the wall with my fingers as they had instructed. What they hadn't told me was that I had to heal a bit before I began. Every time I did these exercises I started bleeding. So I had to stop for a short time to make sure I was healed.

### Did you have anyone who could help you when you went home? What special accommodations did you have to make for yourself?

Being single, I didn't have somebody to ask, "Honey, do this, Honey, make this appointment, or Honey, help me with this." I had to do it all myself. My father was there for the lumpectomy, but after the mastectomy Dad was getting ready to go into surgery himself, so I had no one I could rely on.

It took me a while to convince my plastic surgeon that I was going home alone and nobody would be there to do for me. He kept assuming that I would have help and I kept insisting otherwise. After the third time my message sank in. I said, "Read my lips, I am going home alone; now tell me what to do."

He told me that I should place anything that I normally reach for in my cabinets or above my head on the counter within easy reach. That worked, but the kitchen was a mess for a while. My clothes washer is one that I roll to the sink to hook up, so I had to move it to the middle of the kitchen before surgery so that it could be plugged in easily without my having to exert too much effort. It was in the way, but it did the trick until I was able to lift my arm and move more easily.

### How long did it take you before you returned to your normal level of activity once you got home? How long before you could return to work?

It was about a year before I was totally back to myself, even though my energy level is still not what it was. However, that never interfered with my work. I am stubborn, so I worked half days the whole time. I just did what I had to do to save my life. It was important for me to keep working. It gave me a feeling of accomplishing something every day. Even if I only got one stupid letter typed, it was better than sitting at home vegetating.

### Were they understanding at work about your illness? Were they supportive?

I work for a government agency and have done so for almost 12 years. They were my support system. They had recently started a program that allowed people to donate personal leave time to others. People at work literally supported me for almost 2 years by donating leave to me. I didn't have to worry about bills or where the money was coming from. All I had to worry about was getting better. So many people offered to help. They came out of the woodwork—people that I didn't even know. They gave me a list of people who offered help. If I needed anyone to take me to get groceries, to go to doctors' appointments, or run errands, I could call on these individuals. They bought me a microwave when they learned that I would not be able to raise my arm above my head for a while. They even brought frozen dinners over so I wouldn't have to cook. They were absolutely amazing.

### *What was your reaction to chemotherapy? Did you experience any problems or side effects?*

I had 6 months of chemotherapy. It was given every 3 weeks. It wasn't as bad as I thought it was going to be, even though I did have to adjust to feeling queasy all the time. I enjoyed the nurses; we had a good time. I also enjoyed going to the treatments. I know that sounds crazy, but for me it represented one step closer to getting better.

At the first chemotherapy treatment they had trouble finding good veins. It took a very long time. To avoid having this problem each time, they decided to put a port in. It's a type of tube that is inserted in your chest and goes into your veins or one of your main arteries. It stays in for the whole time. The part that you can feel in your chest is about the size of a quarter, and it's slightly raised. They were able to insert the needle directly into the port rather than into my veins. The port stayed in for 1 year.

I was pleasantly surprised at how far chemo has come since I witnessed my mother's treatment for pancreatic cancer. She was deathly ill and hospitalized for an entire week, throwing up the whole time. I thought, "Oh God, I guess this is what I have to look forward to." But it wasn't that bad. I had a treatment every 3 weeks for a couple of hours. Then I knew that I had about 2 hours before I was going to be sick. So I would get something I enjoyed to eat on the way home, and I would totally indulge myself until I started vomiting. I only became really ill and vomited once during treatment; after that I was just queasy and tired. The fatigue has stayed with me even today. Most of the people I know who had chemo never fully regain their energy. I thought I would. I thought that once the chemicals were out of my system, everything would go back to the way it was—plenty of energy. But it isn't the same.

I also lost all of my hair except for a few strands. I wore turbans until my wig was ready. I had three different turbans and decorated them with various pins and brooches. People started saying, "What's she got on today?" and they would check my turban to see what I had pinned to it that day. That was fun.

### *Did you have your nipple-aerola reconstructed? Did you require any additional adjustments or secondary procedures?*

Yes, I had my nipple and areola redone. That was part of the package. My nipple was rebuilt with the same tissue that they used for the reconstruction—the local tissue on my breast. The areola was created later by tattooing.

Some other adjustments were made during the same outpatient surgery. I had swelling under my arm after the first surgery that felt like a ball of extra tissue. It was really annoying. My plastic surgeon kept assuring me that the swelling would go down, but it didn't. It bothered me a lot. Finally I said, "This swelling needs to go." My plastic surgeon said he could remove it with liposuction when he did the nipple reconstruction. I said, "While you are in there suctioning, could you just slide the suction down and get some of the fat out of my stomach and hip area. He said that a lot of women make that request and he could do it all at the same time. So at the time I was having my nipple reconstructed, they also removed the swelling under my arm and suctioned my stomach area.

When I healed, my areola was tattooed in the office. That was fun. The nurse who was doing the tattooing used the good breast as a palette to match the different colors. We mixed the colors to get as close a match as possible. I chose the final color.

**Did your breast reconstruction meet your expectations? Would you choose to have reconstructive surgery again?**

Yes, I would do it again in a heartbeat. Reconstructive surgery exceeded my expectations; it was much better than I thought it would be. I would also choose the same operation. It was the right one for me.

**Are you satisfied with your breast appearance? Are your breasts symmetric?**

Yes, I am very satisfied. I thought the reconstructed breast would look different from the other one, but it really doesn't. I was just amazed at how careful he was to make sure they are exactly the same. They even droop the same. I couldn't believe it. I really expected some sort of a difference because one is natural. The other one is natural tissue, but it is back tissue. My results are amazing. You can't even tell I had it done. The scars are barely noticeable. My new breast looks just like the other one.

**How does your reconstructed breast feel? Does it have sensation?**

That's the only thing that is different. It's warm like the other one, but there is no feeling in it. It doesn't get hard when I get cold like the natural one does. I can feel pressure, but if I scratch it, I can't feel that.

*What do your scars look like? Where are they located?*

I have one back scar, two breast scars, and one underarm scar. The first time I saw the scars I said, "Whoa!" But now they have faded. There are just little tiny marks. They are not a big deal.

*Did you have any surprises from your breast reconstruction?*

Because they used my back muscle and fatty tissue to make a breast, it still functioned as if it were a back muscle moving my arm. In other words, when I move that arm, my breast moves automatically because it is all connected. It is strange. The first time it happened I went, "Hey, what was that?" It just looks funny and I am going, well maybe it's a good thing I am not married. I guess I had better get used to it because it always happens. No one told me this would happen. I just reached for something one day and all of a sudden that breast went bong. I figured it out, once I stopped laughing. It was really funny. It took me by total surprise. I was going, "Okay, why is my breast doing that?" and then I sat and thought about it and figured it out. It's back tissue; it is still connected, so it seems only natural that when I move my arm the muscle still works.

*Were your doctors helpful to you through this process? Did they provide you with all the information you needed? Did they spend sufficient time with you?*

Yes, I got the information that I needed, but sometimes I had to practically stand in the door to get my plastic surgeon to stay put. He is very busy, I know, but sometimes I just needed to get his attention. I had to say, "Wait a minute, I have some questions." Then he was fine. He would stop and answer whatever questions I had. The oncologist learned early on that I was somebody who wanted to know absolutely everything; I didn't want anything hidden from me at all. Once he realized that, our relationship was a hundred percent better. He was not accustomed to people wanting to know everything. He said most of his patients don't really desire that much information; they just wanted enough to get by, just a little bit. But I said, "I don't want you to hide anything. This is my body, it's my life, and I want to know everything." I went in with questions every time, and after the first two or three visits he realized that this was the pattern. This was who I was, and this was how I worked. Then it was okay. He would do the examination and say, "Okay, hit me with the questions. I'm ready." Then we would go through my list and he would answer every question.

*How could your doctors have been more helpful?*

They talked to me, explained my options, but didn't direct me to any outside resources. I have always felt that every doctor needs to be prepared to hand a patient diagnosed with cancer a booklet with questions and answers and available resources. I didn't have a clue. You have heard this terrible thing, and you go, "I have cancer? What do I do about it?" Somebody needs to be there immediately to tell you. Someone said, "Make sure you ask the right questions." But I didn't know what the right questions were and that's where most people are. Doctors should be a resource for patients.

*Do you think there are special challenges for a single woman coping with something like this?*

Most of my friends who have gone through this experience are married with children. They have family right there—that's both good and bad. It is hard for the family, but at the same time you have people there to help you do things. You have shoulders to cry on, somebody to hug you and tell you it is going to be okay. When you are single and alone, you don't have that; you have to find it elsewhere. I was lucky because I received a lot of that support at work. Also, I wasn't as needy because I just didn't go through the emotional thing at the beginning. I never do anything like anybody else. It was not until I hit my year anniversary that I fell apart.

*How did you fall apart? Why do you think it happened? Were you surprised at the delayed reaction?*

I just fell apart. I was caught completely unaware. At first, after I was diagnosed and then after the surgery I kept waiting for the stages of grief that everyone told me to expect. They said that you have to go through all the steps just like a death." So I waited and I waited, but it never happened. And I really didn't see the point anyway because I never asked, "Why me?" For me, the question was always, "Why not me?" I mean really there is no point in denying cancer. It's just something that happens.

I was sitting in front of my computer at work and one minute I was talking and the next minute I was sobbing for no apparent reason. I was fine; I knew that. I knew I would be cured. I just lost it. I went to one of the ladies I work with and she hugged me and said, "Just let it out. It's all right. You took care of all the technical stuff and now your body is making you listen to it because you have ignored it so far." She was right; she was absolutely right. I needed somebody to tell me it was okay to give in to my emotions. I had been thinking, "This is stupid. I'm fine. What am I doing this for? This is unnecessary. I don't need this." But I was wrong. I had to go through it.

### Was there someone you could talk to about your feelings?

That has proved to be a problem for me. I am an excellent listener and I can help other people, but it is really difficult for me to reach out to somebody when I need help. One of the biggest challenges was confronting this whole disease process by myself. I have lived alone for a long time, and I am accustomed to being the one doing everything for myself and being totally self-sufficient. All of a sudden, however, I wasn't self-sufficient anymore. Cancer has a way of making you dependent. I did not want to admit that and it took a couple of friends sitting me down and saying, "Joan, you have to realize you do need help now. We all need help sometime. We have all these people who want to help you, and when you tell them no, you are not allowing them that chance to feel good because they helped you. It makes them feel good that they can do something." It is such a hopeless feeling when you see someone you care about going through something and there is nothing that you really can do. I try to help others now whenever I can to make this coping process a little easier.

### Have you had any further problems with depression? Is there any warning that this is going to occur? How do you cope?

Although I am feeling positive now, you would have seen another side of me if you had been here 3 weeks ago. Then I was in total depression, crying all the time. I had been that way for about 3 months. I don't really know why I get depressed. The first depression started with the cancer recovery process. I expected to go through a grieving process, which is part of the loss and the cancer experience; however, I never expected that the depression would come back. Since that time, I have found out that this depression recurs for some people. Evidently that's the way it is for me because this is the third or fourth time that I have had this and it got worst. I have seen a therapist and that didn't help. I had to let God help me get through it. After all, he got me through this whole thing in the first place. So I let him handle it and it went away. It comes out of the blue; I can't point to anything in particular that triggers it. Now I realize that this is something I am going to have to deal with. Recently I talked to a few ladies and they said they have also experienced these bouts of depression. That's kind of hard to deal with; you don't function like you should. You aren't happy, but you aren't really sad either. I am fine one minute and the next minute, bam! Kind of like a little gray cloud that follows you around and once in a while drops a little rain on you.

### What contributes to these depressive feelings?

There are so many pressures and stresses to deal with that coping is not always easy. It's difficult when you are single. You only have one income to depend on. My doctors won't let me work a second job anymore. I used to do that, but now, because of the stress I am prone to, they have said no. I don't earn much, and with the additional expense of my illness, I can't pay the bills and creditors are calling. I leave the answering machine on all the time, but I just can't live that way. I also have more pressure at work. They assigned me to a new job 6 months ago; it was either that or no job at all. They have given me a year to learn it. I like it better than I did at first, but it is not what I want to be doing. So there have been a number of pressures that have probably contributed to my depression.

### What do you do to help yourself stay positive and to keep your spirits up?

I try to be good to myself. Sometimes I treat myself to movies or buy something pretty that I might not have purchased before. It is just an extravagance, something that captures my fancy, like a lovely scarf. It's all about enjoying life. I like to get out and walk, to take pleasure in nature, to sit and meditate, to talk to the birds, to read good books, to listen to nice music, to dance, to indulge myself in activities that bring joy. I have joined a singing group: it relaxes me and helps to relieve stress. I have also gotten back into childhood pursuits such as coloring books. Some people say, "At your age, with a coloring book?" But why not? I have found the little child in me again. I had lost that child for a while. But she's back now. So I color sometimes. When I get a chance, I go to a special camp for adult cancer patients; it is just wonderful. It is on a lake in a gorgeous setting. They pamper you there. It is a safe haven. No explanations are ever needed because we are all coming from the same place.

Going back to school has been a big step for me; it is a symbol of my effort to improve my life. It is probably the most significant, positive action I have taken to reverse the pressures that cause my depression. It is both frightening and exciting, but I am committed to it.

### Why are you going back to school? Has the adjustment been difficult?

People ask me, "Why is someone your age going back to college?" My response is, "Why not?" If you are happy with your life, terrific, but I am not and I intend to do something to change it. I am trying to reclaim my opportunities; cancer has given me the second chance that I needed.

I am just starting and there are challenges. I had 2 years of college 30 years ago. I was a sophomore, and believe it or not, after 30 years I am still a sophomore. They accepted almost all of my former credits. It is easier going back now because schools are gearing themselves toward older students. Increasingly they offer special programs to help us and they seem to have respect for older students, so that is good. The problem I am having now is that I have 30 years of catch-up to do. It is also tough finding the money to go to school; I rob Peter to pay Paul. I can't pay the creditors, but I know I have to go to school if I want to have a better life. It is an investment in my future.

### What impact has cancer had on your life?

Cancer has totally turned my life around. I used to consider myself a caterpillar; now I am a butterfly, experiencing the beautiful flowers, the world, and life itself. I used to just inch my way along and watch the world go by. I'd say, "I'd like to try that someday. Oh, well, I'll get to it later." Now I know that there are no guarantees. I seize the opportunity of the moment. If there is something I want to do now, I do it if at all possible. Life is so much better now. I have gone back to school, I have spread my wings, and I am intent on finding a new direction in life.

Cancer made me realize that I was on the wrong path. God wanted me doing something else. I used to sit and wait and wonder why people did not do for me. Now I reach out to others and I do for them. You heal yourself when you help others to heal. It is a process that grows and blossoms. Now I have a goal: I am going to use my education to counsel cancer patients. At this time I am doing it as a volunteer until I have the training to do it as a professional. I get so much joy out of it, much more than I give. It is a gift to be able to help someone in need.

People think of cancer as a negative, but it can become a positive. It has for me. Cancer was a wake-up call. It refocused me and redirected me to the right path, the one I am on now. I don't know where it is going to lead me, but I am going to enjoy the journey.

## SIMONE: A FRENCH PERSPECTIVE

"You know in my country, the French women, we are not like, how would you say, prohibited. You know, not showing yourself. We have a different reaction with our bodies. In France we have the nude beaches and topless beaches. We are more open. We like our bodies and the breasts are for women something special." This charming explanation was given to me by Simone as she described her reasons for wanting breast reconstruction.

Simone is a native of France who has been living in the United States for over 20 years. She is bilingual and works full-time as a French translator at an export company. Even though she apologized during our interview for her inability to communicate because of her lingering accent, I found her to be articulate and intelligent. A small woman with short blond hair, she has the stunning good looks so characteristic of French women and an almost casual sense of style. At 46 years of age she is married, the mother of three, and the grand-mother of four. She prides herself on being health conscious. She eats well, exercises, and loves the outdoors, frequently retreating to the mountains with her husband to hike and contemplate nature. In fact, that is the refuge they sought when her cancer was diagnosed.

Simone's cancer seemed to come out of nowhere. She has no family history and has always been very good about going for physical examinations and mammograms.

Simone describes herself as a strong, even tough, person. She knew she could survive this experience. Fortunately, she didn't have to face it alone. She had her husband. "A wonderful guy . . . he was there with me all the way. The two of us went through it together."

Simone's cancer was treated by mastectomy, followed by 6 months of chemotherapy and then a *TRAM flap breast reconstruction combined with a breast lift on her opposite breast.* She wanted the TRAM reconstruction because her new breast would be created out of her own tissue, not an implant. Originally she had worried that she wouldn't have enough abdominal fat to build a breast. But because of her good eating habits during chemotherapy she gained 18 pounds, leaving her with plenty of abdominal fat to fashion a new breast. Simone's story is an uplifting one and her perspective is uniquely French.

### How did you discover you had breast cancer?

Two years ago in June I was feeling fatigued, so I went to the doctor for a complete physical; all my results came back fine. No sign of anything. Two months later I went to New Orleans with my husband. I was putting on the sexy lingerie I had bought when I felt a lump on the top of my breast. I knew I had fibrocystic disease, so I thought maybe it was just another cyst popping up. I was drinking a lot of caffeinated beverages. I decided to stop drinking so much coffee and I took vitamin E, but it did not go away. When September came, the lump was no smaller. I had company during that time and did not have much time to myself. So I let it ride, just put myself on the back burner and took care of everybody else. In November I decided "that is not right. I have to do something." I went for a mammogram. When I got the mammogram the doctor sent me to a surgeon who did a biopsy and told me I had breast cancer. He advised me to have the breast removed.

### Did the surgeon give you any other options? Did he tell you about lumpectomy and irradiation?

He could tell by the size of the tumor that lumpectomy was not advisable. If he removed the lump, my breast would have been so damaged that even reconstruction would have been difficult. So mastectomy was his recommendation. I trusted this particular surgeon. He was quite special, very caring. I asked him to give me 3 days to think about it.

### What was your reaction to the breast cancer diagnosis?

I was not really shocked because of the size of the lump and the way it felt. But I think every woman must ask, "Why me?" "What is it going to do to my life? How is it going to change?" The breasts are for women something very special. I wanted to be around, so I was going to do whatever was necessary to beat this cancer. I was not really bitter. I am quite strong mentally. I come from a strong family. I have been married before and my first marriage was not a good marriage; I learned to be quite tough. I did not think the breast cancer was the end of the world. I thought I am going to do this and I am going to go on with my life with one breast or two breasts. I am going to have a good time. My husband, he is a great guy, and I think he was more concerned about the way I would react.

When I first found out I had cancer, my husband and I took off for the mountains. When I want to think about something, I have to go where it is quiet. I have to go to nature; I relate with the peace and I guess that is closer to God. We went hiking and talked about it and the things we would have to do. I did not know the extent of the cancer and that concerned me more than having the breast removed. We spent the day in the mountains, talking, and came to the conclusion that the surgery was needed and we would make the best of it. Whatever happened we would make it together.

### How did you tell your children? How did they react?

I just told them like it was. I do not beat around the bushes. That Sunday I decided to call everybody. I called my children and I told them that I had breast cancer and I needed a mastectomy. They were speechless. Nobody knew what to say. I called friends, the people at work, and my family. I got the same reaction from everyone. "No, it is not possible." I said, "You know, it is possible. It happens to one in every eight women and now I am the one of the eight."

### How long did it take you to recover from your mastectomy? Did you experience much pain?

I recuperate quite quickly. I could use my arm right away. My surgeon was totally amazed how much I could do. My husband brought my nice gown and makeup case to the hospital, and the day after surgery I washed my hair and got myself fixed up. I was operated on Wednesday and discharged from the hospital on Sunday. By then I could raise my arm. I really did not have any pain. The drains were probably the most uncomfortable thing I had to endure. I felt good. When the surgeon removed the bandages, my husband and I saw it, and I said, "It is going to be okay. I still have one and I am going to be fine." I was still anxious to find out how far the cancer had gone.

### Did you have any positive lymph nodes? Did you require any additional therapy?

I had three involved nodes. A week later I started chemotherapy.

### When did you return to work?

I stayed off work from December to September. I probably could have gone back after the surgery, but I would have been very fatigued when I was taking chemo. I chose to take a leave of absence to recuperate fully, to get my strength back, to go through chemo. I am a strong believer in nourishing yourself correctly. If I would have gone to work, I probably would not have taken care of myself as well as I did. While I was at home, I went to the market and made a point of buying fresh vegetables and a lot of fresh fruit and prepared special meals. My hus-hand said I was becoming a very good chef. I truly believe eating well helped me quite a bit during chemotherapy. I gained weight during chemo. I had a chance to do some reading, and I got involved with modeling for mastectomy patients.

### How did you start modeling for mastectomy patients?

I went to be fitted for my prosthesis about a month after surgery. The lady at the lingerie shop was very nice. Mastectomy lingerie is not very sexy, and I made a comment to her that somebody needs to come up with much nicer ideas for lingerie. After all, we are still women. It makes you feel better if you have something pretty to wear instead of those ugly bras, heavy-duty looking things. So she said, "Well I know of a company that makes the prostheses and is currently working on a line of bras." Several days later this lady called and said a person from the company wanted to meet me. I came and she showed me this new bra. She said, "What do you think of my product? I need people to try the new bra with their prosthesis and I need feedback. I would like for you to tell me how you feel about it." I said "Great." They were underwire bras, lace with a nice pocket. Much nicer than the regular mastectomy bra. I tried the bra for a few days, and when I returned it, she asked if I would like to be one of their models? "We need someone like you who is not inhibited and can model the bra for the retailers. We like for them to see it on someone who had a mastectomy." I agreed, I even posed in a photo session.

### What was your reaction to having chemotherapy? Did you have any side effects?

Like everyone else, I had heard horror stories about chemotherapy. The oncologist told me exactly what to expect. He said, "I am not going to say that you are not going to lose your hair. Some women do, some women do not. Those are the side effects you may encounter," and he went over them, "but it is very much an individualized type of reaction." The first time I went for chemo his nurse explained what drugs I would be receiving and she stayed with me during the treatment. I went home thinking, "Well, what is this supposed to do to me?" The day went by and I felt fatigue, but they had given me a nausea-type medicine that makes you groggy. That is what I am feeling, more sleepy, nothing happened. No, nothing. No side effect. Second trip, no side effects. So he increased the dosage. We had to do some readjustments, but each time before I would go to chemo, I would always do something special the day before, you know, something to get myself ready and happy. I never took the chemotherapy negatively; I took it positively. I think that has helped me. It was like taking a vitamin, something I had to do to make me feel better. The last treatment was a little bit nauseating, but I did not lose my hair. It only thinned out.

### What did you do to cope with your cancer treatment?

Sometimes I had a good cry, and that kind of clears the air. You let it all out. It takes the tension off. I have been here for 26 years in this country, so you know I have experienced down days missing my home, my country. I always find I can have a good cry and feel better.

My husband was a wonderful help. He would look at me and say, "Okay, let's go hiking. I think it is what you need and here we go." We would pack and go. I feel very close to the earth and to nature, so those trips were very calming.

### How did you learn about breast reconstruction?

I was not ignorant of breast cancer and reconstruction. I had read about it and I had heard about it. You know, you never think it is going to happen to you, but I was aware of some of the techniques available. Before my mastectomy I asked my surgeon what the scar would look like after he removed my breast? I wanted an indication of how big it would be and where it would be. We talked about that and I said, "Now, what do you know about reconstruction? What type of reconstruction would you recommend?" He said, "That is a personal choice; you will have to make your own choice." He had a book on his shelf that talked about the different reconstructive techniques. He told me to read it. It would give me an indication of what to expect and would help me make a decision. He said, "If you have to have chemotherapy, I would suggest you wait until you finish chemo and fully recover."

### Why did you want reconstruction?

I like nice lingerie. I enjoy having a cleavage. With the prosthesis, when you bend down, even with those special bras, it does not feel the same. You never feel complete; it is not attached to you. It does not feel the same in your clothes. I think I had to have it done to feel right, to feel comfortable.

Several years ago I lived in Baton Rouge. After having three children my breasts were sagging. I went to a breast clinic to see about having a breast lift, having the surgeon remove some of the skin and lift the breasts. I always had it in my mind to have my breasts redone. So I was telling my husband when I had the reconstruction, you know, I always wanted a "boob job" and I guess I'll have it now. You have to be careful about what you wish for because it may come true. I had not planned to have my boob job that way.

### How did your husband feel about your reconstruction? Was he supportive?

He knows when I have made up my mind about something I am going to do it. He asked me if I was strong enough to go through it. I said, "Yes I was," and he said, "Okay, you know I will be there. I will be with you every step of the way." We are husband and wife, but we are also best friends. Now he is very complimentary about it. He thinks it is great. Support from your spouse is definitely a plus.

### What reconstructive technique did you select? Why?

I was very impressed when I read about the TRAM flap procedure. I personally believe in taking your own tissue. If that was possible, I wanted to do it. But because I was so thin, only 103 pounds, I did not have much of a stomach there. I said, "Maybe it is not going to be possible." If I do not have enough here, we will have to use a back flap. I didn't want a scar on my back. My second choice was to have tissue expansion. I thought I will go that route. Little did I know then that when I went on chemo, eating the way I was eating, I would gain 18 pounds. I was able to have my TRAM flap after all.

### How did you select your plastic surgeon?

My surgeon recommended him, so I made an appointment. My husband and I spoke with him. He discussed the procedure and I was very pleased with his consultation. There is something very honest about him. I trusted him and I had very good vibes about him. I had heard different stories from different women. Some women had suggested that I go elsewhere. One said, "You are going to be one of many and you are not going to have the attention that you should have." I said, "Possibly, but it is a choice that I have to make." I did not feel that way. He is a very busy man, but I had very good care. He always answered my questions.

### How long were you in the hospital? Did you experience much pain?

I was in the hospital for 6 days. I heard from other women that it would be extremely painful. But the word "painful" means something different for each person. I did not find it painful. I found it uncomfortable, but not painful.

The most discomfort that I encountered was from my back. When you come back from surgery, you are in a "jackknife" position because you have stitches in your abdomen and cannot really stretch. So they position you where you cannot move very well. You do not want to pull anything. I could not find a position in the bed that was comfortable for my back. My lower back was bothering me, but I did not find my abdomen painful; it pulled when I moved, but the pulling was not a pain to me. When I got up from the bed to sit in the chair, I did it very easily. They kept asking me to grade the level of pain, and I really could not tell them. My breast was not painful at all because the nerves had been cut, so there was no feeling.

### Initially, after the first stage of the breast reconstruction, were you satisfied with your breast appearance? Were any adjustments needed?

I was amazed. You see the pictures, but the actual marvel of what the surgeon is able to do to shape a breast can only be understood when you see it in person.

I had the other breast lifted at the same time. My breasts matched pretty well, but the new breast needed to be reshaped a bit. It was a little bit larger and not as round as the normal one. Earlier, he had told me that if I needed any adjustments he would reshape my breast when he did the nipple.

### Did you have any complications or any problems after your breast reconstruction?

I had the other breast lifted at the same time, so I had drains in the abdomen and in both breasts. But I had no complications.

### How long did it take before you could resume your normal activities?

After I got home it took another week to 10 days before I really could walk correctly. I always felt like I was bending down some because the stomach pulls. Within 3 weeks of the surgery I was feeling pretty good. It took a good 6 weeks for my full strength to come back. I did not want to force it, so I was cautious. I took my vitamins again, and I went more slowly regarding activities.

### Why did you decide to have nipple-areola reconstruction?

When I found out I could use the stomach to build my breast, I decided to go all the way, you know. It is like doing half of the job if you don't go for the nipple. Some of the women that I spoke with told me after the initial reconstructive surgery they would not go back for further surgery. But for me, I felt that as soon as I healed enough I wanted to finish the job. I want my breast complete. It turned out great. I am not totally finished with it because we still have to tattoo the nipple.

### What did he use to build your nipple and areola? Did he make any other adjustments at that time?

He took my nipple and areola from the extra tissue left at the end of my abdominal scar (the dog ear) where he cut the flap. When he did the nipple, he trimmed the fat and reshaped the breast. Now it looks great. I am very, very pleased with it.

He also did liposuction around the abdominal scar to flatten it and it turned out great. This was outpatient surgery. I came, had the surgery, and went home.

### How do your scars look?

The reconstructed breast itself has a scar all around it. It is a very thin circular scar. Under the breast, coming from the middle of the breast up, you have a thin scar where they attach the fat. For the nipple, on top of the breast at the point where they attach the areola, there is a little circle scar. My scars were reddish at first, then they turned pink, and now they are beginning to fade and whiten.

The nipple itself is a small piece of your tissue sewn on; you really do not see any scar. It seems like it just grew out, but you can see this very thin scar for the areola.

Now, on the abdomen itself, you have a scar, like a smiley face, and that is where he took the flap for the breast.

### Are any of these scars visible in your clothing?

If I would wear something very low cut, I am maybe a little more restricted now than I will be later when the scar fades. It has only been 7 months. Within a year the scar will fade much more. Then if I wear something lower cut, I can cover it with a bit of makeup, and it will not be that noticeable. My abdominal scar doesn't show even when I wear a bikini, so it was well done.

### Do your breasts match?

Very much. The top of the newer breast may need to be raised a little bit more, but we want to give it a couple more months to let everything settle. Then we may raise that up a bit. If we go that route, my plastic surgeon suggested taking some tissue from under my arm, but it is not an absolute need.

### Do your breasts have sensation?

No. I can touch the breasts. I know my hand is there, but there is no actual feeling. If I pinch myself or if I were to stick a needle in my breast, I do not feel any pain.

### Are your breasts warm? Are they soft?

The temperature is a bit different. The reconstructed breast is sometimes a little colder than the other one. I think it is due to the circulation of the blood because of the way the breast was reconstructed.

The new breast is firm. When I am walking, it does not have the bounce of the normal breast. You feel it moving, but it does not have the feeling of a real breast. When you touch your normal breast, you feel the mammary glands—it's warm and soft. The new breast feels firmer, and I must say it takes a little time to get used to that.

### Did breast reconstruction meet your expectations? Are you satisfied?

Very much. Extremely satisfied. I never went through the reconstruction expecting my new breast to be like the old breast. You go through reconstruction to make you feel better, to help you adjust to the cancer. I like to be able to wear a regular bra and to have my clothes feel better. My new breast has similarities to my old, but it is not like a real breast. I went through reconstruction knowing that. I think that helped me too.

### Did you have any problems or complications with your reconstruction?

No problems whatsoever. I came out of it with flying colors. I would suggest to anyone who wants to go through it to first prepare herself with a good positive attitude. If you are positive, I think you can recover so much better. And you will feel great about yourself.

*If you had it to do over, would you have breast reconstruction again? Would you choose the same technique?*

Oh, yes. For me it was great. If I had cancer again, I would have reconstruction with no hesitation. I would choose the TRAM again. It is a beautiful operation.

*Did your mastectomy or your reconstruction affect the way you feel about yourself? Your feelings of sexuality?*

I am French. You can excuse me please. I like pretty lingerie. Before the mastectomy I was always sleeping in the nude. I would start with a gown, but I never finished that way. In the morning I would never wake up with a gown. When I had the mastectomy done, I came back from the hospital and for the first 2 weeks I was wearing a little gown for protection because of the scar and because I had some drainage. My husband looked at me and said, "Are you going to keep on wearing this gown?" and I said, "Well, what do you think?" He said, "Knowing you, you are going to be uncomfortable. I would not think you would want to be wearing a gown." So I took it off and went back to going without a gown. Because of the scar, I had to be more careful, but that did not stop me. It was still me, you know, and I was not ashamed of me. I have read about women who could not look at themselves, and I know someone like this. I never stopped looking. What I saw in the mirror was me with one breast left, but there was still a whole lot of me left to work with.

*How do you feel now when you look at yourself in the mirror?*

I feel great. I am the type, again, I do not sleep in anything. Many a time when I put on my makeup, I am naked in the bathroom, and I feel comfortable because scar or no scar, it is me and I look good.

## LOUELLA: MAKE THE BEST OF IT

"My philosophy has always been that as long as you feel sorry for yourself, things are not going to get a whole lot better. You will just sink deeper and deeper into those moods, and it will be harder and harder to pull yourself out. You need to break the pattern. Reach out to someone else, get involved, draw on your inner spiritual resources. Do anything to get your mind off yourself. As long as I am on this earth, I will do the best I can to take one day at a time, because that is all we are promised. None of us knows what tomorrow is going to bring. It is time to enjoy life."

Louella expressed these sentiments as she related her breast cancer experience and the series of complications that she weathered during her recovery. Louella is a licensed practical nurse with a big smile and a hearty laugh. She is a striking African-American woman with short, cropped hair, large, expressive eyes, and a full, well-proportioned figure. She came to our interview clad in a bright red sweater and dangling pearl earrings that contrasted beautifully with her dark complexion.

Louella's cancer was discovered during a long-overdue checkup. A routine mammogram was the harbinger of shocking news. Her cancer was advanced and she had one positive node. Treatment involved *lumpectomy with immediate latissimus dorsi breast reconstruction* and then chemotherapy and radiation therapy. She was devastated and angry with herself for having neglected her health care so long that it had led to this. "If I hadn't been so negligent and had checked myself and gotten yearly mammograms, perhaps this could have been caught sooner." As a health care professional, Louella is well aware of the advantages of early detection for breast cancer, and she admonishes herself for being foolish. She knows that breast cancer survival statistics for African-American women are far worse than for the general population, possibly because less attention is paid to routine screening and checkups. She admits she should have known better.

Considering all that Louella has suffered in the past few years, it is truly astounding that she can be so positive about life. She has faced a series of complications, including edema, hematoma, radiation burns, and lymphedema. Most of these were transient problems that have now resolved except for the lymphedema she developed after axillary dissection. The lymphedema is an ongoing reminder of her bout with breast cancer. It is a chronic problem that requires constant care to prevent debilitating fluid buildup. She accepts the problems she encountered philosophically as a small price to pay for the gift of life. As she explains, "I'm grateful to God that I'm here."

### How did you discover your breast cancer?

Realizing I had been negligent about my own health while taking care of others, in July of 1995 I resolved to take care of myself. Three months later I made an appointment with an internist for a full checkup. During that process I had a mammogram that revealed some suspicious areas. Then I had ultrasound and an ultrasound-guided biopsy. These three tests confirmed that I had cancer, and I was referred to one of the cancer surgeons who broke the news to me. It was mind boggling. You just fall apart. You really don't know what to do, what to say, or how to react. My first reaction was let's get it out as soon as possible. I was in a state of shock. Since I thought this was just a routine mammogram, I had no one with me. I pulled myself together long enough to call my husband and he joined me. We then went to see the support nurse. I cried and wept for quite awhile; it was a very emotional time. It was hard pulling myself together, but I had to because I had another doctor to see.

### Did your doctors present you with various treatment options? Which ones did you select and why?

I saw a total of three doctors that day: a cancer surgeon, a radiologist, and a plastic surgeon. The cancer surgeon explained my options to me. I wanted to preserve my breast and requested lumpectomy with radiation therapy if my cancer could be treated with this procedure. Initially they thought that a mastectomy would have to be done because of the type of cancer I had. As it turned out, I was able to have the lumpectomy and radiation that I desired. However, the resulting defect would be large because I had a clump of three tumors. I would need a filler breast reconstruction with a latissimus dorsi back flap if I wanted a normal breast appearance. I also would have to have an axillary dissection so that my lymph nodes could be checked for cancer. With those procedures, my breast was preserved. Once I recovered from surgery, I would have radiation therapy, and if there were positive nodes, I would have chemotherapy. The axillary dissection revealed one positive lymph node, and so I had the full course of chemotherapy. Radiation therapy was given next after my body recovered.

When I first found out that I had cancer, I just wanted to get it out. If I had allowed myself more time to think, I might have explored the alternative of holistic medicine or having chemotherapy first to see if the tumor size could be decreased before I decided on surgery.

### Why did you decide to have a partial breast reconstruction?

I knew I didn't want to wake up with no breast or a partial breast and have to deal with the trauma of a scar. I wanted my body to look as much as possible as it did before surgery.

*Did your doctor inform you of the different options for breast recon-struction? Why did you choose the latissimus dorsi (back) flap?*

I was given several options. I could have implants or tissue expanders or I could have flap surgery with tissue taken from other donor sites. Because I am a heavy, full-figured person, I had abundant tissue in all the right areas. I chose the back as my donor site. If I'm going to hurt, I prefer it to all be in one location—just the chest and back area as op-posed to the chest and stomach area or the chest and the buttock area, which are other areas where donor tissue can be obtained.

*Describe your operation. How long did it take? How long were you hospitalized? Did you experience much pain?*

The surgery took 5 hours. That included the lumpectomy, axillary dis-section, and reconstruction. I was in the hospital for 2 days, which wasn't long enough, but that's the way it is with insurance coverage today. I was sore and stiff and my right arm was swollen and tender. I had two drains, one in my underarm incision and one in my side inci-sion; those drains remained in until I was discharged.

*Did you experience any complications after surgery?*

I had a number of small problems after surgery. Fluid accumulated in my armpit. My drains were removed too soon. They should have re-mained in after I was discharged for a total of 5 days; I paid a price for that. The surgery was done on Wednesday, I was discharged on a Fri-day, and by Sunday fluid had built up in my armpit. It was just jiggling and sloshing around like water in a balloon. I was not physically hurt-ing anymore, but just experiencing a lot of discomfort. I could not lie on that side; my right arm was already swollen and the surgical sites were still painful. I called my plastic surgeon and he told me to come in. For the next 6 weeks, three times a week, I had to have fluid with-drawn every other day. There was no discomfort when the fluid was being withdrawn since I was still numb. I did, however, experience a pulling sensation and pressure in that area. During this time I also felt dizzy and flushed. On two of the trips I was able to walk in but left in a wheelchair because I was so weak. I had to drink liquids each time before I left to ensure adequate fluid replacement. Then I would im-mediately go home to take pain medication, settle down, and let my body adjust to the stress of it all.

I also developed blood clots (hematomas) under one of the inci-sions; those had to be aspirated under local anesthesia. The actual as-piration of those blood clots was deep enough that the local anesthesia didn't numb the area very well. It was painful. I also had an adverse reaction to the antibiotics, which resulted in my losing my sense of taste. Fortunately, it came back after they were discontinued. Those complications lasted about 6 to 8 weeks.

The most serious complication, which developed a few months later, was lymphedema, a swelling of my arm that remains an ongoing concern.

### What caused the lymphedema? What are the symptoms? How is it managed?

Once the lymph nodes were removed (they took 15) and the nerve endings were cut, the lymphatic system in my arm shut down, causing ongoing fluid buildup as well as swelling and tenderness in my arm and hand. Unlike the initial fluid buildup caused by early drain removal, this will not go away. As a result, I must wear a Jobst elastic compression sleeve and do exercises. I also use a sequential sleeve and pump. I put my arm into the sleeve and turn on the machine. It slowly squeezes the arm in segments all the way up to the armpit. It forces the fluid up and out.

When arm fluid starts accumulating, my right arm gets stiff, and the hand and arm swell. It's most uncomfortable. You know it's time for another treatment and so you just do it and get it over with. The fluid is usually excreted through the kidneys, and you feel fine for another 24 or 36 hours before the process starts again. For the most part, it's a minor payment for one's life. Some of the ladies in my support group have a much harder time adjusting to lymphedema. They say it is a terrible inconvenience to have to get into that machine all the time. But you have to make time despite your busy lifestyle. This is a problem that stays with you and you can't neglect it.

### How long did it take before you were performing normal activities? When could you return to work?

I was physically unable to work for some time. I took a hiatus of about 9 months. I had not planned to take that long, but complications and problems kept coming up. Once I recovered from the initial surgery and the complications, then I started chemotherapy.

### What was your reaction to the chemotherapy? Did you experience any side effects? How did your family react?

I started chemotherapy in early December. After the first treatment my hair started coming out in large clumps. That really surprised me.

I didn't expect it to happen so quickly. By Christmas I was completely bald, clean as an onion. I was wearing turbans, berets, scarves, you name it.

Most of us don't appreciate our hair until it is gone. You feel breezes stirring around the ears and the nape of the neck that you didn't know existed. I even had to resort to a sleeping cap. I bought a lacy one; I wanted something fancy. If I have to sleep in this thing, I figured why not wear a pretty one. It would get too hot and I would take it off. Then in the middle of the night I would get chilly again and I would grope for it under my pillow and slip it back on. I don't think any of us ever realize how much heat is lost through the head until your hair is gone. Then you really can appreciate the hair that you have and realize it has a real purpose other than just looks.

During the chemo I also had mood swings, insomnia, upper gastric problems, and minor lesions. My appetite was not good, but the nausea and vomiting were kept to a minimum by medications.

### Why did you need to have radiation therapy?

Radiation is the treatment of choice after lumpectomy. It is just one more treatment to help kill any remaining cancerous cells in the breast area after the tumor has been removed during the lumpectomy. Radiation therapy consists of daily treatments 5 days a week for 5 weeks. I tolerated the first 20 treatments pretty well except that my breast and underarm area became red (like a bad sunburn) and tender. The next treatments did not go as well; I developed problems and painful complications.

### What complications did the radiation therapy cause?

From the twenty-first treatment on the skin rolled off my breast like a peel coming off an onion. It just blistered and burned. There were burned areas across my breast, under it, and in the armpit area. They were treated as if they were thermal burns. My dressings were changed three to five times a day and Silvadine cream applied. My plastic surgeon has pictures documenting all of this. He immediately put me on medication and antibiotics to prevent infection. One of the problems with lymphedema is that you really have to guard against skin irritations and infections because the lymphatic system carries bacteria in and out of the body. If you develop an infection, you're susceptible to much more serious problems.

It took about 6 to 8 weeks for my burns to heal, and during that time I was still taking radiation treatments. I would see the doctor before the treatment, get the treatments, see the doctor afterward so he could change the dressing, and then I'd go home. Then I would repeat the process the next day. That pain was excruciating. If you've ever had a burn, you know how it feels, especially when it affects tender areas such as the breast and armpit. They hurt constantly. I had to shower every day because I didn't want to get it infected. I would take off those slimy dressings, shower, swab on big clumps of Silvadine cream, and put more dressings on. My husband and I dealt with that. I was not a good patient. I cried, screamed, and pulled on his clothes. He'd just hold on to me and we'd do it. Nothing that I took really helped the pain because once you took off the dressing, it started to hurt all over again. It was the same thing if water touched my skin. The pain was terrible.

### How did you cope with the pain from the radiation burns?

I stopped trying to think about anybody else during that time. It was just me, me, and me! I tried to be a good sport about it. I listened to a lot of music and did a lot of praying because at some point it just seemed like the medicine wasn't working. It seemed like the more medication I put on, the more it hurt and the bigger the area got. I was going through dressings right and left. I started buying them in bulk. I recall the day I came in to see my plastic surgeon for a follow-up visit. When he saw what the radiation had done, he closed his eyes, kind of shuddered, and said, "My goodness!" He took pictures and immediately ordered medication. He told me to come back in 2 weeks so he could see how I was healing. He was very pleased once it started to heal.

### Are you on hormonal therapy? Are there any side effects?

I started taking tamoxifen in September. This is one more tool to help fight the cancer. I will take it for 5 years. It increases your hot flashes, but I have developed a solution for that problem. I have a little foldup fan that I pull out and just fan away. No matter what the weather, I can cool down. I keep fans around wherever I am, even at work. I get a big glass of water and fill it with ice. It usually chills me down quickly. I have noticed, however, that sometimes it cools me down so fast I get chills and have to drink some hot tea. Since I work nights nobody is really aware of what I go through to get comfortable. If I were around a lot of folks in the daytime, fanning one minute, chilling the next, they would really have second thoughts about me.

*Were you satisfied with the results of your breast reconstruction?*

My plastic surgeon has done a beautiful job. I'm heavy breasted, and from the beginning he said to me, "Louella, we're not gods, but we will do the best we can to match them up." He did an excellent job. My reconstructed breast is a little larger on the right side, but I can accept that.

*Did you have nipple-areola reconstruction?*

No, I didn't need nipple reconstruction because my nipple was preserved. Everything was done from the side: the muscle was brought from the back through the incision that was in the front and everything was connected. So I never had to have nipple reconstruction, tattoo, or anything of that sort.

*Describe your scars? What do they look like? Are they acceptable?*

The scars are minimal. I wasn't sure they were going to be since I tend to have keloids. I was very concerned about this and told both the cancer surgeon and the plastic surgeon about it. But nothing developed and the scars are fine. Even the places where the drains were inserted have healed beautifully, leaving only hairline incisions.

My reconstructive scar is about 6 inches long. The scar for the axillary area where the lymph nodes were removed and latissimus flap tunneled through is approximately 12 to 14 inches long, extending the full width of the armpit. I also have a tiny, 2 to 2½-inch scar over the top of the nipple. This is where they initially went in to remove the tumors. So I have three scars, all of which are aesthetic. The one in the underarm can't really be seen unless I raise my arms when I have on a swimsuit or a low-cut dress. The one in the latissimus area is in such a spot that it's hidden with a bra, and of course the one over the nipple is also hidden.

*Do you have any sensitivity in your breast and nipple on that side?*

I wouldn't say I have full sensitivity or sexual responsiveness, but it's nearly normal. It's been over a year, and the way it is going I hope to have full sensitivity within the next few months.

*Do you have any other side effects?*

Because my back muscle was transferred to the front of my chest, there is actually a certain little area on my breast I can press and it will push out. I told my plastic surgeon, " I can do things nobody else can do. I think I have a marketing tool here."

I still have a certain degree of numbness in the axillary area where all the lymph nodes were removed and in my arm. The arm numbness used to extend from the elbow to the shoulder, but slowly it's getting better. The numbness in the armpit is still there. I don't perspire in that area anymore.

### Was lumpectomy and breast reconstruction the right choice for you?

I think that was my best choice. I didn't feel that I could deal with the scar or the flat chest after surgery. Psychologically it made a difference to me to have a breast, at least something there, and not have to worry about wearing a prosthesis in my bra.

### Was your husband supportive and helpful during this experience?

My husband did his best to empathize. But he really couldn't understand. That is why I joined a support group. I needed to talk to somebody who could relate to my experience. He kept saying, "Why do you keep crying? Why don't you just cry and get it over with?" I would say, "You don't understand because it is not your breast. It's not your body." He has found strength in talking to the other husbands and boyfriends and loved ones who share their feelings and experiences in dealing with the women they care about.

Initially after the surgery my husband seemed to need to hug and squeeze me all the time. I had a certain way I turned to block him if he squeezed too tight. He would say, "You know I want to hug you, but I always hurt you." Finally, he said, "I'll tell you what, you hug me. You know how tight you can hold me without hurting yourself. Show me how tight to squeeze and I will take your lead." That was what worked. I can remember many days after that when I would look at him and say, "I need my hug, I really do." Then I would squeeze him so he would know how tight to hold me. That solved our problem. We were able to have our little "hug sessions" after all.

Communication is particularly important at a time like this. You need to talk things out because you don't know how he feels and he doesn't understand how you feel. You can yell at each other and have your little temper tantrums, but when that is over, you need to talk to each other, to open up, to share, to say, "Hey, this is how I feel, how do you feel? What do you think about this? What should I do here? I need you to help me. I need you to talk to me. Let's talk this thing through so we can get it resolved and go on." We all have busy schedules and sometimes feel like there just is not enough time in a day, but

30 minutes, even 15 minutes sharing a cup of tea sprinkled with a little conversation goes a long way. That's basically how I have dealt with having cancer and being a cancer patient.

My husband has been a terrific help with my physical recovery. He has never been helpless. He knows how to cook and clean and wash and iron. He was raised by a mom who taught him to do for himself. So that was never a problem for us. He was there every day to fix breakfast, lunch, and dinner. Finally, I said it was too much. "You have to have time away. Why don't you just do breakfast and dinner and I will manage lunch."

### How have your daughters reacted to your breast cancer? Are they concerned for their own health?

There was no history of breast cancer in the immediate family until my cancer was diagnosed. I have two daughters and now they are both edgy. One is in her mid-twenties and has fibrocystic problems. She gets quite anxious. I have encouraged her to check herself regularly and to see her doctor if a problem develops. In the spring of last year she talked to a nurse who reviewed breast self-examination with her and showed her the different techniques for examining her breasts. Then she had my daughter feel a breast form with lumps in it to see if she could detect the breast problems. The nurse was impressed with how thorough my daughter was using the form and in examining her own breasts. She is very vigilant about monitoring herself. She asked the nurse from the hospital to show the ladies at her church how to examine their breasts.

My older daughter needs constant reminders to take better care of herself. She is not in the best of health either. At least once or twice a month I remind her. "Are you talking to your doctor? Are you going to get your mammograms? She is like I was prior to being diagnosed. She doesn't know if she wants to know. She's very reluctant.

### What can people do to help you recover?

One of the most important things people can do is just to listen and be empathetic. I don't say sympathetic because you don't want their sympathy. You just want them to listen and not shy away or be afraid of you. I don't hear from some of my friends anymore; I am not sure why. I think they feel my cancer is contagious. Most people, however, have been caring. Once they found out about my breast cancer, they called, offered suggestions, offered help, and compared experiences. They consoled me when I was hurting and laughed with me when I felt better. It was a wonderful outpouring of love.

### How did your faith help you cope with this experience?

I keep my radio tuned to the gospel station. There is something about music that soothes your soul. If nothing else reaches you, the music does. I meditate to some songs. I also believe in prayer and fasting.

I am a member of the First Christian Fellowship Church, which I joined 2 years ago while visiting my daughter out of town. It is a small church where everybody knows everybody and everybody shares feelings and emotions. They do not yet have a branch church in my city. So I have a long-distance spiritual relationship.

When I learned I had cancer, I called my pastor and he immediately prayed for me and asked to be kept apprised of my progress. Ever since I joined the church and was baptized I had received frequent letters, sometimes six a week, from all of the sisters there. When my cancer was diagnosed, I was flooded with correspondence. They found time to pour out their emotions and offer their prayers. I also got letters from the pastor and I was on the prayer list, on alter call, and in the tape ministry. They send me tapes and I listen to those since I am not physically able to attend church. I feel united with the other church members when I put on the tapes on Sunday, which is the hardest time because that is when everyone goes to church. I have gotten all my strength from these sources of faith and spirituality.

### How has your breast cancer experience affected your relations with others?

It has made me want to reach out to other people and to share my experiences. I have phoned all my relatives and urged them to take care of themselves, to get their daughters to do breast self-examination, and to go for mammograms. I even extended myself to friends, coworkers, and church members. Surprisingly, some of these women were also breast cancer patients who needed to talk about their experiences and to share.

### What advice would you like to share with other women?

We all live in a bubble of sorts. We think that nothing will invade our bodies, and we will always be fine and live forever. We tend to neglect ourselves and it can be harmful. Several people have told me that they don't know how I talk about my experiences and about breast cancer. I find it easy. Keeping things bottled up is a real killer. It just destroys you. I don't say run to every street corner and say, "Guess what I have," but sharing, quiet sharing will heal you.

## FAITH: I COULDN'T FACE BREAST LOSS

"Please be sure to tell your readers that not only people with beautiful bodies are vain. We with the run-of-the-mill-type bodies also want to have the best image of ourselves that we can."

Thus began the letter that I received from Faith several weeks after our interview at her plastic surgeon's office. Faith is a pretty young woman with short dark hair and glasses. She was only 28 when her breast cancer was discovered. She courageously investigated her treatment options. As a young, single woman, Faith was unwilling to face breast loss. Unfortunately, living in a small town, she had few people to consult about reconstructive options. There was only one general surgeon in town and no plastic surgeons. The only women she knew who had had mastectomies were considerably older than she was. Therefore she took it upon herself to write to a Cancer Helpline in a neighboring state and request information on breast cancer and breast reconstruction. The information she received proved a godsend, and she studied everything she could until she found the procedure that she felt was right for her. She used the same research methods to locate a medical center, surgeon, and plastic surgeon to do an immediate breast reconstruction. Faith braved this trauma alone, traveling to the hospital by herself.

She cried through most of our discussion, taking off her glasses to wipe her eyes periodically. This experience was still very fresh and her emotions overwhelming. As she explained, "The doctors and nurses really need to stress that a person is going to be very emotional after any surgery, especially this one. I'd like to see a person assigned to the breast cancer team whose function is to provide emotional support. Because you already have a permanent breast shape in place, people tend to believe you are 'all well.' You are not. You still have to cope with surgery, with having a mastectomy, and with having cancer."

Faith chose the most complex and extensive method of breast reconstruction, an *immediate TRAM free flap*, a microsurgical operation in which her abdominal tissue and muscle were transferred to her breast and the nerves and blood vessels were reconnected under an operating microscope. She was in surgery for approximately 10 hours, and even though she would have liked to have had better information about her operation, she is delighted with the technique that she selected.

### How did you discover your breast cancer?

I found a lump on January 1. Three days later I went to see my family doctor. He felt two lumps and I had a mammogram, but nothing showed up. My doctor said, "It's just fibrocystic disease. It's common in big-busted women. Nothing to worry about." He referred me to a surgeon who also thought they were just cysts. But I wasn't satisfied. My gut told me something was wrong, and I wanted the lumps out. The surgeon tried to discourage me. He said, "You're 28. You'll have a scar." I told him I didn't care; let's get these lumps out and see what they are. So he removed them and he was right. What we had felt were cysts. But when he lifted the cysts, he found extensive intraductal carcinoma.

### How did you get your information about breast cancer and breast reconstruction?

I saw a breast cancer documentary on TV. It was presented by a hospital in North Carolina. They had an 800 number; I called it and they sent me a packet of literature on breast cancer and breast reconstruction. This information was wonderful because it gave me something to read to base my decisions on. I'm a research person. I have to know all the options before I make the decision. I had to make a quick one and they got me the information in 3 days. By the time I got my second opinion I knew what I wanted done.

### Why did you decide to have a mastectomy to treat your cancer?

The doctor in my town suggested a lumpectomy and irradiation, but I went to a neighboring city for a second opinion. That doctor said I needed a mastectomy for the type of cancer I had. I took the pathology slides to this second surgeon, and he had a complete pathology report done on them. I was devious, however; I took the old report out and said, "Here are the slides; tell me what this is." They had another pathologist look at them, and his diagnosis came back word for word as my other pathology report. He told me to have a total mastectomy and get it over with. He said, "If you were my wife, there would be no way I would let you have a lumpectomy. This type of cancer cannot be felt because it is so deep within the tissue." So I said, "Okay, but I want a TRAM flap breast reconstruction done at the same time."

*How did you select the TRAM free flap breast reconstruction?*
*Why did you choose to have microsurgery?*

I knew that's what I wanted done because I had read about it in the material I received from the American Cancer Society; it contained a pamphlet on reconstruction with about a 3-inch paragraph, no pictures or anything, describing the TRAM flap reconstruction technique. I wasn't really sure about the difference between the regular TRAM flap and the free TRAM flap, but I knew that I liked the idea of using my stomach tissue. I have severe allergies, and I was afraid of the implant technique. With my luck, I'd be allergic to them. Anyway, I have plenty of extra abdominal tissue and this seemed to be the right approach for me.

*Why did you want immediate breast reconstruction? What did*
*you do when your surgeon was unwilling to perform an immediate*
*TRAM flap?*

I could not face leaving the hospital without a breast. This surgeon I went to for the second opinion told me to have the mastectomy done and to come back in 3 to 6 months and have the TRAM flap. I said, "No, I want to go home with something. I cannot handle just having a skin flap with an expander underneath to stretch the skin. I want to have a breast when I leave the hospital." He told me that they had never done an immediate TRAM breast reconstruction.

I said it's being done somewhere; I am going to find out where. I called the American Cancer Society and got the name of a good plastic surgeon and cancer surgeon in a nearby city at a major medical center. Then I called my doctor back home and said I want a referral; this was about 4:00 P.M. on a Friday afternoon. He called me back at 4:15 and said be in there Monday morning at 9:00. So I went in and on March 5, 2 months after I found my lump, I had a 10-hour operation.

*Did your plastic surgeon explain the different reconstructive*
*options to you? Did you know that you were having a free TRAM*
*flap and not a pedicle TRAM flap?*

I came in with my mind made up. This was my choice. They saw how hardheaded I was. I came in and told them that I wanted a TRAM flap. I even had my booklet with me with information about TRAM reconstruction. I think they assumed I knew everything about it. They just agreed to do it. I qualified with my weight; I had a stomach for them to use. I heard them refer to it as a free flap, but I didn't really understand that it was a more complicated form of TRAM flap operation. Nobody explained the difference to me, but I think I fooled them; they thought I was much better informed than I really was.

### Did you require blood transfusions?

Yes, I had to have 3 units of blood donated. At first I couldn't think of someone we could trust to give blood and so I had to give my own. They kept telling me, "We'll never get the three out of you in this short period of time." So I called my pastor, and within 3 hours there were 10 people from my church volunteering to give blood for me; it was great! And they all called and came to see me; I saved the cards and counted them. I think I have 900 cards. People just pulled together.

### How long did the operation take?

It took about 10 hours total. The only thing I remember in recovery is the nurse leaning over me and asking, "Can you tell me what they did?" I got so indignant with her because I thought she should have known what they did to me. Then she said, "Send her to her room; she's okay." So I'm sure I had to talk to them before I got to my room.

### Describe your hospital stay. Did you experience much pain?

I was in the hospital 6 days. My surgery was on a Tuesday and I was much better and functioning on my own by Sunday. I came out of surgery with three drain tubes and a catheter; at one time I had nine items going into three needles for IVs. Also I had a morphine pump.

The incisions themselves did not hurt because they were so deep and the nerves had been cut. Most of the pain was through the stomach where they had done the "tummy tuck" to take the tissue. My stomach was very tight. I would try to sit up and I couldn't. I guess my pain resembled the pain of childbirth. A person never realizes how the simplest movements use the stomach muscles. A sneeze will just about kill you. Reaching is impossible. Laying down you don't even think about. I also had trouble from my back. I had hurt it years ago, and it really ached from having to sit and lie in the same position. I had difficulty finding a comfortable position and I had to sleep on my back, propped up with pillows. I'd never have made it without my aunt staying with me during the days and my mother staying at night. After all, the nurses can't be by your side at all times.

I think the main contributor to my pain was the length of surgery. Ten hours is a very long time. I had two major surgeries in one. I remember feeling as if I had been beaten. Every muscle hurt. To help get rid of the aches I did what the doctor advised, I exercised. That meant I shuffled back and forth down the hospital corridor.

I also had trouble with my veins and the IVs. Because I had so many needles in, my veins started rupturing. I was taken back to surgery and had a jugular vein IV inserted. Believe it or not this made me feel much better. It gave me back the use of my one good arm. Until this was done, I couldn't even reach and get my own water or get into bed by myself. I decided that the next time I have major surgery I will have the jugular IV installed during surgery. The larger needle and blood supply in my jugular vein let them draw blood samples directly out of the IV instead of being stuck again when they needed to see if I needed another transfusion. Also, all other medications could be placed directly into the IV.

### Did you require any special monitoring because you had microsurgery?

When you have microsurgery, they need to see if the blood vessels have been connected and that there is blood flow through the tissue. The way they check is to literally take a syringe needle and stick it into the breast tissue, into the flap. If it bleeds, then they know that the blood circulation is good; if it doesn't bleed in an area, they know that the blood vessels have not healed properly and that they may need to do something else. They also touch the reconstructed breast to check it's temperature. If there's a cold spot, they'll know that the blood is not flowing through that area correctly. The first time they checked me I was just about terrified. They were sticking needles in me. I said, "What are you doing?" I didn't understand what they were talking about. They were saying, "Oh, good, it's bleeding." As far as I knew, things aren't supposed to bleed. Later they told me that was the way they checked to see if the blood vessels were connected properly. Once they explained it, I was okay, but they really need to warn a person before they do that.

### Did you have to adjust to any other surprises during your hospital stay?

In a medical center you have to adjust to these young doctors always coming to see you in groups of five or six. I think that's one thing people need to get used to. Even though you have one doctor, he comes attached with five behind him. They were not all students; these were people who already are doctors, but they are studying that particular field and training specifically with someone. It was intimidating at first, but eventually you lose all inhibitions. They just come in and give orders. "Unsnap the top of your gown." You're just sitting there, and the feeling is, "Excuse me, who are you?"

### How long did you recuperate before returning to work?

After my 6 days in the hospital I was at home for 4 weeks before I returned to work. My job requires a lot of lifting. I'm on my feet and it is also hot where I work. So I stayed home for 4 weeks to make sure everything was fine.

### Did you have any problems or complications?

I had an infection; it was the kind you get when you cut yourself and the surrounding area swells. It occurred because the knots from some of the stitches were not dissolving; the stitches dissolved, but the knots didn't. The infection spread. Because I live some distance from the medical center, I went to my family doctor and he gave me an antibiotic for it. The next week when I saw my plastic surgeon for a checkup, the incisions were already looking better. My plastic surgeon told me to continue on that medicine because the infection was healing just fine. It was just a skin infection. There was never any chance of losing the flap, even though that's the first thing that went through my mind. "I can't lose this. I don't have anything else to replace it with, so let's get this infection out of here!"

### How long did it take until you were standing straight again and feeling like yourself?

Everybody kept saying that I was going to walk bent over at first, and they were right. But I thought I would be bent over by choice, not because I couldn't stand up. You should be told that. The muscle is gone. You have to stretch it out in order to be upright again.

At first I was miserable every time I stood up. But I made myself do it. Each time I would try to stand up just a little bit straighter. I noticed by the end of the day as I got tired I also got more slumped over. It was very hard to stand erect. We live on a farm, so I would go out and take walks to try to get my energy back. Within 3 weeks I was standing up straight. It's taken about 5 months to really feel like myself again.

### Did you have nipple-areola reconstruction? Did you have any other adjustments made during that operation?

I came back for the nipple reconstruction 3 months after my initial surgery. My plastic surgeon reconstructed the nipple and areola from the little patches of skin (dog ears) that he left where he made my initial abdominal incision. I felt better before we did the nipple reconstruction than after. The scars were healing. I had some bad scar tissue from the infection. During the nipple reconstruction he cut the skin all over again and took out tissue; so now I have new scars. The nipple looked gross when I first had to start changing the bandages. I was just like, yuck, I shouldn't have had this done. We should have left it the way it was. But now that some time has passed the nipple reconstruction looks better, and the more I see myself in the mirror, the more I like it.

He also did liposuction to smooth my stomach and hip area. That hurt worse than any of the other surgery. I never knew liposuction could hurt so much. My whole hip area was black and blue where they had just rounded and trimmed it off.

### Are you satisfied with your breast appearance? Is it what you expected?

Now that my breast has been shaped and trimmed and my nipple has been reconstructed, it looks pretty normal. As time passes my breast appears more natural. It's not perfect, but I am pleased. My breasts still don't match; they are not exactly the same shape. My new breast is too full in some aspects. My plastic surgeon is not happy with the shape, but I don't want to be put back to sleep again unless it's absolutely necessary to reduce the fullness. When I have a bra on, you can't tell. When I put on a swimsuit for the first time I was like, "Yuck, I can tell it." I could notice that the shapes were not the same. But I'm not in a swimsuit that much, so I don't mind. The surgeon had to cut so low to get part of the breast tissue out that even when I have my bra on you can see the lower part of the scar. I keep thinking I need to pull my bra down.

### What do your scars look like? Where are they placed?

I have a circular scar all the way around the right breast area and underneath the arm. I'm also cut from behind one hip all the way across the abdomen to behind the other one. When you see this scar in the mirror, it's like somebody railroad-tracked you; it looks just like a pair of braces, only it's scar tissue. But my scars are doing better. Every week they seem to fade a little bit more. I'm sure that in a couple years, they will be fine. I have seen pictures of women who had this technique, and I could barely see any scarring. You could tell that their breasts didn't look exactly the same, but who could tell which was the reconstructed breast? I'd have to look on the back of the photographs to see which one was the reconstructed one and which one was the natural breast. Hopefully one day people will look at mine and comment, "I can't tell which one it was. They don't look exactly the same, but. . . ."

### How does your reconstructed breast feel? Is it sensitive?

The new breast is more solid feeling and looks a little different from my other breast. It also has some sensitivity, and as time goes by it is getting more sensitive.

### If you had it to do over again, would you have reconstruction? Was it worth the pain and trouble?

Yes. The results are so important and lasting that the memory of pain fades. I look natural in my clothes. My breast feels natural; it jiggles when I walk. When I had the surgery, it didn't move at all at first, and my plastic surgeon kept telling me when it's healed it'll start jiggling like your other one does. The first time it jiggled, I was so excited! I was like, "It's attached, it works!" My mother said, "What is wrong with you?" and I said, "Watch it, watch it. It jiggles!" It's been worth it, most definitely. I feel more confident because I feel like it is natural. I'm not going to be allergic to it; I'm not going to reject it. I'm not going to have to go back in 2 years to have an implant taken out and another one put in because that one sprang a leak. It's done.

### Are you pleased with the technique that you chose?

Wonderfully. I am very happy. I'm very pleased because now I consider mine finished, whereas some women are still having to go through the process of having the skin stretched and the implant inserted and they're just not finished. Mine's finished.

### Do you think your age had some impact on your desire for immediate reconstruction?

Most definitely. Most people my age are healthy and vibrant. If you've got something wrong or you've got a prosthesis, it makes you a lot more self-conscious. Psychologically I couldn't have handled going home from the hospital with nothing there. I probably would have gone bananas if I had gone home with the scar and a hole.

*Do you feel you were fully informed about the details of your breast reconstruction? Was there more information you could have had? Are there questions you think a woman should ask?*

Personally I wish I had been supplied with all the gory details, not just simple before and after pictures. I would like to see the information written out in simplified medical terms so you can understand what is going on, so that you can anticipate what will happen, and so you will know how your appearance will change. They should tell you that it is going to take three or four surgeries to get your breasts to look right. I was told there would be more than one operation, but it seems like every time I come here there is going to be another one. You should know that you are going to have a year of bad scarring, so when you wake up you will know what to expect. I was able to handle it. I know some women who would be horrified to wake up and see all the stitches and scars. Their response would be, "What did they do to me!" A lot of times, unless you know what you want or are good at asking questions, the doctors won't tell you everything. It simplifies things for them; they just go ahead and do their little procedure and you wake up and that's it. I would like to see the information written out, so if you knew you were going to have the TRAM flap they would explain in detail what they would do. I didn't really understand fully until after I had the surgery what it meant to have the TRAM done with microscopes and to have the blood vessels sewn together. I wish I had known beforehand; I still would have had the procedure done. It was the perfect operation for me. Still . . . I needed more information. After all, these are life-changing decisions.

## MARCY: YOU CAN'T TELL THE DIFFERENCE

"It's amazing! If you didn't know that I had breast cancer and reconstruction, you could never tell. Just look at these pictures; aren't they great? My husband is so proud; he shows them to everyone." Slim and pretty, Marcy's face is framed by bobbed dark hair. This former teacher is married with two small children. She blushes as she pulls several photographs out of her purse and hands them to me. Her delight in her restored appearance is infectious. "These were taken of me wearing the same bathing suit before my mastectomy and after my *tissue expansion reconstruction* and you just can't tell the difference. If anything, I look better now."

Marcy's breast cancer was discovered on her first mammogram, right before her fortieth birthday. Fortunately, it was in its earliest stages, making her prognosis excellent. Nevertheless, decisions about which treatment approach was best for her were not always easy, even though her husband, a cancer specialist, helped her to sort through her options and find the best care possible. She is well informed and the type of woman who wants to know all the facts. Because of her husband's profession, she looks to physicians for expertise and sound advice and does not come to the doctor-patient relationship with the trepidation that many others exhibit. Even so, Marcy frequently found herself puzzled and needing more information and direction in selecting the best treatment for her breast cancer and the right reconstructive technique.

### How did you decide between lumpectomy and mastectomy?

That was frustrating. I kept asking my cancer surgeon what he would recommend. I said, "If I were your wife, what would you do?" All he could say was, "I can't tell you what to do."

I realize it is hard, especially for male doctors, because they feel that breast cancer is a uniquely female problem and they don't know what to make of it. But patients come to doctors for their expertise. I hope that doctors haven't become afraid to recommend a course of action for their patients or to say that mastectomy can cure. I wanted some direction and I persisted in asking him what he would do. He said, "I can't tell you what to do." I protested, "I want you to tell me what is the best thing to do. That's why I am here; you are the expert. You should know." We kept going around in circles; it was frustrating. He said, "You have to do what you feel is right. You have to make that decision." But I was coming to him for an answer, and he wasn't willing to give me one. He said, "You can have a mastectomy or a lumpectomy, or at this point you can choose to do nothing. We can watch it; it is so early."

I said, "Does mastectomy guarantee me better results then a lumpectomy?" He replied noncommittally, "Lumpectomy is an option many people have chosen and they have done well after 5-year and 10-year follow-up. I saw another cancer surgeon for another opinion and he said the same thing.

It was frustrating not to be able to have my doctor tell me what was the best course of action. There is so much controversy surrounding breast cancer, so many different options. I wanted him to say, "This is the way to go." But I guess maybe they really don't know.

### Why did you choose mastectomy over lumpectomy? Are you happy with your choice?

Because I didn't want to worry about a possible recurrence. I knew in my heart that a mastectomy was the best choice for me. I could not put more value on saving a breast than on saving my life. Long-term survival is important; I want to watch my children grow.

I am very happy with my decision. I would do the same thing tomorrow. Knowing that I could have the reconstruction made my decision for mastectomy that much easier. It took away any anxiety. The only anxiety that I experienced throughout the whole ordeal was when I had to wait those 2 days in the hospital before I got the final path report back. My cancer is so early that it would have been 4 to 5 years before I would have felt it on self-exam.

I would recommend what I did to anyone. After the mastectomy they were able to study the whole breast, and they discovered that the cancer was multifocal. Had I had the lumpectomy they would not have gotten every little area of cancer. For me, the procedure I had was the right one. Of course, I didn't know that 100% until after it had been done. But on hindsight it was.

### Why did you seek breast reconstruction?

It is comparable to someone losing a limb and wearing an artificial leg, losing an eye and wanting a glass eye. Your breast is a part of you. It doesn't define who you are sexually, but you want it back. You want to be whole.

Sexual feelings between my husband and me were fine following the mastectomy and prior to reconstruction. I didn't have reconstruction to feel sexy, just to feel complete, to be normal, not necessarily bigger or better than before. I wanted to dress normally . . . to not be concerned with what I could wear and what I couldn't. I felt I was young, just 40, and I wanted to look normal for me, for my husband, and for my children.

### How did you learn about breast reconstruction?

One of my husband's scrub nurses gave him your book to give to me. It turns out she had a double mastectomy and reconstruction. My husband was astounded. He said, "I operate with you every day. I never noticed anything different and you never mentioned it." She said, "Well, I don't talk about it, but this book was a tremendous help to me. I thought it would be a big help to your wife."

I came home that weekend and read the book from cover to cover and said, "Thank goodness, everything is going to be fine." That next week I went in to have my mastectomy and never once gave it a second thought or felt that I was making a mistake.

### How did you select your plastic surgeon?

He was recommended by my husband's surgical colleagues. When I was diagnosed with breast cancer, my husband called everyone he knew and asked, "Where should we go? Who is the best?" They said we had the best right here. It made it easy. My surgeon also recommended the same plastic surgeon. We kept hearing his name so often that it gave us a feeling of confidence and security. We never thought to look elsewhere.

### Have you been happy with your plastic surgeon? Was he responsive to your needs?

He was just wonderful. He went over the different reconstructive options with me, talked about immediate vs. delayed reconstruction, answered my questions, and was very reassuring. He was confident in his ability to reconstruct my breast, and he took away any fear or doubt that I had. His staff was also wonderful, especially the nurses. When I have problems, I call. It has been a terrific experience.

### Why did you decide not to have immediate reconstruction?

My surgeon and plastic surgeon were at two different hospitals, and I felt comfortable with the surgeon at the local hospital; it was where my husband practiced. We were well known there. I wasn't sure what operation I would choose for reconstruction, but I knew I wanted to go ahead with the mastectomy. I decided to get that out of the way and then take time to read the book, talk to other people, and decide what type of reconstruction I wanted. The plastic surgeon also gave me names of former patients and suggested that I call them and talk to them.

### Did your plastic surgeon and general surgeon coordinate your care even though they were at different hospitals?

Yes. They spoke before my cancer surgery, and my plastic surgeon told my cancer surgeon what type of incision would be best for the reconstruction and how much skin to leave.

### What type of reconstructive operation did you choose?

I considered all of the options and decided on tissue expansion with simple reconstruction with an expander implant. During my recovery from the mastectomy I met a woman who had the abdominal flap. She was unhappy with it. She had her reconstructive surgery a number of years ago, and I am sure it was not the state-of-the art operation it is today. Even so, she said that she still can't sit up straight in bed; she can't bend over and pick up a basket of laundry. She has never felt right; she has a very uncomfortable feeling in her mid-chest area where she thinks the flap was turned. She said that if she had it to do over she would not have such an elaborate operation. It was a huge surgery with a long recovery period. I didn't want anything that dramatic. Also, I wasn't rebuilding a huge breast. I didn't need a lot of tissue. I am not that large physically, so I didn't feel they would have a whole lot to work with anyway. So I eliminated the possibility of an abdominal flap.

We talked about the latissimus dorsi back flap. Implants are often used along with that flap. I rejected that option because I figured why subject myself to a major flap procedure with additional scars on my back. I decided I might as well just go with the simple implant.

My husband and I came back to see the plastic surgeon with our decision and said, "What do you think of this; would tissue expansion and an implant be good?" He said he thought it would work in my situation.

### Why did you decide that implant reconstruction was the right choice for you?

I wanted reconstruction; I wanted the breast back, but I didn't want to go through a horrendous process to get it. I wanted the simplest, easiest operation. I wanted a nice cosmetic effect with the least amount of trauma and disruption in my life. My children are small, 7 and 11; I wanted as little time away from them as possible.

### Did you have any surgery on your opposite breast?

Yes, I had an augmentation. We decided to do a small implant on the other side to give that breast the same type of lift and look; plus, since I was going to have implants, I thought it would be a nice bonus if I could go a little bit bigger than I was. My plastic surgeon thought he could do that without any trouble. Augmentation was not what I initially requested, however. Originally I wanted to have a prophylactic mastectomy with an implant on the other side.

### Why did your surgeon dissuade you from having a prophylactic mastectomy? Why did you want a preventive mastectomy?

My surgeon said that my type of cancer is not normally bilateral and he discouraged it. Even so, I knew by just having breast cancer in one breast you have a higher risk of getting it in the other breast, and why would I want that? Why not just do both? But all the doctors said that I was being a little too reactionary because of my type of cancer and the fact that I had no family history. I was not in a high-risk group. I thought, well, if it happened once why would it not happen again. They told me yearly mammograms would be able to catch it soon enough. They said that the pocket for the implant would be already made and it would be a very easy procedure. So I didn't have a prophylactic mastectomy and implant. Instead, I just had an augmentation with an implant. I still think that the prophylactic mastectomy would have given me more peace of mind.

### Describe your hospitalization.

I went in the hospital at 6:00 A.M. and had the procedure done at 8:00 A.M.; I went home at 9:00 the next morning.

### Did you have much pain after reconstruction? How did it compare to the pain you experienced after your mastectomy?

The mastectomy was a breeze. I was in the hospital for three nights, and when I went home I felt almost no pain. I was back doing almost everything I wanted to do within 10 days. I had no complications. It went great. I wanted to start reconstruction as soon as possible. We waited 3 months because my plastic surgeon felt that would allow enough time for my tissues to heal.

I had a lot of pain after reconstruction. That was surprising. None of the patients I spoke with mentioned that reconstruction was painful. When I came for the preoperative workup, I was asked if I generally have a lot of pain. I said no; generally I have a very high tolerance for pain. With the mastectomy, I was pain-free after the first day and then I took Tylenol. So they didn't order any special pain medicine for me, and I agreed with that decision. But I was wrong. I can remember waking up in recovery and not being able to move, not being able to take a breath. I think I was hyperventilating. The nurse kept telling me to calm down. If anyone touched me, I just gasped. I felt a tremendous burning sensation in my chest. I would try to take a breath and it would hurt. Both sides hurt. When the nurse asked if I would like something for pain. I said, "Yes!" She said, "They have nothing ordered for you. They didn't think you would need it." That was my fault. It was very painful and I don't know why. I talked to people who didn't think it was that painful. When I spoke with people later, they admitted that it might have hurt at first, but they really didn't remember anymore, and since I didn't seem to think it would hurt, they hadn't wanted to tell me any different. I thought, oh thanks!

They gave me Darvocet when I went home and that took care of the pain, but it would wear off. It took about 4 days before I felt better. I could move around, but trying to sit up or turn over in bed was painful.

### Did you have much bruising after your reconstruction?

The breasts themselves were not black and blue. But on my side and across the front of my chest there was a little bruising; it healed fairly quickly.

### Did you experience much swelling with the reconstruction and augmentation?

Yes, after my surgery, I was huge and swollen. At first I was petrified. "Oh, my God, I've gone overboard. What am I going to do. This is terrible." My husband says, "This is great." I was like, oh, "This is too much." But then, the swelling started going down and my reaction was, "No, stop—it's going too low—it's not going to be big enough." I went from one extreme to another, but then it leveled out and was fine. It is a nice size although every time I get expanded I am off balance again because they overexpand and overstretch the skin. They do this so that when the permanent implant is in, the breast will fill naturally and appear more normal.

### How long before you could return to normal activity?

After 7 days I started feeling better and I wanted to drive; they said I could try it if I felt up to it. We have a Ford Explorer and the steering wheel was hard to turn with no power steering, but I wanted to drive. I wanted to get back on the road, pick up my children. I knew when I left my driveway it was a mistake. We have a curve in the driveway, and I could barely make the turn. I couldn't turn the wheel. As long as I was going straight I was fine; a turn really hurt. I continued on and then got back home; I didn't drive for another week. I think I set myself back a few days. After the second week I could do just about anything. I don't do aerobics or jog; I am not big into physical activity right now, so I wasn't anxious to get back to something strenuous. For me, normal activity was just regular housework, driving, walking, and riding my bicycle.

### What type of implants do you have? How does the saline implant feel?

I have a saline implant on the right side where my breast was augmented and an expander implant on my left side for my reconstruction.

The saline implant feels normal, not to the touch, but when I walk or move. I don't feel like I have an implant. Now, if I touch or palpate it, it feels like a little water balloon, especially on the underside of my breast. It has more "give." If I push on it, it pops right back out like a balloon. On the top or sides my breast feels like it did before. Underneath I can feel a difference.

### How does the expander implant feel? How does it differ from the saline implant?

It feels fine. The main difference between my expander and my saline implant is the valve. The expander implant has a small fill valve that is positioned under my arm. I can feel it as a small bump in my underarm area, but it is not a problem. The saline was injected through this valve, and if I need any size adjustments later, these can be made through this valve without my having to undergo another operation. This expander just stays permanently in place, and I am happy with it. It is really a good solution for me because I can have control over my breast size with minimal discomfort.

### Describe the expansion process. When did it begin and how often was your expander implant inflated? How long did it take?

I started about 2 weeks after my reconstructive surgery. My skin was expanded about every 3 weeks. I went to the office and it took about 20 minutes. It was very easy. They have a device inside of you, and they plug the syringe into this device that hooks up like an IV. Saltwater is injected to expand it. You just lie on the exam table, and they give you whatever quantity they have determined is needed to expand your breast that day. You can feel it gradually dripping in. One time they were going to put a little more in, but it was feeling tight and a little sore, so I asked to stop for the day. I had a busy weekend coming up. It was nice to have that control.

I had three sessions; then further expansion was delayed because the incision opened up. I started in January and the expansion process was completed by May, so the total process took approximately 4 months. Then during an outpatient procedure my expander implant was converted to a permanent implant.

### Was tissue expansion painful?

It is a full feeling . . . not painful, just tight every time it is expanded. Then after a few days it gives and then feels normal until the next expansion. I guess the tissues stretch so that they will be ready for the permanent implant. Sometimes I took Tylenol right after it was done, but that is all I ever needed.

### Have you had any problems?

No problems on the right side with the augmentation. The only problem I had was on the left side with the expander. My incision opened a little bit; it wasn't a serious problem, but we had to delay the tissue expansion for several weeks.

### Did your surgeon know why that happened?

After the first expansion I still had Steri-Strips covering the incision; we didn't take them off and reapply them. When the tissue stretched, my plastic surgeon thinks the expansion process might have caused a tape burn, causing my incision to open. After a few weeks it healed, and then we left all the Steri-Strips off. I have never had another problem.

### Do you have any restrictions now?

No. We went to Florida after my surgery, and I tried to swim; that was difficult because it was hard to stretch. But everything else I can do fine.

### Are you going to have nipple-areola reconstruction?

Yes. I want my breast to be complete. When we were in Florida, I wore a regular bathing suit. The only time there was a noticeable difference between my breasts was when I came out of the water and was cold, and you could see that I had a nipple on one side and not on the other. I have seen it done on other women and it looks beautiful. Someone described it as "the icing on the cake." If you are going to go this far, why stop? Why not take it through to completion? People who see the pictures think my breast reconstruction is marvelous. I tell them I am a work in progress. I am not finished yet. They are very impressed. A lot of women I have talked to who have seen the bathing suit pictures say now we know that if it happens to us we will not be so afraid because we can see what can happen afterwards.

*Aesthetically, are you pleased with your breast appearance?*

Yes. Here are some pictures of me wearing the same bathing suit before the mastectomy and after the reconstruction. My husband took these to the hospital and showed them to the nurses on the floor who had taken care of me. I was so embarrassed. The results are marvelous.

*Does the reconstructed breast have any feeling or sensation? How does it compare to the opposite breast that was augmented?*

Sensation is normal in the right breast that had no mastectomy and a simple implant. There is feeling in the left reconstructed breast, but it's blunted. When I push on my left breast, I can feel the pressure but not much sensation.

*Is there any sexual feeling or sensitivity?*

To be perfectly honest I have avoided sexual contact on the left side; I don't feel right yet. My husband has no problems with it. But I don't feel finished yet. The shape of the breast still needs some adjustment; it is fuller on the top and below. There is no nipple. I still feel we are working on it.

*If you had to do it over, would you have reconstruction again? Would you have the same kind of reconstructive approach?*

I would do exactly the same thing. It was the right approach for me and I am very happy with what I did.

*Was your husband supportive? How did he react to the idea of your having breast reconstruction?*

He was wonderful. Being a cancer surgeon himself, he understood what we had to face. My husband deals with cancer every day and he has to tell someone they have cancer. The idea of disfigurement never entered into it. The total focus was on the cure.

The minute we found the cancer it was, "We can take care of it," and "If you want, you can have reconstruction." "This isn't the end of the world." He was finding out as much information as he could and as quickly as he could so that we could make the decisions we needed to make.

He supported me all the way and went through the whole learning process with me. I remember one funny incident when my husband and I were looking over the pictures of some patients that the plastic surgeon's nurse was showing us. My husband asked where were the women who had the mastectomies and were re-done? It turned out that was just what we were looking at, but you couldn't tell. It was very reassuring.

It was a learning experience for both of us. Right before I was to have reconstructive surgery one of my plastic surgeon's patients who also had a simple implant reconstruction came to see my husband for a medical problem. As he was taking her history he asked her what other surgeries she had had? When she said that she had a mastectomy and reconstruction, he asked her who her plastic surgeon was and if she was happy. She said she thought he was wonderful. My husband told her that I had just had a mastectomy and was about to have breast reconstruction and she just said, "Well, let me show you!" She was so proud and thrilled with her result. He immediately had her call me on the phone, and she talked to me from his office for 20 minutes, telling me how wonderful everything was, what a positive experience she had, and how terrific my plastic surgeon was. She offered to meet with me and show me how she looked. My husband came home and said, "She looked incredible. She looked wonderful and you would never have known." He said, "I'm a doctor looking and I would never have known. She looked that good."

### What about this experience would you like to share with other women?

I would like to tell women not to risk their lives to save a breast. I was never very big-breasted. That was never the focus of my feelings of self-worth or femininity. Maybe if it had been I would have felt differently. Not all women feel that way. In fact, I talked to a woman doctor who had breast cancer; her husband also was a doctor and he said mastectomy was the way to go for her type of cancer. She said she couldn't or wouldn't have a mastectomy. She couldn't do it; it would be very difficult. I said, "But Susan, when you are faced with the statistics?" She said, "I know but I don't think I could deal with it emotionally." Even her husband admitted that her breasts had always been very important to her and that is why she couldn't face breast loss. I never had that feeling. Anyway, with what can be accomplished with reconstruction today, I would not take the risk of keeping my breast; I would not want to live day in and day out worrying if the cancer is still there? Is it coming back? I would not want to make cancer an everyday part of my life. I would want to take the form of treatment that would be the most definitive and proceed with my life.

*Did knowledge about reconstruction make it easier for you to cope with your cancer surgery?*

Knowing that it could be fixed made all the difference. Knowing that, my attitude was let's get on with it—take care of it, get rid of it, and move ahead as opposed to, "Oh no, this is terrible." I went to my mastectomy almost jubilant; I wanted to get this breast off and rebuilt again. So I coped pretty well because I knew I could have reconstruction. I could do something.

It's the feeling of powerlessness that gets you. Around Christmas we were having company and a string of Christmas lights went off on the tree. When that happened, I just lost it. I decompensated; I panicked. My sister was astounded. She laughed at me and said, "You had cancer, had a mastectomy, and you never said anything. Now you are getting upset about your Christmas tree?" Well, this was important because I couldn't fix it. I had people coming and I couldn't get the lights on. But my breast I could fix. I could take care of it. That made all the difference. I was in control.

*How have your friends reacted to your breast reconstruction?*

They didn't realize how easily breast reconstruction could be accomplished. They never expected me to continue to look so normal throughout the whole procedure, even with the expansion. My friends have just been amazed. They think breast reconstruction is marvelous. Knowing about my experience and about the possibility of breast reconstruction has done wonders for their peace of mind. Now they know that should it happen to them it is not the end of the world.

## INGRID: WE NEED TO TALK ABOUT IT

As I looked at Ingrid, I couldn't believe that this petite blond with her wide smile and ready laugh had undergone a mastectomy and *immediate breast reconstruction with a TRAM flap* only 8 short weeks before our interview. She was not bent over as I would have expected; in fact, she was particularly bouncy and energetic. Her enthusiasm propelled our conversation.

Ingrid, a native of Sweden, has the blond good looks one associates with that part of the world. She is expressive and animated, and her speech is punctuated with short, clipped phrases, a type of verbal shorthand that lends emphasis to her words. A flight attendant working for one of the major airlines, she is 43 years old, married, and has a young daughter and son.

When her cancer was discovered, she and her family had recently relocated, and she knew few people to ask for advice. But for Ingrid, with her outgoing personality, being a stranger in a strange city was not an obstacle. Ingrid, as I was to learn, does not let things get in her way. Accustomed to responding quickly to difficult situations in her job, Ingrid approached her breast cancer and reconstruction with the same no-nonsense attitude. She investigated her options, interviewed everyone she could talk to, and then took the course of action that she felt was best for her and her family.

Because she didn't want anything unnatural in her body, TRAM flap breast reconstruction seemed the best long-term solution. She dealt with each problem as it arose, discussed it, and then solved it. As she explained, "My attitude is to bare it all as soon as possible and see the worst because then it will never be as bad again." That included telling her young children about her cancer and talking to her husband about the impact this surgery would have on their sex life. Her warmth was contagious. Her story is a heartwarming one.

### How did you discover your breast cancer?

I went for a routine mammogram. I had no lump, no indication that anything was wrong. Two days later the doctor called and suggested that I have a biopsy. Right away I thought the worst. "Biopsy equals cancer. Be prepared . . . possible mastectomy." He made an appointment for me to see a general surgeon. I went to see him just to talk and get a general idea of what was going on. He looked at my mammograms and said this doesn't look like cancer, but we need a biopsy. I was not too happy with that particular surgeon. He was brand new. I didn't feel that he had enough experience. I didn't know if I had cancer or if I needed a mastectomy, but I wanted to be prepared—that meant seeing the best doctor possible. I felt that I wanted to get more opinions than just one. I saw another doctor a few days later. That weekend I called some neighbors and told them that I needed a breast biopsy. I was afraid I might have cancer and need a mastectomy. I asked if they knew of anybody in the area who had had a mastectomy. I wanted to find names of surgeons and hospitals. If in fact I had cancer, I had to act quickly. I couldn't sit around for months finding out. By Sunday afternoon people started returning my calls: strangers, friends, friends of friends. I got names of several general surgeons in the area at major hospitals; finally, I selected a woman surgeon.

When I went to the surgeon, she read my previous mammograms and took new ones to verify what she saw. Then she did a fine-needle biopsy. I was at the hospital all day. By the time I left they had diagnosed breast cancer. I was lucky. It was not invasive.

### Did your surgeon offer you a choice between lumpectomy and modified radical mastectomy?

Because a large area of my breast was involved, my surgeon felt a modified radical mastectomy was a better choice for me. I have very small breasts and there wasn't much to work with; I would have very little breast remaining after lumpectomy and irradiation.

### Why did you decide to have immediate breast reconstruction?

When I was diagnosed with cancer, I could only think mastectomy. I did not think immediate reconstructive surgery. That was secondary—for the future. Number one, get rid of the cancer. But when my surgeon said I was an excellent candidate for immediate reconstructive surgery, that was fantastic. I could get rid of my cancer and also walk out of the hospital with something that resembled a breast.

### What were your goals for breast reconstruction? Why did you select a TRAM flap reconstruction?

My cancer surgeon gave me a copy of your book, and I read as much as I could about the different reconstructive options before I met with the plastic surgeon. I learned about implants and possible problems with scar tissue and maintenance and decided that I didn't want an implant if I could avoid it. Also, I didn't want my other breast touched. I wanted to have one that was still intact. I had never wanted to change my breast; I was happy with what I had. My goal was to have my reconstructed breast look and feel as similar as possible to what I had before. Considering my goals, my plastic surgeon suggested a TRAM flap. He saw I had a lot of extra tissue in my abdomen and felt that might be the best method for me. I was delighted when he told me that I wouldn't need an implant; my reconstructed breast could be all my own tissue. That was wonderful.

### Why did you decide on that particular plastic surgeon?

When I discovered I needed a biopsy, I wanted the best, even if I had to go to another state or another country. From the women that kept calling me back that Sunday, I knew that the hospital had a good reputation. I was also confident with the expertise of my cancer surgeon, who was a well-known breast surgeon. She referred me, and I trusted that she would only associate herself with the best plastic surgeon.

When I met with the plastic surgeon, I knew he was right for me. He's very human. As a man, he is surprisingly sensitive to a woman's feelings. He wants to make you feel like a woman. It's important to him to keep you as beautiful as possible and help you stay beautiful. He has a special quality that is hard to put into words. It's not given to everybody; you are born with it. He's a creator, an artist and that came across in our conversation.

### Did he explain to you what he was going to do? Did he give you enough information?

He explained that he was going to use the tissue and muscle from my abdomen and move it up through my body cavity to build a breast. I asked how he would know how much tissue to put in there? He said that when the general surgeon takes out the breast tissue, they weigh and measure it. He would try to put the same amount back in and trim down any excess. He also explained that with the TRAM I could lose a lot of blood; he wanted me to donate 2 units of blood. That took 2 weeks.

### Did you have any reservations about reconstruction?

I was afraid that it would cover up a possible cancer underneath; I also didn't know if it would be more difficult to detect a cancer recurrence after immediate reconstruction. I asked both my surgeons more than once if this was safe. I kept asking. That was my big worry. To me it was more important to live and not worry about the cancer than to look good; that was secondary. My general surgeon and plastic surgeon answered my questions. My surgeon said there was no need to wait because my cancer was caught so early. At a later stage reconstruction would have to be delayed until after chemotherapy and radiation.

### How long were you in the hospital? Did you experience much pain?

The first 2 to 3 days in the hospital were painful and uncomfortable, even though I had the pain pump for the first 2 days. I had oral medication after that. The pain was mostly in the abdomen, not much in the breast at all. I was surprised that I could move my arm on the side of the mastectomy. I was happy with that. I was out of bed on the third day.

### Can you describe the pain that you had in your abdomen?

The first couple of days I ached badly. After that my abdomen felt very, very tight. It is still tight, and it has been 8 weeks since I had my breast reconstruction. It is not uncomfortable; it just feels strange. It's like wearing a belt that is a little too tight. That's how I feel in an area 4 to 5 inches wide from between my breasts down to the pubic area. I can pinch myself and even stick a needle there, but I don't feel anything.

### How long did it take you to recuperate before you could return to work and resume your normal activities?

I'm a flight attendant, and my plastic surgeon didn't want me to go back to work for 3 months. If I had an office job, I probably could have been back at work after 4 weeks. The first day home from the hospital I started doing laundry, dishes, cooking . . . just everything. In the beginning there was a restriction on lifting my arm. The first 2 weeks I could lift it only to shoulder level. Now I have no restrictions; even so, I don't try to lift more than 20 pounds. Otherwise I do everything. I exercise. I take brisk walks. Considering how tight my abdomen is, I am surprised that I still have the control to inhale and exhale.

### Are you satisfied with the appearance of your reconstructed breast? Is it soft? Does it have sensation? Is it warm?

My breast is becoming much softer; I can see it change every week. It still is not quite as soft as the other breast. My breast feels warm to the touch, but it has no sensation; it is numb when you pinch it. Originally my underarm was numb also, but the feeling is coming back. That's probably because they only removed nine lymph nodes; I think if they take more you don't feel as much. It still feels strange when I shave under the arm.

The new breast is a little big right now; I don't know exactly how the finished product with the nipple is going to look. My plastic surgeon is going to make an adjustment when he reconstructs my nipple so my breasts match more closely. But I am happy with what I have right now because I can wear regular clothes. I can wear open sundresses, I can wear bathing suits, I look nice in a bra and underwear.

### What are the scars like?

I have a big scar across my abdomen and a circular scar on my breast where the stomach tissue was inset. I read somewhere that vitamin E oil helps the scars, so I've been putting it on. It softens them. I think that makes them look nicer. I also use it in both areas to alleviate the dryness. I don't think my scars are bad at all; they are pretty good. After 8 weeks I look fine. With this particular incision, my scars don't show in a bathing suit.

### Did you have any problems or complications from your breast reconstruction?

No. Everything has gone very smoothly.

### Are you happy that you had your reconstruction immediately or would you have preferred to have some time to recover between the mastectomy and the breast reconstruction?

I am very happy I did it immediately. After I absorbed the shock of having cancer, it was nice knowing that I would come home with something that looked like a breast. It was summertime and I always like to wear little sundresses and bathing suits; without a breast I couldn't wear those clothes. So it was great to be able to go home right out of the hospital and put on an open sundress and nobody could tell that there wasn't a regular breast there. That was fantastic. Maybe some women would not be as appreciative of a reconstructed breast that isn't quite like the other breast—unless they are without a breast for a time. I felt that whatever I ended up with would be better than nothing. This is much better than nothing; this is almost like the other one. So I am very, very pleased. But I was prepared for the difference. That is important. You are not going to come out with a breast that is identical to what you lost. That will never be. But it will be very good and very acceptable.

### If you had it to do over, would you have a TRAM flap again or would you select another technique?

I know the TRAM flap is major surgery with more potential for problems, but I would still choose it without hesitation. It takes more hours in the operating room, longer to recuperate, and of course my stomach is still stiff. But there is nothing artificial; it's all me. I don't have this maintenance business with an implant to worry about. I am planning to live for many years. In the long run I'm better off with this approach. That's why there was no other choice for me.

### Was your plastic surgeon responsive to your needs?

I don't think that he could have done anything better. I am very satisfied. I chose him because of the way I felt about him. I felt confident that he would do the best possible for me, and he did.

### How did your children react to this experience?

I wanted to tell them what was going on, but I didn't know how. My children are so young. Before I had a chance to talk to them about it, somebody that my husband works with told the mother of a child in my son's class that I had breast cancer. The next day at school the little boy goes to my son and says, "Your mother has breast cancer and she is going to die." That night at the dinner table, my son says, "Mommy, Johnny says that you have breast cancer and you are going to die." I said "Yes, I have breast cancer. That's why I'm going to have surgery. I'm going to have my breast taken off and the cancer removed and I am not going to die." I told them straight out, just like that, and that was fine. The next day I explained further. I said, "One doctor is going to take the old breast off with the cancer in it so that the cancer will be gone; then another doctor is going to make a new breast. And you know Mommy has a little tummy and that is what the doctor is going to use. When I come home from the hospital, I will not have a nipple, but I'm going to get one later. I am going to have a scar on my stomach and a scar on the new breast." I told them this because sometimes when I'm in the shower they come in with "Mommy this, and Mommy that." This way they will not be shocked because they already know about my scars and stomach and that my breast is without a nipple. As soon as I came home from the hospital, my kids asked to see the new breast and the scar on my tummy. So I showed them, and it was fine, because they knew what to expect.

### Was your husband supportive? How did he feel about your having reconstructive surgery?

My husband, Eric, and I looked at a book of pictures of women who had breast reconstruction. He wasn't so worried about the breast; he was more concerned about this big ugly scar on the abdomen. That to him was grotesque. Before the surgery Eric asked me if I was sure I wanted to do this. I wasn't going to worry about what he said. I was going to do what I felt was the right thing. The second day after the surgery when I was in the hospital one of the nurses came in to check on the flap. Eric was sitting right there. She asked if he had seen my surgery yet. She undressed me completely and showed him. I had planned to wait until the scars, especially the one on the stomach, looked a little nicer and not as red as they do the day after surgery. This early unveiling was actually a wonderful idea; he saw the scars at their worst. Now he thinks they looks nice. He says, "Hey, they're looking better."

### Has reconstruction affected your sex life?

Many couples have concerns about their sex life after mastectomy, and they don't talk about it. It is important to talk. Eric and I talked through our worries. After the surgery he was concerned that I would feel rejected if he didn't always want to have sex when I was in the mood for lovemaking. He worried that if he were tired or not in the mood, I would interpret it as a negative and think he didn't find me attractive anymore because of my breast. He felt that he would always have to be on call, responsive to any indications I would give him that I wanted to make love. He didn't know if he could cope with having to make love all the time. Eric was also concerned that I would want to test him, and even when I didn't really want sex I would suggest it just to see what his response would be. So we talked about it, got our concerns out in the open, and now everything is okay. It is essential for couples to discuss these issues.

I think something else helped our initial adjustment. Since I knew that my husband was not too excited about the big scar on my abdomen, I figured that I could still be sexy without being stark naked, at least until the scars looked a little better. I bought some pretty sexy nighties that were revealing but still covered up the scars.

### What advice would you care to share with other women about breast cancer or breast reconstruction?

People came out of the woodwork to provide support to me. Women would come up to me on the street and say, "I know what you're going through. I had breast cancer too, but nobody knows." One woman had a lumpectomy and never even told her husband. Two women on my street told me that they also had mastectomies. There are many women around us who have had breast cancer. I think it is important to talk about it. I share it with everybody because I was very fortunate. I found my cancer because of a mammogram. Many women believe that a mammogram hurts so much that they don't dare go for one.

More information and openness is needed. For a while it was hush-

hush to have a hysterectomy. All of a sudden that's the thing to talk about. Everybody is talking about hysterectomies. You find out every other women has had a hysterectomy and that it's acceptable. Now I think it is time to talk about breast cancer because there are so many of us out there; we are everywhere. So it is important to talk about it and I do. I tell people, "Yes, I had breast cancer. I had a mastectomy, and I was fortunate enough to have had reconstructive surgery." And they want to know more, and then I find out that they haven't had a mammogram for 5 years. They keep running away from it. I must have sent at least 100 women for mammograms because they discovered that's how I found my cancer. I didn't even have a lump. Because the mammogram detected my cancer early, it did not have time to become invasive. My surgeon said if I had come 6 months later my prognosis would have been different. And now it's life after cancer; it's life after a mastectomy, it's life after reconstructive surgery. Life goes on.

## LIBBY: I WOULD NOT BE DISFIGURED!

"I just wanted boobs! I couldn't walk around with a 36C breast on one side and a flat chest on the other. It was inconceivable to me to do that. I had augmentation years ago and it turned out very nice. I am a nurse, a professional, and there was no question in my mind that I would have breast reconstruction so I would not be disfigured." This explanation was given to me by Libby for why she opted for *immediate breast reconstruction with tissue expansion and a latissimus dorsi (back flap) reconstruction* after her breast cancer was discovered.

Libby is married and has a 16-year-old daughter. She has light-brown, curly hair and wears glasses, which lend an air of seriousness to her demeanor. Her carriage is very erect, which I would later learn is partly from her effort to counteract her shoulder falling forward as a result of her transferred back muscle. She had been in nursing for over 20 years; yet she found that she had as many misconceptions about breast cancer as people far less familiar with medicine. She was fortunate, however, in having access at her own hospital to the best possible care from people who knew her and took a personal interest. Even so, she took the time to investigate the different reconstructive options before making a final choice.

Libby is an intelligent woman with a sense of self-confidence and self-assurance. She describes herself as an "involved person who always wants to know more." She is 5 feet 8 inches tall and laughingly admits that "she sees herself as a tall, slender person and probably always will even if she really turns out to be a tall, dumpy person." When she found out she had breast cancer, she was not going to let this disease rob her of her positive body image. She drew on all of the resources she had available, chose the best plastic surgeon to perform her breast reconstruction, and now, 2 years later, is ready to share what she learned in her experience with breast cancer and breast reconstruction.

### How did you discover your breast cancer?

I have a history of fibrocystic breasts. For years my breasts would get sore at the end of my monthly cycle. I used to think one day I would have a prophylactic mastectomy and implant inserted so I would never have to worry about getting cancer, but I never did. Even so, I was always careful about checking my breasts. But you get lax with BSE because of so many lumps and tough spots. A year ago, as I was lying in bed, my hand fell across my chest and my ring finger fell on a spot right below my rib in the middle of my chest, not in a spot that I perceived as being breast tissue, but high on my chest. I felt a lump there; I sat up, put a finger on both sides of it, and could palpate the edges. I went downstairs and had my husband feel it. I said, "That's a lump; it could be cancer." I called an oncologic surgeon the next morning. He examined me that day and told me there was a 50/50 chance that the lump was cancerous. In my mind I knew when I felt it that it probably was.

### Did your surgeon give you a choice between lumpectomy and irradiation and mastectomy and reconstruction? Which did you choose and why?

The surgeon was blunt; he said we're going to have to make some decisions. We need to do a biopsy to see what this is. After the biopsy, if it is cancer, we will need to decide what to do. We can do a lumpectomy; I will make an incision right over the lump and remove it. This will require follow-up radiation therapy. Or you can have a modified radical mastectomy with immediate reconstruction. I will send you to see one of the plastic surgeons I work with. I must tell you that right now the survival statistics are equal for these different therapies.

It was all moving very quickly. I had a mammogram done, but my lump was so high that it was hard to get enough breast tissue to get a picture of it. By the time we did the biopsy I had to know what I wanted to do and what I wanted to do for follow-up because it would make a difference as to how he would cut my chest. I had an appointment with the plastic surgeon and he thought he could do reconstruction at the same time. Then it was a decision as to whether to do lumpectomy or mastectomy with immediate reconstruction. I called another oncologic surgeon and asked her opinion. She said that she was seeing people who had lumpectomy with irradiation come back with cancer in the same breast. She felt that I was just too young, in my early forties, to have a time bomb in my chest. She had seen reconstruction and it was good; she recommended that I get rid of it. That really fit with my surgical background. If it offends you, get rid of it. If I'm going to have a part of my body that's attacking me, then I want it gone. What she said sounded sensible. So I decided to have the mastectomy with immediate breast reconstruction.

### How did you react to the possibility of having breast cancer?

I was under a lot of stress. Another girl in my office had discovered a lump and had already had a mastectomy. Then a third lady in our office developed breast cancer. So out of 35 women in one department three of us had breast cancer. My boss's sister, my age, died 2 weeks earlier from breast cancer. It was as if someone sprinkled breast cancer dust all over and we were caught in the spray.

### Why did you decide to have breast reconstruction?

I did not want to be a victim. I wanted to be in control of this whole process to the best of my ability. By getting the reconstruction I was more in control of my own sense of self. The plastic surgeon I went to gave me a book of pictures of patients who had breast reconstruction. I looked at the pictures and thought there's really little difference between their breasts no matter how they were reconstructed—whether a TRAM flap, a latissimus dorsi flap, or an implant. I would be foolish not to do this. I had augmentation years ago by another plastic surgeon, so I was already familiar with breast surgery. It turned out really nice. I just wanted boobs. I would not be disfigured. There was no question in my mind. And if I could do it immediately, as opposed to having a second surgery, then why not?

### Did your plastic surgeon explain all of the reconstruction options? What type of reconstructive approach did you chose?

My breast was too big for an implant just under the muscle unless I had a breast alteration on the other side. My friends said, "Oh, you can have a tummy tuck and do this all at the same time." But I was too thin for the TRAM flap, so that was not an option. I don't think I would have opted for that anyhow. My best option was a latissimus dorsi flap with tissue expansion. My plastic surgeon thought he could get good balance with a flap.

### Are you happy you had immediate reconstruction?

Yes, it made this experience a whole lot easier to deal with. I came back similar to, although not exactly the same as the way I left. I didn't have to deal with the idea of having cancer and disfigurement and the potential of chemotherapy and my hair falling out. I mean, "Why don't you just cut off my arms, too, or give me a scar across my face?"

### Did you experience much pain from your mastectomy and immediate reconstruction?

There was remarkably little pain. I was tight. They didn't want me to lift my arm higher than elbow or shoulder height. I was afraid that I would have a lot of pain. So I had them hook up a PCA pump after my surgery. That's a pump that is attached to a jug of morphine; every time you hit the pump, you get a little dose, just enough to keep you comfortable as opposed to getting a shot in your hip, which gives you zonk time for 20 minutes to 2 hours until it wears off and you are uncomfortable for another hour until it is time to get your medication. I'm also very sensitive to narcotics and a little bit goes a long way for me. I only used the PCA pump three times after surgery and then I switched to Tylenol.

I also did not have difficulty moving around. It isn't like the TRAM flap where your abdominal muscles are cut and you can't get in and out of bed easily. I could do anything. I had drainage tubes coming from my donor sites and I think I had two coming from my side; one was from the breast tissue somewhere up in the reconstructive site. I could get in and out of the tub with no problem to take a bath, but I couldn't take a shower.

### What was your reaction to your breast reconstruction when you woke after your surgery?

I looked down to see what I looked like, and I was pleased with the immediate picture of this little stretchy thing holding my gauze in place. I was round on both sides. I had a new baby boob and it was nice looking. I didn't have time to incorporate it as part of me yet. It was something new they had built on me; I flashed everybody. I really think women need to see this. People don't know what this looks like; if they could see it, they wouldn't be so frightened of it.

### How did your breasts look and feel after your reconstruction? Did you have any surprises?

When they tunnel under your armpit to drape this tissue into your chest, it leaves a roll of tissue under your arm that resembles a rolled-up washcloth. When I put my arm straight down, it hung forward so it would miss the bulging tissue under my arm. My shoulder fell forward and I didn't like that. I asked the resident why my shoulder was forward. He said it was because the latissimus dorsi muscle had been moved; when it's in its normal position, it pulls your shoulder back. I was constantly having to remind myself to pull my shoulder back. Now I just remember to try and use other muscles to pull my shoulder back.

Also the roll of tissue under my arm was an annoyance. Fortunately, that tissue atrophies and weeks later I realized I wasn't going to have to live with this huge lump under my armpit. It goes away. Now my arm lays flat at my side the way I would want it to.

I didn't expect a roll of back tissue under my armpit, I didn't expect my shoulder to fall forward, and I didn't expect the suture line on my side to be as tight as it is. It felt like somebody had taken a sewing machine and sewn a seam right into my chest wall. It did not move at all. There was no give. And it wasn't until I asked one of the plastic surgeons that he told me that it would become looser as I exercised. I didn't know those things. If I had, I think it would have been easier for me. Also nobody ever told me when I should start exercising. I was told not to exercise because of all that drainage. Just don't move your arm. I probably did a whole lot more than I should have.

### When were you able to resume your normal activities? Did you experience any problems after surgery?

I stayed home from work for 2 weeks. Most people probably stay longer, but I was having problems with drainage and was having to drive 10 miles to the hospital to be drained; it seemed stupid to make this drive when I could just mosey over across the street and be working. So I came back to work. I was a little tired at first and worked half days for the first week.

I drained a lot after my surgery. I went home on a Monday, and I still had all these tubes and the little Jackson Pratt drains in me that I had to keep measuring and draining. I wondered when the drainage would stop. They took the drainage tubes out on a Wednesday or Friday and it still didn't stop. I had to come in three times a week to be drained; they drained 60, 80, sometimes 100 ml.

### Describe the technique that was used for your reconstruction.

They took a big slab of muscle and piece of skin tissue from my back and then tunneled it up under my armpit and laid it across my chest. Then they connected the skin that was left from the mastectomy to this back skin and placed a tissue expander underneath the transferred muscle and skin.

### Did they expand the tissue? If so, when did the expansion process begin?

Approximately 2 months after my surgery they started adding saline solution through the port in the expander. I needed tissue expansion because I didn't have enough skin to accommodate a breast that would match my remaining breast. After the surgery my right reconstructed breast was 34B as compared to my left breast, which was a 36C.

### Was the expansion process uncomfortable? Did you have any pain?

I had a sensory nerve removed with my tissue and the whole breast was numb. But when they put the needle in during my first expansion, it really hurt. I'm a fairly stoic individual, but when the nurse pulled that needle out, I started crying; I turned white and everyone was concerned about me. I said I can't do this and with that I left. Evidently, they stuck a needle into a nerve. Then they started using Novocaine with the injection; I didn't have another bit of trouble.

### What was your primary goal in breast reconstruction? Did you achieve it?

Symmetry. My breasts are perfectly balanced. I wanted to look like I did. And I do. I scar terribly, so I knew I was going to have bad scars. And I do. But I wanted to look good in a bathing suit. I have a pool in my backyard, and people come over. I can't be sitting there in bathing suits that are odd looking because I've had surgery. I wanted to be able to wear whatever I wanted to wear, and I also wanted to jiggle. And I do. So it worked out just fine.

### Where are your scars placed and what do they look like?

My scar starts about 4 inches under my armpit and then it curves down about 2 inches above my waist. I'm a very tall lady. But it's about 10 inches long and it's curved toward the front as opposed to the back. It's totally hidden by my bathing suit. It's also hidden by any backless dress. I also have a scar on my breast that's like a keyhole with two ends; it's an elliptic piece with two straight lines on either end.

### Can you wear the same clothes now or have you changed the way you dress?

I've not had to change anything. That was the nice thing about this whole thing. I didn't have to do anything different. I've always been tall and thin. I weigh around 140 pounds now at 5 feet 8 inches, and this is the most I've ever weighed in my life. I got the best bang for the buck actually. I just can't tell you how good it felt not to bother with a prosthesis and all that. I didn't have to sew a pocket in my bra. I didn't worry about facing the embarrassment when you jump in the pool and the damn prosthesis floats to the surface because you didn't get your little pocket in perfectly. I didn't have to sew elastic pieces onto my bra to prevent my bra sliding up over my suture lines when I raised my arm. I have enough to deal with without having to worry about how to get dressed in the morning, is everything hooked properly, is it going to shift or move, am I going to end up with a boob under my armpit. I don't want to have to deal with those kinds of issues.

### Is your reconstruction complete? Are any adjustments still needed?

I'm not done. I haven't had the final implant yet. I still have the expander.* I haven't had time because of my job. I only stayed out 2 weeks when I had the big surgery; this time I want to stay out 2 weeks for the small surgery to get a real rest. My plastic surgeon said that

---

*Since this interview was conducted, Libby has had her expander removed and replaced with a postoperatively adjustable expander implant during an outpatient procedure. This implant has a small valve in the underarm region to permit future adjustments and to provide long-term control over her breast size.

when you have larger breasts you probably ought to do this slowly and take your time.

### Do you have any concerns about breast implants?

I had implants before, so I have an idea what to expect. I didn't form a capsule the last time and so I said why should I this time. My prior surgeon gave me the name of the implant that was used last time. I thought, well, I'll just have him special order it because it worked the last time.

### Why are you having the nipple-areola reconstruction? When will it be reconstructed?

I told my husband that maybe I won't get a nipple put on. He says, "You can't go to bed without straightening the sheets. Do you really think in the long run you're going to be satisfied with one breast without a nipple?" So I'm going to have that done and just be finished. Get total closure to the whole thing. I also want it for symmetry. I've got a good-size nipple on one side and it leaves an impression; the other side is just smooth. My nipple will be done when my permanent implant is put in.

### How long did it take to incorporate your new breast into your body image?

It took a couple of months. I was so pleased to be symmetric and to be comfortable. But it wasn't incorporated until I started wearing my own bras again. Then I felt back to normal.

### What questions do women need to have answered when they are considering reconstruction?

You get information in small portions. People need to see the whole picture, even if it's just bullet points, so you know what to expect. They need to explain what they mean when they say they are going to overexpand you. Who knows what that means. When my new side got to be equal to my old side, I thought I was done. Then I found out that they were going to put 300 ml more in this sucker. It turned out to be like a watermelon on one side of me. It was huge and it was heavy. I didn't understand that there were other considerations, like having your breasts sag the same. They told me not to wear a bra for a month to let this tissue hang so it would have the same sag as the normal side. After a month of not wearing a bra I had equal droop and equal projection; then I said, now can we take some out? It all made sense, but it would have been better if they had explained it all to me initially.

## BETH ANN: MIND OVER MATTER

"My husband and I have many good memories from our breast cancer experience. I know that sounds crazy, but it's true. Even though breast cancer was a terrible blow, it was not all bad. We managed to enjoy ourselves throughout the whole process and were unwilling to become victims. We took the offensive and attacked the problem. We surrounded ourselves with positive energy, controlled our environment as much as possible, and refused to give in to negativity."

These comments were made to me by Beth Ann as she recounted her experience with breast cancer and the strategies that she and her husband, Dean,* used to cope with her diagnosis and therapy. A striking woman with a peaches and cream complexion and a halo of red hair, Beth Ann's voice is soft and compelling. She is stylishly dressed in a periwinkle suit that shows off a trim figure One would be hard pressed to believe that she is a breast cancer survivor who at 48 years has faced some serious challenges. A loving, participating partner has made her journey easier. It is clear from her story that a positive attitude and a supportive relationship can make all the difference.

Beth Ann and her husband have been together for almost 30 years now, first as friends, then as lovers, and during the last 12 years as married partners. Life seemed complete until 4 years ago when a routine physical examination led to a mammogram, a biopsy, and a diagnosis of DCIS (ductal carcinoma in situ) in her left breast. Two separate surgeons recommended a mastectomy.

Beth Ann opted to have a skin-sparing mastectomy combined with *immediate breast reconstruction with a TRAM (abdominal) flap* to avoid permanent breast loss. Following surgery she had a 6-month course of chemotherapy.

Beth Ann and her husband have a particularly close and sharing relationship. It was only natural that her breast cancer diagnosis should be viewed as their problem, their challenge, their disease. So intent was Dean on becoming actively involved that he initially pushed too hard and assumed too much control. Beth Ann had to tell him to

---

*An interview with Dean is included in Chapter 17.

back off and to allow her do the talking and make the decisions. Despite these initial missteps, Dean's ongoing support served as a lifeline for Beth. As she recalls, "He kept me comfortable and confident. I knew that he loved me, not my breast. He did all of those romantic things that make a difference. He also took care of me when I needed it and provided a shoulder to cry on when my spirits were flagging."

As a former military professional, Dean's instinct was to aggressively attack the problem and that is what he and Beth Ann did. They did extensive research, developed decision trees outlining available options, and laid out "battle plans" to wage their own personal war against breast cancer. Dean was intent on helping Beth Ann maintain a positive attitude. Cheers to rally her spirits, exotic nature posters to help counteract the hospital environment, and motivational tapes to focus energies on recuperation were some of the strategies they adopted to cope with surgery and recovery. They used the same methods during chemotherapy to keep their positive energies flowing and to mitigate the side effects of nausea and hair loss. They refused to let their fears overshadow their zest for life.

As Beth Ann recalls, "I was diagnosed with breast cancer right before the Christmas holidays. My husband gave me the news while I was lying in the recovery room." Maybe I was dopey, but I said, "Well, we'll face it and we'll take care of it." At this point he was more devastated than I was. Then I started to cry. Overall I took it pretty well. I knew that I had no choice. You just have to take care of these things. I'm not the type of person who goes into denial; I face what life holds and move on. I had delayed going to the doctor for a routine Pap smear, so I was probably lucky I went when I did, because my cancer was discovered in its earliest stages.

### Why did you choose to have a mastectomy and breast reconstruction rather than a lumpectomy?

When they removed the tumor, they did not get clean margins. I had a ductal carcinoma in situ (DCIS) and the surgeon recommended a mastectomy. Of course, I wanted a second opinion. A friend sent me to another surgeon for a consultation. He took another mammogram and confirmed my diagnosis and treatment recommendation. You could actually see a golf ball-sized area on the mammogram. If they tried to remove wedges of breast tissue or do a lumpectomy, they would have to remove so much of my breast to get clean margins that I would be deformed and would likely be very unhappy with the aesthetic appearance. Mastectomy seemed the best choice.

### Why did you want to have breast reconstruction?

I didn't want to lose my breast and I let the surgeon know that keeping my breast was important to me. I knew that I would be unhappy without any breast at all. I was too young and enjoyed my sexuality too much to be satisfied with that kind of result. My surgeon recommended a skin-sparing mastectomy and immediate breast reconstruction.

### What is a skin-sparing mastectomy? What are its advantages when combined with immediate breast reconstruction?

With a skin-sparing mastectomy, they leave most of the breast skin intact and only remove the nipple and areola skin and all of the breast tissue underneath. Then they fill the skin in immediately for the breast reconstruction.

### Why did you choose to have immediate breast reconstruction at the time of your mastectomy?

I didn't want to wait. I could see from the pictures the plastic surgeon showed me that the scarring was different when you delayed the breast reconstruction. If I had a standard modified radical mastectomy and delayed the breast reconstruction, they would have to remove a lot more skin and my breast scars would have been longer and more noticeable. With a skin-sparing mastectomy and immediate breast reconstruction, I could minimize my scars and still have a breast. Anyway, I just didn't see any point in having another operation. If my surgeon and plastic surgeon did not see a problem with doing the mastectomy and breast reconstruction at the same time, then that was my preference.

### How did you find a plastic surgeon and decide on the right reconstructive approach for you? Why did you select the TRAM (abdominal) flap?

The surgeon referred me to a plastic surgeon who is part of his breast management team. He called this plastic surgeon and he came over for a consult. After he looked at the mammograms and examined me, the plastic surgeon concurred that mastectomy was the right choice for me. Then he reviewed the various options for reconstructive surgery. When he told me about the possibility of using my own fat to build a new breast without having to use implants, I was delighted. I have allergies and am prone to developing rashes; even Band-Aids tend to irritate my skin. Therefore I did not want anything foreign in me like an implant. When he described the TRAM flap, I knew instantly that it was the approach for me. It was just perfect. I have plenty of fat on my stomach and I could have a totally natural breast. Even though it was a major surgery, I was eager to do it.

### How many hours did your surgery take? How long were you hospitalized?

It's tough surgery. Recovery is slow, but I really didn't have a bad time with it. The operation took about 5 to 6 hours; I needed a blood transfusion during surgery and they used 2 units of my own blood, which I had donated ahead of time at the doctor's suggestion. I was hospitalized a little less than 6 days. I went in on Wednesday and went home the next Monday. I went home with drains hanging out of me because I still had fluid buildup. These stayed in for the next week or two.

### Describe your hospital stay? Did you experience much pain after surgery?

Recovery wasn't bad. I had a private room that had a great view. As I woke up on the first day my husband was putting posters on my wall so people could sign them when they came to visit. I was hot and he placed cold compresses on my forehead to cool me off. I had compression stockings around my legs that were expanding and contracting to keep the blood moving and to prevent blood clots. I also was told to press a pillow against my breast to keep it warm and to maintain good circulation.

I started my period when I was in the hospital. That caught me off-guard because it was early. They tell me it happens all the time and is probably caused by stress. Women need to know that this is likely to happen. I wish I had known ahead of time so I could have planned for it.

I was up sitting in a chair the very next day. I had tubes hanging out of me, but I didn't really have any breast pain; that area was numb because nerve endings are cut when the breast tissue is removed. The pain came from the abdomen. You are very sore in your abdominal area and you are not able to stand up straight, which is very difficult. Everything you do expands and contracts your abdomen. A sneeze or a cough produces a violent pressure. It just hurts. I had an automatic IV drip for pain medicine (PCA), but I didn't need it very often. They'd tell me that I had to "keep ahead of the pain" so I needed to keep using it. I'd say okay, and I'd do it. I didn't take many of the pain pills after they took that out.

The pain was more tolerable than I thought it would be. Some of that was probably due to the positive reinforcement that I got from the motivational tapes that I was listening to and from the positive reinforcement that surrounded me. We made a special effort to control the environment, and I think that helped me to control my pain and to come through this experience with an upbeat attitude.

*How did you take control of your environment? What types of tapes did you listen to? Did they help to make your recovery easier and to keep your spirits up?*

Dean brought in posters to decorate the hospital room. One of the posters had an absolutely gorgeous scene showing a stream rushing through a forest. We used to go backpacking, so I could put myself in this scene. When I went to chemotherapy, we took this poster to hang in front of me. I listened to my tapes and I just tried to chill out and put myself there instead of here. I'd talk to my body and tell it to accept the medicine and kill the cells. I don't know if it works, but I feel I did okay with it so maybe it does.

During surgery, chemotherapy, and throughout this whole process, we took control of our environment and made it as comfortable as possible. We planned the chemotherapy treatments so we could spend the whole afternoon together before I started to feel queasy and had to go home. It really wasn't that bad.

I also listened to motivational audio tapes with a subliminal message to help me remain positive and hopeful. They give you a message that you're going to get well, that you're content with your progress, and that this is for your own good. That positive reinforcement helped me in my recovery. (Beth Ann stops for a minute to wipe her eyes, apologizing for her tears.) I still get emotional thinking about it. I listened to these tapes before I went to surgery and during the operation itself. The whole time I was in surgery I had earphones on. I also listened to them all during my hospital stay. When people weren't around to talk to me, I had them in my ears and Dean and I kept that stuff going. I think that makes a difference.

I later gave the tapes to my sister who had a hysterectomy and everyone was surprised at how fast she recovered. Who knows, maybe we just have good bodies. All I know is that you use what works; the tapes seemed to do the trick for me. The power of suggestion is important when you are feeling so fragile and afraid.

### How soon were you able to move around, to wash your hair, and to shower? Did you need any assistance?

Prior to my surgery I had talked to a friend who had abdominal surgery and she told me that it really wasn't so bad. What I needed to do was to get up and walk as soon as the doctors would let me and that would speed my recovery. That kind of mental preparation helped. I did very well with her advice. At first you can't do much. You can't even stand up straight until your stomach muscles stretch. However, as soon as they told me I could get up and walk, I made an effort to walk as much as I could. I walked around the hospital. I walked to my windows to just watch the birds outside. I did that a lot and it made me feel better.

Dean and I also figured out a way to clean me up a bit and to wash my hair. That was a tremendous help psychologically. I had to pull my knees up and lean my head back so he could wash my hair in the sink. One of the worst parts of recovery is that you feel so sweaty and grungy after surgery. I felt great when I had some makeup on and I toddled over to visit a woman down the hall who was feeling depressed. I mean at that point I was already thinking I need to pass this on to people as much as I can to help people out.

I had a catheter in for the first day or two, which didn't bother me in the slightest, even when they took it out. Then I was able to go in the bathroom and to shower. My first shower turned out to be really funny. Dean helped me wash myself, but he didn't want to get wet, so he took off his long pants and put on a hospital gown and got in with me. In the middle of the shower someone from the pain therapy department came looking for me. You can imagine how shocked he was to see Dean answer the door in a nightgown when he was expecting to see a woman recovering from breast surgery. We had a good laugh about that one.

### Did you need to make any special preparations when you were ready to leave the hospital?

When I tried to get dressed to go home from the hospital, I discovered that I didn't have the right clothes. My waist was swollen from the abdominal surgery and my pants wouldn't fit because they didn't have an elastic waist. I had to leave the hospital in my nightgown. I didn't know to buy anything ahead of time to wear after surgery. That is important information for a woman to have. You need something that buttons up the front because you can't lift your hands above your head for awhile. It also hurts to try to pull something over your head. I went home on Monday and on Thursday my sister took me clothes shopping. I picked two or three things from the rack and then I sat down in the dressing room while my sister brought clothes in for me to try on. I just sat for most of the time because I really didn't have the energy to walk around and shop. I bought clothing that I could get in and out of easily: three pairs of elastic waist pants and three shirts that buttoned up the front. That's what I wore for the next few weeks and months until the swelling in my waist subsided.

### What limitations did you have? Did you need help initially with household chores? How did you cope with them?

During the first few weeks my mother or my sister was there to help me. It is important to have somebody there to assist you when you get home because you really can't do much for yourself. After a while, when I was able to go out to the grocery store, I still could not push my cart to the car, particularly since the lot is situated on a hill. I had to have one of the kids from the store put the stuff in the car. I couldn't carry the bags into the house either. I had to shop when my husband was at home so he could bring them in. I had to pick up the groceries I wanted one item at a time, because you can't lift very much weight. I know you're not supposed to do laundry and things like that, but I just made do. I didn't lift, but I did kick the laundry basket across the room with my foot and then I picked up one piece of clothing at a time for folding. I could still cook, but I had to be careful not to lift anything heavy. You just have to pay attention to what the doctor says you should do. It gets better as time passes.

Because of the pulling in your abdomen, you can't lie flat in bed. We had a big floor pillow (about 2 feet square) that we covered with a sheet, and I propped it behind me and slept in a sitting or partially reclined position. At first you can't even get out of bed, so it helps to have somebody there for the first few days. Then after a little while you start to develop strategies for getting yourself out of bed. I managed by using my leg as a fulcrum. I would pick my knee up and then pull it down; that way I would be able to sit myself up as long as I was holding on to something. Then I could turn my body around and get out of bed. My fulcrum technique is really helpful to know when you are recovering from this operation because you can't pull from your abdomen.

I took a nap every day. You're tired from being bent down and you just have to relax periodically. I would sit on the couch and before long I'd be asleep. For diversion, I went out to lunch with my girl-friends who would pick me up.

**When were you allowed to start exercising?**

Within a few weeks, when I had healed, they let me start doing the hand/arm exercises; I also started walking the parking lot at my apartment complex. I tried to walk as much as I could. One time I walked too far and I had to call a cab to get me back to the apartment for a $2.00 fare. I was so embarrassed, but I was just too worn out to get back on my own. You have to learn your endurance; you can't walk for very long at a time because you get worn out easily, partly because you are not standing up straight. After the tummy tuck your stomach is pulled really tight and you lean over to counteract the pulling. It hurts to straighten up. It takes a while for your skin and muscles to stretch back out so that you can stand upright.

**How long was it before you could drive? When were you able to go back to work?**

It took about 6 or 7 weeks before I could drive. I have a stick shift, so it might have been even more difficult for me. You can't drive at first because you need to be more flexible and to be able to turn your abdomen a bit along with your head to see better. Things like that slow you down. I went back to work after 7 weeks, which I think is probably an average time. I worked only part-time for the first 2 weeks because it was very tiring for me.

**Did you have any problem or complications after your breast reconstruction?**

Several weeks after I was home I felt a hardness in my breast. The weight of my husband's body hurt me when we were close to one another. The doctor said that a part of the flap had died and my body had formed a capsule around it. It was a little hardened area, the size of a marble, but it hurt so I decided to have it removed. This was done at the same time I had my nipple reconstructed.

**Why did you decide to have your nipple-areola reconstructed? What was done? Were any other adjustments made at the same time?**

Before I had the nipple done, my reconstructed breast was just a round shape formed with abdominal skin. I just didn't feel done. A lot of women decide not to go any further, but I wanted to do it. The plas-tlc surgeon created a nipple from the available skin on my breast. I know that some women worry that a reconstructed nipple will look funny because it sticks out prominently, but the projection goes down and it looks quite natural after a time.

My plastic surgeon also used liposuction to smooth out the hip area where it was still a little puffy around the ends of the abdominal incision. That hurt. You are bruised after the liposuction and it hurts to even scrape against things for the first few days. It takes about 10 days for the bruising to go down. Once I had the nipple tattooed, I felt like I was done.

### Are you happy with the aesthetic appearance of your reconstructed breast? Is the contour good? Is it symmetric with your natural breast?

Aesthetically, my new breast looks very good now. It has a wonderful shape. It's not perfect, but it is very similar to the one I have and it hangs symmetrically. If I gain weight it sort of swells and is tender, so it is important for me to keep my weight down as much as I can. That's harder to do now because I am not as good about exercising as I once was.

The nipple-areola tattooing did not produce a very good color match. The colors are just not the same as those on my natural breast; they keep fading. I had the color put on twice. During the second time there was a lot of scar tissue and it was difficult to get the color to take. It's not the same beige-brown tone as my normal breast. In my eyes, however, it's perfectly fine and I don't think it makes a difference to my husband. So I don't consider it a problem.

### How many scars do you have? Where are they located? What do they look like?

I have a scar under my arm that comes up across the breast in the middle and then goes around the nipple. That has faded to such a fine white line that it's barely noticeable. (I also applied cocoa butter and vitamin E oil to help the healing process). There's a small pucker under the arm where things were put together again, but it's not much of anything. I have a bigger scar on my abdomen. It extends from hip to hip and looks like a big smile. It's redder, but I'm sure that's because it's still healing. As soon as the doctors said it was okay, I massaged my abdominal scar to improve the blood flow to that area and to help me recuperate faster.

*Do you have any sensation in the breast? Is your nipple sensitive
to touch? Is it responsive to sexual stimulation?*

Oh, I have regained a lot of the sensitivity. I even have sensitivity in
the nipple. The nerves have grown back. It's never going to be the
same as the other side; it certainly isn't going to have the sexual responsiveness. I can still tell that someone's touching it. I can tell I
have clothes on. But it is still not complete sensory return and I doubt
that it ever will be. Even so it is definitely getting better as the nerves
grow back. The same is true for my abdomen. I lost a lot of feeling in
that area, but it is coming back.

*What impact did the loss of sexual sensitivity in your breast
and nipple have on your sex life? Did you have to make any special
accommodations?*

Actually this didn't change my sex life at all, other than having to be
careful of positioning to avoid undue weight or pressure in the beginning.

*How long did you have to wait before you could resume
sexual relations? Was it awkward? Were you worried about
your husband's reaction?*

You don't have to wait a particular length of time; it's a comfort issue
more than a privacy issue. My husband was careful not to pressure me
about sex. In fact, I pushed him into having sexual relations again. He
would say, "Do you want to right now?" and I would say, "Sure." He
was very funny about it at first because he didn't want to hurt me. I
also had to shift around a bit until I found a comfortable position; it
was a little awkward that way. I didn't feel less of a sexual woman because of it, however.

My husband's a special man. He had told me long before any of
this came up that he really liked my breasts, but it wasn't my breasts
he wanted or that he was married to. He wanted me not just them. So
I was not totally fearful of that. You always have some doubt because
you don't know how people will really react. But I felt his background
would make him understanding. My breast also looked good. It looks
so real, so much like the other one and it's got the same feel. From
that perspective and because I did go the distance and do the nipple
reconstruction, I look pretty much the way I did. It's not perfect, but
it's very nice for both of us.

*Have you had to change your clothing because of the reconstruction? Can you still wear the same things?*

I really haven't had to make major changes. I wasn't supposed to wear an underwire bra, and I thought that would be an inconvenience in the beginning because I have been wearing underwire bras for years now. However, I was starting to feel a little pinch around the side, and I thought I should do what they recommended if it would be more comfortable. So I bought one that doesn't have an underwire and I do believe that I'll be happy with that. Other than that, all my other clothes are about the same. I've always kept in shape and done my arm exercises so I haven't had problems with arm swelling

*Was breast reconstruction worth the pain, time away from work, and recovery? Did it meet your expectations?*

I tell women who ask me about breast reconstruction that it is a personal decision. It made a difference to me. It made me feel like I was complete. You know your reconstructed breast is different when you look in the mirror, but that is okay because I love the way it turned out. I'm very happy, very content with the result and it makes a difference in my attitude and in all of the things that I do.

*If you had the decision to do over would you choose the same treatments? Would you have immediate reconstruction again? What would you advise other women about this approach?*

I would do it in a minute with the same techniques. The younger you are, the more likely you are to choose this approach. It is hard surgery and there's a lot of recovery time; some people might not be up to it. I know I have talked to women on the phone whose husbands and boyfriends say, "Why would you want to do any thing that takes so long to recover from." I know it's not right for everybody. However, I can honestly say it was right for me. If I develop another breast cancer, I couldn't use my abdomen again, but I would use my back (the latissimus dorsi flap) or another donor area. I would do it again because I like the effect; I like the way it looks and I like getting it over at the same time as the cancer surgery. I also knew that I didn't want to deal with putting a prosthesis in every day in order to feel matched. I also didn't want to cope with looking at myself in the mirror without a breast. For some women that wouldn't be a problem, but I was young, in my forties, and to me the thought of it was shocking.

*Were your doctors responsive to your needs? Did they communicate well? What could they have done better?*

Every doctor is in a hurry; that is why we must take responsibility for our own health care. If a doctor is talking while starting to walk out and I'm not done, I say, "Please, I have more questions," and I make him come back in. Some of them can't help it because they're just in a hurry, and they look at you and tell you that you are doing just fine. My advice is always to make them sit back down. And they will, they always do. I now have a great relationship with my surgeons and my oncologist. I feel secure in their knowledge and their abilities. It made a difference to me knowing that these doctors are respected in the medical community and that they have wonderful reputations. I knew that I was getting the best of everything. I felt in good hands. Plus, with my husband's medical background, he was always looking at my charts and trying to keep track of what was happening. A lot of people aren't going to be able to do that, but I would suggest that you take the time to go to the medical library and get some information so that you feel like you know the topic and you're not totally befuddled by what the doctor is telling you. I realize that may be a younger person's attitude. My mother doesn't do that; she just listens to what the doctor has to say. She doesn't want to know any more. But you miss things that way. You need to educate yourself. There is a lot of information out there to help you feel that you can gain control of your situation and make an informed decision. This is your life and you need to make the best of it.

*What kind of advice would you give other women about breast cancer and breast reconstruction?*

First, I'd tell them to get periodic checkups. It's important not only to do breast self-exams, but also to have your doctors examine your breasts and to get routine mammograms. Do not be an ostrich with your head in the sand, afraid of finding things. The sooner you find something, the earlier you can take care of it.

The second thing I would say is that a cancer diagnosis is not a death sentence. You can recover from this. You need to go into this experience with a mindset that says that you can do this; you can take care of it. Then you'll come through it. Breast cancer is not the end of anything. I do as much as I have ever done before. I've done a lot of things in my life and now I am able to continue to do them. I flew home 2 days after my biopsy; I did that as soon as I could go. Within a year, while I was still wearing my wig, I took trips to Florida and took a vacation inner-tubing down a river. I realize that's no big deal, but it has a symbolic meaning. It shows that you can do a lot; cancer is no reason to stop living and to stop enjoying yourself.

### How can a man be supportive of a woman during this experience? What works and what doesn't?

The first thing a man is going to have to realize is that he can't make all the decisions for you. Men tend to want to be problem solvers and they, like my husband, want to gather all the information, make a decision, and then provide the direction. "Let's do it this way." But you can't do that. The woman has to take the lead. This is a woman's body we are talking about and a woman's prerogative. She has to be the one to say this is what I want to do or not do. And in the end the man needs to be able to go along with what she decides.

I was very happy that my husband could actually be with me in the hospital the whole time. He cheered me up and helped me keep a positive attitude. We actually had fun, and I don't think many people could say that. He spent the night there every night and he did a lot of things for me. He was just there and took care of things; he brought me flowers and he was always showing my breast to everybody. It was great just having him there when I needed him to put cold compresses on my head or to help me shower or wash my hair or just get out of bed. The nursing staff can't run to you the second you want a glass of water and you can't reach it. They are busy. Having someone in the room with you, a husband, a relative, a friend, makes a big difference and is very helpful. You need someone you are comfortable with who will be there with you to let you talk and cry if you need to—someone who will also give you the freedom to choose your own options.

# APPENDICES

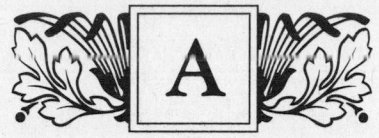

# BREAST CANCER
# RESOURCE GUIDE

One of the major advances in the care of cancer patients in recent years has been the development of effective and widely available cancer information and support services. The American Cancer Society and the National Cancer Institute have both been instrumental in improving the quality of communication and overall care for patients with breast cancer.

Today, a woman who seeks information on breast care, breast cancer, or breast reconstruction has a variety of sources to investigate. Updated literature written for patients can be obtained from physicians' offices, hospitals, cancer information services, and local American Cancer Society offices or by telephone from the National Cancer Institute. The popular literature has also grown to meet information needs, and a plethora of books and articles are now available in bookstores and libraries.

Many hospitals or communities have established cancer information centers that provide a variety of publications, audiocassettes, and videotapes for easy patient access. These centers are usually staffed by nurses, social workers, or volunteers who are knowledgeable about breast cancer and the many emotional and physical effects of this illness and its treatment. Support services are often coordinated with or through these cancer information (or support) centers.

Computer networks are another source of information. One of the best of these is the Physician Data Query (PDQ), an international computer network supported by the National Cancer Institute and its International Cancer Information Service, that helps to coordinate and update the information provided to patients and health care professionals. The computer system contains material written for patients and their families, physicians, and nurses. The content of the computer files is updated regularly, and research studies are also listed by disease, stage, and even geographic area. PDQ may be reached by online computer, telefax (CancerFax No. 301-402-5874), or telephone (800-422-6237 or 800-4-CANCER). Another valuable resource is the American Institute for Cancer Research, which provides information on diet, nutrition, and cancer. This organization can be reached by telephone (800-843-8114).

While factual information is critical to a woman confronting breast cancer and its treatment, she needs more than facts to cope with the trauma that accompanies this disease. Support groups of women who have experienced similar problems provide an enormous service and their value has become increasingly evident with time. Several years ago David Spiegel, a psychiatrist at Stanford University, published the results of a study that examined the value of support groups on the survival of women with metastatic breast cancer. His study confirmed what many have long suspected. He found that the value of these groups extended beyond ministering to a woman's emotional needs—women who participated in the support groups survived almost twice as long as those who had not participated.

Support groups are now available to address a variety of needs of women and their loved ones. Although not all women avail themselves of these groups, those who do praise them for their educational value and the opportunity they provide to learn from others who have had similar experiences and from the experts that they recruit to educate them about the latest developments in research and treatment. As one woman explained during an interview, "When I am with my group, I can express my fears openly because these women know what I am talking about. They have walked in my shoes. We can discuss sex, children, anything. It is a wonderfully liberating and empowering experience."

Some groups such as the I Can Cope program, developed by the American Cancer Society, emphasize cancer information and introduce the range of support services. Reach to Recovery, one of the original and most successful efforts, has emphasized the practical and emotional aspects of supporting women who have had mastectomies. CanSurmount is another patient support mechanism from the American Cancer Society.

Organized breast cancer support groups have developed across this country and internationally and are often coordinated by hospitals, treatment centers, the American Cancer Society, or even free-standing community-based centers. Support groups are usually led by a health care professional such as a nurse or social worker but are dependent on those women who attend for the daily activities. There is a trend toward the development of groups that are targeted to women or family members with specific needs. Mastectomy and lumpectomy patients, individuals interested in reconstructive surgery, women with young children, patients with metastatic disease, or even spouses may each have their own support groups.

Some women require emotional support and counseling that cannot be provided by a support group, gynecologist, oncologist, or oncology nurse. Those individuals may be best served by referral to psychologists, social workers, and counselors who have developed expertise with cancer patients. Patients with specific emotional or psychiatric problems might be helped by referral to psychiatrists as well.

As physicians study and refine the scientific aspects of treating cancer with drug therapy, surgery, and radiation, there is an increasing amount of research being done on the supportive care needs of the cancer patient. Recent work has emphasized the emotional aspects of cancer treatment and even evaluated improvements in the quality of life possible with treatment. New drugs have been introduced that help to control anxiety, pain, and nausea. All of these efforts have improved the ability to comfortably treat cancer and best support the patient through a difficult illness.

The following appendix incorporates a range of supportive services and facts and suggestions that may be helpful to a woman and her loved ones as they seek to cope with this disease.

# BREAST CANCER INFORMATION AND SUPPORT SERVICES
LOIS HOWLAND, R.N., B.S.N.

## 800 Numbers/Hotlines

AMC Cancer Information and
Counseling Line
800-525-3777

American Cancer Society
800-ACS-2345
800-227-2345

American College of Radiology
703-648-8900

American Institute for Cancer
Research
800-843-8114

American Society of Plastic and
Reconstructive Surgeons
(ASPRS)
800-635-0635

Cancer Care Line
800-622-8922

Cancer HelpLink
800-999-LINK
800-999-5465

Cancer Information Service
800-422-6237
800-4-CANCER

Food and Drug Administration
Breast Implant Information Line
800-532-4440

Hospice Link
800-331-1620

Look Good, Feel Better
800-395-LOOK

National Alliance of Breast Cancer
Organizations (NABCO)
888-80-NABCO

National Cancer Institute (NCI)
800-4-CANCER

National Coalition of Cancer
Survivorship (NCCS)
301-650-8868

National Health Information
Clearinghouse
800-336-4797

National High-Risk Registry for
Women
800-521-9356 or 212-794-4900

National Hospice Organization
800-658-8898

National Insurance Consumer
Help Line
800-942-4242

National Lymphedema Network
800-541-3259

National Rehabilitation Information
Center
800-346-2742

National Surgical Adjuvant Breast
Project (NSABP)
412-624-2666

National Woman's Health
Organization
800-532-5383

Susan G. Komen Breast Cancer
Foundation
800-IMAWARE

Y-ME National Breast Cancer Hotline
800-221-2141
(24 hours, 7 days a week)

## National Cancer Support Services

*American Cancer Society (ACS)*
National Office
1599 Clifton Rd., NE
Atlanta, GA 30329
800-ACS-2345
404-320-3333
Web address: http://www.cancer.org
The ACS is the nationwide community-based voluntary health organization dedicated to eliminating cancer as a major health problem by preventing cancer, saving lives from cancer, and diminishing suffering from cancer through research, education, and service. Services include:

1. Public and professional information
2. Service and rehabilitation
   - Nutritional supplements
   - Nonsterile dressings
   - Road to Recovery—transportation services
   - Reach to Recovery—support program for breast cancer patients
   - Guest room services
   - Durable medical equipment for loan
   - Wigs, breast prostheses
   - Ostomy supplies—reimbursement available for 3 months
   - Pain-relieving medications

The ACS has a variety of excellent programs for cancer patients and their families, such as I Can Cope, CanSurmount, Reach to Recovery, and Look Good, Feel Better. Patients can call the national office or their local ACS for further information on where to obtain low-cost mammograms and breast self-examination training.

### Cancer Response System
The CRS, sponsored by the ACS, provides telephone information and publications on cancer and refers callers to local chapters of the society for support services. Call 800-ACS-2345.

### CanSurmount
CanSurmount is a one-on-one hospital visitation program in which a newly diagnosed patient is matched to a trained volunteer with the same kind of cancer to offer emotional support.

### I Can Cope
This information seminar is sponsored by the ACS through area hospitals and offers (free of charge) eight sessions for cancer patients and their families on living with various aspects of cancer. The local ACS can be contacted for times, dates, locations, and registration information.

### Reach to Recovery

The Reach to Recovery program sponsored by the ACS is a one-on-one visitation program in which a trained volunteer who has had breast cancer is matched with a newly diagnosed patient to provide support and share concerns. The goal of the program is to provide an outlet for the patient to express anxieties and concerns and help improve the quality of life by facilitating physical, emotional, and social adjustment.

- A carefully selected volunteer is contacted to meet with the patient either prior to surgery or, if this is not possible, following surgery in the patient's room.
- The volunteer provides the patient with a kit containing information on breast cancer, the type of procedure the patient is undergoing, exercises, and a temporary prosthesis, ball, and rope.
- A follow-up phone call is made by the volunteer 2 to 3 weeks following surgery to check on the patient's progress.
- Any questions or concerns brought up during the Reach to Recovery visit will be directed to the nurse coordinator for appropriate follow-up.

For more information on this program, contact your local ACS chapter.

### Reconstruction Education for National Understanding (RENU)

RENU is a breast reconstruction support group sponsored by the ACS that provides volunteers who will discuss reconstruction options and related issues. Call 216-356-2683.

### Road to Recovery

This group enlists volunteers to drive cancer patients to and from medical facilities for treatment and rehabilitation. For information, contact your local ACS chapter.

## American Institute for Cancer Research (AICR)

1759 R St., NW
Washington, DC 20009
800-843-8114 (Nutrition Hotline)
202-328-7744
Fax: 202-328-7226
Web address: http://www.aicr.org

AICR focuses exclusively on the link between diet and cancer. In addition to supporting research in this field nationwide, AICR provides a wide range of educational publications.

**Blood and Marrow Transplant (BMT) Newsletter**
1985 Spruce Ave.
Highland Park, IL 60035
847-831-1913
Fax: 847-831-1943
Web address: http://www.bmtnews.org
e-mail: help@bmtnews.org
BMT publishes a quarterly newsletter for bone marrow and peripheral stem cell transplant patients and a 157-page book describing blood and marrow transplant and peripheral stem cell transplants. Offers attorney referral services to help resolve insurance problems and a "patient to survivor telephone link."

**Cancer Care, Inc.**
1180 Avenue of the Americas
New York, NY 10036
212-302-2400
800-813-HOPE
Fax: 212-719-0263
Web address: http://www.cancercare.org
e-mail: info@cancercare.org
This organization provides free professional counseling, support groups, education and information, and referrals to cancer patients and their families to help them cope with the psychological and social consequences of cancer.

**Cancer Research Council**
4853 Cordell Ave., Ste. 11
Bethesda, MD 20814
301-654-7933
This organization will send information regarding new medical treatments currently in the experimental stage.

**Cancer Research Institute**
681 Fifth Ave.
New York, NY 10022
212-688-7515
800-99-CANCER
Fax: 212-832-9376
Web address: http://www.cancerresearch.org
This independent organization directs its efforts to selecting and supporting the most significant advances in cancer immunology research aimed at preventing, treating, and curing cancer. It is a good resource for medical and research questions.

**Coping, Living With Cancer Magazine**
P.O. Box 682268
Franklin, TN 37068-2268
615-790-2400
Fax: 615-794-0179
e-mail: Copingmag@aol.com
*Coping* magazine is a consumer magazine for people whose lives have been touched by cancer. The magazine's primary purpose is to provide readers with the knowledge they need to cope with the many issues confronting their daily lives. *Coping* aims to inspire patients and survivors to assume greater responsibility for, and participation in, the many facets of their disease. A 1-year subscription (six issues) is $18.00 ($24.00 Canadian/foreign) and a 2-year subscription (12 issues) is $32.00 ($44.00 Canadian/foreign).

**Corporate Angel Network**
10604 Westchester County Airport
Bldg. #1
White Plains, NY 10604
914-328-1313
Fax: 914-328-3938
Web address: http://www.corpangelnetwork.org
e-mail: info@corpangelnetwork.org
This nationwide volunteer program provides free long-distance air transportation by using available space on corporate and private jets for cancer patients (and one accompanying family member) who need to travel for their treatment. To inquire about the availability of flights, a patient should call at least 5 days before she needs to travel.

**Encore Plus**
YWCA of the USA
Office of Women's Health Initiative
624 9th St. NW, 3rd Floor
Washington, DC 20001-5303
202-628-3636
Fax: 202-783-7123
Web address: http://www.ywca.org
e-mail: HN2205@handsnet.org
This program is aimed at medically underserved women in need of early detection education, breast and cervical cancer screening, and support services. This group provides supportive discussion and rehabilitative exercise for women who have been treated for breast cancer. To find the location of the nearest program, contact the national office.

**The Hereditary Cancer Institute**
P.O. Box 3266
Omaha, NE 68103-9990
800-648-8133

The Hereditary Cancer Institute at Creighton University is a nonprofit institution dedicated to research about hereditary cancers. It also disseminates information on cancer genetics and research and evaluates families to identify hereditary cancer and to predict cancer risk to family members and their offspring. This group maintains a registry of families with a pattern of familial cancer.

*National Alliance of Breast Cancer Organizations (NABCO)*
9 East 37th St., 10th Floor
New York, NY 10016
212-889-0606
Fax: 212-689-1213
Web address: http://www.nabco.org
e-mail: NABCOinfo@aol.com

NABCO is the leading nonprofit central resource for information and education about breast cancer and a network of more than 375 organizations providing detection, treatment, and care to hundreds of thousands of women in the United States. NABCO provides assistance and referral to anyone with questions about breast cancer, educates the public about the disease, and links underserved women to medical services. In addition to NABCO's role as a source of up-to-date, accurate information on all aspects of breast cancer, this organization spends time locally, on the state level, and nationally as an advocate for regulatory change and legislation to benefit breast cancer patients and survivors and women at risk.

NABCO has successfully collaborated with public and corporate partners on educational and medical programs such as the October National Breast Cancer Awareness Month, a partnership program with the Liz Claiborne Foundation providing breast care education and screening mammography to underserved women, and Avon's Breast Cancer Awareness Crusade, a national campaign to promote breast cancer education and access to early detection. NABCO is also active in efforts to influence public and private health policy on issues that pertain directly to breast cancer, such as insurance reimbursement, health care, and funding priorities. Individuals and organizations who join NABCO receive the quarterly *NABCO News*, resource lists, and other important information such as *Breast Cancer: Your Best Protection . . . Early Detection and Partner's Guide*, which is available free of charge on written request. NABCO is an excellent resource organization for any breast cancer patient. (Membership fee to join.)

**National Breast Cancer Coalition**
1707 L St. NW, Ste. 1060
Washington, DC 20036
202-296-7477
Fax: 202-265-6854
Web address: http://www.natlbcc.org
This grass roots advocacy movement includes over 400 member organizations and thousands of individuals working through the National Action Network dedicated to wiping out breast cancer.

**National Cancer Institute (NCI)**
Publications Order—Office of Cancer Communications
National Cancer Institute
Bldg 31, Room 10 A 24
Bethesda, MD 20892
301-496-5583
800-422-6237 (cancer information specialist)
800-4-CANCER (pub order line)
Web address: http://cancernet.nci.hih.gov.
The NCI is the federal government's principal agency for research on cancer prevention, diagnosis, treatment, and rehabilitation and for dissemination of information for the control of cancer. This organization offers free information to the general public and to professionals about cancer detection, diagnosis, and treatments, NCI-supported clinical trials, and research programs. NCI supports treatment centers around the country and conducts research on the causes, prevention, diagnosis, and treatment of breast cancer. In addition to its Cancer Information Service, NCI also conducts clinical studies. If a woman wishes to learn more about participating in these clinical studies, she can ask her physician, write NCI, or call the Cancer Information Service. Free literature is available on request.

### Cancer Information Service
The NCI conducts its own breast cancer research. Especially useful and valuable to breast cancer patients and their families is NCI's information and referral service. This service is called the Cancer Information Service (CIS). The toll-free phone numbers are:
  800-4-CANCER (continental U.S., except Washington, DC)
  808-524-1234 (local in Oahu, Hawaii; call collect from neighboring islands)
  202-636-5700 (Washington, DC, and suburbs in Maryland and Virginia)
  800-638-6070 (Alaska)

When you call the CIS number, you are connected with the regional office serving your area. They can give you accurate, personalized answers to your breast cancer questions and can tell you about various community agencies and services available. In many places the CIS offices are affiliated with Comprehensive Cancer Centers (specialized research and treatment centers designated by the NCI) and with the American Cancer Society.

### CancerFAX 301-402-5874
(From fax handset)
Provides treatment summaries with current data on prognosis, relevant staging and histologic classifications, and news and announcements of important cancer-related issues.

### Cancer Net
e-mail address: cancernet@icicc.nci.hih.gov
To get the CancerNet contents list, send an e-mail message that says "help" in the body of the message.

### Physician Data Query (PDQ)
The CIS's PDQ system is a computer system that gives up-to-date information on treatment for over 80 types of cancer. This NCI service is for doctors and for people with cancer and their families. PDQ tells about the current treatments for most cancers. The information in PDQ is reviewed each month by cancer experts and is updated when there is new information. PDQ also tells about clinical trials (research on treatments) and lists doctors who treat cancer and hospitals with cancer programs. For the latest information, call:

> 800-4-CANCER
> 808-524-1234 (local in Oahu, Hawaii; call collect from neighboring islands)
> 800-638-6070 (Alaska)*

### National Cancer Survivors Day (NCSD) Foundation
P.O. Box 682285
Franklin, TN 37068-2285
615-794-3006
Fax: 615-794-0179
NCSD is America's nationwide celebration for cancer survivors, their families, friends, and health care providers. NCSD is celebrated on the first Sunday in June of each year.

---

*Spanish-speaking staff are available to callers from California, Florida, Georgia, Illinois, New Jersey (area code 201), New York, and Texas.

**National Coalition for Cancer Research (NCCR)**
425 C St., NE
Washington, DC 20002
202-544-1880
Fax: 202-543-2565
This group is devoted to furthering the cause of cancer research. It provides a forum for organizations to promote cancer research through cooperative efforts in public education and advocacy leading to the eradication of cancer.

**National Coalition for Cancer Survivorship (NCCS)**
1010 Wayne Ave, Ste. 505
Silver Spring, MD 20910
Toll free: 888-650-9127
Fax: 301-565-9670
Web address: http://www.cansearch.org
e-mail: info@cansearch.org
The NCCS is a network of independent groups and individuals offering support to cancer survivors and their loved ones. It provides information and resources on support for those persons diagnosed as having cancer. This organization publishes a quarterly newsletter, *The Networker*, for its members.

**National Consortium of Breast Centers (NCBC)**
c/o Robert Wood Johnson Medical School
Comprehensive Breast Center
1 Robert Wood Johnson Place CN-19
New Brunswick, NJ 08903-0019
NCBC is a professional membership organization of comprehensive breast centers throughout the nation. To locate a comprehensive breast center near you, write for further information or check local phone listings. Comprehensive breast centers are full-service facilities that offer detection, diagnosis, and treatment services.

**The National Health Information Center**
P.O. Box 1133
Washington, DC 20013-1133
800-336-4797
301-565-4167 (Maryland)
This center is a health information referral organization that puts people with health questions in touch with those organizations best able to answer them. The center's main objectives are to identify health information resources, channel requests for information to these resources, and develop publications on health-related topics of interest to health professionals, the health media, and the general public.

**National Hospice Organization (NHO)**
1901 N. Moore St., Ste. 901
Arlington, VA 22209
800-658-8898
Fax: 703-525-5762
Web address: http://www.nho.org
e-mail: drsnho@cais.com
This organization's hospice helpline assists callers in locating a hospice in their area.

**National Lymphedema Network, Inc. (NLN)**
2211 Post St., Ste. 404
San Francisco, CA 94115-3427
415-921-1306
800-541-3259
Fax: 415-921-4284
Web address: http://www.hooked.net/-lymphnet
e-mail: lymphnet@hood.nct
This organization publishes a newsletter providing referrals, presents a biennial national conference on lymphedema, and offers educational materials for purchase.

**National Marrow Donor Program**
3433 Broadway St., NE, Ste. 500
Minneapolis, MN 55413
800-MARROW-2
Fax: 612-627-8125
Web address: http://www.marrow.org
This network maintains a data bank of available tissue-typed marrow donor volunteers nationwide and provides information and support to patients in search of an unrelated marrow donor.

**National Patient Air Transport Helpline (NPATH)**
P.O. Box 1940
Manassas, VA 20108-0804
800-296-1217
Fax: 757-318-9107
Web address: http://www.npath.org
e-mail: npathmsg@aol.com
This group makes referrals to charitable, charitably-assisted, and special discounted patient medical air transport services based on an evaluation of patients' needs.

**The National Women's Health Network**
1325 G St., NW
Washington, DC 20005
This organization is a national consumer group devoted to women and their health needs and concerned with protecting the rights of women in areas of health care. This group acts as a strong advocate for legislative and medical issues, including breast cancer. They have produced pamphlets on breast cancer and diet-related issues. They also produce newsletters (*Network News*) providing current information on a variety of women's health issues. Anyone may join this group, but there is a membership fee to join. Staff personnel will answer questions on the phone or send out an information package on breast cancer for $5.

**R.A. Bloch Cancer Foundation Inc.**
The Cancer Hotline
4435 Main St.
Kansas City, MO 64111
800-433-0464
816-932-8453
Fax: 816-931-7486
This foundation provides a hotline that matches newly diagnosed cancer patients with someone who has survived the same kind of cancer. Offers free information, resources, and support groups. Also supplies three books at no charge: *Fighting Cancer, Cancer . . . There's Hope,* and *Guide for Cancer Supporters.*

**Susan G. Komen Breast Cancer Foundation**
5005 LBJ Freeway, Ste. 370
Dallas, TX 75244
800-IMAWARE (800-462-9273)
Fax: 972-855-1605
Web address: http://www.breastcancerinfo.com
The Komen Foundation offers a comprehensive program for the research and treatment of breast disease. Information on screening, BSE, treatment, and support is available by telephone. Works through chapters and Race for the Cure events fighting to eradicate breast cancer as a life-threatening disease by funding national breast cancer research, project grants, and local education, screening, and treatment projects in communities nationwide.

**The Wellness Community**
10921 Reed Hartman Highway, Ste. 215
Cincinnati, OH 45242
513-794-1116
Fax: 518-262-1822
e-mail: wellnessnational@fuse.net
This group provides free psychosocial support to people fighting to recover from cancer as an adjunct to conventional medical treatment; 18 facilities nationwide.

**Y-ME National Breast Cancer Organization**
National Headquarters
212 W. Van Buren St.
Chicago, IL 60607
312-986-8338
National 24-hour hotline: 800-221-2141
Spanish hotline: 800-986-9505
Fax: 312-294-8597
Web address: http://www.y-me.org
e-mail: help@y-me.org
Y-ME is a nonprofit consumer-driven organization that provides information, referral, and emotional support to individuals concerned about or diagnosed with breast cancer. Its national toll-free hotline is staffed by trained counselors and volunteers who have experienced breast cancer. Several men whose partners have breast cancer are also available.

Y-ME national and its chapters conduct support and educational meetings in many states. Y-ME provides free written materials and publishes a bimonthly award-winning newsletter, as well as booklets directed toward single women, partners, and women with metastatic disease. A wig and prosthesis bank is available for those in need. Contact the Y-ME hotline for information about their local chapters.

## SOURCES FOR CERTIFIED SPECIALISTS AND CANCER FACILITIES

*American Cancer Society*
800-ACS-2345
Will provide the names of breast and cancer specialists and approved hospital programs.

*American College of Radiology*
1891 Preston White Dr.
Reston, VA 22091
703-648-8900
Will provide names of certified radiologists for mammography and a list of accredited mammography facilities by geographic area as well as the ACR resource materials listed previously. A fee is charged for bulk orders. Contact 800-ACR-LINE (8:30 A.M. to 5 P.M., EST, Monday-Friday)

*American College of Surgeons*
55 East Erie St.
Chicago, IL 60611
312-202-5000
Will provide names of certified surgeons specializing in breast surgery by geographic area.

**American Medical Association**
535 N. Dearborn St.
Chicago, IL 60610
312-464-5000
Will provide a list of member doctors in your area or refer you to a local service that can do the same. Can also give you information on the educational background and credentials of any doctor who is a member.

**American Psychological Association**
1200 17th St., NW
Washington, DC 20036
202-863-1648
Will put you in touch with a local group.

**American Society of Plastic and Reconstructive Surgeons**
444 East Algonquin Rd.
Arlington Heights, IL 60005
312-228-9900
800-635-0635 (referral message tape only)
Referral operators provide listings of up to 10 certified plastic surgeons within the caller's geographic area; also provide written materials.

**International Cancer Lines**
4853 Cordell Ave., Ste. 11
Bethesda, MD 20814
301-654-7933
Will send information regarding new medical treatment concepts currently in the experimental stage.

## NATIONAL CANCER INSTITUTE CANCER CENTERS PROGRAM

The National Cancer Institute (NCI) Cancer Centers Program* comprises more than 50 NCI-designated cancer centers engaged in multidisciplinary research to reduce cancer incidence, morbidity, and mortality. Through Cancer Center Support grants, this program supports three types of centers:
- Comprehensive Cancer Centers conduct programs in all three areas of research—basic research, clinical research, and prevention and control research—as well as programs in community outreach and education.

*Information on NCI Cancer Centers Program is being reprinted with permission from the National Cancer Institute.

- Clinical Cancer Centers conduct programs in clinical research and may also have programs in other research areas.
- Cancer Centers (formerly called Basic Science Cancer Centers) focus on basic research or cancer control research, but do not have clinical oncology programs.

Each type of cancer center has special characteristics and capabilities for organizing new programs of research that can exploit important new findings and address timely research questions. All NCI-designated cancer centers are reevaluated each time their cancer center support grant comes up for renewal (generally every 3 to 5 years).

To attain recognition from NCI as a Comprehensive Cancer Center, an institution must pass rigorous peer review. Under guidelines revised in 1997, a Comprehensive Cancer Center must perform research in three major areas: basic research; clinical research; and cancer prevention, control, and population-based research. It must also have a strong body of interactive research that bridges these research areas. In addition, a Comprehensive Cancer Center must conduct activities in outreach, education, and information provision, which are directed toward and accessible to both health care professionals and the lay community.

Clinical Cancer Centers have active programs in clinical research and may also have programs in another area (such as basic research or prevention, control, and population-based research). Clinical Cancer Centers focus on both laboratory research and clinical research within the same institutional framework. This interaction of research and clinical activities is a distinguishing characteristic of many Clinical Cancer Centers.

The general term "Cancer Center" refers to an organization with scientific disciplines outside the specific qualifications for a comprehensive or clinical center. Such centers may, for example, concentrate on basic research, epidemiology and cancer control research, or other areas of research.

Since the passage of the National Cancer Act of 1971, the Cancer Centers Program has continued to expand. Today NCI-designated Cancer Centers continue to work toward creating new and innovative approaches to cancer research. Through interdisciplinary efforts, Cancer Centers can effectively move this research from the laboratory into clinical trials and into clinical practice.

Patients seeking clinical oncology services (screening, diagnosis, or treatment) can obtain those services at Clinical Cancer Centers or Comprehensive Cancer Centers. They can also participate in research studies (clinical trials) at these types of cancer centers. Most Cancer Centers are engaged almost entirely in basic research and do not provide patient care.

Below is a list of the NCI-designated Cancer Centers. Additional information about the Cancer Centers Program can be found at the Cancer Centers Branch Website at http://www.nci.nih.gov/extra/dcbdc/ccbmain.htm on the World Wide Web.

## Comprehensive* and Clinical** Cancer Centers Supported by NCI

Information about referral procedures, treatment costs, and services available to patients can be obtained from the individual cancer centers listed below.

*Alabama*
University of Alabama at Birmingham
  Comprehensive Cancer Center*
Wallace Tumor Institute
Room 237
1824 Sixth Ave. South
Birmingham, AL 35294-3300
205-934-5077

*Arizona*
University of Arizona Cancer Center*
Department of Hematology/Oncology
1525 North Campbell Ave.
Tucson, AZ 85724
520-626-6044

*California*
City of Hope National Medical
  Center**
Beckman Research Institute
1500 East Duarte Rd.
Duarte, CA 91010
800-826-HOPE (800-826-4673)

Jonsson Comprehensive Cancer
  Center*
University of California at
  Los Angeles
10920 Wilshire Blvd., Ste. 1010
Los Angeles, CA 90024-6502
800-825-2631

USC/Norris Comprehensive Cancer
  Center*
University of Southern California
1441 Eastlake Ave.
Los Angeles, CA 90033-0800
800-522-6237
213-764-3000

Irvine Comprehensive Cancer
  Center*
University of California at Irvine
Bldg. 23, Route 81
101 The City Drive
Orange, CA 92868
714-456-8200

University of California at
  San Diego Cancer Center**
200 West Arbor Dr.
San Diego, CA 92103-8421
619-543-3456

*Colorado*
University of Colorado Cancer
  Center*
Campus Box E190
4200 East Sixth Ave.
Denver, CO 80262
800-473-2288

*Connecticut*
Yale Cancer Center*
Yale University School of Medicine
333 Cedar St.
New Haven, CT 06520-8028
203-785-4095

*District of Columbia*
Lombardi Cancer Research Center*
Georgetown University Medical
  Center
3800 Reservoir Rd., NW
Washington, DC 20007
202-784-4000

**Florida**
H. Lee Moffitt Cancer Center
& Research Institute**
University of South Florida
12902 Magnolia Dr.
Tampa, FL 33612-9497
813-972-4673

**Hawaii**
Cancer Research Center of Hawaii**
University of Hawaii at Manoa
1236 Lauhala St.
Honolulu, HI 96813
808-586-3013

**Illinois**
Robert H. Lurie Cancer Center*
Northwestern University
Olson Pavilion 8250
303 East Chicago Ave.
Chicago, IL 60611
312-908-5250

University of Chicago Cancer
    Research Center**
5841 South Maryland Ave.
Chicago, IL 60637-1470
800-289-6333
773-702-9200

**Maryland**
The Johns Hopkins Oncology
    Center*
600 North Wolfe St.
Baltimore, MD 21287-8943
410-955-8964

**Massachusetts**
Dana-Farber Cancer Institute*
44 Binney St.
Boston, MA 02115
617-632-2155

**Michigan**
University of Michigan
    Comprehensive Cancer Center*
CCGC 6303
1500 East Medical Center Dr.
Ann Arbor, MI 48109-0942
800-865-1125
313-936-2516

Barbara Ann Karmanos Cancer
    Institute*
Wertz Clinical Cancer Center
4100 John R. St.
Detroit, MI 48201-1379
800-527-6266
313-745-4400

**Minnesota**
Mayo Cancer Center**
200 First St., SW
Rochester, MN 55905
507-284-9589

**New Hampshire**
Norris Cotton Cancer Center*
Dartmouth-Hitchcock Medical
    Center
One Medical Center Dr.
Lebanon, NH 03756-0001
603-650-5527

**New Jersey**
Cancer Institute of New Jersey**
Robert Wood Johnson Medical
    School
195 Little Albany St.
New Brunswick, NJ 08901
908-235-6777

*New York*

Albert Einstein Cancer Center*
Montefiore Medical Center
Department of Oncology
111 East 210th St.
Bronx, NY 10467
718-920-4826

Roswell Park Cancer Institute*
Elm and Carlton Streets
Buffalo, NY 14263-0001
800-ROSWELL (800-767-9355)

Herbert Irving Comprehensive
    Cancer Center*
Columbia University
Room 435, Sixth Floor
Milstein Hospital Bldg.
177 Fort Washington Ave.
New York, NY 10032
212-305-8610

Kaplan Cancer Center*
New York University Medical Center
550 First Ave.
New York, NY 10016
212-263-6485

Memorial Sloan-Kettering Cancer
    Center*
1275 York Ave.
New York, NY 10021
800-525-2225

University of Rochester Cancer
    Center**
Box 704
601 Elmwood Ave.
Rochester, NY 14642
716-275-4911

*North Carolina*

UNC Lineberger Comprehensive
    Cancer Center*
University of North Carolina
    Chapel Hill School of Medicine
Campus Box 7295
102 West Dr.
Chapel Hill, NC 27599-7295
919-966-3036
919-966-1101

Duke Comprehensive Cancer
    Center*
Duke University Medical Center
Box 3843
Durham, NC 27710
919-684-3377

Comprehensive Cancer Center at
    Wake Forest University*
Bowman Gray School of Medicine
Medical Center Blvd.
Winston-Salem, NC 27157-1082
910-716-2255

*Ohio*

Case Western Reserve University
    Hospitals
Ireland Cancer Center*
11100 Euclid Ave.
Cleveland, OH 44106-5065
800-641-2422
216-844-5432

Ohio State University
    Comprehensive Cancer Center*
Arthur G. James Cancer Hospital
300 West 10th Ave.
Columbus, OH 43210-1240
800-293-5066
614-293-5066

### Oregon

Oregon Health Sciences University**
3181 Southwest Sam Jackson
 Park Rd.
Portland, OR 97201-3098
503-494-9000

### Pennsylvania

Fox Chase Cancer Center*
7701 Burholme Ave.
Philadelphia, PA 19111
215-728-6900

Kimmel Cancer Center**
Thomas Jefferson University
College Bldg., Ste. 1014
1025 Walnut St.
Philadelphia, PA 19107
800-1-CNETWORK (800-426-3895)

University of Pennsylvania Cancer
 Center*
Sixth Floor, Penn Tower
3400 Spruce St.
Philadelphia, PA 19104-4383
800-383-UPCC (800-383-8722)
215-662-6364

University of Pittsburgh Cancer
 Institute*
Information & Referral Service
Iroquois Bldg., Ste. 206
3600 Forbes Ave.
Pittsburgh, PA 15213-3410
800-237-4PCI (800-237-4724)

### Tennessee

St. Jude Children's Research
 Hospital**
332 North Lauderdale St.
Memphis, TN 38105-0318
901-495-3300

Vanderbilt Cancer Center**
Vanderbilt University
649 Medical Research Bldg. II
Nashville, TN 37232-6838
800-811-8480
615-936-1782

### Texas

The University of Texas M.D.
 Anderson Cancer Center*
1515 Holcombe Blvd.
Houston, TX 77030
800-392-1611

San Antonio Cancer Institute*
8122 Datapoint Dr., Ste. 250
San Antonio, TX 78229-3264
210-616-5590

### Utah

Huntsman Cancer Institute**
University of Utah
Room 70410
15 North 2030 East
Salt Lake City, UT 84112-5330
800-488-2422

### Vermont

Vermont Cancer Center*
University of Vermont
One South Prospect St.
Burlington, VT 05401-3498
802-656-4414

### Virginia

Cancer Center at University of
 Virginia**
P. O. Box 334
Charlottesville, VA 22908
800-223-9173
804-924-2562

Massey Cancer Center**
Virginia Commonwealth University
Box 980037
401 College St.
Richmond, VA 23298-0037
804-828-0450

*Washington*
Fred Hutchinson Cancer Research
Center*
1100 Fairview Ave. North
P.O. Box 19024
Seattle, WA 98109-1024
800-804-8824
206-667-5000

*Wisconsin*
University of Wisconsin
Comprehensive Cancer Center*
600 Highland Ave.
Madison, WI 53792-0001
608-263-8090

## Cancer Centers Supported by the National Cancer Institute

The Burnham Institute
La Jolla, CA

Armand Hammer Center for Cancer
Biology, Salk Institute
La Jolla, CA

Purdue Cancer Center, Purdue
University
West Lafayette, IN

The Jackson Laboratory
Bar Harbor, ME

Center for Cancer Research,
Massachusetts Institute of
Technology
Cambridge, MA

Eppley Institute, University of
Nebraska Medical Center
Omaha, NE

Cold Spring Harbor Laboratory
Cold Spring Harbor, NY

American Health Foundation
New York, NY

Wistar Institute
Philadelphia, PA

Drew-Meharry-Morehouse
Consortium Cancer Center
Nashville, TN

McArdle Laboratory for Cancer
Research, University of Wisconsin
Madison, WI

## SOURCES OF NATIONAL CANCER INSTITUTE INFORMATION

Cancer Information Service
Toll-free: 1-800-4-CANCER (1-800-422-6237)
TTY: 1-800-332-8615
NCI Online
*Internet*
NCI's main Website at http://www.nei.nih.gov or NCI's Website for patients, public, and the mass media at http://rex.nci/nih.gov
*Cancer Mail Service*
To obtain a contents list, send e-mail to cancermail@icicc.nci.nih.gov with the word "help" in the body of the message.
CancerFax® fax on demand service
Dial 301-402-5874 and listen to recorded instructions.

## SOURCES FOR LOCAL AND REGIONAL SUPPORT GROUPS

### *National Self-Help Clearinghouse*
Any individual who is looking for a self-help group in their region can find it by calling this organization at 212-642-2944. Also check for listings of statewide self-help clearinghouses. Call 800-555-1212 for information. If you cannot locate a convenient support group from this listing or from the National Self-Help Clearinghouse:

- Call NABCO and inquire about local groups in your area. They maintain a list of groups located in your area. Call Y-ME to inquire if they have a local chapter in your area.
- Inquire at a local major hospital's Breast Center or Departments of Social Work or Psychiatry.
- Call NCI's Cancer Information Service at 800-4-CANCER for names of American College of Radiology (ACR)–accredited mammography providers in your area and ask these providers for support group suggestions.
- Contact your local American Cancer Society office for local groups that they or others sponsor.
- Call a group on the list in your state and ask if they know of any groups located nearer to you.

For information on starting your own support group, contact your local American Cancer Society office or call Y-ME (see p. 587).

# LOCAL AND REGIONAL BREAST CANCER SUPPORT GROUPS*
*(alphabetical order by state/city)*

### Alabama
Woman to Woman
Gadsden, AL
205-543-8896

SISTAs CanSurvive Coalition
Montgomery, AL
334-277-5224

UPFRONT Support Group
Tuscaloosa, AL
205-759-7000

### Alaska
The Anchorage Women's Breast
  Cancer Support Group
Anchorage, AK
907-261-3607

### Arizona
Bosom Buddies
Phoenix, AZ
602-231-6648

Good Samaritan Medical Center
Phoenix, AZ
602-239-3250

New Beginning/Maryvale Samaritan
  Hospital
Phoenix, AZ
602-848-5588

Y-ME Breast Cancer Network of
  Arizona
Scottsdale, AZ
602-231-6666

Arizona Cancer Center
Tucson, AZ
520-626-6044

### Arkansas
Northwest Arkansas Cancer Support
  Home
Fayetteville, AR
501-521-8024

Phillips Cancer Support House
Fort Smith, AR
501-782-6302

CARTI Cancer Answers
Little Rock, AR
800-482-8561

### California
Anaheim Memorial Medical Center
Anaheim, CA
714-999-3880

Alta Bates Hospital
Berkeley, CA
510-204-1591

Woman's Cancer Resource Center
Berkeley, CA
510-548-9272

Beyond Breast Cancer Support
  Group
Chico, CA
916-892-6888

WIN Against Breast Cancer
Covina, CA
818-332-2255

Vital Options and "The Group
  Room" Cancer Radio Talk Show
Encino, CA
818-508-5657

Pallmar Pomerado Health System
Escondido, CA
619-737-3960

St. Agnes Medical Center
Fresno, CA
209-449-5222

Scripps Memorial Hospital
La Jolla, CA
619-626-6756

UCSD Cancer Center
La Jolla, CA
619-543-6650

Y-ME Bloomers of Orange County
La Palma, CA
714-560-7444

Y-ME Ladies of Courage/Antelope
Valley
Lancaster, CA
805-266-9109

Long Beach Memorial Breast Center
Long Beach, CA
310-933-7880

Y-ME South Bay/Long Beach
Long Beach, CA
310-984-8456

Rhonda Flemming Mann Resource
Ctr. for Women w/Cancer
Los Angeles, CA
310-794-6644

Sisters Network for African-American
Women
Lynwood, CA
310-639-6511

Bosom Buddies
Napa, CA
707-257-4047

The Breast Care Center
Orange, CA
714-541-0101

The Desert Comprehensive Breast
Center
Palm Springs, CA
619-323-6676

Community Breast Health Project
Palo Alto, CA
415-342-3749

Discovery Breast Cancer Support
Group/YWCA
Palo Alto, CA
415-494-0972

Breast Cancer Networking Group
Pasadena, CA
818-796-1083

Y-ME, Save Ourselves
Sacramento, CA
800-422-9747

WIN Against Breast Cancer
San Diego, CA
619-488-6300

Y-ME San Diego Chapter
San Diego, CA
619-569-9309

Bay Area Lymphedema Support
Group
San Francisco, CA
415-921-2911

The Cancer Support Community
San Francisco, CA
415-648-9400

UCSF–Mt. Zion Cancer Center
The Breast Care Center
San Francisco, CA
415-476-3678

Y-ME Bay Area Breast Cancer
  Network
San Jose, CA
408-261-1425

Wellness Community
Santa Monica, CA
310-314-2555

Center for Attitudinal Healing
Sausalita, CA
415-331-6161

The Breast Center
Van Nuys, CA
818-787-9911

John Muir Medical Center
Walnut Creek, CA
510-933-4107

Queen of the Valley
West Covina, CA
818-814-2479

*Colorado*
AMC Cancer Research Center
Colorado Springs, CO
303-239-3424

Penrose Cancer Center
Colorado Springs, CO
719-776-5273

Lesbian Cancer Support Services
Denver, CO
303-448-5558

Rose Medical Center—Men's
  Discussion Group for Male
  Partners
Denver, CO
303-320-7142

Rose Medical Center Patient Care
  Services
Denver, CO
303-320-7142

*Connecticut*
Y-ME of New England
Branford, CT
203-483-8200 or 800-933-4963

I Can
Danbury, CT
203-790-6568

St. Francis Hospital and Medical
  Center
Hartford, CT
860-714-4866

Cancer Care, Inc.
Norwalk, CT
203-854-9911

The Revivers
Ridgefield, CT
203-438-5555

Building Bridges
Stamford, CT
203-325-7447

*Delaware*
Looking Ahead Support Group
Wilmington, DE
302-421-4161

*District of Columbia*
George Washington University
Washington, DC
202-994-4589

Georgetown University Medical
  Center Lombardi Cancer Center
Washington, DC
202-784-4309

The Mary-Helen Mautner Project
  for Lesbians with Cancer
Washington, DC
202-332-5536

**Florida**
Halifax Medical Center Women's
  Services
Daytona Beach, FL
904-254-4211

Bosom Buddies
Jacksonville, FL
904-633-8246

Bosom Buddies Breast Cancer and
  Lymphedema Support Group
Naples, FL
941-514-3845

Bosom Buddies
Orlando, FL
407-281-8663

Florida Hospital
Orlando, FL
407-897-1617

Ann L. Baroco Center for Women's
  Health
Pensacola, FL
904-474-7878

Sarasota Memorial Hospital
Sarasota, FL
941-917-1375

FACTORS/H. Lee Moffit Cancer
  Center
Tampa, FL
813-972-8407

**Georgia**
Northside Hospital
Atlanta, GA
404-851-8635

Bosom Buddies
Tucker, GA
770-455-7637

**Hawaii**
Queens Medical Center
Honolulu, HI
808-547-4243

**Idaho**
Women's Life Center
Boise, ID
208-381-2764

The Wellness Group
Ketchum, ID
208-726-8464

**Illinois**
CARE-Alton Memorial Hospital
Alton, IL
618-463-7150

Good Shepherd Hospital
Barrington, IL
847-381-9600 ext. 5336

St. Elizabeth Hospital
Belleville, IL
618-234-2120 ext. 1260

Moving Towards Recovery
Chicago, IL
773-205-2017

Y-ME National Breast Cancer
  Organization
Chicago, IL
800-221-2141

Decatur Memorial Hospital
Decatur, IL
217-876-2380

Elmhurst Memorial Hospital
Elmhurst, IL
708-782-7900

St. Joseph's Medical Center
Joliet, IL
815-741-7560

McDonough District Hospital
Macomb, IL
309-836-1584

Pekin Hospital—Mastectomy
  Support Group
Pekin, IL
309-353-0807

OSF St. Francis
Peoria, IL
309-655-3293

Breast Cancer Support Group for
  Younger Women
Rockford, IL
815-971-7115

Sangamon Breast Cancer Support
  Group
Springfield, IL
217-787-7187

*Indiana*
Women's Cancer Support Group
Bluffton, IN
219-824-6493

Methodist Hospital, Northlake
  Campus
Gary, IN
800-952-7337

Uplifter's Breast Cancer Support
  Group
Indianapolis, IN
317-355-4848

Y-ME of Central Indiana
Indianapolis, IN
317-240-3331

American Cancer Society
South Bend, IN
219-234-4097

Y-ME of the Wabash Valley
Terre Haute, IN
812-877-3025

Women Winning Against Cancer
Warsaw, IN
219-269-9911

*Iowa*
"ESPECIALLY FOR YOU" After
  Breast Cancer
Cedar Rapids, IA
319-398-6265

Quad City's Breast Cancer Survivors
Davenport, IA
309-764-2888

Marshalltown Support Group
Marshalltown, IA
515-752-6486

ABC—After Breast Cancer Support
  Group
Sioux City, IA
712-252-0088

Breast Cancer Support Group
Waterloo, IA
319-292-2100

*Kansas*
Monorah Medical Park
Overland Park, KS
913-498-7742

Breast Cancer Care Group
Wichita, KS
316-262-7559

*Kentucky*
Breast Cancer Support Group
Ashland, KY
606-327-4535

St. Elizabeth Women's Center
Edgewood, KY
606-344-3939

The Thursday Group
Lexington, KY
606-269-4836

After Breast Cancer
Louisville, KY
502-589-6000

American Cancer Society
Owensboro, KY
502-584-6782

Breast Cancer Support Group
Prestonsburg, KY
606-886-8511 ext. 7575

*Louisiana*
West Jefferson Medical Center
Marrero, LA
504-349-1640

Center For Living With Cancer
Metairie, LA
504-454-4500

Breast Cancer Support Group
New Orleans, LA
504-897-4223

Ochsner Breast Cancer Support
   Group
New Orleans, LA
504-842-4251

Tulane Medical Center
New Orleans, LA
504-587-2120

North Shore Regional Medical
   Center
Slidell, LA
504-649-7070

*Maine*
Campus Support Group
Orono, ME
207-581-3433

Breast Cancer Support Group
Portland, ME
207-773-1919

*Maryland*
Arm In Arm
Baltimore, MD
410-494-0083

Y-ME of the Cumberland Valley
Hagerstown, MD
800-963-0101

Shady Grove Adventist Hospital
Rockville, MD
301-279-6619

*Massachusetts*
Margaret Gozlin Counseling Center
Amherst, MA
413-256-4600

Beth Israel Hospital Support
Boston, MA
617-667-2661

Dana Farber Cancer Institute
Boston, MA
617-632-3459

Faulkner Breast Centre Support
   Group
Boston, MA
617-983-7967

New England Medical Center
Boston, MA
617-636-9227

Lahey Clinic Breast Cancer
   Treatment Center
Burlington, MA
617-273-8989

Faculty and Staff Assistance Program
   Harvard University
Cambridge, MA
617-495-4357

Metro West Medical Center
Framingham, MA
508-383-1378

Y-ME of the Berkshires
Pittsfield, MA
413-499-2486

Baystate Medical Center
Springfield, MA
413-784-8010

**Michigan**
Diane Z. Breast Cancer Support
   Group
Ada, MI
616-676-1748

University Hospital
Ann Arbor, MI
313-936-9425

Barbara Anne Karmanos Cancer
   Institute—Unique Breast Cancer
   Support Group
Detroit, MI
313-966-0761

Cancer Counseling Program
Detroit, MI
313-493-6507

McLaren Mastectomy Support Group
Flint, MI
810-342-2375

St. Mary's Breast Center
Grand Rapids, MI
616-774-6756

Sparrow Regional Cancer Center
Lansing, MI
517-483-2689

Marquette General Hospital
Upper Michigan Cancer Center
Marquette, MI
906-225-3500

Midland Community Cancer Services
Midland, MI
517-835-4841

Just For Us
Petoskey, MI
616-347-8443

Breast Cancer Support Group
St. Clair Shore, MI
313-343-3684

**Minnesota**
Mercy Unity Oncology Services
Coon Rapids, MN
612-780-7780

Duluth Clinic—Breast Diagnostic
   Center
Duluth, MN
218-725-3195

Virginia Piper Cancer Institute
Minneapolis, MN
612-863-3150

Methodist Hospital
St. Louis Park, MN
612-932-6086

**Mississippi**
Biloxi Regional Medical Center
Biloxi, MS
601-432-1571 ext. 1691

UNMC Cancer Center
Tupelo, MS
601-841-4077

**Missouri**
St. Mary's Hospital
Jefferson City, MO
573-896-5583

The Cancer Institute of Health
   Midwest
Kansas City, MO
816-751-2929

Reach Together
Springfield, MO
417-269-6170

St. John's Breast Center
Springfield, MO
417-885-2565

St. Joseph Health Center—
Hospital West
St. Charles, MO
314-947-5424

Barnes Jewish Hospital
St. Louis, MO
314-454-7500

Missouri Baptist Medical Center—
I Can
St. Louis, MO
314-567-1105

Missouri Baptist Hospital—We Can
St. Louis, MO
314-996-5669

St. John's Mercy Cancer Information
Center
St. Louis, MO
314-569-6400

St. Luke's Hospital—Focus Breast
Cancer Support Group
St. Louis, MO
314-205-6090

Wellness Community Breast Cancer
Support Group
St. Louis, MO
314-993-4333

*Montana*
The Women's Center
Billings, MT
406-657-8730

Breast Cancer Support Group
Missoula, MT
406-251-3995

Bosom Buddies
Sidney, MT
406-482-2423

*Nebraska*
St. Elizabeth Community Health
Center
Lincoln, NE
402-486-7567

Breast Cancer Support Group &
Men's Support Group
Omaha, NE
402-345-6555

Breast Cancer Recovery Group
Scottsbluff, NE
308-630-1348

*New Hampshire*
Breast Cancer Support Group
Concord, NH
603-224-2051

Norris Cotton Cancer Center
Lebanon, NH
603-650-5789

Elliot Hospital
Manchester, NH
603-628-4130

*New Jersey*
Bayonne Hospital
Bayonne, NJ
201-858-8848

Brick Hospital
Brick, NJ
908-206-8340

Northwest Covenent Health Care
System
Dover, NJ
201-989-3106

Breast Cancer Support Group
Flemington, NJ
908-782-6112

Health Awareness Center
Freehold, NJ
732-308-1850

Hackensack Medical Center
Hackensack, NJ
201-996-5800

Mid-Monmouth County Recurrence
　Support Group
Little Silver, NJ
908-933-1333

St. Barnabas Medical Center
Livingston, NJ
201-533-8414

Monmouth Medical Center
Long Branch, NJ
908-870-5360

Cancer Care, Inc.
Millburn, NJ
201-379-7500

Jersey Shore Breast Care Center
Neptune, NJ
908-776-4440

Cancer Institute of New Jersey
New Brunswick, NJ
732-235-6792

Atlantic City Medical Center
Pomona, NJ
609-652-3500

Beyond Cancer
Princeton, NJ
609-683-0692

Breast Cancer Resource Center
　(for men and women)—
　Princeton YWCA
Princeton, NJ
609-497-2126

Riverview Regional Cancer Center
Red Bank, NJ
908-530-2382

Cancer Care, Inc.
Ridgewood, NJ
201-444-6630

Valley Hospital
Ridgewood, NJ
201-447-8557

Somerset Medical Center
Somerville, NJ
908-685-2953

WISE-Women's International
　Support Environment
South River, NJ
908-257-6611

Pathways
Summit, NJ
908-277-3663

Community Medical Center
Toms River, NJ
908-240-8148

After Breast-Cancer Surgery
Wash. Township, NJ
201-666-6610 ext. 202

CHEMOcare
Westfield, NJ
800-55-CHEMO/908-233-1103

*Nevada*
St. Mary's Regional Medical Center
Reno, NV
702-786-4421

*New Mexico*
People Living Through Cancer
Albuquerque, NM
505-242-3263

The Four Corners Breast Cancer
Support Group
Farmington, NM
505-326-0743

Y-ME of Southern New Mexico
Las Cruces, NM
505-521-4794

*New York*
SHAREing and CAREing
Astoria, NY
718-777-5766

Cancer Institute of Brooklyn
Brooklyn, NY
718-283-6599

Long Island College Hospital
Brooklyn, NY
718-780-1139

Breast Cancer Network of Western
New York
Buffalo, NY
716-631-8665

St. John's Queens Hospital
Elmhurst, NY
718-558-1000 ext 2250

Flushing Hospital Medical Center
Flushing, NY
718-670-5636

Adelphi New York Statewide Breast
Cancer HOTLINE and Support
Program
Garden City, NY
516-877-4444/800-877-8077
(statewide)

Men With Breast Cancer
Garden City, NY
516-877-4314

Sisters Network for African-
American Women
Garden City, NY
516-538-8086

Glens Falls Hospital
Glens Falls, NY
518-761-2204

Huntington Hospital
Huntington, NY
516-351-2568

Cayuga Medical Center
Ithaca, NY
607-274-4011

Ithaca Breast Cancer Alliance
Ithaca, NY
607-277-9410

Women's Health Connection—
United Health Services
Johnson City, NY
607-763-6546

Benedictine Hospital
Kingston, NY
914-338-2500 ext 4453

North Shore University Hospital
Manhasset, NY
516-926-HELP

Beth Israel Medical Center,
Cancer Center
New York, NY
212-844-6022

Beth Israel Medical Center
(North Division)
New York, NY
212-870-9502

Breast Examination Center of Harlem
New York, NY
212-864-0600

Cancer Care, Inc.
New York, NY
212-302-2400

Creative Center for Women With
   Cancer
New York, NY
212-868-4766

Gilda's Club
New York, NY
212-647-9700

Memorial Sloan-Kettering Cancer
   Center
New York, NY
212-717-3527

Mount Sinai Medical Center
New York, NY
212-987-3063

SHARE: Support Services for
   Women with Breast or
   Ovarian Cancer
New York, NY
212-719-0364/
212-719-4454 (Spanish)

Live Love & Laugh Again
Pt. Jefferson, NY
516-473-1320 ext 4246

Cancer Action, Inc.
Rochester, NY
716-423-9700

Cancer Support Team, Inc.
Rye Brook, NY
914-253-5334

FEGS/Jewish Community Services
Syosset, NY
516-364-8040

Franklin Hospital
Valley Stream, NY
516-256-6012

Cancer Care, Inc.
Woodbury, NY
516-364-8130

### North Carolina
Life After Cancer/Pathways, Inc.
Asheville, NC
704-252-4106

Chapel Hill Support Group
Chapel Hill, NC
919-929-7022

Presbyterian Hospital
Charlotte, NC
704-384-5223

Women Living With Cancer
Charlotte, NC
704-355-7283

Duke Comprehensive Cancer Center
Durham, NC
919-684-4497

Breast Cancer Support Group
Raleigh, NC
919-787-2637 ext. 147

Rocky Mount Area Breast Cancer
   Alliance
Rocky Mount, NC
919-443-8607

Kathy Farris Memorial Mastectomy
   Group
Wilson, NC
919-237-0439

Pink Broomstick—Cancer Services,
   Inc.
Winston, Salem, NC
910-725-7421

**North Dakota**

Great Plains Rehabilitation
  Services—Mastectomy Support
  Group
Bismarck, ND
701-224-7988

Roger Maris Cancer Center
Fargo, ND
701-234-6161

**Ohio**

Bethesda Oak Hospital Breast
  Center
Cincinnati, OH
513-569-5152

Cancer Family Care
Cincinnati, OH
513-731-3346

University of Cincinnati Hospital
Cincinnati, OH
513-558-8567

Cleveland Clinic Foundation
Cleveland, OH
216-444-3770

Arthur G. James Cancer Hospital
Columbus, OH
614-293-3237

Riverside Cancer Institute
Columbus, OH
614-566-4321 or
800-752-9119

Franciscan Breast Center
Dayton, OH
937-229-7474

Y-ME of the Greater Dayton Area
Dayton, OH
513-833-5414

Fort Hamilton Hughes Hospital
Hamilton, OH
513-867-2700

SOAR/Strength, Optimism &
  Recovery
Kettering, OH
937-298-4331 ext 7318

Marietta Memorial Hospital
Marietta, OH
614-374-1450

Mercy Medical Center
Springfield, OH
513-390-5030

Cancer Care Center
Youngstown, OH
330-740-4176

**Oklahoma**

Central Oklahoma Cancer Center
Oklahoma City, OK
405-636-7982

University of Oklahoma, Institute of
  Breast Health
Oklahoma City, OK
405-271-4514

Y-ME of Northeastern Oklahoma
Tulsa, OK
918-481-4839

**Oregon**

St. Vincent Hospital and Medical
  Center
Portland, OR
503-215-4673

Community Health Resource Center
Springfield, OR
541-744-6123

Meridian Park Hospital
Tualatin, OR
503-692-2113

*Pennsylvania*
John and Dorothy Morgan Cancer
 Center
Allentown, PA
610-402-0500

Lower Bucks Hospital
Bristol, PA
215-785-9818

Bryn Mawr Hospital
Bryn Mawr, PA
610-526-3073

Brandywine Hospital and Trauma
 Center
Coatesville, PA
610-383-8549

Abington Memorial Hospital
Dresher, PA
215-646-4954

Milton S. Hershey Medical Center
Hershey, PA
717-531-5867

Wyoming Valley Health Care System
Kingston, PA
717-283-7851

Lancaster Breast Cancer Network
Lancaster, PA
717-393-7477

Montgomery Breast Cancer Support
 Program
Norristown, PA
610-270-2703

Fox Chase Cancer Center
Philadelphia, PA
215-728-2668

Linda Creed Breast Cancer
 Foundation
Philadelphia, PA
215-545-0800

Thomas Jefferson University Hospital
Philadelphia, PA
215-955-8370

Burger King Cancer Caring Center
Pittsburgh, PA
412-622-1212

Magee-Women's Hospital
Pittsburgh, PA
412-641-4255

Taylor Hospital
Ridley Park, PA
610-595-6537

Breast Cancer Support Services of
 Berks County
West Reading, PA
610-478-1447

York Cancer Center
York, PA
717-741-8100

*Rhode Island*
Hope Center for Life Enhancement
Providence, RI
401-454-0404

Roger Williams Medical Center
Providence, RI
401-456-2284

*South Carolina*
Bosom Buddies and Man to Man
Columbia, SC
803-771-5244

Breast Cancer Support Group
Columbia, SC
803-434-3378

McLeod Resource Center
Florence, SC
803-667-2888

Breast Cancer Support Groups
Greenville, SC
864-455-7591

Supporting Sisters
Lexington, SC
803-796-6009 or 951-2088

**South Dakota**
After Breast Cancer Survivor's
  Program
Sioux Falls, SD
605-333-5244

**Tennessee**
Y-ME of Chattanooga
Chattanooga, TN
423-495-7724

Breast Cancer Networker
Knoxville, TN
423-546-4661

EMBRACE—Memphis Cancer
  Center
Memphis, TN
901-763-0446

Memphis Area Mastectomy/
  Lumpectomy Association
Memphis, TN
901-382-9500

**Texas**
Together We Will
Arlington, TX
817-548-6400

Between US
Dallas, TX
214-521-5225

Common Cares
Dallas, TX
214-692-8893

Medical City Hospital
Dallas, TX
972-566-4997

Patient to Patient
Dallas, TX
214-648-8969

Presbyterian Hospital of Dallas
Dallas, TX
214-345-2600

Sammons Cancer Center
Dallas, TX
214-820-2608

Sisters Network for African-
  American Women
Dallas, TX
214-637-7451

Breast Reconstruction Educational
  Support Group
Ft. Worth, TX
817-335-6363

M.D. Anderson Cancer Network—
  Tarrant County
Ft. Worth, TX
817-820-4863

The Rose Garden
Houston, TX
281-484-4708

The Rosebuds
Houston, TX
713-665-2729

Sisters Network
Houston, TX
713-781-0255

Sisters Network for African-
  American Women
Lake Jackson, TX
409-297-4419

North Texas Cancer Center
Plano, TX
972-867-3577

Bosom Buddies/Women's Center
Baylor-Richardson Medical Center
Richardson, TX
972-498-4000

Coping With Breast Cancer
Woodlands, TX
800-450-0026

*Utah*
Salt Lake Regional Breast Care
  Center
Salt Lake City, UT
801-350-4973

St. Mark's Hospital
Salt Lake City, UT
801-268-7599

Ashley Valley Medical Center
Vernal, UT
801-789-3342

*Vermont*
Breast Care Center
Burlington, VT
802-656-2262

*Virginia*
National Capital Area Y-ME
Alexandria, VA
800-970-4411

Martha Jefferson Hospital
Charlottesville, VA
804-982-8407

University of Virginia Cancer Center
Charlottesville, VA
804-243-6444

Fairfax Hospital
Falls Church, VA
703-698-3201

Rockingham Memorial Hospital
Harrisonburg, VA
540-249-5200

Sentara Leigh Hospital
Norfolk, VA
757-466-5738

Sentara Norfolk General
Norfolk, VA
757-668-4268

Massey Cancer Center
Richmond, VA
804-828-0450

Lewis-Gale Regional Cancer Center
Salem, VA
800-543-5660

*Washington*
Overlake Hospital
Bellevue, WA
206-688-5248

Breast Cancer Support Group of
  Kitsap Co.
Bremerton, WA
360-373-1057

Puget Sound Tumor Institute
Edmonds, WA
206-640-4300

Providence General Medical Center
Everett, WA
206-258-7255

Evergreen Hospital
Kirkland, WA
206-899-2265

St. Peter Hospital Regional Cancer
Center
Olympia, WA
360-493-4111

Highline Community Hospital
Seattle, WA
206-439-5577

Northwest Hospital, Seattle Breast
Center
Seattle, WA
206-368-1457

Providence
Seattle, WA
206-320-2100

Swedish Hospital Tumor Institute
Seattle, WA
206-386-2323

**West Virginia**
Women & Children's Hospital
Charleston, WV
304-348-9712

**Wisconsin**
Women Who Care
Holmen, WI
608-526-3348

Meriter Hospital Women's Center
Madison, WI
608-258-3750

Sheboygan Memorial Medical Center
Sheboygan, WI
414-451-5536

Breast Cancer Support Group &
Partners of Women With Breast
Cancer
Waukesha, WI
414-548-9148

**Wyoming**
United Medical Center
Cheyenne, Wy
307-633-7991

# INTERNATIONAL BREAST CANCER SUPPORT GROUPS

**Australia**
Anti-Cancer Council of Victoria
1 Rathdowne St.
Carlton South VIC 3053
(03) 9279-1111 or 131120

New South Wales Cancer Council
P.O. Box 572
153 Dowling St.
Woolloomooloo 2011
(02) 9334-1900 or 131120

ACT Cancer Society, Inc.
159 Maribyrnong Ave.
Kaleen ACT 2617
(02) 6262-2222

Cancer Council of the Northern
Territory, Inc.
P.O. Box 42719
Unit 2/3 Casl House
23 Vanderlin Dr.
Casuarina 0811
(08) 8927-4888

Queensland Cancer Fund
P.O. Box 201
Spring Hill QLD 4004
1300 361 366
553 Gregory Terrace
Fortitude Valley 4006

Cancer Council of Tasmania
140 Bathurst St.
Hobart 7000
(03) 6233-2030

Cancer Foundation of Western
Australia
1029 Wellington St.
West Perth 6008

Anti-Cancer Foundation of South
Australia
202 Greenhill Rd.
Eastwood 5063
(08) 8291-4111 or 131120

*Austria*
Frauenselbsthilfe nach Krebs
Obere Augartenstr. 26-28
A-1020 Wien

*Brazil*
Instituto do Cancer
Praca Cruz Vermelha, 23
(021) 221-7375/221-4131

Kora Group
Rua Madalena, 99
(011) 813-3340/813-0927/210-2360

Fundacao Oncocentro
Rua Oscar Freire, 2396
(011) 280-5622

Hospital do Cancer-Fundacao
Antonio Prudente
Rua Professora Antonio Prudente,
211
(011) 242-5000

Instituto Brasileiro do Controle
do Cancer
Av. Alcantara Machado, 2576
(011) 291-6988/692-1381

*Canada*
Breast Cancer Action
Montreal
514-483-1846

Burlington Breast Cancer Support
Services
Burlington, Ontario
905-634-2333

Breast Cancer Action
Ottawa, Ontario
613-736-5921

Niagara Breast Cancer Support
Group
St. Cath. Ontario
905-687-3333

*England*
Breast Care and Mastectomy
Association
London 071-867-1103

*Germany*
Deutsches Krebsforschungszentrum
(German Cancer Center)
Krebsinformationsdienst für
den Bürger
Im Neuenheimer Feld 280
D-69120 Heidelberg
06221-410121) (24-hour hotline)

Deutsche Krebsgesellschaft e.V.
Paul-Ehrlich-Str. 41
D-60596 Frankfurt/Main

Deutsche Arbeitsgesellschaft
Selbsthilfegruppen
Friedrichstr. 28
D-35392 Giessen

Bundeszentrale für gesundheitliche
  Aufklärung
Postfach 910152
D-51071 Koln

Vereinigung der Deutschen
  Plastischen Chirurgen e.V.
Bleibtreustr. 12a
D-10623 Berlin

**Japan**
Akebono-kai
1-27-1-102 Higashiyama
Meguro-ku, Tokyo 153-0043

**Scotland**
Breast Care and Mastectomy
  Association
Edinburgh
031-458-5598

Glasgow
041-353-1050

**Switzerland**
Leben wie zuvor
Untere Rebergstr. 96
CH-4135 Reinach

## SECOND OPINION CENTERS

A number of major hospitals throughout the country offer second opinion consultation services at varying costs. A multidisciplinary team of specialists will meet with the patient and the family to review the diagnosis and other diagnostic tests to provide the patient with a recommended second opinion for the course of treatment. Call the Cancer Information Service at 800-4-CANCER to locate the center nearest you.

## INFORMATION ON HEALTH INSURANCE

*The Health Insurance Association of America*
Fulfillment Department
P.O. Box 41455
Washington, DC 20018
202-866-6244
This association will answer questions concerning insurance coverage as it applies to breast cancer prevention and treatment.

*Local Social Security Office*
A patient's local Social Security office distributes single copies of a "Guide to Health Insurance for People With Medicare," which explains what Medicare does not pay for and what to look for in private health insurance.

**Medicaid/Medicare**
Health Financing Administration
Department of Health and Human Services
Washington, DC 20201
202-245-0312
The home office can provide women with the address and telephone number of
their regional office.

**The National Insurance Consumer Organization**
121 North Payne St.
Alexandria, VA 22314
703-549-8050
This nonprofit public interest advocacy and educational organization promotes
the interests of insurance buyers and helps consumers buy insurance wisely.

**The People's Medical Society**
14 East Minor St.
Emmaus, PA 18049
This society acts as a consumer advocate in the health care field; it also helps
consumers evaluate and select health insurance.

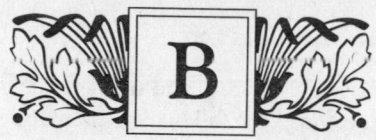

# THE PATIENT'S RIGHTS

The three documents that follow confirm the rights and standard of care that women should expect from their doctors and from the medical personnel who treat them.

## A BREAST CANCER PATIENT'S OPTIONS AND RIGHTS*

- To receive a simple and clear diagnosis of her condition.
- To receive all available diagnostic procedures and a complete workup prior to surgery.
- To have the consent form clearly explained to her before she signs it.
- To have the biopsy performed first (under local anesthesia), including the right to see the pathologist's report and have it explained to her. Surgery may be performed at a later date.
- To be aware that for certain patients the future option of reconstructive plastic surgery exists and to have the surgeon take that option into consideration.
- To receive consideration from the surgeon and other medical personnel for the physical and emotional trauma she is undergoing.
- To receive an explanation of any viable alternative treatments—including biopsy with radiation therapy as primary treatment, chemotherapy, mastectomy, etc.—risks, disadvantages, and advantages of each treatment.
- To receive a satisfying explanation as to why the surgeon has decided on a particular surgical procedure rather than a less mutilating one.
- To be referred to a therapist for physical or psychiatric therapy following surgery.
- To receive competent follow-up care after surgery and to know who is going to be responsible for that care.
- To be referred to a support group for information and assistance with her personal concerns.
- To be always treated as an adult.

*Prepared by Women for Women, a nonprofit West Coast organization.

## A PATIENT'S BILL OF RIGHTS*

During the 1970s the board of trustees and house of delegates of the American Hospital Association developed the following statement on patients' rights with the expectation that observation of these rights would contribute to more effective patient care and greater satisfaction for the patient, her physician, and the hospital organization. It defines the responsibilities of the physicians and medical staff. Implicitly, it expects the patient to share in her own health care by first knowing her rights, then exercising them.

1. The patient has the right to considerate and respectful care.
2. The patient has the right to obtain from her physician complete current information concerning her diagnosis, treatment, and prognosis in terms the patient can be reasonably expected to understand. When it is not medically advisable to give such information to the patient, the information should be made available to an appropriate person on her behalf. She has the right to know, by name, the physician responsible for coordinating her care.
3. The patient has the right to receive from her physician information necessary to give informed consent prior to the start of any procedure and/or treatment. Except in emergencies, such information for informed consent should include, but not necessarily be limited to, the specific procedure and treatment, the medically significant risks involved, and the probable duration of incapacitation. Where medically significant alternatives for care or treatment exist, or when the patient requests information concerning medical alternatives, the patient has the right to such information. The patient also has the right to know the name of the person responsible for the procedures and/or treatment.
4. The patient has the right to refuse treatment to the extent permitted by law and to be informed of the medical consequences of her action.
5. The patient has the right to every consideration of her privacy concerning her own medical care program. Case discussion, consultation, examination, and treatment are confidential and should be conducted discreetly. Those not directly involved in her care must have the permission of the patient to be present.
6. The patient has the right to expect that all communications and records pertaining to her care should be treated as confidential.
7. The patient has the right to expect that within its capacity a hospital must make reasonable response to the request of a patient for services. The hospital must provide evaluation, service, and/or referral as indicated by the urgency of the case. When medically permissible, a patient may be transferred to another facility only after she has received complete information and ex-

*Prepared by the American Hospital Association.

planation concerning the need for and alternatives to such a transfer. The institution to which the patient is to be transferred must first have accepted the patient for transfer.

8. The patient has the right to obtain information as to any relationship of her hospital to other health care and educational institutions insofar as her care is concerned. The patient has the right to obtain information as to the existence of any professional relationships among individuals, by name, who are treating her.

9. The patient has the right to be advised if the hospital proposes to engage in or perform human experimentation affecting her care or treatment. The patient has the right to refuse to participate in such research projects.

10. The patient has the right to expect reasonable continuity of care. She has the right to know in advance what appointment times and physicians are available and where. The patient has the right to expect that the hospital will provide a mechanism whereby she is informed by her physician of the patient's continuing health care requirements following discharge.

11. The patient has the right to examine and receive an explanation of her bill, regardless of source of payment.

12. The patient has the right to know what hospital rules and regulations apply to her conduct as a patient.

## CANCER SURVIVORS' BILL OF RIGHTS*

The American Cancer Society has presented "Cancer Survivors' Bill of Rights" to call attention to the needs of survivors and to enhance cancer care:

1. Survivors have the right to assurance of lifelong medical care, as needed. The physicians and other professionals involved in their care should continue their constant efforts to be:
   - sensitive to the cancer survivors' lifestyle choices and their need for self-esteem and dignity;
   - careful, no matter how long they have survived, to have symptoms taken seriously, and not have aches and pains dismissed, for fear of recurrence is a normal part of survivorship;
   - informative and open, providing survivors with as much or as little candid medical information as they wish, and encouraging their informed participation in their own care;
   - knowledgeable about counseling resources, and willing to refer survivors and their families as appropriate for emotional support and therapy which will improve the quality of individual lives.

*Prepared by the American Cancer Society.

2. In their personal lives, survivors, like other Americans, have the right to the pursuit of happiness. This means they have the right:
   - to talk with their families and friends about their cancer experience if they wish, but to refuse to discuss it if that is their choice and not to be expected to be more upbeat or less blue than anyone else;
   - to be free of the stigma of cancer as a "dread disease" in all social relations;
   - to be free of blame for having gotten the disease and of guilt for having survived it.
3. In the workplace, survivors have the right to equal job opportunities. This means they have the right:
   - to aspire to jobs worthy of their skills, and for which they are trained and experienced, and thus not to have to accept jobs they would not have considered before the cancer experience;
   - to be hired, promoted and accepted on return to work, according to their individual abilities and qualifications, and not according to "cancer" or "disability" stereotypes;
   - to privacy about their medical histories.
4. Since health insurance coverage is an overriding survivorship concern, every effort should be made to assure all survivors adequate health insurance, whether public or private. This means:
   - for employers, that survivors have the right to be included in group health coverage, which is usually less expensive, provides better benefits, and covers the employee regardless of health history;
   - for physicians, counselors, and other professionals concerned, that they keep themselves and their survivor clients informed and up-to-date on available group or individual health policy options, noting, for example, what major expenses like hospital costs and medical tests outside the hospital are covered and what amount must be paid before coverage (deductibles).

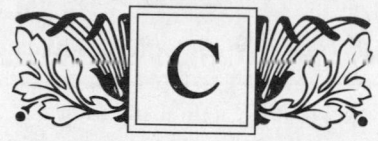

# THE BREAST CANCER INFORMED CONSENT SUMMARY

Currently, several states require physicians to inform their patients of alternative treatments for breast cancer. In California physicians must provide that information in printed form: a seven page pamphlet written in simple, nonmedical language, describing the various options (advantages and disadvantages) for breast cancer treatment with surgery, radiation, and chemotherapy.

The form is reprinted below.

## BREAST CANCER TREATMENT: SUMMARY OF EFFECTIVE METHODS, RISKS, ADVANTAGES, DISADVANTAGES
### Introduction

Breast cancer is a treatable disease, and you should know about the treatment options that are available, including surgical treatment, x-ray (radiation) therapy, and chemical and hormone treatment procedures. This brochure has been written to help you understand the various treatments with their advantages, disadvantages, and risks.

The treatment of breast cancer is complex and must be individualized. Choosing the best therapy for you may be difficult. It is important for you to have basic information about the methods of treatment so that you may discuss them with your physician. Using this information, you and your physician will be able to make the best choice for your stage or extent of the disease.

It may be appropriate for either you or your physician to seek additional opinions if either of you desire. Your consent is required before any treatment is carried out, and you have the right to make the final choice of the treatment procedure(s). Your physician has a corresponding right to withdraw from the case if the two of you cannot agree on a treatment plan.

Although a long delay may interfere with the ultimate success of your treatment, it is very important to take two to four weeks to obtain enough medical information and consultation to make a final and informed decision. Once that final and informed decision is made by you and your physician, you will be ready to begin treatment. A positive attitude will help you as you and your physician work together to carry out the treatment of your cancer. Because progress is being made in the management of breast cancer, your doctor may have new suggestions that have not been included in this brochure.

Plans and procedures to try out new methods of treatment are called protocols or clinical trials. Such trials often compare the current standard of care (the best treatment widely available) to a new treatment that is expected to increase the number of persons cured. The new treatment method is put into general use only after long-term evaluation by cancer experts shows that the new treatment is better than the current ones. The National Cancer Institute endorses the participation of patients and their physicians in clinical trials of new treatments.

## Management of Breast Cancer

Management of breast cancer is achieved with the cooperation of appropriate specialists in the field which include:

- The primary (personal) physician for diagnosis, support, and coordination.
- The surgeon for diagnosis by biopsy and specific surgical procedures for removal of the breast tumor and/or axillary lymph nodes.
- The pathologist for examining the biopsy tissue under the microscope.
- The radiation oncologist for supervising and administering radiation treatment.
- The medical oncologist for administering and monitoring chemotherapy.

These health professionals proceed fairly independently once a treatment plan has been decided, but maintain communication with each other by telephone and written correspondence.

## Diagnosis

While signs and symptoms of abnormal breast conditions such as presence of a lump, skin dimpling, red discoloration of the nipple, or thickening in the breast felt by self-examination or seen in a mammogram all may be suggestive of cancer, the final diagnosis is the scientific determination made by the pathologist of the nature of the tumor. It is done by examining biopsied material from the breast lump under a microscope.

A breast biopsy is the procedure performed to find out (diagnose) if the abnormal breast tissue (lump or change on a mammogram) is cancer. Biopsies can be performed by inserting a needle into the lump, if it can be felt, and removing a small piece of tissue or opening the skin and removing all or part of the abnormal tissue. The pathologist then examines the biopsy material under a microscope. In addition to making a diagnosis of cancer, the pathologist may also prepare the tissue for analysis of other characteristics of the cancer such as hormone receptor concentration (proteins inside cancer cells that link up with the female hormones estrogen and progesterone), genetic studies, DNA analysis, epidermal growth factors, and others.

When the diagnosis of breast cancer can be made with a needle aspiration of the lump (through the skin), you and your doctor can discuss the various treatment options before any surgery is performed. If the biopsy requires surgery, the cancer operation may be done at the same time (one-step procedure) or at a later date (two-step procedure). The twostep procedure is considered preferable by many professionals in the field. Because your final choice for treatment may influence the biopsy technique to be used, you and your surgeon should discuss your decision for cancer treatment prior to the biopsy.

Prior to any surgical procedure, a general medical evaluation should be performed. It may include your medical history (including family history of cancer), physical examination, blood tests that evaluate the function of various systems (e.g., liver, kidney, etc.), chest x-ray and breast x-ray (mammography). Additional tests to assess the spread of the disease may be indicated, such as radioisotope scan (bones, liver, etc.), computerized tomographic (CT) or magnetic resonance (MRI) body scans (specialized views of internal organs and bones), or sonograms (pictures of internal organs made with ultrasound waves).

## Surgery

Surgery for breast cancer can be divided into two parts: (1) operations to remove part or all of the diseased breast and (2) operations to remove the lymph nodes under the arm. The portion of the operation performed on the breast is designed to treat the cancer. The portion of the operation performed on the lymph glands in the armpit (axilla) is designed to evaluate whether or not the cancer has spread, as well as to remove the nodes into which the cancer has spread. This information is needed for further treatment decisions.

## Segmental Mastectomy, Partial Mastectomy, Lumpectomy

These operations are designed to remove the breast cancer and preserve the breast shape. To be effective in controlling cancer in the breast, radiation therapy lasting five to six weeks is often given after any of these breast-preserving operations, but particularly after a lumpectomy, which is not adequate in most cases.

**Advantages.** There is only partial loss of breast tissue. No reconstruction is required. The chances of cure for certain types and stages of breast cancer, when combined with radiation therapy, are equal to having a total mastectomy.

**Disadvantages.** This method of treatment requires an operation and also five to six weeks of radiation therapy. Partial surgery may not be an option for all women, depending on the type and size of the cancer, the location of the tumor in the breast, and the size of the breast. Sometimes the cancer is in a part of the breast that cannot be removed without significantly changing the shape and appearance of the breast (for example, right under the nipple). Radiation therapy does not eliminate the possibility of a new or recurrent cancer in the treated breast. In addition, sensations in the breast may change or be experienced differently than before treatment.

### Modified Radical Mastectomy, Total Mastectomy

The term "mastectomy" includes many different types of operations. In general, all breast tissue and the skin over the breast including the nipple and lymph nodes from the armpit are removed. Sometimes the smaller muscle of the chest wall (pectoralis minor) is removed or cut, but the larger muscle (pectoralis major) is left in place.

**Advantages.** This operation provides treatment for the cancer in the breast and evaluates the armpit lymph nodes for removing additional tumor tissues if present. There is minimal loss of arm strength or mobility due to muscle weakness. No radiation exposure is required.

**Disadvantages.** Some women experience shoulder stiffness, numbness of the skin on the inner side of the upper arm, and arm swelling. The entire breast is removed, and reconstructive surgery or an external prosthesis is required for those who wish to rebuild the breast form.

### Radical (Halsted) Mastectomy

This operation is reserved for patients with extensive cancers of the breast that invade the underlying large muscle of the chest (pectoralis major). In addition to the entire breast, the lymph nodes in the armpit, the muscle of the chest wall, and large amounts of skin are also removed.

**Advantages.** In selected cases, this operation may increase the chances of controlling the cancer on the chest wall.

**Disadvantages.** Compared to the other operations already described, the radical mastectomy does not increase cure rates for most stages of breast cancer. This operation removes the entire breast and underlying chest muscles. It leaves a long scar and a hollow area where the muscles were removed. The operation may result in arm swelling, some loss of muscle power in the arm, and restricted shoulder motion and numbness in some individuals. Reconstructive (plastic) surgery and fitting of a breast prosthesis are more difficult.

### Lymph Node Dissection

This procedure is the removal of some (lymph node sampling) or most (lymph node dissection) of the lymph nodes in the armpit and behind the large muscles of the chest. It is done to find out if the cancer has spread and for further treatment to prevent recurrence of the cancer in the axilla. When this operation is combined with a segmental mastectomy, a separate incision may be used.

## Radiation (X-Ray) Therapy

Radiation treatment of local tissues of the body, known as radiotherapy, can destroy cancer cells while producing minimal injury to surrounding tissues. The radiation may come from a number of devices (e.g., linear accelerator, betatron, cobalt-60, and radioactive isotopes). The source and type of radiation are chosen to suit the requirements of the individual. Radiation to the breast does not cause loss of hair from the head.

## Breast-Preserving Treatment of Early Breast Cancer

This approach has been used for about 20 years in the United States and 30 years in Europe for the treatment of early breast cancer. Recent scientific studies involving thousands of breast cancer patients in the United States and in Europe demonstrate that the breast-preserving treatment is as effective as either modified radical mastectomy or radical mastectomy for tumor control and survival. Breast-preserving treatment involves both surgery (segmental mastectomy, partial mastectomy, lumpectomy) and radiation therapy to achieve the best possible results. Initially, surgery is performed to remove the tumor in the breast (and usually the lymph nodes in the armpit). Following healing from surgery, external radiation therapy is used to treat the breast and the chest wall. In some patients, the lymph nodes behind the collarbone and the breastbone may need treatment. Treatment usually consists of a few minutes each day, four or five days a week, for approximately six to seven weeks. Following this, some patients will need a radiation "boost" to the biopsy site. This can be accomplished by continuing treatment for approximately one to two weeks with external radiation or a temporary placement of radioactive seeds (implants) in the breast at the biopsy site. The implant requires a minor procedure under general anesthesia in the operating room and a hospital stay of two to three days.

**Advantages.** The breast is preserved, though it may be mildly to moderately firmer. Usually, there is minimal or no visible deformity of surrounding tissues. After completion of the treatment, the skin usually regains a nearly normal appearance. In early breast cancer, lumpectomy or segmental resection, with radiation as the primary treatment, has demonstrated results that are equal to more extensive, long-established surgical procedures.

**Disadvantages.** A full course of treatment requires daily outpatient visits for five to eight weeks. Treatment may produce mild tiredness and a skin reaction similar to a mild to severe sunburn. If the lymph nodes behind the breastbone are treated, there may be a temporarily mild swallowing discomfort. Radiation therapy may affect the bone marrow where blood cells are made. This usually occurs only to a mild degree and is temporary. If chemotherapy is given at the same time, a small area of the bone marrow may be affected to a greater degree and may, in some cases, limit the dosage of chemotherapy that can be given. This is rarely a significant problem. A small portion of the lung behind the breast and chest wall will develop scar tissue from radiation therapy. This may be visible on x-ray examination but usually causes no breathing difficulties or other problems.

### Radiation Therapy as a Supplement (Adjuvant) to Surgery

Following modified radical mastectomy or radical (Halsted) mastectomy, examination of the surgical specimen by the pathologist may show that all of the cancer cells were not completely removed. Postoperative radiation therapy may be recommended in this instance, particularly if the cancer is large, or the cancer has spread beyond the tumor which was removed. Radiation therapy will usually control cancer cells remaining in these areas. The treatment of advanced cancer requires the consultation and coordination of efforts of the surgeon, radiation oncologist, and medical oncologist.

**Advantages.** The goal of radiation therapy is to destroy cancer cells in the tissue of the irradiated area. Modern equipment gives precise control of the x-ray treatment. Radiation therapy may be used to treat the spread of cancer to a specific part of the body, for example, the bones.

**Disadvantages.** The major side effects are the same as those listed under radiation (x-ray) therapy. When cancer is treated by radiation therapy as a supplement to surgery, there may be wide variations in the extent of the treatments required, depending on the problem or site of the disease being treated.

### Chemotherapy (Anti-Cancer Drug Therapy)

The medical oncologist is an internal medicine specialist who plans and administers the chemotherapy or hormone therapy and may coordinate the patient's management with other physicians. Anti-cancer drugs or hormone drugs are given orally or by injection into the vein (intravenous) to destroy cancer cells that cannot be removed by surgery, by radiation, or by their combination.

In recent years, important and effective advances in breast cancer treatment have been made in the area of medical oncology, especially in treatment of patients with advanced cancer. Each treatment, however, must be selected to the individual patient. The decision to treat a patient with either hormonal therapy, chemotherapy, or a combination is complex and can be made only after a thorough medical evaluation.

### Adjuvant (Supplemental) Chemotherapy

In this type of treatment, chemotherapy and/or hormone drugs supplement the initial surgical or radiation treatment when it is likely or possible that the cancer will recur. Certain characteristics may predict a higher risk of spread: involvement of the axillary lymph nodes with cancer, the microscopic characteristics of the cancer cells, the patient's age, and the lack of sensitivity of the cancer to female hormones. In certain groups of women with breast cancer, supplemental therapy may reduce the likelihood or recurrence slightly. Adjuvant chemotherapy may continue for six months to two years or longer, depending on several factors, including the cancer being treated and the drug program being used. It is almost always given on an outpatient basis.

**Advantages.** Adjuvant treatment may increase the effectiveness of surgery or radiation therapy and reduce or delay the recurrence of breast cancer. Because the drugs are blood borne and have a systemic (total body) effect, they work to stop cancer growth at distant sites (bones, lungs, liver) in the body. Every drug has specific effects (benefits) that vary for each patient.

**Disadvantages.** Most chemotherapy drugs have temporary side effects. Some are minimal while others can cause discomfort, including nausea, temporary loss of hair, blood count suppression (resulting in temporary susceptibility to infection, bleeding tendency, and anemia), loss of appetite, fatigue, and rarely, damage to heart muscles. The medication may also depress reproductive function and cause change of life (menopause) symptoms. Newer techniques of administration and more precise dosage reduce the side effects of chemotherapy. Most side effects are tolerable and do not interfere greatly with daily activities.

## Chemotherapy for Recurrent or Metastatic (Widespread) Breast Cancer

Anti-cancer drugs, taken alone or in combination with other treatment, can arrest cancer growth or shrink the tumors, thereby helping to relieve symptoms and prolonging the life of a patient who has recurrent or metastatic breast cancer.

## Hormonal Therapy

Some breast cancers are sensitive to and can be affected by the female hormones estrogen and progesterone. A fresh piece of the tissue from the tumor biopsy can be tested to measure hormone sensitivity (estrogen or progesterone receptor assay). In some breast cancer patients, beneficial effects can be produced by hormonal therapy. Treatment may consist of oral administration of hormones or anti-hormone pills that counteract the effects of hormones produced by the body or by surgically removing female hormone–secreting glands (ovaries).

Hormonal therapy can be effective by itself in recurrent or metastatic disease or may be used following primary therapy as an adjuvant treatment to decrease the likelihood of cancer recurrence.

## Unproven Treatments

Although the great majority of the therapies offered to patients with breast cancer have well-recognized benefits, some practitioners offer and promote unproven therapies which are ineffective and possibly dangerous.

If you are offered a treatment which you suspect is unproven, you may consult either the American Cancer Society at 1-800-227-2345, or the California Department of Health Services' Food and Drug Branch for information and assistance. The two national organizations available for guidance are the National Council Against Health Fraud and the U.S. Food and Drug Administration.

## Restoration of the Breast Forms

External prostheses are worn beneath clothing to restore the bustline. They either fit in a brassiere or adhere to the skin. They are made of a variety of substances such as silicone, foam rubber, glycerin, or other viscous fluid.

## Reconstructive Surgery

Reconstructive surgery is an option a patient may choose to assist in restoring the form of the breast. It may begin either at the time of mastectomy or at a later date. Achieving an optimal result usually requires more than one surgery, done in stages. The opposite breasts may be reshaped to improve the match between the two breasts. Prior radiation may impair or prevent breast reconstruction and must be brought to the attention of the surgeon. You should investigate the extent of financial coverage available through your health insurance while plans for treatment are being formulated.

## Internal Prostheses

Internal prostheses are placed in the soft tissue in front of the ribs to replace the volume of removed breast. They are composed of silicone, salt water, or polyurethane and are of the same style as the implants used for cosmetic breast enlargement over the last 25 years. So far, there is no evidence to show that they cause cancer.

**Advantages.** Internal prostheses may be placed at the time of mastectomy. The overlying skin usually regains much of its sensation and is the same color as the other breast. A one-step procedure may make further surgery unnecessary.

**Disadvantages.** Some patients develop a thick "peel" (capsule) around the implant which can distort the implant and result in a breast mound which may become firmer. This capsule, which is not a cancer, may have to be treated surgically and, in rare cases, requires the removal of the implant. While an implant does not impair the physician's ability to detect the return of cancer, it may require special techniques for both x-ray examination and any future biopsies.

## Flap Procedures (Autogenous Reconstruction Graft)

This operation is accomplished by transferring skin, fat, and muscle to the mastectomy site from a nearby area of the body such as the back, abdomen, or buttock. Depending on the size of tissue transferred and the other breast, an internal prosthesis may also be used. Since the tissue is from the patient's own body, there is no possibility of a rejection of the transplant

**Advantages.** Since the tissue is your own, it will usually grow with you (i.e., if you gain or lose weight, it will do the same). Many reconstructions can be done without an implant, so once reconstruction is complete, there is no concern with artificial material in your body.

**Disadvantages.** Successful grafting requires adequate blood supply to the tissue. If blood flow problems develop, part or all of the tissue may be lost. There may be temporary or permanent weakness in the area from which the tissue was taken. There are additional scars (usually hidden by clothing). This surgery and recovery take longer than placement of an internal prosthesis, and can be considerably more complicated and difficult.

## Nipple/Areolar Reconstruction

This is a final option which one may consider after the breast has been reconstructed. There are many techniques used which can be discussed with your surgeon.

**Advantages.** Offers greater similarity to the other breast, especially under clothing.

**Disadvantages.** There is often a change in color of the areola and the size of the nipple may decrease. The sensations present in normal nipple/areola are not restored.

## Follow-up

The success of cancer treatment depends on early detection, effective treatment, and a careful, consistent follow-up program. Regular visits to your physician and monthly self-examination are essential. Yearly mammograms (breast x-rays) may detect new cancers in the opposite breast, and may reveal a return of the cancer, if it occurs in the remaining breast tissue on the treated side. New methods of detection and treatment are being continually developed and may be used to your advantage.

Many very helpful and thoughtful women who have been through a similar experience can lend you their support and guidance. They can be contacted through your physician, your hospital, your local unit of the American Cancer Society, or the National Cancer Institute's Cancer Information Service.

## Summary

The purpose of this brochure is to increase your knowledge of the effective methods of treating breast cancer, and to emphasize the importance of your role in choosing the best method to be used.

There are three basic forms of therapy that are utilized in the management of breast cancer. *Surgical procedures* are undertaken to establish the diagnosis (biopsy), to remove the local disease in the breast (lumpectomy, mastectomy), and to estimate the extent of the disease and treat the remaining cancer if it has spread to the lymph nodes (lymph node dissection). *Radiation therapy* is administered to control local disease in the breast or to treat specific sites of spread. *Chemotherapy and hormone therapy* may be used to treat cancer in the breast, to reduce likelihood of recurrence, and to treat known spread of breast cancer to other body sites. In most situations, effective therapy involves use of more than one form of treatment.

In order to reach a decision of the best treatment method for you, it is important for you to understand the nature of the disease, the extent of your problem, the treatment needed, the method or methods of providing that treatment suitable to your particular situation, and finally the results that reasonably may be expected. This is best done by having a complete evaluation followed by a thorough discussion with your physician(s). The brochure will assist you in participating in these discussions. It provides background information that will prepare you to ask questions about your individual treatment, its advantages, disadvantages, and risks.

Many important details are necessarily left out. You should ask your personal physician for complete and current information. Being well informed and having thoroughly discussed the options with your doctor will make it easier for you to reach an informed decision. Knowledge of all the optional treatments will give you a justified confidence that you have made the best possible choice. This confidence will be a tremendous help to you and your physician as you carry out your treatment and establish your follow-up program.

## Second Opinion Centers

A number of major hospitals throughout the country offer second-opinion consultation services at varying costs. A multidisciplinary team of specialists will meet with the patient and the family to review the diagnosis and other diagnostic tests in order to provide the patient with a recommended second opinion for the course of treatment. Call the Cancer Information Service at 800-4-CANCER to locate the center nearest you.

# HISTOPATHOLOGIC TNM CLASSIFICATION OF BREAST CARCINOMA

The following classification was prepared by the American Joint Committee on Cancer (AJCC) and the International Union Against Cancer (UICC). It describes the tumor, the condition of the lymph nodes, and the presence of metastasis individually and then combines that information to classify breast cancer into four stages.

## Primary Tumor (T)

**TX**  Primary tumor cannot be assessed

**T0**  No evidence of primary tumor

**Tis**  Carcinoma in situ: Intraductal carcinoma, lobular carcinoma in situ, or Paget's disease of the nipple with no tumor

**T1**  Tumor 2 cm or less in greatest dimension

    **pT1mic**  Microinvasion 0.1 cm or less in greatest dimension

    **T1a**  Tumor more than 0.1 cm but not more than 0.5 cm in greatest dimension

    **T1b**  More than 0.5 cm but not more than 1 cm in greatest dimension

    **T1c**  More than 1 cm but not more than 2 cm in greatest dimension

**T2**  Tumor more than 2 cm but not more than 5 cm in greatest dimension

**T3**  Tumor more than 5 cm in greatest dimension

**T4**  Tumor of any size with direct extension to (a) chest wall or (b) skin, only as described below

    **T4a**  Extension to chest wall

    **T4b**  Edema (including peau d'orange) or ulceration of the skin of breast or satellite skin nodules confined to the same breast

    **T4c**  Both (T4a and T4b)

    **T4d**  Inflammatory carcinoma

## Regional Lymph Nodes (N)

NX    Regional lymph nodes cannot be assessed (e.g., previously removed)
N0    No regional lymph node metastasis
N1    Spread to movable ipsilateral axillary lymph node(s)
N2    Spread to ipsilateral axillary lymph node(s) fixed to one another or to other structures
N3    Spread to ipsilateral internal mammary lymph node(s)

## Pathologic Classification (pN)

pNX   Regional lymph nodes cannot be assessed (e.g., previously removed or not removed for pathologic study)
pN0   No regional lymph node metastasis
pN1   Metastasis to movable ipsilateral axillary node(s)
    pN1a    Only micrometastasis (none larger than 0.2 cm)
    pN1b    Metastasis to lymph node(s), any larger than 0.2 cm
    pN1bi   Metastasis in 1 to 3 lymph nodes, any more than 0.2 cm and all less than 2 cm in greatest dimension
    pN1bii  Metastasis to 4 or more lymph nodes, any more than 0.2 cm and all less than 2.0 cm in greatest dimension
    pN1biii Extension of tumor beyond the capsule of a lymph node metastasis less than 2 cm in greatest dimension
    pN1biv  Metastasis to a lymph node 2 cm or more in greatest dimension
pN2   Metastasis to ipsilateral axillary lymph nodes that are fixed to one another or to other structures
pN3   Metastasis to ipsilateral internal mammary lymph node(s)

## Distant Metastasis (M)

MX    Distant metastasis cannot be assessed
M0    No distant metastasis
M1    Distant metastasis (includes metastasis to supraclavicular lymph node[s])

## R Classification

The absence or presence of residual tumor after treatment may be described by the symbol R. The definitions of the R classification are:

RX    Presence of residual tumor cannot be assessed
R0    No residual tumor
R1    Microscopic residual tumor
R2    Macroscopic residual tumor

## AJCC/UICC Stage Grouping of Primary Tumor, Regional Lymph Nodes, and Distant Metastasis

The descriptions are combined to define four stages:

| Stage 0 | Tis | N0 | M0 |
|---|---|---|---|
| Stage I | T1 | N0 | M0 |
| Stage II | T2 | N0 | M0 |
| Stage III | T3 | N0 | M0 |
| | T1 | N1 | M0 |
| | T2 | N1 | M0 |
| | T3 | N1 | M0 |
| Stage IV | T4 | N0 | M0 |
| | T4 | N1 | M0 |
| | Any T | N2 | M0 |
| Stage IVB | Any T | N3 | M0 |
| Stage IVC | Any T | Any N | M1 |

## Histopathologic Grade (G)

**GX**  Grade cannot be assessed
**G1**  Well differentiated
**G2**  Moderately differentiated
**G3**  Poorly differentiated
**G4**  Undifferentiated

## Histopathologic Type

The histologic types are as follows:

*Carcinoma, NOS*
   (not otherwise specified)

*Ductal*
   Intraductal (in situ)
   Invasive with predominant intraductal component
   Invasive, NOS (not otherwise specified)
   Comedo
   Inflammatory
   Medullary with lymphocytic infiltrate
   Mucinous (colloid)
   Papillary
   Scirrhous
   Tubular
   Other

*Lobular*
   In situ
   Invasive with predominant in situ component
   Invasive

*Nipple*
   Paget's disease, NOS
      (not otherwise specified)
   Paget's disease, with intraductal carcinoma
   Paget's disease with invasive ductal carcinoma
   Other

*Undifferentiated carcinoma*

# GLOSSARY

For a physician reading a medical journal or consulting with another colleague, medical terminology is a familiar part of the communication process. Consequently, it is natural for doctors to continue using technical language when speaking to patients, not realizing the confusion and anxiety it may cause. For the woman seeking information on breast cancer and breast reconstruction, it is a source of frustration. Before a woman is able to make an intelligent decision about her health care, she must be able to decipher the terminology. This glossary defines some of the more commonly used medical terms that women need to understand when consulting doctors about breast problems.

## A

**adjunctive (adjuvant) therapy**  A secondary treatment in addition to the primary therapy. For example, chemotherapy is often an adjunctive therapy to mastectomy.

**adjuvant chemotherapy**  The use of anticancer drugs after surgery to prevent a recurrence of cancer. For women with breast cancer, the most important indication for adjuvant chemotherapy is the spread of the cancer to the lymph nodes in the woman's underarm (axillary lymph nodes).

**advanced breast cancer**  Stage of cancer in which the disease has spread from the breast to other body systems by traveling through the bloodstream or lymphatic system.

**anterior axillary fold**  Fold created where the breast and arm meet at the front of the armpit area. The large chest muscle (pectoralis major), which extends from the chest to the upper arm, is the main component of this fold.

**areola**  The circle of pigmented skin on the breast that surrounds the nipple.

**aspirate**  To remove or withdraw fluid or tissue from a cavity by applying suction.

**aspiration**  Withdrawal of fluid or tissue from a cyst or lump through a needle.

**asymmetric**  Off balance. When one side does not match the other.

**asymptomatic**  Without obvious signs or symptoms of disease.

**atypical cells** Not usual; abnormal.

**atypical hyperplasia** Excessive growth of cells, some of which are abnormal.

**augmentation mammaplasty (breast augmentation)** An operation to enlarge a woman's breast, usually by placing a silicone breast implant behind the breast.

**autologous** From the same person. An autologous blood transfusion is blood removed and then transfused back into the same person at a later date.

**autologous bone marrow transplantation** Removal of a person's bone marrow to allow for high-dose chemotherapy; the same marrow is replaced after chemotherapy.

**autologous flap breast reconstruction** Breast reconstruction with a woman's own natural tissues. Common donor sites for flaps are the abdomen, back, buttocks, and thigh.

**axilla** The underarm area behind the anterior axillary fold. It contains the axillary lymph nodes.

**axillary dissection** Surgical removal of lymph nodes from the armpit. This tissue is then sent to a pathologist to determine if the breast cancer has spread.

**axillary lymph nodes** Lymph nodes in the armpit area that drain the breast.

## B

**baseline mammogram** A woman's first mammogram to use as a standard reference for evaluating changes in future mammograms.

**benign** Opposite of cancerous or malignant. A benign tumor is a noncancerous growth. It is self-limiting and does not spread to other areas of the body.

**bilateral** Involving both sides, such as both breasts.

**bilateral mastectomy** Surgical removal of both breasts.

**biopsy** Removal of tissue with a needle or scalpel for the purpose of examining it under a microscope to determine whether it is cancerous or benign.

**blood count** Test to measure the number of red blood cells, white blood cells, and platelets in a blood sample.

**bone marrow** Soft inner part of large bones that makes blood cells.

**bone scan** Test to determine if there is any sign of cancer in the bones.

**brachial plexus** A bundle of nerves in the underarm area that supply sensation to the arm.

**BRCA1 and BRCA2** Breast cancer genes that have been linked to familial breast cancer.

**breast-conserving surgery and irradiation** Treatment option for breast cancer whereby the tumor and axillary lymph nodes are surgically removed. Most of the breast is preserved, and the remaining tissue is then treated using a course of radiation therapy.

**breast implant** A soft, silicone form that can be placed in the body to simulate a breast.

**breast reconstruction**   An operation to create or rebuild a natural-looking breast shape after a mastectomy.

**breast self-examination (BSE)**   Monthly self-examination of the breasts in which a woman becomes familiar with the normal look and feel of her breasts.

## C

**calcifications**   Small calcium deposits in the breast tissue that can be seen by mammography.

**cancer**   A general term for the more than 100 diseases characterized by abnormal and uncontrolled growth of cells.

**cancerophobia**   An exaggerated fear of cancer.

**capsular contracture**   A capsule or shell of scar tissue that may form around a woman's breast implant, giving it a feeling of firmness, as her body reacts to the implant.

**carcinogen**   A substance that can cause cancer.

**carcinoma**   Most cancers are carcinomas. These are cancers arising in the epithelial tissue, including the skin, glands, and lining of the internal organs.

**cathepsin-D**   An enzyme present in breast tissue and in other cells that helps break down tissue. Large quantities of this enzyme in breast tissue may indicate a high degree of invasion into surrounding healthy tissue.

**catheter**   A tube implanted or inserted into the body to inject or withdraw fluid.

**cells**   Individual living units of which all organisms are composed. Cells are organized into tissues and organs.

**centigray**   Measurement of radiation dose.

**chemotherapy**   Treatment of cancer with powerful anticancer drugs capable of destroying cancer cells.

**clavicle**   Collarbone.

**clinical trials**   Studies designed to evaluate new cancer treatments.

**core biopsy**   Type of needle biopsy in which a small core of tissue is removed from a lump without surgery.

**cyst**   A sac arising within the body that is filled with liquid or semisolid material.

**cytology**   Study of cells under a microscope.

## D

**designer estrogens**   A class of drugs such as raloxifene developed to replace traditional estrogen therapy without some of the associated risks.

**differentiated**   Clearly defined. Differentiated tumor cells are similar in appearance to normal cells.

**DNA (deoxyribonucleic acid)**   Genetic material contained in the nucleus of the cell.

**donor site**   A part of the body from which tissue is taken and transferred to another part of the body for reconstruction.

**drain** Tubes or suction devices inserted after mastectomy or breast reconstruction to drain the fluids that accumulate postoperatively. Drains may be left in place for several days as needed.

**duct** In the female breast, milk travels through a system of tubelike ducts from milk glands to milk reservoirs in the nipple area. The duct is the site of most breast cancers.

**ductal carcinoma in situ (DCIS)** Ductal cancer cells that have not grown beyond their site of origin; sometimes referred to as precancerous.

**E**

**early-stage breast cancer** When cancer is limited to the breast and has not spread to the lymph nodes or other parts of the body. Also called in situ, or localized, breast cancer.

**edema** Excess fluid in the body or a body part that usually causes puffiness or swelling.

**endoscopic surgery (or minimally invasive surgery)** Operating through short incisions using special long instruments. The operative cavity is visualized through small video cameras attached to the endoscope; these cameras project a video image of the tissues beneath the skin on the video monitor via fiberoptic light. This technique is commonly used in many general surgery operations and can also be used for plastic surgery operations to obtain distant tissue for breast reconstruction.

**engorgement** An area of the body that is filled and stretched with fluid or distended with blood.

**epidermal growth factor receptors** Indirect measurements of the rate of tumor growth. They along with hormone receptor tests can be used to predict how a patient will respond to hormone therapy.

**estrogen** A female hormone produced mainly by the ovaries.

**excisional biopsy** Surgical removal of tissue by opening the skin and removing the suspected tissue for pathologic examination.

**F**

**familial cancer** Cancer occurring in families more frequently than would be expected by chance.

**fascia** A sheet or broad band of fibrous or connective tissue that covers muscles and various organs of the body and attaches the breasts and other body structures to underlying muscles.

**fat necrosis** Area of dead fat, usually following some form of trauma or surgery. May appear as lumps or thickened areas.

**fibroadenoma** A benign, firm, identifiable breast tumor commonly found in the breasts of young women.

**fibrocystic breasts** A recurring benign condition characterized by breast tenderness, pain, swelling, and the appearance of cysts or lumps.

**fibrous**   Gristlelike strands of tough tissue that can grow in the body. In breast reconstruction this usually refers to shell or scar tissue formation sometimes found around implants.

**flap**   A portion of tissue with its blood supply moved from one part of the body to another. Flaps of muscle, fat, and skin are frequently used to provide additional tissue for reconstructing a woman's breasts. Common donor sites for flap reconstruction are the abdomen (transverse rectus abdominis musculocutaneous, or TRAM, flap), back (latissimus dorsi flap), buttocks (gluteus maximus flap), and thigh.

**flow cytometry**   Test that measures DNA content in tumors and indicates the aggressiveness of the tumor.

**frozen section**   A tissue sample removed in a biopsy and quick frozen prior to thin-slicing for microscopic examination.

**frozen shoulder**   Shoulder stiffness that causes pain and limits the ability to lift the arm.

## G

**gene**   A unit of DNA that specifies the manufacture of a particular protein.

**genetic code**   A code contained in genes that determines the manufacture of proteins.

**genetic material**   Genes and the DNA from which they are made.

**gluteus maximus musculocutaneous flap**   Breast reconstruction operation that uses a distant flap of the patient's own tissue (autologous) from the buttock area to build a new breast.

**grading**   Classification of cancers according to the appearance of cancer cells under the microscrope. Low-grade cancers often grow more slowly than high-grade cancers.

**growth rate factors**   Markers used to predict the growth rate of cancerous cells and the likelihood that the cancer will spread.

## H

**Halsted radical mastectomy**   Surgical removal of the breast, skin, pectoralis muscles (both major and minor), all axillary lymph nodes, and fat for local treatment of breast cancer.

**harvest**   To obtain distant tissue for use in reconstructive surgery such as breast reconstruction.

**hematoma**   A collection of blood that can form in a wound after an injury or operation.

**HER-2/*neu* gene (or *erb* B-2/*neu* gene)**   Name of oncogene that is often associated with a poor breast cancer prognosis. These genes are known to have a high growth rate.

**heterogeneous**   Composed of many different elements. For breast cancer, heterogeneous indicates numerous different types of breast cancer cells within one tumor.

**hormone** A chemical substance produced by the body that can turn organs on and off, thus regulating many body functions such as growth and sexual functions. Synthetic forms of many hormones are used to treat hormone deficiencies such as those cause by menopause.

**hormone receptor assay** Diagnostic test to determine whether a breast cancer's growth is influenced by hormones or can be treated with hormones.

**hormone therapy** Treating cancer by removing or adding hormones to alter the hormonal balance; some breast cancer cells will only grow in the presence of certain hormones.

**hot flashes** Sensation of heat and flushing that occurs suddenly. May be associated with meonopause or occur as a side effect of some medications.

**hyperplasia** Excessive growth of cells.

**hysterectomy** Removal of the uterus (not necessarily the ovaries).

# I

**immune system** System by which the body is able to protect itself from foreign invaders.

**in situ cancer** Localized or noninvasive cancer that has not begun to spread.

**incisional biopsy** Operation to remove a portion of tissue for pathologic examination that is suspected of being abnormal.

**inert** Does not react or cause a reaction.

**infiltrating (invasive) cancer** Cancer that can grow beyond its site of origin into neighboring tissue.

**infiltrating ductal cell carcinoma** Cancer that begins in the mammary duct and spreads to areas outside the duct.

**informed consent** Legal standard that states how much a patient must know about the potential risks and benefits of a therapy before being able to undergo it knowledgeably. Many states have informed consent laws regarding breast cancer that require physicians to provide treatment options to patients before any medical treatment is given.

**infraclavicular nodes** Lymph nodes lying beneath the collarbone.

**inframammary crease** The crease where a lower portion of the breast and chest wall meet.

**intraductal** Within the duct. Intraductal can describe a benign or malignant process.

**intraductal carcinoma in situ (DCIS)** This preinvasive cancer is located in the milk ducts of the breast.

**intravenous (IV) line** A needle inserted into a vein to administer blood products, nutrients, and medications directly into the bloodstream through a tube.

**invasive cancer** Cancer that has spread outside its site of origin to infiltrate and grow in surrounding tissue.

**inverted nipple**   The turning inward of the nipple. Usually a congenital condition, but if the nipple was projecting and suddenly becomes inverted, it can be a sign of breast cancer.

**irradiation**   A form of ionizing energy that can destroy or damage cells. Cancer cells tend to be more easily destroyed than the normal cells in the surrounding tissue. For breast cancer treatment, this therapy can be used as an adjunct to breast-conserving surgery to reduce the chance of cancer recurrence.

## L

**latissimus dorsi muscle**   Triangular back muscle that is transferred with some overlying skin as donor flap tissue for reconstructing a breast after mastectomy.

**lobular**   Having to do with the lobules of the breast.

**lobular carcinoma in situ (LCIS)**   Abnormal cells within the lobule that do not form lumps but can serve as a marker of future cancer risk.

**local treatment of cancer**   Treatment only of the tumor.

**localized cancer**   Cancer confined to its site of origin.

**lump**   Mass of tissue found in the breast or other parts of the body; 80% of breast lumps are benign.

**lumpectomy**   Surgical removal of a cancerous tumor along with a small margin of surrounding tissue.

**lymph**   Fluid that flows through the body much like the blood, but in a separate system of vessels called the lymphatic system. Lymph fluid contains some waste products that are filtered through the lymph nodes and then this tissue fluid is returned to the blood.

**lymph nodes**   Structures in the lymphatic system that act as filters, catching bacteria and cancer cells, and contribute to the body's immune system, which fights infection and disease.

**lymphedema**   A condition characterized by the collection of excess fluid in the hand and arm after lymph nodes are removed or blocked.

## M

**malignant**   Cancerous.

**mammaplasty**   Breast operation to alter breast size.

**mammogram**   Breast x-ray film detailing the structure of breast tissue; requires only low doses of radiation.

**mammography**   Process of taking breast x-ray films to detect breast cancer.

**margins**   The area of tissue surrounding a tumor when it is removed by surgery. Positive margins indicate that this area of tissue is not clear of tumor.

**mastectomy**   Surgical removal of the breast, usually for treatment of cancer.

**mastitis** Infection of the breast.

**mastodynia** Pain in the breast.

**mastopexy** Breast lift to tighten the breast by removing sagging skin caused by the forces of gravity and the effects of aging.

**mediport** A temporary device that is surgically implanted in the chest or arm to accept an IV during chemotherapy.

**menopause** The cessation of menstruation, usually as a result of aging. The level of female sex hormones is reduced in menopausal women.

**metastasis** Spread of cancer from one part of the body to another. It can spread through the lymphatic system, the bloodstream, or across body cavities.

**microcalcification** Tiny calcifications in the breast tissue usually seen only on a mammogram. The presence of clusters may be a sign of ductal carcinoma in situ.

**micrometastasis** Microscopic and as yet undetectable but presumed spread of tumor cells to other organs.

**microsurgical breast reconstruction** Method of breast reconstruction whereby a flap of a woman's own tissue is moved from a distant area of the body such as the abdomen, back, thigh, or buttocks to the chest wall area to build a breast. Once this tissue is transferred, the blood vessels are sutured and reattached under the magnification of the operating microscope.

**modified radical mastectomy** Surgical removal of the breast, some fat, and most of the lymph nodes in the armpit, leaving the chest wall muscles largely intact.

**multicentric** More than one origin. Cancer cells may grow in several locations within the breasts and not be related to each other.

**muscle flap** A muscle or portion of muscle that can be transferred with its blood supply to another part of the body for reconstructive purposes.

**musculocutaneous (myocutaneous)** Muscle and skin.

**mutation** An alteration in the structure of a gene.

# N

**necrosis** Death of a tissue.

**needle aspiration** Diagnostic method of removing fluid or tissue from a breast tumor or cyst with a fine needle for microscopic examination.

**needle biopsy** Removal of a small sample of tissue with a wide-bore needle and suction.

**needle localization** Procedure to pinpoint a lump before biopsy.

**negative nodes** Lymph nodes that are free of cancer cells.

**nipple** The pigmented, central projection on the breast containing the outer openings of the breast ducts.

**nulliparous** Never having given birth to a child.

## O

**oncogenes** Growth-regulating genes that can cause tumors when activated (onco comes from Latin root meaning "tumor").

**oncologist** A physician who specializes in treating cancer. (There are medical, surgical, and radiation oncologists.)

**oncology** The study and treatment of cancer.

**one-step procedure** Breast biopsy and mastectomy performed in a single operation.

**oophorectomy** Surgical removal of the ovaries, sometimes performed as a part of hormone therapy.

**orange peel skin** Skin that has the appearance of an orange peeling. This pitting and coloration is caused from inflammation and edema and may be a sign of cancer.

**osteoporosis** Softening of bones that occurs with age, calcium loss, and hormone depletion. After menopause, women are particularly suceptible to this condition without some form of hormone supplement.

## P

**palliative** Affording relief of symptoms such as pain but not a cure.

**palpable** Distinguishable by touch.

**palpate** To feel.

**palpation** Examining with the hand.

**partial or segmental mastectomy** Breast surgery that removes only a portion of the breast, including the cancer and a surrounding margin of breast tissue.

**pathologist** A physician who specializes in the diagnosis of disease via the study of cells and tissue.

**pathology** The study of disease through the microscopic examination of body cells and tissues. Any tumor suspected of being malignant must be diagnosed by pathologic examination.

**pathology report** The pathologist's written record of the analysis of tissue.

**patient-controlled anesthesia (PCA)** Advance in pain control that allows the patient to be in charge of her own pain relief. When pain relief is needed, the patient pushes a button on the PCA machine that delivers a predetermined dose of pain medication.

**pectoralis muscles** Muscular tissues attached to the front of the chest wall and extending to the upper arms. These are divided into the pectoralis major and pectoralis minor muscles. The pectoralis muscles usually are removed during a standard radical mastectomy, leaving a large deformity. They are preserved in a modified radical mastectomy.

**pedicle** A connection of nourishing blood vessels from the body to a flap of tissue.

**permanent section** A tissue sample removed in a biopsy and embedded in wax or paraffin prior to thin-slicing and staining for microscopic examination.

**ploidy**  Measurement of the amount of DNA in a tumor cell that helps to predict tumor behavior.

**positive nodes**  Lymph nodes that have been invaded by cancer cells.

**postmenopausal**  After menopause.

**precancerous (premalignant)**  Abnormal cellular changes that are potentially capable of becoming cancer.

**predisposition**  A latent susceptibility to disease that may be activated under certain conditions.

**Premarin**  A form of estrogen sometimes given to women after menopause.

**primary**  The first.

**progesterone**  Female hormone produced by the ovaries during the menstrual cycle.

**prognosis**  Forecast as to the expected outcome of disease.

**prophylactic mastectomy**  Removal of high-risk breast tissue to prevent the development of a cancer. This procedure usually is combined with breast reconstruction. Also called preventive mastectomy and risk-reducing mastectomy.

**prosthesis**  Any artificial body part. A breast-shaped form may be worn outside the body after a breast has been removed because of cancer. It fits into the woman's brassiere in a specially designed pocket. Prostheses are made of different materials.

**protein**  A substance found in all cells. Different proteins are used to drive different types of events in cells. The manufacture of each protein is specified by a different gene.

**Provera**  A form of progesterone that is sometimes given to women in combination with Premarin after menopause.

**ptosis**  Sagging. Breast ptosis is usually the result of normal aging and the pull of gravity or changes caused by pregnancy or weight loss.

## Q

**quadrant mastectomy (quadrantectomy)**  Removal of one fourth of the breast.

## R

**radiation oncologist**  A physician who specializes in treating cancer patients with radiation therapy.

**radiation oncology (radiation therapy)**  Treatment of disease by x-rays or other ionizing energy.

**radical mastectomy**  Removal of the breast, underlying muscles, and underarm (axillary) lymph nodes.

**radiologist**  A physician with special training in diagnosing disease by studying x-ray films and other images and using these procedures to facilitate treatment.

**radiolucent**    Allows x-rays to pass through.

**radiopaque**    Blocks x-rays; appears as white on an x-ray film.

**raloxifene (Evista)**    Selective estrogen receptor modulators (SERMs), also called designer estrogens, are drugs developed to replace traditional estrogen therapy. Provide protection against osteoporosis, potentially without the associated risk of breast cancer. May have some benefit in breast cancer protection, but further study is needed.

**randomized**    Chosen at random. In a randomized research study, subjects are chosen to receive a particular treatment by means of a computer programmed to randomly select names.

**reconstructive mammaplasty (breast reconstruction)**    Rebuilding of the breast by plastic surgery techniques.

**rectus abdominis muscles**    The vertical paired muscles on either side of the midline of the abdomen. These muscles can be used as donor tissue for breast reconstruction (see TRAM flap breast reconstruction).

**recurrence**    Return of a tumor after the initial treatment of the primary tumor.

**reduction mammaplasty**    Operation for reducing the size of the breasts by removing glandular and fatty tissue.

**remission**    Complete or partial disappearance of the signs and symptoms of disease in response to treatment. The period during which a disease is under control.

**retraction**    Often referred to as skin dimpling; describes process of skin pulling in toward breast tissue.

**risk factors**    Anything that increases an individual's chance of getting a disease.

**risk reduction**    Techniques used to reduce chances of getting a certain cancer.

## S

**saline solution**    Saltwater; sometimes used in breast implants.

**sentinel node(s)**    The first draining node or nodes in the axilla.

**sentinel node biopsy**    A promising but unproven procedure in which only the first draining node or nodes are removed through a small incision instead of an entire axillary node dissection.

**seroma**    A fluid mass caused by the localized accumulation of lymph fluid within a body part or area. This condition sometimes occurs after an operation. In breast surgery it may occur after an axillary dissection.

**side effects**    Reactions to drugs or treatments that are usually temporary and reversible.

**silicone**    A chemical polymer that is used to replace numerous body parts. Breast implant envelopes are made of silicone.

**silicone gel**    Silicone produced in a semisolid, semiliquid state used as a filling in breast implants; similar in consistency to a normal breast.

**simple or total mastectomy**    Removal of the breast only; the lymph nodes and pectoralis muscles are preserved.

**skin-sparing mastectomy** Removal of the breast with less skin removal and shorter incisions; only the nipple and areola are excised as well as the overlying skin in those areas. Only appropriate for individuals who have no tumor involvement of the skin area to be spared. Usually combined with immediate breast reconstruction.

**sloughing** The process in which the body rids itself of dead tissue. Frequently this happens when the tissue being used does not have an adequate blood supply.

**S-phase fraction** Measurement of how fast a tumor is growing.

**spiculated** Appearing on mammography as small projections into surrounding tissues from a mass.

**staging** System for classifying cancer according to the size of the tumor, its stage of development, and the extent of its spread.

**statistical probability** The mathematically determined likelihood that some event (such as survival from breast cancer) will occur.

**stereotactic (minimally invasive) biopsy** Newer closed-needle or minimally invasive biopsy method using three-dimensional computer imaging for removing suspicious areas seen on mammograms but not able to be felt for analysis by a pathologist.

**subcutaneous mastectomy** Preventive mastectomy that removes most of the breast tissue but leaves the nipple intact.

**subcutaneous tissue** The tissue under the skin.

**supraclavicular nodes** The lymph nodes located above the collarbone.

**survival rate** The percentage of people who live a period of time after a surgical procedure or the diagnosis of a disease as opposed to the percentage of those who die.

**symmetric** Balanced. When one side matches the other. One of the chief goals of the patient and plastic surgeon for breast reconstruction.

**systemic** Involving the entire body.

**systemic treatment** Treatment involving the whole body, usually with drugs.

## T

**tamoxifen (Nolvadex)** An anti-estrogen (estrogen blocker) drug commonly used as a hormonal therapy for breast cancer. Tamoxifen is often prescribed as an alternative to chemotherapy in postmenopausal women. Initial clinical studies indicate that this drug may have some benefit in breast cancer protection, but further study is needed.

**tissue expander** An adjustable implant that can be inflated with saltwater to stretch the tissues at the mastectomy site.

**toremifene (Fareston)** An anti-estrogen (estrogen blocker) drug used in hormonal therapy for breast cancer. Toremifene is prescribed as an alternative to chemotherapy in postmenopausal women.

**total mastectomy with axillary dissection**   A mastectomy in which the breast tissue and most of the axillary lymph nodes are removed. Another name for modified radical mastectomy.

**TRAM flap breast reconstruction**   Breast reconstruction operation that uses a flap of the patient's own lower abdominal tissue (transverse rectus abdominis musculocutaneous flap) to build a breast. The TRAM flap can be a pedicle flap in which the tissue is moved while still attached to its blood supply, or it can be a free flap in which the flap is totally separated from its donor site and moved to its new location and the vessels reattached microsurgically.

**tumor**   An abnormal growth of tissue that can be benign or malignant.

**tumor markers**   Substances released by the tumor or in response to the presence of a tumor. They are studied as potential diagnostic and prognostic tools.

**two-step procedure**   Breast biopsy and breast cancer treatment performed as two steps, allowing diagnosis of cancer and treatment to be separated by hours, days, or even longer periods of time.

## U

**ultrasound**   A special technique using high-frequency sound waves for generating images of organs in the body. It is particularly useful for determining whether a lump is liquid or solid and for use in minimally invasive biopsy techniques.

**ultrasound-guided biopsy**   The use of ultrasound to guide a biopsy needle to remove a sample of tissue from a suspicious area (seen on mammography but not able to be felt) for analysis by a pathologist.

**unilateral**   Involving one side, such as one breast.

## X

**x-ray**   High-energy radiation used in high doses to treat cancer or in low doses to diagnose the disease.

# BIBLIOGRAPHY

This bibliography contains materials that we found helpful to us in preparing this book. Many of the pamphlets cited are available free through the American Cancer Society (ACS), the National Alliance of Breast Cancer Organizations (NABCO), and the National Cancer Institute (NCI). To allow our readers to explore these topics in whatever depth they feel is appropriate, we have included a mixture of articles and books; some are written for a general audience and others are written for a professional audience. Some books or pamphlets were particularly valuable to us, and these have been indicated by bullets throughout the reference listings.

## Detection and Diagnosis of Breast Lumps, Breast Problems, and Breast Cancer
### General

Black ST. Specter of breast cancer: Don't sit home and be afraid. McCall's, Feb, 1973.

Castleman M. Early detection: The best defense. Family Circle 105:107, Oct 13, 1992.

Castleman M. What's normal, what's not. Family Circle 105:101, Oct 13, 1992.

Chances are . . . you need a mammogram. Pub No PF4730, Washington, DC: AARP, 1991. (Contact AARP, 601 E St, Washington, DC 20049.)

Kneece JC. Finding a Lump in Your Breast: Where To Go . . . What To Do. Seattle: EduCare, 1996.

- Understanding breast changes: A health guide for all women. Pub No 97-3536, Washington, DC: National Cancer Institute, 1997.

### Breast Examination

- Breast exams: What you should know. Pub No 91-2000, Washington, DC: National Cancer Institute, 1992.

Dispelling myths about self-examination. USA Today 126:14, Feb, 1998.

Examining your breasts: How to do it right. Ladies' Home J 103:59, Aug, 1986.

- Foster RS Jr, Costanza M. Breast self-examination practices and breast cancer survival. Cancer 53:999, 1984.

How to examine your breasts. Pub No 2088-LE, Atlanta: American Cancer Society, 1990.

McGuinn KA. The Informed Woman's Guide to Breast Health. Palo Alto, CA: Bull Publishing, 1992.

## Mammography and Other Imaging Methods

Burns RB, McCarthy EP, Freund KM, et al. Black women receive less mammography even with similar use of primary care. Ann Intern Med 125:173, 1996.

• Ellerbee L. Our 50s: Yes! Mammography saved my life; It can save yours, too! New Choices Magazine, Oct, 1996.

Feig SA. Mammographic screening of elderly women. JAMA 276:446, 1996.

• Godbey F, George SC. Sooner screening: Why women under 50 need mammograms. Prevention 49:32, April, 1997.

Good news about mammograms. US News & World Report 103:17, Sept, 1987.

The lessons from Mrs. R's case: Early detection through mammography greatly reduces the risks of breast cancer. Newsweek 110:30, Oct, 1987.

Mammograms: A must. Weight Watchers 19:10, Oct, 1986.

• Mammography guidelines for asymptomatic women. Atlanta: American Cancer Society, March 23, 1997.

• National Alliance of Breast Cancer Organizations (NABCO) fact sheets and news articles (available free of charge from NABCO; see Appendix A).

The older you get, the more you need a mammogram. Pub No 5020, Atlanta: American Cancer Society, 1993.

Questions and answers about choosing a mammography facility. Pub No 94-3228. Atlanta: American Cancer Society, 1994.

• Seppa N. Mammograms get boost for women over 40. Science News 153:12, Jan 3, 1998.

## Biopsy

Acosta JA, Greenlee JA, Gubler D, et al. Surgical margins after needle-localization breast biopsy. Am J Surg 170:643, Dec, 1995.

Albertini JJ, Lyman OH, Cox C, et al. Lymphatic mapping and sentinel node biopsy in breast cancer. JAMA 277:791, 1997.

Breast biopsy: What you should know. Pub No 90-657, Washington, DC: National Cancer Institute, 1993.

Burns RP. Image-guided breast biopsy. Am J Surg 173:9, 1997.

Hatada T, Aoki L, Okada K, et al. Usefulness of ultrasound-guided fine-needle aspiration biopsy for palpable breast tumors. Arch Surg 131:1095, 1996.

Lee CH, Egglin TK, Philpotts L, et al. Cost-effectiveness of stereotactic core needle biopsy: Analysis by means of mammographic findings. Radiology 202:849, 1997.

• Lein BC, Alex W, Zebley M, et al. Results of needle localized breast biopsy in women under age 50. Am J Surg 171:356, 1996.

Morrow M. When can stereotactic core biopsy replace excisional biopsy? Breast Cancer Res Treat 36:1, 1995.

Pettine S, Place R, Babu S. Stereotactic breast biopsy is accurate, minimally invasive, and cost effective. Am J Surg 171:474, 1996.

• Sterns EE. Changing emphasis in breast diagnosis: The surgeon's role in evaluating mammographic abnormalities. J Am Coll Surg 184:297, 1997.

Thompson WR, Bowen JR, Dorman BA, et al. Mammographic localization and biopsy of nonpalpable breast lesions—A 5-year study. Arch Surg 126:730, 1991.

• Wallace JE, Sayloer C, Mcdowell NG. The role of stereotactic biopsy in assessment of nonpalpable breast lesions. Am J Surg 171:471, 1996.

## Genetics, Risk, and Prevention

Altman R. Every Woman's Handbook For Preventing Cancer: More Than 100 Simple Ways To Reduce Your Risk. New York: Pocket Books, 1996.

Anderson DE. Breast cancer in families. Cancer 40:1855, 1977.

• Baker NC. Relative Risk: Living With a Family History of Breast Cancer. New York: Viking Press, 1991.

• Brownlee S, Cook GG, Hardigg V, et al. Tinkering with destiny. U.S. News & World Report 117:58, June 23, 1997.

Castleman M. Are you at risk for breast cancer? Family Circle 105:103, Oct 13, 1992.

Davies K, White M. Breakthrough: The Race to Find the Breast Cancer Gene. New York: John Wiley & Sons, 1995.

Dranov P. Do I have the gene? Harper's Bazaar 3431:232, Oct, 1997.

• Driedger SD. The genetic debate: Screening for breast cancer is controversial. Maclean's 109:66, Oct 21, 1996.

Eades MD. If It Runs in Your Family. Breast Cancer: Reducing Your Risk. New York: Bantam Books, 1991.

FitzGerald MG, MacDonald DJ, Krainer M, et al. Germ-line BRCA1 mutations in Jewish and non-Jewish women with early-onset breast cancer. N Engl J Med 334:143, 1996.

Gilson E, Vaidya J, Baum M, et al. Benefits and risks of screening mammography in women with BRCA1 and BRCA2 mutations. JAMA 278:289, 1997.

• Hawkins D. Dangerous legacies: New gene tests provide fresh grounds for discrimination. U.S. News & World Report 123:99, Nov 10, 1997.

• Healy B. A New Prescription for Women's Health. New York: Penguin Books, 1995.

• Kelly PT. Understanding Breast Cancer Risk. Philadelphia: Temple University Press, 1991.

King MC. Zeroing in on a breast cancer susceptibility gene. Science 259:622, 1993.

• Kodish E, Wiesner GL, Mehlman M, et al. Genetic testing for cancer risk: How to reconcile the conflicts. JAMA 279:179, 1998.

Lerman C, Narod S, Schulman K, et al. BRCA1 testing in families with hereditary breast-ovarian cancer: A prospective study of patient decision making and outcomes. JAMA 275:1885, 1996.

Macdonald KG, Doan B, Kelner M, et al. A sociobehavioural perspective on genetic testing and counselling for heritable breast, ovarian, and colon cancer. Can Med Assoc J 154:457, 1996.

Marshall E. The battle over BRCA1 goes to court: BRCA2 may be next. Science 278:1874, Dec 12, 1997.

Miki Y, Swensen J, Shattuck-Eidens D, et al. Isolation of BRCA1 the 17q-linked breast and ovarian cancer susceptibility gene. Science 266:66, 1994.

Rosin H. Family misfortune. Vogue, Sept, 1996.

Royak-Schaler R, Benderly BL. Challenging the Breast Cancer Legacy. New York: Harper Collins, 1993.

Seppa N. Obesity poses cancer risk for older women. Science News 152:294, Nov 8, 1997.

Shapiro L, Springen K. Zeroing in on breast cancer. Newsweek, Sept 26, 1994.

Smith-Warner SA, Spiegelman D, Yaun S, et al. Alcohol and breast cancer in women: A pooled analysis of cohort studies. JAMA 279:535, 1998.

Visser A, Bleiker E. Genetic education and counseling. Patient Educ Couns 32:1, 1997.

• Waldholz M. Curing Cancer: Solving One of the Greatest Medical Mysteries of Our Time. New York: Simon & Schuster, 1997.

• Waldholz M. A cancer survivor's genetic time bomb. The Wall Street Journal, Nov 10, 1997.

Weber B. Breast cancer susceptibility genes: Current challenges and future promises. Ann Intern Med 124:1088, 1996.

• Weber B, Collins F. Genetic counseling: A prefix of what's in store. Science 259:624, 1993.

Wooster R, Neuhausen SL, Mangion Y, et al. Localization of a breast cancer susceptibility gene, BRCA2, to chromosome 13Q12-13. Science 265:2088, 1994.

## Preventive (Prophylactic) Mastectomy for the Woman at Risk

Berman C. Breast surgery to prevent cancer: The big dispute. Good Housekeeping 192:151, March, 1981.

Buchler P. Patient selection for prophylactic mastectomy: Who is at high risk? Plast Reconstr Surg 72:324, 1983.

Clark M, Shapiro D. Breast surgery before cancer. Newsweek 96:100, Dec 1, 1980.

Jarrett JR, Cutler RG, Teal DF. Subcutaneous mastectomy in small, large, or ptotic breasts with immediate submuscular placement of implants. Plast Reconstr Surg 62:381, 1978.

Love S. Discussion of patient selection for prophylactic mastectomy: Who is at high risk? Plast Reconstr Surg 72:326, 1983.

Sureck N. Vanity fear. Modern Maturity, Sept-Oct, 1996.

## Breast Cancer Information

• Cancer facts and figures, 1998. Pub No 5008.98. Atlanta: American Cancer Society, 1998.

Castleman M. Medical breakthrough! The new ways to detect and treat breast cancer. Redbook 169:180, Sept, 1987.

Castleman M. News about breast cancer that could save your life. Family Circle 110:60, May 13, 1997.

Cockburn J, Redman S, Kricker A. Should women take part in clinical trials in breast cancer? Issues and some solutions. J Clin Oncol 16:354, 1995.

Dees EC, Schulman LN, Souba WW, Smith BL. Does information from axillary dissection change treatment in clinically node-negative patients with breast cancer? An algorithm for assessment of impact of axillary dissection. Ann Surg 226:279, 1997.

Degner LF, Kristjanson LJ, Bowman D, et al. Information needs and decisional preferences in women with breast cancer. JAMA 277:1458, May 14, 1997.

Everything doesn't cause cancer, but how can we tell which things cause cancer and which ones don't? Pub No 87-2039, Washington, DC: National Cancer Institute, 1992.

• Friedewald V, Buzdar AU, Bokulich M. Ask the Doctor: Breast Cancer. Kansas City: Andrews & McMeel, 1997.

Harris JR, Hellman S, Henderson IC, et al. Diseases of the Breast. Philadelphia: JB Lippincott Co, 1995.

• Harris JR, Lippman ME, Veronesi U, et al. Breast cancer [first of three parts]. N Engl J Med 327:319, 1992.

• Harris JR, Lippman ME, Veronesi U, et al. Breast cancer [second of three parts]. N Engl J Med 327:390, 1992.

• Harris JR, Lippman ME, Veronesi U, et al. Breast cancer [third of three parts]. N Engl J Med 327:473, 1992.

• Hirshaut Y, Pressman P. Breast Cancer: The Complete Guide, revised ed. New York: Bantam Books, 1996.

Journal of the American Medical Women's Association: Special edition on breast cancer. (Contact JAMWA, 801 N Fairfax St, Alexandria, VA, 22314 for a single copy.)

• Lange D. Making sense of breast cancer treatments. New York Times, June 22, 1997.

LaTour K. The Breast Cancer Companion. New York: William Morrow, 1994.

- Lauersen NH, Stukane E. The Complete Book of Breast Care. New York: Fawcett Columbine, 1996.

  Love SM, Lindsey K. Dr. Susan Love's Breast Book, 2nd ed. Reading, MA: Addison-Wesley Publishing Co, 1995.
- National Alliance of Breast Cancer Organizations (NABCO) fact sheets and NABCO news articles (see p. 581 for ordering information).

  Questions and answers about metastatic cancer. Pub No 91-3194, Washington, DC: National Cancer Institute, 1991.

  Rosenthal MS. Breast Sourcebook: Everything You Need To Know About Cancer Detection, Treatment, and Prevention. Los Angeles: Lowell House, 1996.

  Seligson M. Breast cancer: Report from the research front. Lear's 5:46, Dec, 1992.

  Seltzer VL. Every Woman's Guide to Breast Cancer Prevention, Treatment, and Recovery. New York: Penguin Books, 1987.

  Swirsky J, Balaban B. The Breast Cancer Handbook. Staten Island, NY: Power Publications, 1998.

  What you need to know about cancer of the breast. Pub No 93-1556, Washington, DC: National Cancer Institute, 1993.
- When cancer recurs: Meeting the challenge again. Pub No 93-2709, Washington, DC: National Cancer Institute, 1993.

  When someone in your family has cancer. Pub No 92-2685, Washington, DC: National Cancer Institute, 1992.

### Lymphedema

  Carter BJ. Women's experiences of lymphedema. Oncol Nurs Forum 24:875, 1997.

  Swirsky J, Nannery DS. Coping With Lymphedema. New York: Avery Publishing Group, 1998.

### Personal Accounts of Breast Cancer and Breast Reconstruction

  Bren E, Bren J, Jaworski M. A man, a woman, and breast cancer: One couple's story. Redbook 190:106, Dec, 1997.
- Brinker N. The Race Is Run One Step at a Time: My Personal Struggle and Every Woman's Guide to Taking Charge of Breast Cancer, 2nd ed. New York: Simon & Schuster, 1995.
- Cerquozzi A. I'm too young to have breast cancer. Mademoiselle 103:164, Oct, 1997.

  Conway K. Ordinary Life: A Memoir of Illness. New York: WH Freeman, 1997.
- Dunnavant S. Celebrating Life: African American Women Speak Out About Breast Cancer. Dallas: USFI, 1995.
- Ellerbee L, Veselka V. Hello dear; I have cancer. Good Housekeeping 225:74, Oct, 1997.

Ford B. The Times of My Life. New York: Harper & Row, 1978.

Greene E. A woman of valor. Good Housekeeping 226:74, Jan, 1998.

Gross A, Ito D. Women Talk About Breast Surgery. New York: Harper Perennial, 1990.

Hargrove A. Getting Better: Conversations With Myself and Other Friends While Healing From Breast Cancer. Minneapolis: CompCare Publishers, 1988.

Kushner R. My side. Working Woman 8:160, May, 1983.

Lamberg L. Back to business: Surviving the biggest crisis of all. Working Woman 6:85, April, 1981.

• McCarthy P, Loren JA. Breast Cancer? Let Me Check My Schedule! 2nd ed. Boulder: Westview Press. 1997.

Morris H. My Adventure With Breast Cancer. The Atlanta Journal, Oct 29, 1997.

Murdock S, Ziv L. I gave up my breasts to save my life. New York: Cosmopolitan 223:186, Aug, 1997.

• Orenstein P. Twenty-five and mortal: A breast cancer diary. The New York Times Magazine, June 29, 1997.

Pepper CB. The victors—Patients who conquered cancer. The New York Times, Jan 29, 1984.

Riter R. I have breast cancer; Yes, men as well as women can get and survive this terrible disease. Newsweek 130:14, July 14, 1997.

Rogers J. One woman's battle against cancer. 50 Plus 26:34, 1986.

Rollin B. First You Cry. Philadelphia: JB Lippincott Co, 1976.

• Sheehy G. They fought and won: Surviving breast cancer. Family Circle 105:94, Oct 13, 1992.

Simons A. My story: A doctor's personal battle. Family Circle 105:118, Oct 13, 1992.

• Zalon J. I Am Whole Again: The Case for Breast Reconstruction After Mastectomy. New York: Random House, 1978.

## Treatment Options (*see also* Breast Cancer Information)
### General

Balch CM. Clinical decision making in early breast cancer. Ann Surg 217:207, 1993.

• Breast cancer: Understanding treatment options. Pub No 91 86-2675, Washington, DC: National Cancer Institute, 1990.

• Brownlee S, Guttman M. Closing in on breast cancer. Reader's Digest, Feb, 1996.

Castleman M. Good news: Treatment breakthroughs. Family Circle 105:114, Oct 13, 1992.

Morra M, Potts E. Choices: Realistic Alternatives in Cancer Treatment. New York: Avon Books, 1994.

NIH Consensus Conference statement: Treatment of early stage breast cancer. (Contact Office of Medical Applications of Research, National Institutes of Health, Bldg 1, Room 260, Bethesda, MD 20892 or NABCO.)

• Nowack EJ, Vikhanski L. The Well-Informed Patient's Guide to Breast Surgery. New York: Dell Publishing, 1992.

Rubin R, Beddingfield KT, Brink S. Plugging into the clinical trials. U.S. News & World Report 121:81, June 23, 1997.

• Snyderman N. Breakthroughs in battling breast cancer. Good Housekeeping 225:44, August, 1997.

Spletter MA. A Woman's Choice: New Options in the Treatment of Breast Cancer. Boston: Beacon Press, 1982.

What are clinical trials all about? A booklet for patients with cancer. Pub No 88-2706, Washington, DC: National Cancer Institute, 1993.

### Surgery: Lumpectomy, Mastectomy, and Axillary Lymph Node Dissection

Axillary dissection. The Steering Committee on Clinical Practice Guidelines for the Care and Treatment of Breast Cancer. Can Med Assoc J 158(Suppl 3): S22, Feb 10, 1998.

Bedwani R. Management and survival of patients with "minimal" breast cancer. Cancer 47:2769, 1981.

• Bedwinek J. Breast cancer: Primary treatment. In Gilbert H, ed. Modern Radiation Oncology: Classic Literature and Current Management, vol 2. Philadelphia: Harper & Row, 1984.

Bedwinek J. Treatment of stage I and II adenocarcinoma of the breast by tumor excision and irradiation. Int J Radiat Oncol Biol Phys 7:1553, 1981.

Carlson GW, Bostwick J III, Styblo TM, et al. Skin-sparing mastectomy: Oncologic and reconstructive considerations. Ann Surg 225:570, 1997.

Fisher B. Five-year results of a randomized clinical trial comparing total mastectomy and segmental mastectomy with or without radiation in the treatment of breast cancer. N Engl J Med 312:665, 1985.

Kroll SS, Schusterman MA, Tadjalli HE, et al. Risk of recurrence after treatment of early breast cancer with skin-sparing mastectomy. Ann Surg Oncol 4:193, 1997.

Lynden P. Your breasts or your life. American Health for Women 16:29, June, 1997.

Mastectomy: A treatment for breast cancer. Pub No 91-658, Washington, DC: National Cancer Institute, 1991.

More or less? Lumpectomy and radiotherapy found as effective as mastectomy on breast cancer. Sci Am 253:59, Aug, 1985.

• Schain WS, Edwards BE, Garrell CR, et al. Psychosocial and physical outcomes of primary breast cancer therapy: Mastectomy versus excisional biopsy and irradiation. Breast Cancer Res Treat 3:377, 1983.

Singhal H, O'Malley EP, Tweedie E, et al. Axillary node dissection in patients with breast cancer diagnosed through the Ontario Breast Screening Program: A need for minimally invasive techniques. Can J Surg 40:377, Oct, 1997.

The Steering Committee on Clinical Practice Guidelines for the Care and Treatment of Breast Cancer. The palpable breast lump: Information and recommendations to assist decision-making when a breast lump is detected. Can Med Assoc J 158(Suppl 3):S3, Feb 10, 1998.

Veronesi U, Paganelli G, Galinberti V, et al. Sentinel-node biopsy to avoid axillary dissection in breast cancer with clinically negative lymph-nodes. Lancet 349:1864, 1997.

Winchester DJ, Menck HR, Winchester DP. The National Cancer Data Base report on the results of a large nonrandomized comparison of breast preservation and modified radical mastectomy. Cancer 80:162, July 1, 1997.

Wohlberg WH. Mastectomy or breast conservation in the management of primary breast cancer: Psychological factors. Oncology 4:101, 1990.

### Chemotherapy

Bone marrow transplantation and peripheral blood stem cell transplantation. Pub No 91-1178, Bethesda, MD: National Cancer Institute, 1994.

Breast cancer: When chemotherapy works. Ms Magazine 16:70, Nov, 1987.

Brenner DJ, Hall EJ. Making the Radiation Therapy Decision. Los Angeles: Lowell House, 1996.

Bruning N. Coping With Chemotherapy, revised ed. New York: Ballantine, 1997.

Chemotherapy: Your Weapon Against Cancer. New York: Chemotherapy Foundation (212-213-9292).

Chemotherapy and you: A guide to self-help during treatment. Pub No 94-1136, Washington, DC: National Cancer Institute, 1993.

Dodd M. Managing the Side Effects of Chemotherapy & Radiation Therapy: A Guide for Patients and Their Families, 3rd ed. San Francisco: University of California, 1996.

Drum D. Making the Chemotherapy Decision. Los Angeles: Lowell House, 1996.

Gelber RD, Cole BF, Goldhirsch A, et al. Adjuvant chemotherapy plus tamoxifen compared with tamoxifen alone for postmenopausal breast cancer. Lancet 347:1066, 1996.

Gradishar WJ, Tallman MS, Abrams JS. High-dose chemotherapy for breast cancer. Ann Intern Med 125:599, 1996.

Kennedy MJ. Systemic therapy for breast cancer. Curr Opin Oncol 9:532, 1997.

• National Alliance of Breast Cancer Organizations (NABCO) fact sheets and NABCO news articles (see Appendix A).
    Autologous bone marrow transplantation (ABMT) information package
    Metastatic breast cancer: Treatment update

Questions and answers about adjuvant therapy for breast cancer. Bethesda, MD: National Cancer Institute, Aug 14, 1997.

Ragaz J, Jackson SM, Nhu Le IH, et al. Adjuvant radiotherapy and chemotherapy in node-positive premenopausal women with breast cancer. N Engl J Med 337:956, Oct, 1997.

Smigel K. Women flock to ABMT for breast cancer without final proof. J Natl Cancer Inst 87:952, 1995.

### Hormonal Therapy

• Burton TM. New drugs give cause for hope in fight against breast cancer: Preventive therapies show promise, but the testing has a long way to go. The Wall Street Journal, April 20, 1998.

Grey AB, Stapleton JP, Evans MC, et al. The effect of the antiestrogen tamoxifen on bone mineral density in normal late postmenopausal women. Am J Med 99:636, 1995.

Henderson BE, Ross RK, Pike MC. Hormonal chemoprevention of cancer in women. Science 259:633, 1993.

O'Shaughnessy JA. Chemoprevention of breast cancer. JAMA 275:1349, 1996.

### Radiation Therapy

Beadle GF, Silver B, Botnik L, et al. Cosmetic results following primary radiation therapy for early breast cancer. Cancer 54:2911, 1984.

Brenner DJ, Hall EJ. Making the Radiation Therapy Decision. Los Angeles: Lowell House, 1996.

• Radiation therapy and you: A guide to self-help during treatment. Pub No 91-2227, Washington, DC: National Cancer Institute, 1990.

## Breast Reconstruction (*see also* Breast Cancer Information; Treatment Options)

• Bostwick J III. Plastic and Reconstructive Breast Surgery. St Louis: Quality Medical Publishing, 1990 (new edition in press).

Breast Reconstruction Following Mastectomy. (Contact American Society of Plastic and Reconstructive Surgeons, 444 East Algonquin Rd, Arlington Heights, IL 60005; 708-228-9900.)

Charavel M, Bremond A, Courtial I. Psychosocial profile of women seeking breast reconstruction. Eur J Obstet Gynecol Reprod Biol 74:31, 1997.

Chen L, Hartrampf CR, Bennett GK. Successful pregnancies following TRAM flap surgery. Plast Reconstr Surg 91:69, 1993.

Goin MK. Discussion: The psychological impact of immediate breast reconstruction for women with early breast cancer. Plast Reconstr Surg 73:627, 1984.

Goin MK, Goin JM. Midlife reactions to mastectomy and subsequent breast reconstruction. Arch Gen Psychiatry 38:225, 1981.

Goin MK, Goin JM. Psychological reactions to prophylactic mastectomy synchronous with contralateral breast reconstruction. Plast Reconstr Surg 70:355, 1982.

Hartrampf CR. Breast reconstruction with a transverse abdominal island flap: A retrospective evaluation. Perspect Plast Surg 1(1):123, 1987.

Hartrampf CR, Scheflan M, Black PW. Breast reconstruction following mastectomy with a transverse abdominal island flap: Anatomical and clinical observations. Plast Reconstr Surg 69:216, 1982.

Kasper AS. The social construction of breast loss and reconstruction. Women's Health 1(3):197, 1995.

• Levinson J. Breast reconstruction: A patient's view. Plast Reconstr Surg 73:703, 1984.

Little JW, Spear SL. The finishing touches in nipple-areolar reconstruction. Perspect Plast Surg 2(1):1, 1988.

Nahai F. Breast reconstruction with a free gluteus maximus musculocutaneous flap. Perspect Plast Surg 6(2):65, 1993.

• National Alliance of Breast Cancer Organizations (NABCO) fact sheets and articles on breast reconstruction (available free; see Appendix A).

Noone RB, Murphy JB, Spear SL, et al. A 6-year experience with immediate reconstruction after mastectomy for cancer. Plast Reconstr Surg 76:258, 1985.

Schain WS. Reconstructive mammoplasty: Reversibility of a trauma. In Western States Conference on Cancer Rehabilitation. Palo Alto, CA: Bull Publishing Co, 1982.

Schain WS, Edwards BK, Gorrell CR, et al. The sooner the better: A study of psychological factors of women undergoing immediate versus delayed breast reconstruction. Am J Psychiatry 142:40, 1985.

Schain WS, Jacobs E, Wellisch DK. Psychosocial issues in breast reconstruction: Intrapsychic, interpersonal, and practical concerns. Clin Plast Surg 2:237, 1984.

Serletti JM, Moran SL. Free versus the pedicled TRAM flap: A cost comparison and outcome analysis. Plast Reconstr Surg. 100:1418, 1997.

Stevens LA, McGrath MH, Druss RG, et al. The psychological impact of immediate breast reconstruction for women with early breast cancer. Plast Reconstr Surg 73:619, 1984.

Strom SS, Baldwin BJ, Sigurdson AJ, et al. Cosmetic saline breast implants: A survey of satisfaction, breast-feeding experience, cancer screening, and health. Plast Reconstr Surg 100:1553, 1997.

Teimourian B, Adham MN. Survey of patients' responses to breast reconstruction. Ann Plast Surg 9:321, 1982.

To be whole again: Mastectomy treated Peggy McCann's cancer, but breast reconstruction made her well. Life 10:78, May, 1987.

Zalon J. I Am Whole Again: The Case for Breast Reconstruction After Mastectomy. New York: Random House, 1978.

## Breast Implants

American Cancer Society Documents 002197 & 003068 (1-800-ACS-2345).

American College of Rheumatology Statement on Silicone Breast Implants. Oct, 1995.

The American disease [editorial]. The Wall Street Journal, Jan 20, 1992.

American Society of Clinical Oncology. American Society of Clinical Oncology and cancer patients seek to ease FDA restrictions on silicone breast implants [press release]. Sept 19, 1996.

Angell M. Breast implants—Protection or paternalism? N Engl J Med 326:1695, 1992.

Angell M. Do breast implants cause systemic disease? Science in the courtroom. N Engl J Med 330:1748, 1994.

Angell M. Evaluating the health risks of breast implants: The interplay of medical science, the law, and public opinion [Shattuck lecture]. N Engl J Med 334:1513, 1996.

Angell M. Science on Trial: The Clash of Medical Evidence and the Law in the Breast Implant Case. New York: WW Norton & Co, 1996.

Berkel H, Birdsell DC, Jenkins H. Breast augmentation: A risk factor for breast cancer? N Engl J Med 326:1649, 1992.

Birdsell DC, Jenkins H, Berket H. Breast cancer diagnosis and survival in women with and without breast implants. Plast Reconstr Surg 92:795, 1993.

Breast implants—An information update. Rockville, MD: U.S. Food and Drug Administration, Department of Health & Human Services, July, 1997.

The breast implant tragedy. Review & outlook. The Wall Street Journal, May 19, 1995.

Brinton LA, Malone KE, Coates RJ, et al. Breast implants and subsequent breast cancer risk. Am J Epidemiol 141:S85, 1995.

Brinton LA, Malone KE, Coates RJ, et al. Breast enlargement and reduction: Results from a breast cancer case-control study. Plast Reconstr Surg 97:269, 1996.

Brody GS, Conway DP, Deapen DM, et al. Consensus statement on the relationship of breast implants to connective-tissue disorders. Plast Reconstr Surg 90:1102, 1992.

Brown SL, Silverman BG, Berg WA. Rupture of silicone-gel breast implants: Causes, sequelae and diagnosis. Lancet 350:1531, 1997.

Bruning N. Breast Implants: Everything You Need To Know. Alamed, CA: Hunter House, 1992.

Bryant H, Brasher PMA. Breast implants and breast cancer—Reanalysis of a linkage study. N Engl J Med 332:1535, 1995.

Bryant H, Brasher PMA, van de Sande JH, et al. [Alberta Cancer Board]. Review of methods in breast augmentation: A risk factor for breast cancer? N Engl J Med 330:293, 1994.

Burns CJ, Laing TJ, Gillespie BW, et al. The epidemiology of scleroderma among women: Assessment of risk from exposure to silicone and silica. J Rheumatol 23:1904. 1996.

Burton TMA. Harvard study finds no major link between implants and immune illnesses. The Wall Street Journal, June 22, 1995.

Burton TMA, Woo J. Lawyers contest implant class action. The Wall Street Journal, March 16, 1992.

Chandler PJ Jr. An outcome analysis of 100 women after explanation of silicone gel breast implants and connective tissue disease and other rheumatic conditions following breast implants in Denmark. Ann Plast Surg 40:103, 1998.

Cook RR, Delongchamp RR, Woodbury M, et al. The prevalence of women with breast implants in the United States—1989. J Clin Epidemiol 48:519, 1995.

Council on Scientific Affairs, American Medical Association. Silicone gel breast implants. JAMA 270:2602, 1993.

Deapen DM, Bernstein L, Brody GS. Are breast implants anticarcinogenic? A 14-year follow-up of the Los Angeles study. Plast Reconstr Surg 99:1346, 1997.

Deapen DM, Brody GS. Augmentation mammoplasty and breast cancer: A five-year update of the Los Angeles study. J Clin Epidemiol 48:551, 1995.

Deapen DM, Pike MC, Casagrand JT, et al. The relationship between breast cancer and augmentation mammoplasty: An epidemiologic study. Plast Reconstr Surg 77:361, 1986.

Destouet JM, Monsees BS, Oser RF, et al. Screening mammography in 350 women with breast implants: Prevalence and findings of implant complications. Am J Roentgenol 159:973, 1992.

Duffy MJ, Woods JE. Health risks of failed silicone gel breast implants: A 30-year clinical experience. Plast Reconstr Surg 94:295, 1994.

Elkund GW, Busby RC, Miller SH, et al. Improved imaging of the augmented breast. Am J Roentgenol 151:469, 1988.

Englert HJ, Brooks P. Scleroderma and augmentation mammoplasty—A causal relationship? Aust NZ J Med 24:74, 1994.

Englert HJ, Morris D, March L. Scleroderma and silicone gel breast prostheses—The Sydney study revisited. Aust NZ J Med 26:349, 1996.

FDA Talk Paper. TDA and polyurethane breast implants. June 28, 1995.

Feder BJ. A war baby, versatile silicone now shows up everywhere. The New York Times, Dec 29, 1991.

Fee-Fulkerson K, Conway MR, Winer EP, et al. Factors contributing to patient satisfaction with breast reconstruction using silicone gel implants. Plast Reconstr Surg 97:1420, 1996.

Ferguson JH. Silicone breast implants and neurologic disorders—Report of the practice committee of the American Academy of Neurology. Neurology 48:1504, 1997.

Firestone S. Challenging the fear industry again. San Diego Tribune, June 11, 1997.

Fisher JC. The silicone controversy—When will science prevail? N Engl J Med 326:1696, 1992.

Fisher JC, Brody GD. Breast implants under siege: An historical commentary. J Long Term Effects Med Implants 1:243, 1992.

Fisher JC, Potchen EJ, Sergent J. Office communication with breast implant patients: Radiologic and rheumatologic concerns. Perspect Plast Surg 6(2):79, 1992.

Friis S, McLauglin JK, Mellemkjaer L, et al. Breast implant and cancer risk in Denmark. Int J Cancer 7:956, 1997.

Gabriel SE, O'Fallon WM, Kurland LT, et al. Risk of connective-tissue diseases and other disorders after breast implantation. N Engl J Med 330:1697, 1994.

Gabriel SE, Woods JE, O'Fallon WM, et al. Complications leading to surgery after breast implantation. N Engl J Med 336:677, 1997.

Giltay EJ, Moens HJB, Riley AH, et al. Silicone breast prostheses and rheumatic symptoms: A retrospective follow up study. Ann Rheum Dis 53:194, 1994.

Goldman JA, Greenblatt J, Joines R, et al. Breast implants, rheumatoid arthritis, and connective tissue diseases in a clinical practice. J Clin Epidemiol 48:571, 1995.

Goldrich SN. Restoration drama: A cautionary tale by a woman who had breast implants after mastectomy. Ms Magazine 16:20, June, 1988.

Gorczyca DP, Sinha S, Ahn CY, et al. Silicone breast implants in vivo: MR imaging. Radiology 185:407, 1992.

Green S. A woman's right to choose breast implants. The Wall Street Journal, Jan 20, 1993.

Gumucio CA, Pin P, Young VL, et al. The effect of breast implant on the radiographic detecting of microcalcification and soft-tissue masses. Plast Reconstr Surg 84:772, 1989.

Gutowski KA, Mesna GT, Cunningham BL. Saline-filled breast implants: A Plastic Surgery Educational Foundation multicenter outcomes study. Plast Reconstr Surg 100:1019, 1997.

Handel N, Jensen JA, Black Q, et al. The fate of breast implants: A critical analysis of complications and outcomes. Plast Reconstr Surg 96:1521, 1995.

Handel N, Wellisch D, Silverstein MJ, et al. Knowledge, concern, and satisfaction among augmentation mammaplasty patients. Ann Plast Surg 30:1, 1993.

Hart D. The psychological outcome of breast reconstruction. Plast Surg Nurs 16(3):167, 1996.

Hazelton R. The tort monster that ate Dow Corning. The Wall Street Journal, May 17, 1995.

Hennekens CH, Lee I-M, Cook NR, et al. Self-reported breast implants and connective-tissue diseases in female health professionals. JAMA 275:616, 1996.

Hochberg MC, Perlmutter DL, Medsger TA Jr, et al. Lack of association between augmentation mammoplasty and systemic sclerosis (scleroderma). Arthritis Rheum 39:1125, 1996.

Huber P. Galilio's Revenge: Junk Science in the Courtroom. New York: Basic Books, 1991.

Huber P. A woman's right to choose. Forbes 149:138, Feb 17, 1992.

Implants and the press [editorial]. The Wall Street Journal, Jan 27, 1992.

Junk science and judges. The Wall Street Journal, Nov 8, 1995.

Karns ME, Cullison CA, Romano TJ, et al. Breast implants and connective-tissue disease. JAMA 276:100, 1996.

Kessler DA. The basis of the FDA's decision on breast implants. N Engl J Med 326:1713, 1992.

Kessler DA, Merkatz RB, Schapiro R. A call for higher standards for breast implants. JAMA 270:2607, 1993.

Kolata G. Legal system and science come to differing conclusions on silicone. New York Times, May 16, 1995.

Kolata G. Will the lawyers kill off Norplant? New York Times, May 28, 1995.

Kolata G, Meier B. Implant lawsuits create a medical rush to cash in. New York Times, Sept 18, 1995.

Laing TJ, Gillespie BW, Lacey JV Jr, et al. The association between silicone exposure and undifferentiated connective tissue disease among women in Michigan and Ohio. Arthritis Rheum 39:S150, 1996.

Macdonald KL, Osterholm MT. A case control study to assess possible triggers and cofactors in chronic fatigue syndrome. Am J Med 100:548, 1996.

McLaughlin JK, Fraumeni JF, Nyren O. Silicone breast implants and risk of cancer? JAMA 273:116, 1995.

McLaughlin JK, Fraumeni JF, Olsen J, et al. Re: Breast implants, cancer, and systemic sclerosis. J Natl Cancer Inst 86:1424, 1994.

National Cancer Institute. What are clinical trials all about (92-2706). 1992 (800-4-CANCER).

Noone RB. A review of the possible health implications of silicone breast implants. Cancer 79:1747, 1997.

Park AJ, Black RJ, Watson ACH. Silicone gel breast implants, breast cancer and connective tissue disorders. Br J Surg 80:1097, 1993.

Park AJ, Chetty U, Watson ACH. Patient satisfaction following insertion of silicone breast implants. Br J Plast Surg 49:515, 1996.

Park AJ, Walsh J, Reddy PSV, et al. The detection of breast implant rupture using ultrasound. Br J Plast Surg 49:299, 1996.

Peters WJ, Smith DC, Fornasier V, et al. An outcome analysis of 100 women after explantation of silicone gel breast implants. Ann Plast Surg 39:1, 1997.

Petit JY, Le MG, Mouriesse H. et al. Can breast reconstruction with gel-filled silicone implants increase the risk of death and second primary cancer in patients treated by mastectomy for breast cancer? Plast Reconstr Surg 94:115, 1994.

Reed ME. Daubert and the breast implant litigation: How is the judiciary addressing the science? Plast Reconstr Surg 100:1322, 1997.

Risk assessment of polyurethane breast implants. Department of Health & Human Services, Food and Drug Administration, July 1, 1991.

Romanelli JN, Solomon G, Silverman S, et al. More on breast implants and connective-tissue diseases. N Engl J Med 332:1306, 1995.

Rose NR. The silicone breast implant controversy: The other courtroom. Arthritis Rheum 39:1615, 1996.

Sanchez-Guerrero J, Colditz GA, Karlson EW, et al. Silicone breast implants and the risk of connective-tissue diseases and symptoms. N Engl J Med 332:1666, 1995.

Sanchez-Guerrero J, Liang MH. Silicone breast implants and connective tissue diseases: No association has been convincingly established. Br Med J 309:822, 1994.

Schusterman MA, Kroll SS, Reece GP, et al. Incidence of autoimmune disease in patients after breast reconstruction with silicone gel implants versus autogenous tissue: A preliminary report. Ann Plast Surg 31:1, 1993.

Science abdicates [editorial]. The Wall Street Journal, Jan 9, 1992.

Strom BL, Reidenberg MM, Greundlich B, et al. Breast silicone implants and risk of sytemic lupus erythematosus. J Clin Epidemiol 47:1211, 1994.

Taubes G. Silicone in the system. Discover, The World of Science 16:64, Dec 1994.

U.S. survey clears implants of role in breast cancer. New York Times, Nov 17, 1997.

Wigley FM, Miller R, Hochberg MC, et al. Augmentation mammoplasty in patients with systemic sclerosis: Data from the Baltimore scleroderma research center and Pittsburgh scleroderma data bank. Arthritis Rheum 35:S46, 1992.

Williams HJ, Weisman MH, Berry CC. Breast implants in patients with undifferentiated connective tissue disease. Arthritis Rheum 40:437, 1997.

Wolfe F. Silicone breast implants and the risk of fibromyalgia and rheumatoid arthritis. Arthritis Rheum 38:S265, 1995.

Wong O. A critical assessment of the relationship between silicone breast implants and connective tissue diseases. Regulatory Toxicol Pharmacol 23:74, 1996.

Woods JE, Arnold PE. Fiction obscures the facts of breast implants. The Wall Street Journal, April 7, 1992.

## Psychological and Sexual Considerations After Breast Cancer

• Dackman L. Up Front: Sex and the Post-mastectomy Woman. New York: Viking Press, 1990.

Dackman L. Affirmations, Meditations, and Encouragements for Women Living With Breast Cancer. Los Angeles: Lowell House, 1991.

- Greenberg M. Invisible Scars: A Guide to Coping With the Emotional Impact of Breast Cancer. New York: Walker & Co, 1988.

  Jobin J. How men respond to mastectomy. Woman's Day, Nov, 1977.
- Kahane DH. No Less a Woman: Femininity, Sexuality & Breast Cancer, 2nd ed. Alameda, CA: Hunter House, 1995.

  Kaye R. Spinning Straw Into Gold: Your Emotional Recovery From Breast Cancer. New York: Simon & Schuster, 1991.

  Lee K. Facing breast cancer before 50. Essence 28:36, Oct, 1997.
- Morra M, Potts E. Triumph—Getting Back to Normal When You Have Cancer. New York: Avon Books, 1990.
- Murcia A. Man to Man: When the Woman You Love Has Breast Cancer. New York: St Martin's Press, 1989.

  Nessim S, Ellis J. Cancervive—The Challenge of Life After Cancer. Boston: Houghton Mifflin Co, 1991.

  Randolph LB. Breast cancer. Confronting a major killer of black women. Ebony 52:148, Oct, 1997.

  Royak-Schaler R. Challenging the Breast Cancer Legacy: A Program of Emotional Support and Medical Care for Women at Risk. New York: Harper Collins, 1992.

  Schain WS. Sexual and intimate consequences of breast cancer treatments. Cancer J Clinicians 38:154, 1988.
- Schover L. Sexuality and Fertility After Cancer. New York: John Wiley & Sons, 1997.

  Schover L, Schain WS, Montague DK. Sexual problems of patients with cancer. In DeVita VT Jr, Hellman S, Rosenberg SA, eds. Principles and Practices of Oncology, 3rd ed. Philadelphia: JB Lippincott Co, pp 2206-2219, 1989.

  Tarrier N. Living With Breast Cancer and Mastectomy: A Self-Help Guide. Wolfeboro, NH: Longwood Publishing Group, 1987.
- Wellish DK. Psychosocial aspects of mastectomy: II. The man's perspective. Am J Psychiatry 135:543, 1978.

## Family and Friends and Breast Cancer

Babcock EN. When Life Becomes Precious: A Guide for Loved Ones and Friends of Cancer Patients. New York: Bantam, 1977.

Braddock S, Edney JJ. Straight Talk About Breast Cancer From Diagnosis to Recovery: A Guide for the Entire Family. San Diego: Addicus Press, 1994.

Harpham WS. When a Parent Has Cancer: A Guide To Caring for Your Children. New York: Harper Collins, 1997.

Pederson LM, Trigg JM. Breast Cancer: A Family Survival Guide. Westport CT: Greenwood, 1995.

Virag I, Berger E. We're All in This Together: Families Facing Breast Cancer. Kansas City: Andrews & McMeel, 1995.

### Recovery, Rehabilitation, and Survival

Altman R. Waking Up/Fighting Back: The Politics of Breast Cancer. Boston: Little Brown & Co, 1996.

Belkin L. How Breast Cancer Became This Year's Cause. The New York Times Magazine, Dec 12, 1996.

• Charting the Journey: An Almanac of Practical Resources for Cancer Survivors. The National Coalition for Cancer Survivorship. New York: Consumer Reports Books, 1990.

• Clifford C. Not Now . . . I'm Having a No Hair Day. Duluth, MN: Pfeifer-Hamilton, 1996.

Domar AD, Dreher H. Healing Mind, Healthy Woman: Using the Mind-Body Connection to Manage Stress and Take Control of Your Life. New York: Holt Rhinehart & Winston, 1996.

Fabian C, Warren A. Recovering From Breast Cancer: A Doctor's Guide for Women and Their Families. New York: Harper Paperbacks, 1992.

Facing forward: A guide for cancer survivors. Pub No 90-2424, Washington, DC: National Cancer Institute, 1990.

Gray R, Fitch M, Davis C, Phillips C. A qualitative study of breast cancer self-help groups. Psychooncology 6:279, 1997.

• Hoffman B. A Cancer Survivor's Almanac: Charting Your Journey, 2nd ed. Washington, DC: National Coalition for Cancer Survivorship, 1996.

Mickley J, Soeken K. Religiousness and hope in Hispanic and Anglo-American women with breast cancer. Oncol Nurs Forum 20:1171, 1993.

• Porter ME. Hope Is Contagious: The Breast Cancer Treatment Survival Handbook. New York: Fireside, Oct, 1997.

Rosenfeld R. Dr. Rosenfeld's Guide to Alternative Medicine: What Works, What Doesn't—And What's Right for You. New York: Random House, 1996.

Runowicz CK, Haupt D. To Be Alive: A Woman's Guide to a Full Life After Cancer. New York: Holt, Rhinehart & Winston, 1995.

Taking time: Support for people with cancer and the people who care about them. Pub No 91-2059, Washington, DC: National Cancer Institute, 1992.

• Weiss MC, Weiss E. Living Beyond Breast Cancer: A Survivor's Guide for When Treatment Ends and the Rest of Your Life Begins. New York: Times Books, 1997.

Woodman S. Life after breast cancer; 1,000 women speak out. McCall's, Oct, 1995.

### Hormone Replacement Therapy

Breast cancer and hormone replacement therapy: Collaborative reanalysis of data from 51 epidemiological studies of 52,705 women with breast cancer and 108,411 women without breast cancer. Lancet 350:1047, 1997.

Brinton LA, Schairer C. Postmenopausal hormone-replacement therapy—Time for a reappraisal? N Engl J Med 336:1821, 1997.

Castlemen M. Hormonious heart: Hormone replacement therapy helps prevent heart disease—A major killer. Mother Jones 22:21, July-August, 1997.

Davidson NE. Is hormone replacement therapy a risk? Sci Am 275:101, 1996.

Hillard T. Evaluation and management of the hormone replacement therapy (HRT) candidate. Int J Fertil Women's Med 42(Suppl 2):347, 1997.

Hormone replacement therapy: Weighing the benefits and risks. Harvard Health Letter 22:1, Oct, 1997.

Mestel R. Redesigning women: Breast cancer and estrogen. Health 11:70, March, 1997.

National Women's Health Network. Hearts, Bones, Hot Flashes, and Hormones. Washington, DC: National Women's Health Network, 1994.

Stanford JL, Weiss NS, Voigt LF, et al. Combined estrogen and progestin hormone replacement therapy in relation to risk of breast cancer in middle-aged women. JAMA 274:137, 1995.

## Nutrition, Exercise, and Beauty Aids

Bernstein L, Henderson BE, Hanisch R, et al. Physical exercise and reduced risk of breast cancer in young women. J Natl Cancer Inst 86:1403, 1994.

Breast cancer and diet. Maclean's 111:64, March 2, 1998.

Buyer's guide to wigs and hairpieces. (Contact Ruth L. Weintraub Co, Inc, 420 Madison Ave, Ste 406, New York, NY 10017; 212-838-1333.)

Calhoun S, Bradley J. Nutrition, Cancer and You: What You Need To Know and Where To Start. Lenexa, KS: Addax Publishing Group, 1997.

Darion E. Exercises for mastectomy patients. McCall's 109:44, April, 1982.

Diet, nutrition & cancer prevention: A guide to food choices. Pub No 87-2878, Washington, DC: National Cancer Institute, 1993.

• Eating hints: Recipes and tips for better nutrition during cancer treatment. Pub No 91-2079, Washington, DC: National Cancer Institute, 1990.

Eating smart. Pub No 87-2042, Atlanta: American Cancer Society, 1989.

Emmer J. The pink ribbon: On breast cancer, new hair, first running steps and hope. Runner's World 30:32, May, 1995.

Good news, better news, best news . . . Cancer prevention. Pub No 84-2671, Washington, DC: National Cancer Institute, 1984.

Graham S. Alcohol and breast cancer. N Engl J Med 316:1211, 1987.

Kaplan J. Does alcohol increase the risk of breast cancer? Vogue 177:174, Nov, 1987.

Krucoff C. Exercise and breast cancer. Saturday Evening Post 267:22, Nov-Dec, 1995.

Lieberman S, Bruning N. Design Your Own Vitamin and Mineral Program. New York: Avery, 1990.

Liebman B. Can exercise beat breast cancer? Nutrition Action Healthletter, 24:1, July 1997.

Michnovicz J, Klein DS. The anti-breast cancer diet. Ladies' Home Journal, July, 1994.

Noyes D, Mellody P. Beauty and Cancer. Los Angeles: AC Press, 1988.
* Spear R. Low Fat and Loving It. New York: Warner Books, 1990.
* Time to take five: Eat 5 fruits and vegetables a day. Pub No 95-3862, Washington, DC: National Cancer Institute, 1995.

## Insurance and Other Resource Information

Cancer: Your job, insurance and the law. Pub No 4585-PS, Atlanta: American Cancer Society, 1987.
* Cancer treatments your insurance should cover, Rockville, MD: Association of Community Cancer Centers (11600 Nebel St, Ste 201, Rockville, MD 20852; 301-984-9496).
The consumer's guide to disability insurance. Pub No C104, Washington, DC: Health Insurance Association of America, 1991.
The consumer's guide to health insurance. Pub No C103, Washington, DC: Health Insurance Association of America, 1991.
The consumer's guide to long-term care insurance. Pub No C101, Washington, DC: Health Insurance Association of America, 1991.
The consumer's guide to medicare supplement insurance. Pub No C102, Washington, DC: Health Insurance Association of America, 1991.

## Cancer Resources on the Internet

Ferguson T. Health online and the empowered medical consumer. Joint Comm J Qual Improv 23:251, 1997.
Haines J. Breast cancer resources online. Can Nurse 93(9):49-50, 1997.
Korn K. Cancer information on the Internet. J Am Acad Nurse Pract 9(8):385, 1997.
Mizsur G. Helping patients find support on the Internet. Nursing 27(8):28, 1997.
Nally M. Patient power in the net. Nurs Time 92:31, Nov 6, 1996.
Sharf BF. Communicating breast cancer online: Support and empowerment on the Internet. Women's Health 26(1):65, 1997.
* Sharp R, Sharp VF. Web Doctor: Your Online Guide to Health & Wellness. St. Louis: Quality Medical Publishing, 1988.
Woodworth M, Loochtan A. A road map to cancer resources on the Internet. Cancer Pract 4:160, 1996.

## Resources, References, and Additional Reading

Many of the cancer-related pamphlets listed previously are from one of the following three major organizations.
*American Cancer Society* (ACS). For materials listed contact your local American Cancer Society unit or state chartered division. If the material is not available locally, contact the ACS National Office, 1599 Clifton Road NE, Atlanta, GA 30329; 404-320-3333 (800-ACS-2345).

*National Alliance of Breast Cancer Organizations* (NABCO). Order all NAB-CO fact sheets and NABCO news articles from The National Alliance of Breast Cancer Organizations, 9 East 37th St., 10th Floor, New York, NY 10016; 212-889-0606.

*National Cancer Institute* (NCI). Order all materials from Public Inquiry Section, Office of Cancer Communications, National Cancer Institute, Bldg 31, Room 10 A 24, Bethesda, MD 20892; 1-800-4CANCER.

### References for Locating Articles in the Popular Literature

Articles appearing in the popular literature are listed in the *Readers' Guide to Periodical Literature* or in the *Public Affairs Information Service,* available in most public libraries. Look in the index under the subject in which you are interested or under the author's name.

### References for Locating Articles in Health Science Journals

For articles appearing in the scientific literature, check the *Index Medicus,* which is found in medical libraries, most university and college libraries, and some public libraries. This book lists articles appearing in over 2500 science journals. The National Library of Medicine has a series of medical databases called MEDLARS, which are also helpful. These include the following:

MEDLINE. A database with over 4 million citations and abstracts taken from approximately 3200 medical journals published in the United States and throughout the world.

Physician Data Query (PDQ) A database providing current cancer information. PDQ is discussed in Appendix A.

CANCERLIT. A database containing approximately 550,000 citations and abstracts of articles published since 1978 on all aspects of cancer.

# INDEX